Stevens & Lowe's
HUMAN
HISTOLOGY

SIXTH EDITION

Stevens & Lowe's
HUMAN HISTOLOGY

James S. Lowe, BMedSci, BMBS, DM, FRCPath
Emeritus Professor of Neuropathology
School of Medicine
University of Nottingham
Nottingham, UK

Peter G. Anderson, DVM, PhD
Professor, Department of Pathology
Heersink School of Medicine
University of Alabama at Birmingham
Birmingham, AL, USA

Susan I. Anderson, BSc, MMedSci, PhD, FRMS, FHEA
Professor of Anatomy and Pathology
Deputy Head of School of Life Sciences
Faculty of Medicine & Health Sciences
University of Nottingham Medical School
Nottingham, UK

ELSEVIER

Notice

Practitioners and researchers must always rely on their own experience and knowledge in evaluating and using any information, methods, compounds or experiments described herein. Because of rapid advances in the medical sciences, in particular, independent verification of diagnoses and drug dosages should be made. To the fullest extent of the law, no responsibility is assumed by Elsevier, authors, editors or contributors for any injury and/or damage to persons or property as a matter of products liability, negligence or otherwise, or from any use or operation of any methods, products, instructions, or ideas contained in the material herein.

ISBN: 978-0-443-10970-6

Editorial Assistant: Susana Sainz Garcia
Senior Content Development Manager: Somodatta Roy Choudhury
Senior Content Strategist: Alexandra Mortimer
Content Development Manager: Ranjana Sharma
Publishing Services Manager: Shereen Jameel
Project Manager: Vishnu T. Jiji
Design Direction: Ryan Cook

Printed in India

Last digit is the print number: 9 8 7 6 5 4 3 2 1

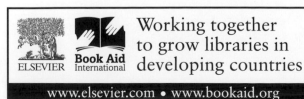

Working together
to grow libraries in
developing countries

www.elsevier.com • www.bookaid.org

It is easy to become completely immersed in interesting projects afforded to us in our work. What saves us are the family, friends and others who tolerate our mental absences, support us and make our lives complete. To these we dedicate this book, with love and gratitude.

To our significant others: Joan Anderson, Susana Sáinz García and Brendan Devaney
To our children: Nicholas and William Lowe, Robert and Lindsey Anderson and first grandson Robert Charles Anderson, Matthew Anderson and Katherine and Emily Devaney

To those who brighten our lives in other ways:
The musicians, cyclists, colleagues and students who have sustained the sunny disposition of one of the authors (SA) throughout this revision
The welcoming owners and staff of the establishments in Cambados, Galicia, who provided fine Albariño, seasonal local seafood and the occasional glass of a Ribera del Duero to one of the authors (JL) during the revision of this book

JL, PA, SA

PREFACE TO THE SIXTH EDITION

We are delighted to present this sixth edition of *Human Histology* and hope that it will provide the knowledge required to allow recognition of structures in histological images and link this to wider understanding in relation to structure and function.

The beliefs which are behind writing this textbook remain as follows:

Studying histology equips students with vocabulary, knowledge and insights that improve their learning and understanding of cell biology, anatomy, physiology, pathology and medicine.

Students benefit from using a textbook which is user-friendly, nicely organized and well-illustrated (despite the wide availability of learning resources on the Web).

There is a lot that could go into a textbook, and it is easy to overburden the reader. When faced with the conflict between being comprehensive and being comprehensible, we have chosen comprehensible.

We have stuck with our principles of only using human material and aligning the text to that which happens in humans. The book is not aimed at those wanting to know about rodents, fish or flies.

Things continue to change as biological discoveries are made and new concepts emerge. How cells are characterized and classified continues to evolve. Single-cell RNA sequencing (scRNA-seq) technology, with its ability to characterize individual cells, has led to the definition of different cell types and their functions within tissues. When coupled with access to resources such as the Human Protein Atlas, insights from histology continue to be essential components of modern cell biology. This revision, as with the previous editions, has had a main aim of updating the text and images accordingly.

The place of histology in curricula also continues to change. We have again reviewed the text to match with the changes in teaching in medicine, dentistry, biomedical sciences, nursing and midwifery courses. While maintaining a systematic approach to presentation, we have included more links to clinical contexts where knowledge of histology helps clinical understanding. It continues to be our experience that the students who demonstrate a good understanding of histology stand out in their wider, contextualized understanding of their subject.

Digital imaging and virtual microscopy are transforming many aspects of practical microscopy. It was always evident that for many people acquiring skills in looking down a microscope was a barrier to learning. Now, with virtual microscopy, students of histology can concentrate on images and understanding the structure of cells and tissues rather than struggling with lenses, focus and illumination. This edition has been revised with this in mind, and we hope will be a valued companion to learning when reviewing histology using all types of microscopy.

The fact that computer-based imaging and high-throughput systems for histology are being routinely applied in clinical diagnosis and in biomedical research implies a need for people who have knowledge of what they are looking at. A core competence in histology is increasingly in demand.

We have enjoyed revising the book, and we hope you enjoy using it.

JL, PA, SA, 2023

ACKNOWLEDGEMENTS TO THE SIXTH EDITION

Sadly, Dr Alan Stevens, one of the original authors of this textbook, died from non–small cell carcinoma of the lung on 10 April 2019. Steve, as he was known by his friends and colleagues, supported and contributed to many textbooks on histology, pathology, dermatopathology and histotechnology throughout his professional career. We gratefully acknowledge his contribution to this textbook and remember Steve as teacher, author, friend and wine consultant.

Once again, we take this opportunity to give our thanks to the many colleagues who made contributions to the five previous editions of the book.

In the preparation of the sixth edition, we want to thank the following organisations and people for their generous help.

We gratefully acknowledge the Human Protein Atlas (www.proteinatlas.org) for the ability to use material under a Creative Commons License (https://creativecommons.org/licenses/by-sa/3.0/). The atlas includes tissue microarray-based immunohistochemistry with virtual microscopy images that localize a vast range of proteins in human tissues (see Uhlén M et al. Tissue-based map of the human proteome. *Science.* 2015. PubMed: 25613900; doi: 10.1126/science.1260419).

Professor Philip Quirke leads the Leeds Institute of Medical Research Division of Pathology and Data Analytics at the University of Leeds, UK. Amongst his many areas of work is the application of digital microscopy and artificial intelligence in pathology. We are grateful for permission to use images using digital slides hosted in the University of Leeds Virtual Pathology Project. The Virtual Pathology team at Leeds is dedicated to high-quality digital slide scanning, hosting and research, with their data centre containing 167.5 terabytes of digital slide data. Those interested in experiencing digital microscopy and histopathology are recommended to have a look at https://www.virtualpathology.leeds.ac.uk/.

Images for this book were also obtained from the Pathology Education Instructional Resource website developed by one of the co-authors, Peter Anderson, and hosted by the University of Alabama at Birmingham, USA. This website contains over 30,000 curated pathological images and hundreds of virtual histology slides of normal and pathologic tissues, which can be found at https://peir.path.uab.edu.

Technological advances continue to be made in the field of histology, and without the involvement of manufacturers of equipment, they would not be in wide use. Tissue microarray technology, digital slides and analytical software are proving to be important tools in applying histological techniques in diagnosis and research. We are grateful to Peter Murad Anwar and the team at 3DHISTECH (https://www.3dhistech.com/) Budapest, Hungary for discussion and for images of their equipment.

Dr Ian Scott works as a clinical neuropathologist at The Walton Centre NHS Foundation Trust, Liverpool, UK. On a day-to-day basis he spends his time looking at histological preparations to make diagnoses of diseases of the brain, nerve and muscle. We are grateful for his assistance in sourcing ultrastructural images of peripheral nerve for the chapter on the nervous system and images of the equipment used for slide scanning in the Queen's Medical Centre in Nottingham.

Professor Mohammad Ilyas works as a research clinician in the University of Nottingham Medical School, UK, and applies molecular and cell biological methods to further understanding of diseases of the gastrointestinal system. As a diagnostic clinical histopathologist, he was an early adopter of image analysis and digital systems in histology. We are grateful for his help in providing images related to tissue microarray and digital microscopy.

Dr Marian Pigera is a consultant histopathologist who works at Lincoln County Hospital, UK, and has a special interest and expertise in breast disease. We are very grateful to her for review of the section on breast histology and for providing histological images of both normal breast and common disorders.

Several images in the book have been reproduced from original publications, cited in the relevant captions. We thank the authors and their publishers for permission to reproduce these images using the RightsLink service of the Copyright Clearance Centre (http://www.copyright.com).

In a digital age, continuous access to communication is vital. Many thanks go to Manuel and Chus, our dear neighbours, for letting us use their Internet when we needed it.

We would especially like to extend our sincere thanks to the team from Elsevier, especially Alexandra Mortimer, Ranjana Sharma and TJ Vishnu who greatly assisted in our work and were very patient if things got a bit slow.

COPYRIGHT INFORMATION

CONTENTS

HUMAN HISTOLOGY ONLINE VIDEOS

The authors of *Human Histology* have created a series of online videos to support learning. Each chapter is backed by several brief videos that can be viewed online.

Chapter Overview – a brief summary of what is covered in the chapter, useful to view before reading and studying a chapter.

Topic Videos – covering a key histology topic from the chapter such as:

- Basic structure – summary of key histological features
- Walk-through of a complex diagram, with explanation of the concepts involved
- Virtual microscopy – one of the authors demonstrating practical histology: "What can you see in an H&E?"

Visit eBooks.Health.Elsevier.com to see the Human Histology Online Videos.

Histology

INTRODUCTION

Histology is the study of the microscopic structure of biological material and the ways in which individual components are structurally and functionally related.

> Histology is central to biological and medical sciences, standing at the crossroads between a range of disciplines.

- Anatomy: sometimes referred to as microscopic anatomy or microanatomy, histology places gross anatomy into context, enabling the understanding of cell and tissue microstructure and how it relates to function.
- Physiological and life sciences: physiology, pharmacology, cell biology and biochemistry, among others; histology links them together, providing a point of reference that is between gross anatomy and these disciplines and explains the structure underpinning function and treatment.
- Pathology: knowledge of histology makes it easier to predict, understand and treat the functional deficits that are brought about by structural changes resulting from physiological adaptations or disease.

Knowledge of normal histological appearance is essential if abnormal or diseased structures are to be recognized and to understand how abnormal biochemical and physiological processes result in disease. Samples of human biological material can be obtained from many areas of the body by quick, safe biopsy techniques (Fig. 1.1), using instruments such as:

- Scalpels for directly accessible tissues such as the skin, mouth and nose.
- Needles into solid organs.
- Endoscopic tubes into the alimentary tract or body cavities.
- Special flexible cannulae inside blood vessels.

In modern medicine, despite sophisticated imaging and genetic testing, a histological diagnosis is still the mainstay, or the 'gold standard', of clinical practice. This is illustrated via two case studies in Fig. 1.2.

> Histology is a dynamic and evolving science.

Modern investigative techniques have revolutionized our understanding of cells and tissues. The techniques of electron and confocal microscopy, cloning of cells in culture, protein sequencing and molecular genetics have also given unprecedented insight into the working of cells. In the past 10 years, the application of single-cell RNA sequencing (scRNA-seq) has allowed

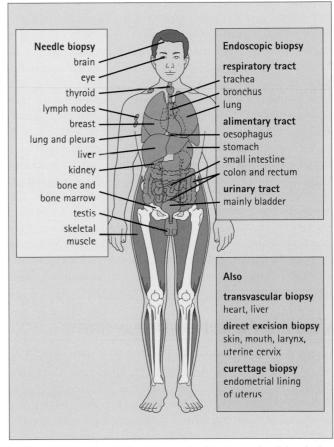

Fig. 1.1 Histology in Clinical Diagnosis. Small samples (biopsies) are obtained from different areas of the body by various techniques. Histological examination of such biopsies is an important and direct way of diagnosing disease.

new cell types to be discovered in tissues and new functions to be ascribed to known cell types. This research has been translated into clinical practice, enabling significant advances in diagnostic pathology and in developing new and targeted treatment (for an example see Advanced Concept: Tissue Microarray, page 8).

These studies are giving new insights into normal tissue function and how these are altered in disease. An understanding of the dynamics of cell populations in the respiratory system and the kidney is stimulating research into new targets for treatment. In tumour biology, there is a shift to personalized medicine in the understanding that even similar-looking tumours are unique: two breast tumours can have different expression of oncogenes and markedly different receptor expression (see Fig. 18.27). Knowing the detailed cellular characteristics of a tumour enables targeted treatment of individuals in a bespoke manner, appropriate to their tumour biology, rather than treating all tumours of an organ as one disease. Knowledge of normal tissues, including through histology, is the starting point for wider applications in both research and diagnosis.

> **Some histological terminology persists from a time before cell and tissue function was understood.**

The first microscopic investigations of biological material were carried out by Robert Hooke in his seminal publication *Micrographia,* just over 300 years ago. The study of histology began with the development of simple light microscopes and techniques for preparing thin slices of biological material to make them suitable for examination.

Such studies led Virchow to propound his cellular theory of the structure of living organisms that established the **cell** as the basic building block of most biological material. Each cell was considered an individual unit surrounded by a wall called the **cell membrane** and containing within it all the machinery for its function. Early microscopists had limited understanding of physiology and function and named features by their appearance or eponymously; for example, the microscopic connections running through bone and linking osteocyte cells are called *canaliculi* and the macrophage-like cells in the liver *Küppfer cells.* This can be frustrating, as there is a lot of vocabulary to learn and the system does not easily accommodate new information; however, it is slowly evolving.

CELLS ARE BASIC FUNCTIONAL UNITS

The cell is the basic unit of structure of most living organisms, and cells vary considerably. Although all cells in the human body are ultimately derived from a single fertilized ovum, each cell develops structural attributes to suit its function through the process of differentiation. Cell biology has shown that cells of diverse morphological appearance can be grouped together because of common functional attributes or interactions.

The general structural and biological properties of cells are discussed in Chapter 2.

Some cells are adaptable. It has also become apparent that even in adults, there are populations of highly adaptable, uncommitted stem cells, which can modify both their structure and their functional activity to adapt to changing environmental demands. This facility is of vital importance in adaptation to internal or external stress and is seen in normal and disease processes, for example, enlargement (hypertrophy) of a skeletal muscle cell in response to exercise, a reduction in size (atrophy) caused by inactivity or increasing numbers of cells (hyperplasia) in a gland because of excess stimulation. Some cells are constantly being replaced by this population of stem cells and are able to repopulate tissues after injury, for example, the outer layers of skin. Other cells cannot regenerate in a meaningful way; loss of such cells leads to the formation of a replacement tissue that fills the defect but is non-functional (e.g. replacement of damaged heart muscle by strong fibrous tissue after a heart attack).

⚕ CLINICAL EXAMPLE
Histology in Disease Diagnosis

Case Study 1 A 20-year-old student develops kidney failure, and the cause is not apparent from blood tests or imaging findings. The renal physician therefore removes a piece of kidney via a needle biopsy so that the diagnosis can be made by histological examination, immunohistochemical staining and electron microscopy. Special staining methods highlight subtle structural abnormalities by light microscopy (see Fig. 1.2). Electron microscopy provides valuable information about abnormalities at a subcellular level, and immunohistochemical staining allows the detection of immune complex deposition contributing to the pathogenesis of the disease. Based on the abnormalities that are revealed, an accurate histological diagnosis is determined and the renal physician can institute appropriate treatment. Clinical management of this patient's condition requires knowledge of the microanatomy of the kidney. Assessment of progress and the effectiveness of treatment can be monitored by repeat biopsy.

Case Study 2 A 15-year-old girl has swollen lymph nodes in her neck. A surgeon removes one so that it can be examined histologically, and microscopy reveals that the swelling is caused by a form of cancer. The classification of tumours is determined by histology and immunohistochemistry. Accurate histological assessment of tumours is the cornerstone of modern cancer treatment, because the treatment given to this girl depends on the histological type of the tumour (i.e. whether it is derived from muscle, lymphoid cells or endocrine cells). Thus the pathologist's report, which depends on the histological assessment of that specific tumour being accurate, will determine the type of chemotherapy deemed to be most efficacious for each cancer patient's treatment protocol. Increasingly, an initial histological diagnosis is the gateway to further molecular analysis of the tumour, which can give prognostic or therapeutic information used in patient management.

Fig. 1.2 Kidney. (a) Percutaneous needle biopsy histological sections from a diagnostic case. **(b)** High-power view of these needle biopsy specimens of kidney (paraffin section, martius scarlet blue trichrome [MSB] stain). The special stain shows the nature and location of the main abnormality, destruction of the afferent arteriole of the glomerulus by a disease process called fibrinoid necrosis *(arrow).*

Cell group	Epithelial cells	Support cells	Contractile cells	Nerve cells	Germ cells	Blood cells	Immune cells	Hormone-secreting cells
Example	gut and blood vessel lining, covering skin	fibrous support tissue, cartilage, bone	muscle	brain	spermatozoa	circulating red and white blood cells	lymphoid tissues and white cells (nodes and spleen)	thyroid and adrenal
Function	barrier, absorption, secretion	organize and maintain body structure	movement	direct cell communication	reproduction	oxygen transport, defence	defence	indirect cell communication
Special features	tightly bound together by cell junctions (see Chapter 3)	produce and interact with extracellular matrix material (see Chapter 4)	filamentous proteins cause contraction (see Chapter 5)	release chemical messengers on to surface of other cells (see Chapter 6)	half normal chromosome complement (see Chapters 16 and 17)	proteins bind oxygen, proteins destroy bacteria (see Chapter 7)	recognize and destroy foreign material (see Chapter 8)	secrete chemical messengers (see Chapter 14)

Fig. 1.3 Functional Cell Classification.

Cells are classified according to their main function.

The following groupings are used in this book: epithelial cells, support cells, contractile cells, nerve cells, germ cells, blood cells, immune cells and hormone-secreting cells (Fig. 1.3). It is important, however, to recognize that a cell may have several functions and be a member of more than one cell group. For example:

- Many of the hormone-producing cells are also epithelial in type, being tightly bound together by specialized junctions to form a gland.
- Many immune cells are also blood cells.
- Some support cells are also contractile.

The structural and functional specializations delineating each type of cell group are broadly outlined in Chapters 3–8 and are discussed in more detail throughout the book.

Tissues are functional arrangements of cells.

Tissues are discrete, organized collections of cells having similar morphological characteristics. These were traditionally subdivided into four types:

- Epithelial tissues, or cells that cover surfaces, line body cavities or form solid glands such as salivary glands.
- Muscular tissues, or cells with contractile properties.
- Nervous tissues referred to cells forming the brain, spinal cord and nerves.
- Connective tissue, a term used widely to describe a wide range of living material characterized by a dominant extracellular matrix component and the associated cells that produce the matrix. In theory, its function is to act as a supporting stroma, serving more highly specialized cell types.

The original group of 'connective tissues' included cell/matrix combinations, such as bone, cartilage, tendon, fibrous tissue, adipose tissue, bone marrow and blood. It has also been traditional to use the term *loose areolar connective tissue* to describe tissue that is partly made up of support cells that produce an extracellular matrix but which also contains cells belonging to the immune system (e.g. lymphocytes and macrophages), nerve cells and blood vessels.

In this book, the term *connective tissue* has been avoided because it underemphasizes the structural organization involved in this group of highly developed tissues. Instead, the concept of **support cells** is used, which emphasizes the importance of interactions between extracellular matrix and cells.

Support cells and their specializations are discussed in Chapter 4, and bone, cartilage, tendons and ligaments are discussed in Chapter 13.

In some cases, the cells forming a tissue are all of the same structure, forming **simple tissues**; for example, fat cells forming adipose tissue. However, most apparently distinct tissues contain a mixture of cells with different functions, which may be termed **compound tissues** (Fig. 1.4). For example, 'nervous tissue' contains nerve cells (neurons), support cells (astrocytes), immune cells (microglia) and epithelial cells (ependyma).

The concept of simple and compound tissues is useful in descriptive histology, but for brevity, the unqualified term *tissue* is used to imply either type.

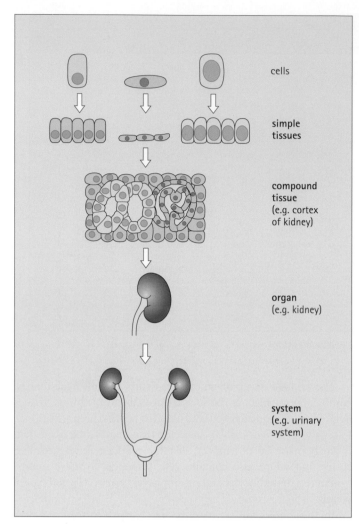

Fig. 1.4 Cells, Tissues, Organs and Systems.

cells

simple tissues

compound tissue (e.g. cortex of kidney)

organ (e.g. kidney)

system (e.g. urinary system)

Tissues form organs and systems.

An **organ** – for example, the heart, liver or kidney – is an anatomically distinct group of tissues, usually of several types, that perform specific functions. For example, in the organ skin, the tissue types involved are an outer epithelium – the epidermis – overlying the dermis, made of supporting connective tissue and containing the mechanical, immunological and nutrient support, and nerve endings, and housing the skin appendages. Deep to this is the subcutis, which is composed primarily of adipose tissue. In the intestines of the gastrointestinal (GI) tract, these organs are composed of layers of tissues from the lumen outward, including a lining epithelium, layers of underlying support tissue followed by external smooth muscle arranged to facilitate peristalsis. Peristalsis (the coordinated muscle contractions propelling food along the intestine) and glandular secretions are controlled by a range of nerve plexi.

The term **system** can be used to:
- Describe cells with a similar function but widely distributed in several anatomical sites.
- Describe a group of organs that have similar or related functional roles.

The specialized hormone-producing cells scattered in the gut and lung (diffuse endocrine system) cannot be an organ, as they do not form an anatomically distinct mass, whereas the tongue, oesophagus, stomach, intestines, exocrine pancreas and rectum are components of the 'alimentary system', and the kidney, pelvicalyceal system, ureters and bladder are part of the 'urinary system'.

The relationships between cells, tissues, organs and systems are shown in Fig. 1.4.

TECHNIQUES USED IN HISTOLOGY AND CELL BIOLOGY

The most common way to study cells is by light microscopy. Tissues are mounted on glass slides as thin preparations, stained with appropriate dyes, illuminated by light and viewed using glass lenses. This is called **histology**, or **histopathology** if biopsy material from diseased tissue is being investigated. The analysis of the fine structure of cells – for example, blood cells or those obtained via cervical smear – by light microscopy is referred to as **cytology**.

There is a limit to the detail that can be resolved using light microscopy, with very small structures within cells being invisible. Electron microscopy uses a beam of electrons instead of light, which greatly increases resolution, allowing the subcellular composition of cells to be defined.

These techniques are complemented by the increasing use of immunohistochemical methods. Antibodies are applied to specific cell constituents to visualize details within cells at the light microscopic level that are not visible by other techniques. For example, the location of specific proteins or subcellular components can now be defined in light microscopic preparations by using immunohistochemical staining techniques. Complementary to this, immunofluorescence techniques enable molecules to be visualized using antibodies linked to fluorescent probes. Use of a fluorescence microscope with the appropriate filters to produce a wavelength of light that excites the fluorescently tagged antibody facilitates viewing of a range of dyes, and the advent of confocal microscopy has greatly enhanced the resolution possible with light microscopy (Fig. 1.5) It is also possible to demonstrate specific DNA and RNA sequences by the technique of in situ hybridization, thereby gaining fundamental insight into the molecular working of cells.

Light Microscopy

Light microscopy using wax-embedded sections is the main technique used in histology.

Routine light microscopy uses thin sections of tissue to study cell morphology. Resolution of structures by light microscopy is of the order of 0.2 µm, but in routine practice with paraffin sections, resolution seldom exceeds 0.6 µm. Sections are usually obtained from paraffin wax-impregnated tissues (see box on p. 6 for detail) using a cutting instrument called a *microtome*. Sections are mounted on a glass microscope slide for staining. In routine laboratory practice, it generally takes 24 hours to produce a wax section for histology.

In some cases (e.g. diagnostic biopsies), it is necessary to look at fresh tissues that have not been exposed to protein cross-linking in fixation. In this situation, tissue is made sufficiently firm to cut by freezing, a technique referred to as *preparing a frozen section* (see box on p. 6 for detail).

Fig. 1.5 Comparison of microscopic techniques using a kidney glomerulus visualized by different microscopic methods: **(a)** wax histology, **(b)** resin histology, **(c)** scanning electron microscopy, **(d)** transmission electron microscopy and **(e)** confocal microscopy. Different methods show different levels of detail. In the wax section **(a)** can be seen arterioles (EA and AA), Bowman's capsule lined by epithelium (BC), the space where urine flows (US) and the tubule down which it leaves the glomerulus (TP). The resin section **(b)** shows more detail with red blood cells (RBC) seen in glomerular capillaries and details of mesangial cells (M) not easily seen in the wax section. The scanning EM image **(c)** shows the three-dimensional shape of glomeruli (G) and tubules (T) in the renal cortex but not much fine detail. A transmission EM **(d)** shows very high resolution and additional detail revealing the fine structure of podocytes (EP), which have foot processes (P1, P2) lying on a basement membrane (GBM), with very thin endothelial cells (EnC) on the other side. The confocal image **(e)** has been stained by immunohistochemistry and shows basement membrane components in green with cell nuclei in purple.

◎ ADVANCED CONCEPT
Paraffin Embedding

Paraffin embedding is the standard method of preparing thin sections of biological material for histological examination by light microscopy. It is cheap, comparatively simple and lends itself to automation.

The sample is preserved by immersion in a fixative, usually in an aqueous formalin-based fixative solution, which cross-links or precipitates proteins and prevents degradation of the tissue. It is then progressively dehydrated by passage through a series of alcohol solutions (e.g. 60%, 70%, 90% and 100%) until all water (intrinsic tissue water and fixative water) has been removed and the specimen is thoroughly permeated with absolute alcohol. The alcohol is then replaced by an organic solvent (e.g. xylene), which is miscible both with alcohol and with molten liquid paraffin wax (alcohol is not miscible with paraffin wax). The resulting specimen is immersed in paraffin wax at a temperature just above the melting point of the wax, which is solid at normal working room temperature. When the biological material is thoroughly permeated by the molten wax, it is allowed to cool so that the wax solidifies. The wax acts as a physical support to the sample, allowing thin sections (2–8 μm) to be cut using a microtome, without deformation of the cellular structure and architecture.

◎ ADVANCED CONCEPT
Frozen Sections

The process of fixation and embedding of biological material in paraffin and other media may destroy certain components, particularly enzymes, fats and some antigenic sites. If frozen water is used as the supporting medium, these components are better preserved and can be demonstrated by suitable techniques. Fresh (unfixed) material is rapidly frozen to −150°C to −170°C by immersion in, for example, liquid nitrogen, so that it hardens to a solid mass owing to freezing of tissue water. Thin sections (5–10 μm) are then cut on a special microtome housed in a refrigerated cabinet (a cryostat) and stained without exposure to alcohol or other organic solvents.

Frozen sections are used to demonstrate the cellular localization of enzymes and soluble lipids and in the identification of substances using immunofluorescence and immunocytochemical methods. There are obvious advantages to preparing frozen sections, including speed and retention of antigenicity, although without appropriate consideration, ice crystal damage can damage the tissue, thereby reducing resolution.

Further use is made of frozen sections in diagnostic histopathology, when an urgent tissue diagnosis is required of, for example a suspected tumour while the patient is still on the operating table. In skilled hands, a frozen section of a sample of human tissue stained with haematoxylin and eosin (H&E) can be prepared and examined under the microscope within 5 minutes of its removal from the body. In this way, a rapid and accurate histological diagnosis can be established while the patient is in the operating theatre, enabling the appropriate surgical room procedure to be performed.

Tissue Staining

> **To see tissue detail, it is necessary to stain the tissue components in a histological section.**

Cells are virtually colourless, and thus sections need to be stained for light microscopy. To enable staining, the wax is removed from the sections with an organic solvent before the section is rehydrated through increasing dilutions of alcohol in water. When fully rehydrated, the sections are stained with any of a number of stains, some of which are listed here. There are four main types of staining:

- Empirical
- Histochemical
- Enzyme histochemical
- Immunohistochemical

> **Empirical stains are widely used and form the basis of most routine stains in histology and histopathology.**

Many of the stains have been discovered by trial and error over a period of 100 years or more, and many methods use dyes and principles (e.g. use of mordants to fix a dye in a material) that were developed by the textile industry. In many cases, the precise details of the mechanism of the specific linkage between dye and tissue is not fully understood: sometimes it appears to be related to the sizes of the dye molecules used and sometimes the result of ionic charges on the dye molecules. The most common empirical stain is **haematoxylin and eosin (H&E),** a simple, reliable and inexpensive method of producing sections with blue nuclei and pink/red cytoplasm. Most of the micrographs in this book are stained with H&E. Other empirical stains include van Gieson's and trichrome methods (see Advanced Concept box on p. 7).

> **In histochemical methods, specific chemical compounds within the tissue can be localized.**

In some cases, staining is the result of a specific chemical reaction between a tissue component and a component of the stain solution; these methods are called *histochemical methods*. A commonly used example of a simple histochemical staining method is the periodic acid–Schiff (PAS) reaction, which demonstrates a wide range of tissue carbohydrates, including cytoplasmic glycogen and complex carbohydrate–containing substances, such as epithelial mucins. The rationale of the method is that carbon-to-carbon bonds in 1,2-glycols are cleaved using an oxidative agent, periodic acid. This produces dialdehydes, which then react with the colourless Schiff's reagent (fuchsin–sulphurous acid) to produce a vivid magenta-coloured compound.

◎ ADVANCED CONCEPT

Commonly Used Histological Stains

Haematoxylin and Eosin (H&E)
The combination of the two dyes, haematoxylin (blue) and eosin (red), is the most useful stain for the examination of biological material; the staining is simple to perform, reliable, inexpensive and informative. Cell nuclei stain blue (depending on section thickness and the formulation of haematoxylin used), and most components of the cell cytoplasm stain pink/red.

Van Gieson Method
The simple van Gieson method stains collagen pinkish-red and muscle yellow (see Fig. 10.23); it is commonly used in combination with a stain for elastic fibres. The elastic van Gieson (EVG) stain is valuable for demonstrating and differentiating the common support cell fibres, particularly elastic fibres, which stain brown-black, and collagen fibres, which stain pinkish-red; muscle is stained yellow (see Fig. 9.5).

Trichrome Methods
The trichrome methods employ a mixture of three dyes to stain different components in different colours. There are many trichrome methods, and they can be used to demonstrate general architecture, to emphasize support fibres or to distinguish support fibres from muscle fibres. An important use of a trichrome method is the demonstration of the cellular, osteoid and mineralized components of bone in non-decalcified bone embedded in acrylic resin (see Figs 13.17a and 13.19b).

Silver Methods
Under appropriate conditions, certain biological components, both within cells and in intercellular materials, reduce silver nitrate to form black deposits of metallic silver at the site of chemical reduction. By modifying the conditions of the silver nitrate solution used, these methods can demonstrate a wide range of structures, including reticular fibres (see Fig. 4.5).

Periodic Acid–Schiff (PAS) Method
The widely used PAS method has many applications, particularly in the demonstration of various carbohydrates, either alone (e.g. glycogen; Fig. 1.6) or combined with other molecules, such as proteins (e.g. glycoproteins), which are stained magenta. It can therefore be used to delineate basement membranes (see Fig. 4.13a) and some neutral mucins secreted by various secretory epithelial cells. The mucous cells of the stomach are strongly PAS-positive.

Alcian Blue Method
The Alcian blue dye method is used mainly to demonstrate acidic mucins secreted by some epithelial cells (see Fig. 11.44b) and can be combined with the PAS reaction to distinguish between acidic and neutral epithelial mucins. Through control of pH or other variables in the staining solution, the Alcian blue method can be used to demonstrate the extracellular glycosaminoglycan matrix (see Fig. 4.16d) of support cells.

May–Grünwald–Giemsa Method
The use of the May–Grünwald–Giemsa method is confined mainly to the examination of smear preparations of blood and bone marrow cells. Most of the micrographs in Chapter 7 show red and white blood cells stained by this method.

Myelin Methods
Several staining techniques can be used to demonstrate normal myelin. The dye Luxol Fast Blue is used frequently to demonstrate myelin in paraffin sections (see Fig. 6.21). Other methods use modified haematoxylin or osmium tetroxide.

Fig. 1.6 Liver – Paraffin Section: PAS Stain. This high-power photomicrograph shows intense red staining of the liver cell cytoplasm by the PAS stain, demonstrating the large amounts of glycogen present.

> **Enzyme histochemical techniques identify and localize the sites of activity of particular enzymes.**

As most biological enzyme systems are labile, they may be destroyed by fixation and tissue processing; thus, most enzyme histochemical methods are carried out on frozen sections.

To look at the tissue distribution of specific enzymes, sections of fresh tissue prepared on a cryostat are placed in an incubating solution containing the specific substrate for the enzyme or group of enzymes to be demonstrated, together with any necessary cofactors or inhibitors. The enzyme in the tissue reacts with the substrate to form an insoluble primary reaction product. This is then visualized by its reaction with a visualizing agent, which may be included with the incubating medium or applied as a separate second step.

This technique can be used to show the localization of a vast number of enzymes, including acid and alkaline phosphatases, dehydrogenases and ATPases, and is used routinely to detect abnormalities in certain diseased tissue, particularly muscle (see Fig. 13.4).

> **Immunocytochemistry uses antibodies to localize specific proteins in tissue sections.**

Immunocytochemistry is one of the most important innovations in histology. Antibodies to specific cell molecules are used to detect their presence in tissue sections. These are tagged either directly or indirectly with a product enabling visualization of the labelled molecules. For light microscopy, this is a brown-coloured product such as 3,3′-diaminobenzidine (DAB); for fluorescence microscopy, the tag emits fluorescence when excited by an appropriate wavelength of light. In immuno-electron microscopy, electron-dense particles of gold are used. Primary antibodies are either polyclonal or monoclonal. Polyclonal antibodies to a substance are obtained by inoculating an animal (commonly rabbits or sheep) with the purified protein and then harvesting serum from which a specific antibody can be extracted. Alternatively, monoclonal antibodies may be produced by inoculating a mouse and fusing suitable antibody-producing cells with immortal mouse myeloma cells to continually produce antibodies in tissue culture.

There are many examples of the use of immunohistochemistry throughout this book. Those wishing to explore further can explore the Human Protein Atlas (https://www.proteinatlas.org/) and by using the 'tissue' tag to see immunostaining of most human tissues using a huge set of antibodies to a vast number of proteins.

◎ ADVANCED CONCEPT

Tissue Microarray

Tissue microarray (TMA) is a way of examining many tissue samples at once. Instead of having to cut sections from hundreds of wax blocks from different cases, a single wax block is constructed which contains cores taken from hundreds of existing paraffin-embedded blocks. The method is shown in Fig. 1.7. This technique has revolutionized histological screening of tissues in research studies, as it is usual to use digital microscopy to view stained TMA slides and apply computer image analysis to achieve a high-throughput system.

The construction of a TMA starts with a person with a knowledge of histology selecting the area in a H&E slide from which the tissue donor block core will be taken for the array (see Fig. 1.7).

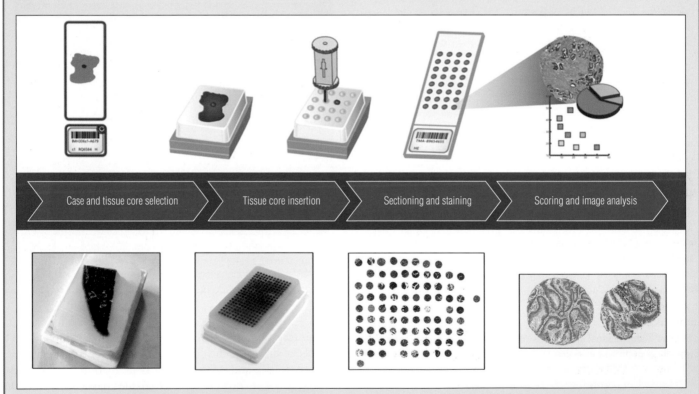

Case and tissue core selection   Tissue core insertion   Sectioning and staining   Scoring and image analysis

Fig. 1.7 Tissue Microarray. There are several stages in making a tissue microarray (TMA). First, the donor blocks, often many hundreds for a study, are selected from archives, and from each one, an H&E section is created and examined by a competent histologist to mark the areas of interest, which will be extracted as a core. A donor block is shown here which has had three core samples removed – the rest of the tissue is available for future studies or further diagnostic use. Next, each core is inserted into a recipient TMA block. The position in the block is recorded. Using computerized robotic systems to create a TMA block automates such record keeping and starts with bar-coding the donor blocks. A completed TMA block is shown, and a section is cut and stained. A H&E-stained TMA section is shown and is made up of a regular array of circular tissue cores. The most common application of TMA is in screening using immunohistochemistry, for example, to see what proportion of a type of cancer expresses a novel growth factor receptor, with such information being used in drug discovery. (Image modified with permission from 3DHISTECH, https://www.3dhistech.com.)

Fig. 1.8 Tissue Microarrayer. Many of the processes involved in preparing tissues for histology are now automated. Computer-controlled robotics systems are now used for processing, embedding and staining sections. The creation of a tissue microarray, which used to be a time-consuming task, can now be performed using a robotic system. This example is a TMA Master I, a high-speed, fully automated machine. Such equipment is transforming the application of histology in bioscience by facilitating large-scale high-throughput studies. (Image modified and used with permission from 3DHISTECH, https://www.3dhistech.com.)

Tissue blocks used in diagnosis are kept as part of the patient record for many decades and, with consent or approval, can be used in research. Tissue embedded in paraffin blocks is stable and retains its antigenicity for at least 60 years. TMA studies on such archival samples are increasingly used in large-scale studies and correlated with known treatment response and outcome for the patients. Because each section from a TMA block contains many small tissue cores (e.g. 0.6–2 mm diameter), resources are saved in only sectioning and staining one block to get information about hundreds of cases. A practical advantage of all cores being arrayed on one slide is that there is no variation in staining technique between samples. Small cores also mean that precious tissue is used sparingly and can therefore be available for other studies. Even though cores are small, validation in cancer studies has suggested they are suitably representative when two cores per biopsy are included in a TMA.

The construction of TMA blocks used to be performed manually but increasingly computerized robotic systems take cores from donor blocks, insert them into the TMA block and also keep track of the location of each sample during readout of the results after staining (Fig 1.8).

> **High-resolution light microscopy can be performed with tissue embedded in resin.**

Resolution of structures by light microscopy using paraffin sections is seldom better than 0.6 μm, the resolution being limited by the thickness of the section, which is rarely thinner than 3 μm. Much better resolution can be obtained by using thinner

ADVANCED CONCEPT
Resins and Histological Embedding Media

Acrylic Resin Embedding

Certain acrylic resins are used in a manner similar to paraffin wax as embedding media. When set, the resins are harder than paraffin wax and offer more support to the tissue than wax. They have two main advantages over paraffin wax for light microscopy:

- With the use of a special microtome, much thinner sections (i.e. 1–2 μm thick) can be obtained than with paraffin wax, giving greater resolution with the light microscope and enabling much more detail to be seen.
- They cause very little tissue shrinkage and enable good-quality sections of very hard material to be cut and are therefore used in the histological examination of mineralized bone (see Figs 13.17a and 13.19b).

Epoxy Resin Embedding

Epoxy resins are the hardest supporting media for biological material. With special sectioning machines, sections as thin as 0.5–1 μm can be cut for high-resolution light microscopy, and ultrathin sections, typically 70–90 nm, can be prepared for transmission electron microscopy.

The transmission electron micrographs in this book were prepared from ultrathin epoxy resin sections. These resins are resistant to the damaging effects of the electron beam in the electron microscope and continue to support the biological material, whereas other embedding media volatilize in the electron beam.

Most of the staining methods used with paraffin and acrylic resin sections cannot penetrate epoxy resins. Fortunately, the stain toluidine blue is an exception and differentially stains biological components in various shades of blue. The greatest cellular detail obtainable by conventional light microscopy is attained with the use of 0.5–1 μm epoxy resin sections stained with toluidine blue (see Figs 15.5d and 15.5e).

Toluidine Blue Stain

Toluidine blue is used to demonstrate cells and fibres in very thin epoxy resin sections. Toluidine blue is one of the very few dyes that will penetrate the dense epoxy resin to stain the tissue section. It provides considerable cellular detail, staining the various components of the cells and fibres in the shades of blue in a way that represents their relative electron density; hence the resulting blue picture closely resembles a low-power electron micrograph but is blue instead of black. Before preparation of ultrathin sections for electron microscopy, a toluidine blue–stained survey section is obtained from the epoxy resin block to enable the microscopist to trim down the appropriate area of tissue for ultrathin sectioning.

sections – about 0.5–2 μm – but these cannot be achieved consistently with wax as the embedding medium and using a standard microtome. The use of harder acrylic and epoxy resins as embedding media allows thinner tissue sections to be cut, thereby allowing increased cellular detail to be seen by increasing resolution (see Figs 15.5d and 15.5e).

> **Acrylic resins are a suitable embedding medium for the production of histological sections of non-decalcified bone.**

Bone, unless severely diseased, is usually too hard to produce thin histological sections using standard paraffin wax as the embedding medium and normal microtome knives. This is because the difference in hardness between the bone and the wax in which it is embedded is too great, so the bone shatters when the microtome knife blade passes through it, rendering the histology uninterpretable. Bone can be examined histologically in this way only if it is first softened by complete removal of the calcium salts by immersing the fixed bone sample in dilute acid until all the calcium has disappeared; sections can then be produced, but the histology is inevitably modified by the acid treatment. Furthermore, any distinction between mineralized bone and unmineralized osteoid is destroyed by the acid decalcification; this can be important in the diagnosis of some important bone diseases.

The problem can be overcome by embedding the bone in an acrylic resin embedding medium (e.g. methylmethacrylate) which, when set (polymerized), has a hardness that is the same as calcified bone, and good sections can be obtained without fragmentation or distortion. Examples are shown in many of the photomicrographs in Chapter 13; for example, see Figs 13.17, 13.19 and 13.25.

ELECTRON MICROSCOPY

> **An electron microscope uses parallel beams of electrons instead of light waves.**

In light microscopy, the degree of magnification and resolution achievable is limited by the wavelength of light. Parallel beams of electrons have a much shorter wavelength and, if used instead of light, much greater magnification can be achieved. This allows resolution of structures as small as 1 nm, thus permitting the study of subcellular morphology. Two main types of electron microscopy are used in the study of biological material: **transmission electron microscopy (TEM)** and **scanning electron microscopy (SEM)**.

To get the best results in both types of electron microscopy, fixation must be as perfect as can be achieved; this means that a different fixative solution (glutaraldehyde) is used. This must act on the tissues as soon as possible after the tissue sample has been obtained, as subcellular structures can be structurally altered as soon as they become anoxic. For TEM, this is achieved by using very small tissue fragments (<2 mm^3) to allow the fixative to penetrate all parts of the tissue as quickly as possible.

> **Transmission electron microscopy allows resolution of subcellular structures in very thin tissue sections.**

In TEM, the electrons in a vacuum chamber pass through a very thin section of fixed tissue, some components of which absorb all the electrons ('electron dense'), whereas others allow the passage of all electrons through the tissue sections ('electron lucent'). Some tissue elements allow only a percentage of electrons through, with the remainder being absorbed by the tissue. The electrons that do pass through strike a phosphorescent screen, allowing direct vision of the image, or a camera chip, which renders the image as a permanent record in black, white and various shades of grey.

The fixed tissue is embedded in an epoxy resin, which is harder than paraffin wax, and therefore allows thinner sections to be prepared (typically 70–90 nm) with a special machine, an 'ultramicrotome', using either diamond knives or special glass knives. These ultrathin epoxy resin sections are then placed in the electron microscope on a supporting copper mesh grid. The ultrathin section allows the passage of the electron beam to pass through the tissue section (except where it is in contact with the copper mesh support).

The natural variations in electron density and electron lucency of the tissue components are emphasized with the use of 'stains', such as osmium tetroxide, which has an affinity for lipid components, and other solutions of heavy metal salts, which makes them more electron dense and provides contrast.

> **A scanning electron microscope generates a three-dimensional view of a sample surface.**

The SEM uses a moving electron source, which scans the surface of a solid piece of tissue in a square raster pattern. Low-energy secondary electrons bounce back from the interaction of the incident electrons with atoms in the surface layer of the specimen. The detection system converts these low-energy secondary electrons into a three-dimensional image of the surface.

SEM uses solid pieces of tissue rather than ultrathin tissue sections. Tissue is fixed, dehydrated and dried to remove all liquid. It is coated with a thin even layer of metal such as gold to prevent the build-up of charge on the surface. SEM gives excellent detail of isolated cells or subcellular components such as villi and, in fractured cells, cytoskeletal elements or organelles. Because the x-rays given off by the tissue can also be detected, it can give information about the elemental composition of structures; for example, it can be used to locate and identify asbestos fibres in lung tissue (see Figs 7.3b, 7.15b, 11.11, 11.12b and 11.37).

> **Light and electron microscopes have similar components, with similar functions.**

Both types of microscopes have four major systems:
- An **illuminating system,** which includes a source of radiation.
- A system to hold the specimen in the radiation beam.
- An **imaging system,** which consists of a number of lenses to produce the final magnified image of the specimen.
- An **image translating system,** which allows the magnified image to be visualized and recorded.

Fig. 1.9 illustrates the similarities between the two microscopes.

In the **light microscope,** the illuminating system comprises a low-voltage electric lamp, with an adjustable **condenser lens** that focuses and concentrates the light into the plane of the object. After passing through the specimen, the light passes into the **objective lens,** the function of which is to collect the light rays and form a magnified intermediate image within the body tube above the objective lens. The **projector lens** in the microscope eyepiece further magnifies the intermediate image and presents the retina of the eye with a magnified virtual image, which appears to the microscopist to be in the plane of the tissue specimen.

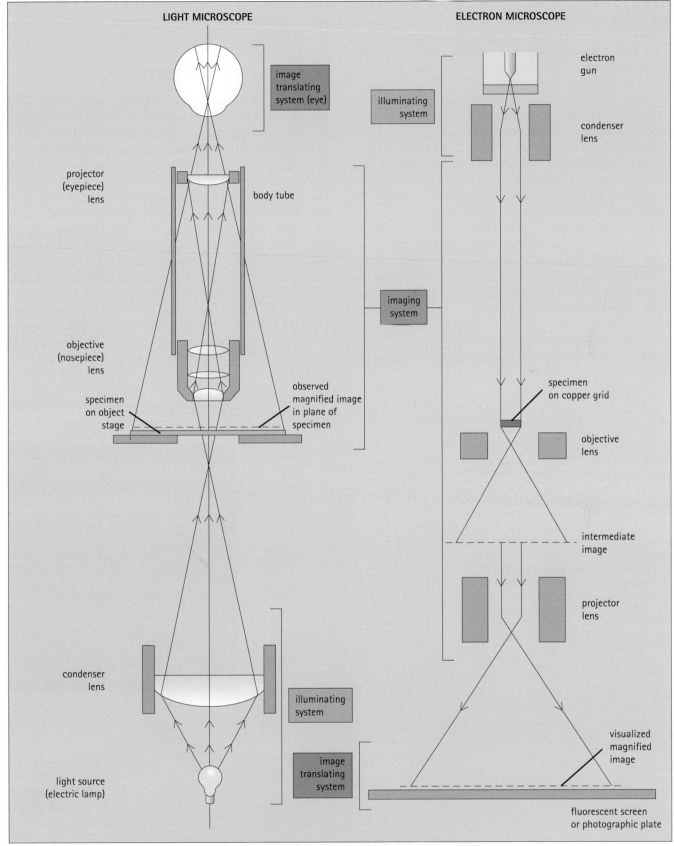

Fig. 1.9 Comparison of Light and Transmission Electron Microscopes.

In the **electron microscope,** the 'illuminating' system comprises the source of radiation (an electron gun) and a condenser lens system, which focuses the electrons on to the specimen. Like all lenses in an electron microscope, the condenser lens is an electromagnetic coil, which creates a magnetic field, the strength of which can be controlled to deflect electrons. To focus an electron beam onto a given plane (e.g. the specimen), the current passing through the electromagnetic coil is changed. Most electron microscopes have two condenser lens systems, the first of which reduces the electron beam from about 50 μm to 1 μm, and this narrow beam is then focused onto the specimen by the second condenser lens. When the focused electrons strike the specimen, many of the electrons pass through without deviation, but some are scattered by heavy atoms present in the stained specimen and are knocked out of the beam. This forms a pattern in the emergent beam, which is converted into an image by the objective lens, thereby bringing the emergent electrons to focus a few millimetres below the plane of the section. Below the focal point, a magnified intermediate image is formed, which is then magnified by the projector lens or lenses (there are often two or three, one after the other). The final magnification is controlled by the amount of current passing through these projector lenses. The magnified image is produced by the electrons passing on to a fluorescent screen, where it can be viewed through a binocular microscope, or onto a camera chip to make a permanent image (see Fig. 1.9).

CONFOCAL MICROSCOPY

Fluorescence microscopy has the benefit of being able to visualize specific receptors in a cell or tissue; however, the disadvantage is that the fluorescence signal from above and below the plane of focus is weakly incorporated into the image, affecting resolution and termed *out-of-focus blur.* By incorporating aligned pinholes into the optical path, confocal microscopy eliminates this out-of-focus blur and greatly improves resolution. Acquiring such a thin image allows optical sections to be generated by simply changing the plane of focus. Thin optical sections allow the localization or co-localization of multiple targets to the cell membrane or organelles, and this can also be achieved in live cells, so that the response of targets can be measured longitudinally; for example, the movement of receptors in response to increasing doses of treatment. These may then be rendered to form a three-dimensional image. It is even possible to carry out correlative techniques where the probe has both a fluorescence and immunogold tag, enabling a sample to be visualized (Fig. 1.10).

Fig. 1.10 Principle of confocal laser scanning microscopy (CLSM). CLSM uses lasers of a specific wavelength to excite fluorescence. These are scanned over the tissue, and an image is generated. **(a)** Confocally aligned pinholes in the light path exclude out-of-focus information from the image. The emitted fluorescence is collected using photomultiplier tubes and each channel (i.e. each colour) can be separately optimized. By changing the plane of focus, optical slices can be generated **(b)** and a three-dimensional image reconstructed **(c). (b)** A single optical slice of brain showing the interaction of astrocyte processes *(red)* with blood vessels *(green).* **(c)** A three-dimensional reconstruction of a live *Schistosoma.*

Laser

Confocal pinholes

Detector

Objective

Object
in Focal Plane
not in Focal Plane

VIRTUAL MICROSCOPY

> **Virtual microscopy uses high-resolution slide scanners to digitize the histological image.**

In the same way that computerized and robotic equipment has transformed many aspects of preparation and staining of slides (see Fig. 1.8), the viewing and examination of histological sections are being transformed by the use of digital microscopy. This now allows histological images to be examined on a computer screen using software that re-creates the use of the stage and objectives of a light microscope.

Histological slides, prepared and stained as previously described, are digitized and the digital images stored in such a way that they can be examined using a specialized digital microscopy workstation, as may be used in a clinical laboratory by a pathologist, in addition to through the Internet using a laptop, tablet or even a smartphone, as might be used by students of histology.

In order to replicate the resolution of a good light microscope, glass slides are scanned with specialized high-speed slide scanners (Fig. 1.11a). It has largely been the development of such high-speed, high-resolution scanning machines that has enabled virtual microscopy to be developed (see Fig. 1.11b). The digital image data for each slide are very large, and a system for virtual microscopy is only possible thanks to the availability of very high-capacity data storage systems and file servers. The digital data are processed and stored using compression and tiling algorithms that allow full-resolution images to accessed over a local network in a laboratory or over the Internet. These virtual slides can be magnified, panned and zoomed, to recreate the functionality of a conventional light microscope.

> **Virtual microscopy is increasingly used in teaching, learning and assessment.**

The teaching and learning of histology is being transformed by the use of virtual microscopy. It is often said that one of the barriers to learning histology was having to learn how to use a microscope, with student microscopes not always being of good quality. Now, students can focus on histology rather than microscopy technique.

Fig. 1.11 Slide Scanner. (a) High-throughput slide scanners operating in a clinical histopathology laboratory. **(b)** The scanner is loaded with batches of bar-coded histology slides, and a scanning run is started in which all slides are scanned at high resolution. Software links the digital image from each slide to the correct patient record. A computer monitor allows the operator to see which slide is being processed during a scanning run. Once scanned, digital slides are viewed from a workstation running dedicated software (see Fig. 1.13).

Fig. 1.12 Student Learning. (a) Students engaged in a histology class using a virtual microscope in place of glass slides and microscopes. The focus is on the microanatomy, rather than microscopy technique, and students work collaboratively, enhancing understanding. **(b)** An example of a student-generated virtual microscopy screenshot for notes. **(c)** An example of a staff-generated image for a multiple-choice formative assessment.

In most virtual microscopy systems, a thumbnail image on the screen shows where the location of a high-magnification image is in a slide. Studies have shown that students work collaboratively around the virtual microscope screen and remain engaged (Fig. 1.12).

Fig. 1.13 Histology reporting station in use in a histopathology department in a hospital.

This way of learning allows students to focus on acquiring knowledge and recognition skills and enables better engagement with instructors because the images are displayed in the familiar environment of a screen. A virtual microscopy system enables generation of personalized revision aids by students, who can use annotated screenshots to make notes (see Fig. 1.12b), and also facilitates generation of assessment items by instructors for both formative and summative purposes (see Fig. 1.12c).

For those who wish to experience and learn from online collections of histological images, several sites are available to experience virtual microscopy; doing an Internet search for 'virtual microscope' can be a good start.

> **Virtual microscopy is being used by histopathology staff in clinical diagnostic work.**

Such has been the pace of development of equipment to deliver virtual microscopy that histopathology is increasingly being provided as a digital pathology service. The histology of clinical diagnostic cases is viewed and reported using computer screens, using software which links to file servers holding the digitized slides (Fig. 1.13). Studies have been performed which underpin the use of digital histopathology in clinical practice based on reliability, reproducibility and quality assurance compared with conventional light microscopes.

Virtual microscopy has the advantage of enabling histologists to examine and review virtual microscopic images remotely and so collaborate in clinical diagnostic work.

In terms of professional training and development, virtual microscopy allows for the wide sharing of rare and unusual slides, without the limitations and risks associated with sending glass slides through the mail, as had to be done before. Clinical diagnostic quality assurance schemes are increasingly delivered using virtual microscopy.

For online review questions, please visit https://studentconsult. inkling.com.

The Cell

INTRODUCTION

Cells of all types have several common defining attributes and are composed of a fluid material (**cytosol**) that contains smaller elements, termed *subcellular structures,* which provide the framework for cellular activities.

Each cell is contained within a cell wall composed of a specialized cell membrane.

The fluid inside the cell, the **cytosol,** is a dense proteinaceous liquid that contains many of the essential enzymes and metabolites. The genetic material, in the form of chromosomes, is contained in the nucleus, and energy for cellular activity is largely generated by **mitochondria**. There is a constant generation of new structural elements within the cell, and this takes place in the membrane systems of the **endoplasmic reticulum** (ER) and **Golgi**.

Equally, cells must take in substances from outside and break them down using a system of small organelles called **lysosomes** that contain digestive enzymes. The shape of cells and much of the movement that takes place within cells are organized by an internal scaffolding of proteins known as the **cytoskeleton.**

This chapter describes the main building blocks of cells and the functional relationships that exist between them.

> **Cells have a common basic structure.**

Cells have many common features, which are independent of any specialized function (Fig. 2.1):
- An outer membrane surrounds each cell and separates it from its environment and from other cells.

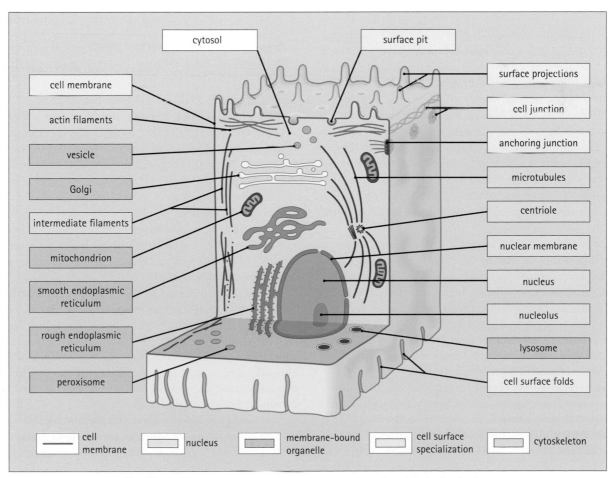

Fig. 2.1 Cell Structure. The main constituents of a cell and their distribution.

- Cells are composed of a solution of proteins, electrolytes and carbohydrates (cytosol), divided into specialized functional compartments (organelles) by inner membrane systems.
- Their shape and fluidity are determined partly by the arrangement of internal filamentous proteins (intermediate filaments, actin and microtubules) that form the cytoskeleton.

Cell membranes delineate several compartments within cells, each with a specialized function.

The main membrane-bound compartments are:

- The nucleus, which contains the cellular DNA.
- Mitochondria, which provide energy and act as sensors for the health of the cell.
- ER, which is involved in the biosynthesis of protein and some lipids.
- Golgi, which is involved in processing biosynthetic products for incorporation into the cell or for secretion.
- Vesicles, which act as temporary packages of material undergoing transport around the cell.
- Lysosomes, which contain hydrolytic enzymes to digest macromolecules within the cell.
- Peroxisomes, which contain enzymes involved in fatty acid metabolism.

CELL MEMBRANES

> **Cell membrane structure is based on a lipid bilayer.**

The outer membrane surrounding each cell and the membranes surrounding internal cellular organelles have a common basic structure of a lipid bilayer containing specialized proteins in association with surface carbohydrates.

The most important determinant of membrane structure is the lipid component. Each type of membrane lipid molecule has one hydrophilic end and one hydrophobic end (Fig. 2.2); thus they are amphipathic. Such lipids spontaneously form a bilayer in water, with the hydrophobic ends forming an inner layer between the outwardly directed hydrophilic groups.

This basic cell membrane structure, into which membrane proteins are inserted (Fig. 2.3), confers important functional attributes:

- The membrane is a fluid, allowing lateral diffusion of membrane proteins and facilitating cell mobility by curving.
- The polar lipid composition leads to a variable permeability to different substances, it being highly permeable to water, oxygen and small hydrophobic molecules such as ethanol, but virtually impermeable to charged ions, such as Na^+ and K^+.
- Breaks and tears are sealed spontaneously, as the polar nature of lipids eliminates free edges where hydrophobic groups would meet the aqueous environment.
- Membrane proteins are placed to perform functional roles in processes such as transport, enzymatic activity, cell attachment and cell communication. Membrane curvature is, in part, also determined by the local concentration of specialized membrane proteins. Insertion of specific proteins into parts of the membrane facilitates and, in some cases, drives curving or folding.

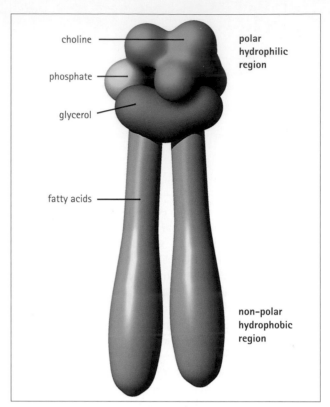

Fig. 2.2 Membrane Phospholipid Molecule. A membrane phospholipid molecule, which is the main component of cell membranes and determines the fundamental properties of the cell membrane as a whole.

> **There are three major types of membrane lipids: phosphoglycerides, cholesterol and glycolipids.**

Lipid forms 50% of the mass of cell membranes.

Phosphoglycerides (phospholipids) make up about 50% of the lipid component and tend to surround membrane proteins, often specifically anchoring proteins with enzyme or transport functions. There are three major phosphoglycerides in the cell membrane:

- Phosphatidylcholine
- Phosphatidylserine
- Phosphatidylethanolamine

Cholesterol in the cell membrane limits the movement of adjacent phospholipids and makes the membrane less fluid and more mechanically stable.

Glycolipids are found in the outer face of cell membranes, with their associated sugars exposed to the extracellular space, where they may be involved in intercellular communication.

The sphingolipids are the main type of glycolipid in cell membranes. An important membrane glycolipid is galactocerebroside, which is a major component of myelin, the fatty insulation layer around nerves (see Chapter 6). Another group of important glycolipids is the gangliosides, which constitute up to 10% of the lipid in nerve cell membranes.

The composition of inner and outer lipid layers is not the same. For example, high concentrations of certain phospholipids in the inner face may be needed to complement the presence of an inner membrane protein because certain proteins need to be

Fig. 2.3 Cell Membrane Structure. The cell membrane is composed of a lipid bilayer with phospholipid hydrophobic groups facing inward and hydrophilic groups facing outward. Protein molecules float within this basic structure, with projecting carbohydrate groups being attached to glycolipids or proteins.

linked with specific phospholipids. Islands of high concentration of sphingolipids and cholesterol can form in the membrane to produce **lipid rafts,** which are typically 50 nm in size and carry specific proteins or cell-signalling molecules and act as a specialized membrane domain. Membrane stiffness and fluidity can be altered by dynamically changing lipids in different layers of the cell membrane, and this is key to allowing the formation of different structures derived from the cell membrane within the cell.

> **Membrane proteins carry out many of the specialized functions of cell membranes.**

The types of membrane protein encountered vary according to cell type. Integral membrane proteins are those that span the lipid bilayer of the cell membrane, whereas peripheral membrane proteins are associated with either the inner or the outer half of the lipid bilayer. Membrane proteins have several functions:

- Attach cytoskeletal filaments to cell membrane
- Attach cells to extracellular matrix (e.g. adhesion molecules)
- Cause the cell membrane to curve or fold to form subcellular specialized structures
- Transport molecules in or out of cells (e.g. carrier proteins, membrane pump proteins, channel proteins)
- Act as receptors for chemical signalling between cells (e.g. hormone receptors)

- Act as antigens as part of the system for immune surveillance
- Possess specific enzymatic activity

Some membrane proteins can diffuse laterally over the surface of the cell. Others appear fixed in the cell membrane.

> **Membrane carbohydrates are mostly present on the membrane surfaces that are not in contact with cytosol.**

Membranes have associated carbohydrate residues, usually as a component of glycoproteins and glycolipids, which are mainly confined to the membrane surface that faces away from the cytosol. They are therefore found on the luminal aspect of inner membrane systems and on the cell surface, where they have been termed the **glycocalyx.**

Membrane-associated carbohydrates can be demonstrated by staining with lectins, proteins extracted from plants with binding capabilities for specific carbohydrate groups.

These membrane carbohydrates, as a component of glycoproteins or glycolipids, are important in cell–cell interactions. The oligosaccharide moieties of glycolipids and glycoproteins are also important as antigens involved in tissue compatibility in blood transfusion or organ transplantation. Given the understanding that complex sugar residues determine many functional aspects of cells, the study of glycobiology has been identified as an important area of investigation.

TRANSPORT IN AND OUT OF CELLS

> Transport of material in or out of a cell takes place by the processes of diffusion, active transport, endocytosis and exocytosis and in extracellular vesicles.

Substances may diffuse through cell membranes, or they may be transported by special membrane protein transport systems (pumps, carriers or channels). Other material from the extracellular space, in addition to the surface membrane, may be incorporated into the cell by invagination of the cell surface in a process termed **endocytosis** (Fig. 2.4a). The invaginated cell membrane fuses to form an **endocytotic vesicle** or **endosome**, which is a small, sealed, spherical membrane-bound body. The membrane and any material incorporated into such a vesicle can then be processed within the cell.

The terms **pinocytosis** (Fig. 2.4b) and **potocytosis** are used when cells take up fluid and small molecules to form small vesicles about 50 nm in diameter. The terms **endocytosis** and **phagocytosis** (Fig. 2.4c) are used when cells ingest large particles to form endosomes more than 250 nm in diameter.

Fig. 2.4 Endocytosis, Macropinocytosis, Phagocytosis and Exocytosis. Specific proteins mediate the process of membrane integration in endocytosis and exocytosis. **(a) Endocytosis.** The invaginated cell membrane fuses to form an endocytotic vesicle (endosome), which is a small, sealed, spherical, membrane-bound body. The membrane and any material incorporated into such a vesicle can then be processed within the cell. **(b) Macropinocytosis.** In this process, the cell extends as a sheet to envelop and enclose a large amount of extracellular fluid. Membrane fusion internalizes this within the cell. Unlike endocytosis and phagocytosis, the process is not stimulated by binding of a membrane surface receptor to a cargo. **(c) Phagocytosis.** In phagocytosis, a particle outside the cell has proteins on its surface that are recognized by receptors on the cell surface. In the case of a foreign particle, such as a bacterium, the protein may be antibody bound to its surface, and the receptor recognizes the Fc portion of the antibody. The binding of the receptor leads to activation of cell-signalling systems that cause processes to extend from the cell to progressively engulf the particle. Subsequent fusion of the cell membrane leads to internalization of the particle within the cell, contained in a membrane-bound vesicle. **(d) Exocytosis.** This is the fusion of a membrane-bound vesicle with the cell surface to discharge its contents into the extracellular space. This allows the secretion of products manufactured by the cell. In addition, fusion of vesicles with the cell membrane allows new membrane to be incorporated into the cell surface.

Exocytosis is the reverse of endocytosis and describes the fusion of a membrane-bound vesicle with the cell surface to discharge its contents into the extracellular space (Fig. 2.4d). This mechanism allows the secretion of products that have been manufactured by the cell. Fusion of vesicles with the cell membrane also allows new membrane to be incorporated into the cell surface.

It is increasingly recognized that buds of the cell membrane can pinch off to form spherical membrane-bound vesicles containing cytosol, which leave the cell surface to form extracellular vesicles (EVs). The following three main classes of EVs have been described, but the functional relationship between these is still under investigation:

- Exosomes (40–120 nm)
- Ectosomes (100–1000 nm)
- Large oncosomes (1–10 μm diameter)

Once formed, EVs act as transport vesicles that can move between cells in the extracellular space. EVs can transport a range of cargo material (especially proteins, lipids and other metabolites) in addition to nucleic acids, including different RNA species and DNA. EVs can fuse and internalize their cargo into a target cell. It is believed that cargo delivered to other cells can have effects in cell signalling, growth regulation, cell motility and immune recognition. Exosomes can also form to eliminate toxic or waste products from the cell, ejecting the material in membrane-bound vesicles into the extracellular space, where they are believed to be taken up and processed by 'professional' phagocytic cells such as macrophages. There is great interest in these structures involved in cell signalling in the study of immunity and cancer biology.

> The two main vesicles involved in the transport of substances into cells are derived from surface membrane invaginations called *coated pits* and *caveolae*.

Small invaginations of membrane constantly form at the surface of most cells to ingest extracellular material, which is then processed by the cell. The invaginations are drawn down to form vesicles; once the contents have been processed, the vesicle membrane returns to the cell surface. Thus there is a constant shuttle of membrane between the cell surface and cell interior (membrane trafficking). These vesicles originate in two main types of specialized areas of the cell membrane termed *coated pits* and *caveolae*.

Coated pits are invaginations braced by special membrane-associated proteins and are used to bring material into the cell for further processing (Fig. 2.5). In many instances, special receptor proteins are present in the cell membrane that can bind to specific substances outside the cell and draw them inside in a process termed **receptor-mediated endocytosis**. Coated vesicles may also develop from other internal membrane systems inside cells.

Fig. 2.5 Ultrastructure and Coated Pit Formation. (a) A coated pit is braced by a coat of protein *(orange)* and bears surface receptors *(blue)* that bind specific extracellular ligands *(red)*, for example, a substance that needs to enter the cell, such as iron. In many cases, the coat protein (visible ultrastructurally as a fuzzy membrane thickening) is clathrin, which forms a hexagonal lattice around the pit membrane. **(b, c, and d)** Assembly of the coat protein lattice drives progressive invagination of the pit to form a coated vesicle. The protein dynamin forms a collar around the neck of the vesicle and assists in budding. **(e)** Once internalized, the coat protein is shed from the vesicle and returns to the cell surface to form new *coated pits*. This form of transport into cells is termed *receptor-mediated endocytosis* and is a feature of the internalization of iron, low-density lipoprotein and some growth factors.

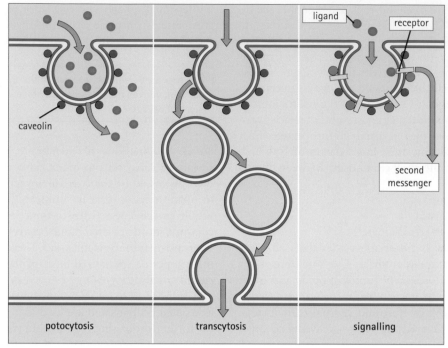

Fig. 2.6 *Caveolae.* There are three functions of *caveolae*. First, receptors on *caveolae* can concentrate substances from the extracellular space, and these can then move into the cytosol. This is termed *potocytosis,* and such *caveolae* remain as invaginations and do not form vesicles. Second, some *caveolae* form vesicles and internalize material, which is then transported across the cell and released from the other side in a process termed *transcytosis.* Third, some *caveolae* are the site of concentration of surface receptors that influence intracellular secondary messenger signal systems, thereby making *caveolae* an important structure in signal transduction.

Caveolae are also invaginations of the cell surface membrane but, in contrast to *coated pits*, are braced by proteins termed *cavins*, one of which is caveolin. *Caveolae* have three important cellular roles (Fig. 2.6):

• The surface of *caveolae* may carry receptor proteins that bind to molecules in the extracellular space. They can concentrate substances from the extracellular space and transport them into the cell in a process termed **potocytosis.**

• *Caveolae* are used to transport material from the extracellular space on one side to the extracellular space on the other in a process termed **transcytosis.** This happens in cells such as the flat cells that line blood vessels (endothelial cells).

• These invaginations are also believed to have roles in **intracellular signalling.** The cell membrane associated with *caveolae* is enriched with many of the cell surface proteins that have functions as receptors. *Caveolae* are believed to allow extracellular events to trigger intracellular secondary cellular messenger systems.

⊚ ADVANCED CONCEPT

There are two types of secretory mechanisms. In some cells, secretion occurs by a constant fusion of vesicles with surface membrane, termed the **constitutive secretory pathway.** In other cells, fusion of secretory vesicles with the surface must be triggered by a signal to the cell, termed the **regulated secretory pathway.**

Several proteins have been defined that mediate the processes of membrane fusion. The Rab family of GTPases controls the specificity of trafficking and docking and recruits tethering factors and fusion factors. So-called 'SNARE' proteins (from SNAp REceptor) are responsible for tethering and docking of the vesicle to the membrane. Different members of the SNARE family are specific to different vesicle systems and cell compartments, allowing specificity of fusion events.

⊚ ADVANCED CONCEPT

Clathrin

Clathrin is an example of a membrane-bracing protein. It forms a hexagonal lattice structure that develops as a coat around the outside of the vesicle and accounts for the fuzzy layer seen ultrastructurally.

Assembly of this lattice is believed to drive the invagination of the surface membrane. A protein called *dynamin* forms a collar around the neck of the invaginating vesicle and is believed to be important in facilitating budding and separation of the formed vesicle from the surface. Several different adapter or assembly proteins are associated with the coat and target the clathrin-coated vesicle to the correct place for docking and transport. The clathrin scaffolding is broken down by a series of proteins in an uncoating reaction once the vesicle is internalized.

Macropinocytosis and phagocytosis internalize large particles into the cell.

Cells internalize material from the extracellular environment by two additional processes:

In **macropinocytosis** the cell membrane curves out to extend a crescent-like thin fold of membrane to encapsulate a pool of extracellular fluid, which is then incorporated into the cell by invagination of the derived membrane-bound vesicle (see Fig. 2.4b).

In **phagocytosis**, an area of the cell surface bears receptors that recognize proteins attached to a – generally – foreign particle in the extracellular space. The proteins that are recognized may be antibodies: for example, antibodies bound to a disease-causing bacterium. The binding of receptor and protein triggers extension of the cell membrane to engulf the particle, followed by fusion of the membrane to internalize the particle into the cell, where it then fuses with other vesicles (see Fig. 2.4c). This mechanism is also believed to operate in the internalization of extracellular vesicles involved in the transfer of cargo material between cell types.

CYTOSOL

The cytosol is the fluid matrix of the cell.

The cytosol of the cell is a concentrated, dense fluid. This fluid matrix contains the following important components:

- Much of the machinery involved in protein synthesis, posttranslational modification, protein degradation and carbohydrate metabolism, including glycolysis (it is therefore rich in enzyme systems).
- Proteins involved in cell signalling and cell death pathways.
- Filamentous proteins that form the cytoskeleton (see p. 33).
- Some products of metabolism, such as glycogen and free lipid, for which the cytosol acts as a storage compartment.
- Numerous ribosomes, both free in the cytosol and associated with the cytosolic surface of rough ER. RNA is associated with these structures. mRNA also forms RNA–protein complexes termed **P bodies** which are involved in mRNA sequestration, modulation and degradation.
- Free ions involved in cell signalling in addition to regulating the oncotic balance between the cell and the extracellular space.

⊚ ADVANCED CONCEPT

Nanotubes allow direct communication and transfer of material between cells. Direct cell-to-cell communication can occur through extremely thin tubes of membrane called *tunnelling nanotubes* (TNTs). These protrusions can connect cells that may be a significant distance away from each other: up to several cell diameters (Fig. 2.7). The formation of such nanotubes is assisted by actin filaments. The cell membrane of the nanotubes may include specialized structures such as communication gap–junction complexes. Once formed, TNTs are believed to deliver a range of cargo from one cell to another, including mitochondria, DNA, and a range of RNA species including microRNA (miRNA). The importance of the recent recognition of this mode of cell-to-cell communication is that it is likely to be involved in the spread of certain pathogens, in the modulation of immunity and in control of cell growth, including in cancer biology.

Fig. 2.7 Tunnelling Nanotubes. These structures allow direct communication and exchange of material between cells. **(a)** To show transport between cells by nanotubes, trabecular meshwork cells were cultured. **(b)** Half were labelled with DiD *(red)* and half with DiO *(green)* and then mixed 1:1. After culturing overnight, a long cell process has extended from the red cell to the green cell representing a nanotube **(c)** at a higher magnification. Red DID-labelled vesicles can be seen in a green DiO-labelled cell *(arrows)* showing that there has been direct communication and transport of cargo between cells via the nanotube. (Image courtesy of Kate Keller, PhD, Casey Eye Institute, Oregon Health & Science University, Portland, Oregon.) (Further reading: Keller KE, et al. Tunneling nanotubes are novel cellular structures that communicate signals between trabecular meshwork cells. *Invest Ophthalmol Vis Sci.* 2017;58:5298–5307.)

Fig. 2.8 Ribosomes. Electron micrograph showing free ribosomes in the cytosol. They are small, electron-dense particles 20–30 nm in diameter, present either singly or in chains called polyribosomes.

Although many proteins are uniformly distributed within the cytosol, other proteins are locally concentrated to facilitate specific interactions and metabolic processes. It is therefore possible to consider different cell regions within the cytosol of a cell according to functional activity.

> **Ribosomes are involved in the synthesis of proteins.**

Ribosomes are a key structure in protein synthesis. They synchronize the alignment of both messenger RNA (mRNA) and transport RNA in the production of peptide chains during protein synthesis. Ribosomes are small electron-dense particles (Fig. 2.8) that impart a blue colour (basophilia) to the cytoplasm of protein-producing cells on light microscopy. Each ribosome is composed of a small subunit that binds RNA and a large subunit that catalyses the formation of peptide bonds. They are made up of specific ribosomal RNA and specific proteins. Ribosomal RNA is manufactured in the nucleolus (see p. 24).

THE NUCLEUS

> **The nucleus contains the cellular DNA and the nucleolus.**

The nucleus is the largest single membrane-bound compartment in the cell and contains the cellular DNA together with many different proteins that are involved in organizing and regulating DNA function (Fig. 2.9).

In light microscopic preparations, nuclei are spherical or ovoid, generally measuring 5–10 μm in diameter; they stain strongly with basic dyes, such as haematoxylin (i.e. basophilic)

Fig. 2.9 Nucleus. Electron micrograph showing typical cell nucleus. It is bounded by a double nuclear membrane (NM). The nucleolus (N) is clearly visible as an electron-dense circular area. Nucleus chromatin is divided into two types: heterochromatin (H) is dense-staining and euchromatin (E) is light-staining.

and contain a smaller spherical structure, the nucleolus, which synthesizes ribosomal subunits.

Nuclei are bound by two concentric membranes with different functional roles. The inner nuclear membrane contains specific membrane proteins that act as attachment points for filamentous proteins, termed **lamins**, which form a scaffolding to maintain the spherical shape. The outer nuclear membrane bounds the perinuclear space, which is continuous with the lumen of the ER; it may be associated with ribosomes in a similar manner to rough ER.

The nuclear membrane is perforated by numerous pores, which establish continuity between the cytosol and the nuclear lumen containing the chromatin (Fig. 2.10). The nuclear pore is one of the most complex structures within the cell, being ringed by many proteins involved in governing traffic in and out of the nucleus. Many aspects of cell signalling involve transport of a signalling factor from the cytosol via the nuclear pore to the nucleus to control specific gene expression.

> **Nuclear DNA is tightly packed by association with special proteins and forms the chromatin.**

The nucleus contains DNA wound around proteins called *histones* to form nucleosomes, which are regularly repeating globular structures like beads on a string. The nucleosome string is then wound into filaments 30 nm in diameter, which make up the structure of chromatin. Further condensation into distinct chromosomes is possible during cell replication, when

Fig. 2.10 Nuclear Pore. (a) The double nuclear membrane (NM) bounding the perinuclear space (PNS) is perforated by nuclear pores (P), which appear as gaps in transmission electron micrographs. **(b)** Structurally, the pores are formed by concentric rings of subunits to form the nuclear pore complex shown in this diagram. Above and below the large protein units are rings from which filaments radiate into nuclear and cytoplasmic spaces. The structure formed by rings and filaments in the nuclear space is termed the nuclear basket. **(c and d)** The high resolution of protein subunits in the nuclear pore has been determined, allowing construction of an accurate model of its structure. The pores form channels, which allow the transport of small molecules but restrict the movement of large molecules between the cytosol and the nucleus. Movement of some proteins into the nucleus is desirable, however, and the nuclear pore complex recognizes and actively transports specific peptide sequences in proteins destined for the nucleus. In a similar fashion, large ribosomal subunits produced in the nucleus are actively transported into the cytosol. The central granules seen by electron microscopy in the pore complex are believed to be large proteins or components of ribosomes in transit between different cell areas. (Image courtesy of Jan Kosinski and Martin Beck, Structural and Computational Biology Unit, European Molecular Biology Laboratory, Heidelberg, Germany.)

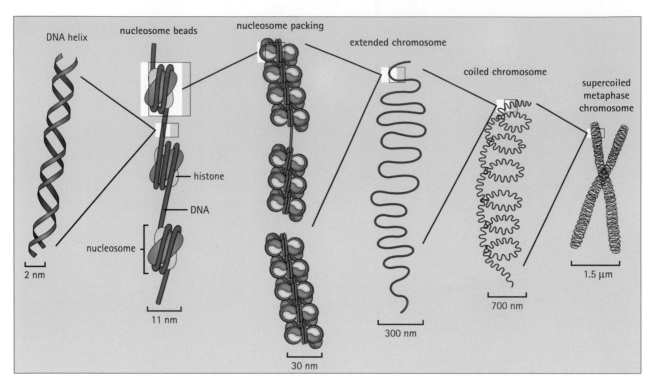

Fig. 2.11 Chromatin Structure. DNA is organized around histones into nucleosomes. The nucleosomes are wound into a helix to form chromatin. In chromosomes, this is then wound again into a supercoiled structure.

chromatin forms large, looped domains by attachment to DNA-binding proteins. This relationship is shown in Fig. 2.11.

The distribution of chromatin is not uniform, and this reflects varying degrees of unfolding according to whether genes are being transcribed. **Euchromatin** is seen as light-staining electron-lucent areas and represents actively transcribed cellular DNA. **Heterochromatin** is seen as a dense-staining area, often adjacent to the nuclear membrane, and is the highly condensed, transcriptionally inactive form. A possible function of converting between euchromatin and heterochromatin is to regulate gene expression. Cells with a high proportion of euchromatin, often encountered in a large nucleus, can be interpreted as cells with active processing of DNA, and hence actively functioning. Cells with a uniformly dense-stained, compact and small nucleus with a high proportion of heterochromatin can be interpreted as having little active DNA processing, and hence functionally inactive. In all cells, however functionally inactive, a small proportion of chromatin will undergo transcription as part of essential maintenance of the cell. Such genes have been termed *housekeeping genes*. In disease states, housekeeping genes may be switched off and instead a system of so-called *cell stress genes* become transcribed, and these function to protect the cell and limit any damage.

> **The nucleolus is the site of formation of ribosomal RNA in the nucleus.**

The nucleolus is an example of a self-assembling non–membrane-bound cellular body, which forms to maximize interactions between specific DNAs, RNAs and proteins involved in common processes within the nuclear space. The nucleolus is a roughly spherical structure within the nucleus measuring 1–3 μm in diameter. This region forms to contain

and organize the areas of DNA that code for ribosomal elements termed *nucleolar organizing regions*. The binding of ribosomal DNA (rDNA) by cohesin proteins is important in the forming of the nucleolus. During the cell cycle there is disassembly and then reassembly of the nucleolus, which forms when RNA polymerase I–mediated transcription takes place in the cell. Nucleoli increase in size with active gene transcription so that inactive cells have indistinct nucleoli, whereas metabolically active cells have large or multiple nucleoli. In haematoxylin and eosin preparations, nucleoli stain blue-pink because of their affinity for both acidophilic and basophilic dyes.

The most recognized function of the nucleolus is as the site of production of ribosomal RNAs, which are packaged with proteins to eventually form ribosomal subunits; these are later exported to the cytosol via the nuclear pore complexes. The nucleolus also produces signal recognition particles, involved in threading nascent proteins as they form on ribosomes into the ER. The nucleolus is also understood to have roles in the processing of different forms of RNA, in cell cycle regulation and as a sensor for certain types of DNA damage.

Three regions of the nucleolus can be distinguished by electron microscopy (Fig. 2.12):
- Pale fibrillar centres (**pars amorpha**) correspond to large loops of transcribing rDNA containing the ribosomal RNA genes associated with RNA polymerase I (Pol I) transcription factors.
- Dense fibrillar regions (**pars fibrosa**) correspond to early pre-RNA processing factors and transcripts of ribosomal RNA genes beginning to form ribosomes.
- Granular regions (**pars granulosa**) correspond to RNA-containing maturing ribosomal subunit particles and signal recognition particles.

Fig. 2.12 Nucleolus. Electron micrograph showing the nucleolus from a cell actively producing protein. The pale fibrillar centre (pars amorpha) (A), dense fibrillar region (pars fibrosa) (F) and granular regions (pars granulosa) (G) are clearly visible.

CLINICAL EXAMPLE

Nucleolar Size: Significance in Histology

In histological diagnosis, changes in the size, shape and morphology of the nucleus are used to help diagnose malignancy (cancerous change). Amongst other features, malignant cells tend to have more prominent nucleoli compared with normal cells. In malignant cells, nucleoli may be much larger than normal, or a cell may contain multiple large nucleoli (Fig. 2.13). In malignant cells, a distinct area has been seen around the nucleolus, termed the *perinucleolar cap*, and this has been linked to more aggressive forms of tumours.

Fig. 2.13 Nucleoli In Cancer Cells. The nucleoli (arrows) in these cancer cells are large and show irregular shapes, and some cells have multiple nucleoli appearing as many granules.

> The nuclear lamina is a scaffolding that maintains the shape of the nucleus.

The nuclear lamina is a network of protein filaments 20 nm thick that lines the internal nuclear membrane. It is composed of three proteins termed *nuclear lamins A, B and C*, which are organized into filaments and form a regular square lattice as a scaffold beneath the nuclear membrane (Fig. 2.14).

Fig. 2.14 Nuclear Lamina. Micrograph of kidney immunostained to show one of the proteins of the nuclear lamina *(brown)*. There is staining on the inner side of the nuclear membrane corresponding to the location of lamin B, one of the cytoskeletal proteins responsible for organizing the structure of the nucleus. (Image used under Creative Commons License https://creativecommons.org/licenses/by-sa/3.0/ from the Human Protein Atlas Antibody to nuclear lamin B1 HPA050524 https://www.proteinatlas.org/ENSG00000113368-LMNB1/tissue/kidney#img.)

It is thought that this nuclear lamina network interacts with nuclear membrane proteins and acts as a nuclear cytoskeleton, possibly interacting with chromatin in the spatial organization of the nucleus.

MITOCHONDRIA

The mitochondria are the most important sites of energy production through oxidative phosphorylation and adenosine triphosphate (ATP) production in the cell but also have several other important functions in cells:

- Metabolism of amino acids and lipids
- Biosynthesis of haem and iron–sulphur clusters
- Act as a sensor for the health of the cell and able to trigger cell death through apoptosis

Mitochondria are membrane-bound organelles (Fig. 2.15), typically measuring 0.5–2 μm in length. Although mitochondria are often depicted as bean-shaped structures, they can adopt a range of shapes in different cell types from spherical, finger-like, to irregular globular and bean-shaped forms.

Mitochondria are believed to have evolved in human cells as symbiotic prokaryotic organisms like bacteria. In support of this hypothesis, each mitochondrion has its own DNA and systems for protein synthesis independent of the cell nucleus. Although only less than 1% of mitochondrial proteins are encoded by mitochondrial genes, those that are formed within mitochondria are mainly subunits of the oxidative phosphorylation machinery and are imported into the inner membrane by specific translocation proteins.

Fig. 2.15 Mitochondrion. (a) The structural organization of a mitochondrion showing different compartments. The cristae link to the inner boundary membrane at circular pores termed crista junctions. **(b)** Electron micrograph of a mitochondrion. Note the *black arrowheads* showing the outer membrane (OM), inner boundary membrane (IM) and cristae (C).

Each mitochondrion is constructed with two membranes, an outer and an inner, which define inner mitochondrial spaces, the intermembranous space and the matrix space. The intermembranous space contains metabolic substrates, which diffuse through the outer membrane.

The outer membrane contains specialized transport proteins such as porin, which allow free permeability of molecules up to about 10 kDa molecular weight from the cytosol into the intermembranous space. The outer membrane is also the site of proteins whose role is to transport proteins encoded by nuclear genes into the mitochondrion from where they are made in the cytosol. It has been estimated that around 1000 structural proteins encoded by nuclear genes are recruited to mitochondria in this way.

The outer mitochondrial membrane also contains transmembrane pores which, with special triggers, can assemble and open to release large mitochondrial proteins into the cytosol. This action is triggered by a variety of cell stimuli and leads to activation of cell death mechanisms (apoptosis). In this way, the mitochondrion acts as an important transducer for certain stimuli that lead to death of the cell.

The inner membrane is very different from the outer membrane and is highly impermeable to small ions owing to a high content of the phospholipid cardiolipin. This feature is essential to mitochondrial function, as it permits the development of electrochemical gradients during the production of high-energy cell metabolites. The inner membrane is the location of respiratory chain enzymes in addition to ATP synthetase, which is responsible for energy generation.

The inner membrane is folded into pleats and tubular structures (cristae), thereby increasing its surface area. The folding of the inner membrane defines a further space within the mitochondrion termed the *intracristal space*. The intracristal space

communicates with the intermembranous space at crista junctions and contains:

- ATP generated within the mitochondrion
- Ions pumped out of the matrix space during oxidative phosphorylation

The matrix space surrounds the intracristal space bounded by the crista membrane structures and contains enzymes to oxidize fatty acids and pyruvate and for the citric acid (or tricarboxylic acid, TCA) cycle. It also contains mitochondrial DNA and the specific mitochondrial machinery for mitochondrial DNA transcription, including ribosomal structures and mitochondrial RNA.

As noted previously, the morphology of mitochondria varies with cell type. In cells with a high oxidative metabolism, mitochondria are commonly large and serpiginous. In steroid hormone–secreting cells, such as those of the adrenal cortex, the cristae are tubular structures rather than flat plates.

It is more useful to consider the cellular mitochondria as a fluid dynamic cell compartment, rather than as individual organelles. Mitochondria function as an integrated membrane-bound compartment that is continually remodelled by both fusion and fission events. Mitochondria replicate within each cell by a process of division through fission (mitochondrial biogenesis). It is also known that mitochondria can fuse together to create larger structures. Mitochondrial biogenesis is regulated by well charactered genes and proteins to ensure that cellular energy demands are met.

Turnover of mitochondria is important in cells, and aged or damaged mitochondria are degraded by a process termed **mitophagy**. In this process, effete mitochondria are wrapped in membrane derived from the ER and enter the autophagic system (see p. 32). Defects in this system have been linked to neurodegenerative diseases such as Parkinson's disease in addition to ageing.

◎ ADVANCED CONCEPT

Crista Form From the Inner Membrane at Pore-Like Structures Termed Crista Junctions

Mitochondria examined in normal tissues by electron microscopy show differences in structure from that seen in isolated mitochondria, from which many original observations were made. In tissues, mitochondria are seen to have a large matrix volume relative to the other spaces, and this space compresses the inner membrane up against the outer membrane with only a very small space between them; this outer part of the inner membrane that follows the contour of the mitochondrion is called the **inner boundary membrane (IBM)**. There is therefore a minimal intermembranous space around the margins of the organelle. At sites around the periphery of the IBM, the inner and outer membranes form contacts, and it has been shown that these sites are characterized by the location of defined protein complexes, some involved in protein translocation systems. The three-dimensional arrangement of cristae had originally been proposed to be flat sheets of membrane folding in from the inner membrane, similar to baffles; however, study of mitochondria (Fig. 2.16) has shown that the inner membrane is not simply folded to form the cristae. The cristae, which divide up the matrix compartment, have been shown to form at the IBM from regularly sized circular structures resembling pores called **crista junctions** (Fig. 2.17) and not by folds and pleats. A large protein complex is found at the crista junctions, termed *MICOS* (mitochondrial contact site and cristae organizing system), and is also involved in the formation of the defined membrane contact sites between the inner and outer mitochondrial membranes.

This model of crista structure defines the intracristal space as a space that is continuous but distinct from the intermembranous space, with a boundary at the site of the crista junctions. The structure of individual crista away from the crista junction can be finger-like, flat plates or less regular shapes. There may be multiple crista junctions associated with a single intracristal space.

The importance of this concept is that the IBM and cristae membrane systems, although connected at crista junctions, have different protein compositions and functions. For example, protein translocases and components of the mitochondrial fusion system are localized in the IBM, whereas ATP synthase and respiratory chain complexes are found in the cristae membranes.

(a) (b) (c) (d)

Fig. 2.16 (a) Electron micrograph of mitochondria taken using the special technique of electron micrograph tomography that allows three-dimensional reconstructions to be made. *Arrows* show the circular profiles corresponding to crista junctions, where crista form from the inner boundary membrane. **(b)** One section of the electron tomogram of the mitochondrion shown in **(a)**; the *vertical arrows* show cross-sections of crista junctions. The inset at the lower left is a vertical section in which the *horizontal arrows* point to two circular crista junctions. **(c)** A three-dimensional model built from serial sections; the outer membrane is displayed in translucent *dark blue*, the IBM in translucent *light blue* and the cristae in *yellow*. **(d)** A three-dimensional model of the tomogram in **(b)** with only four cristae shown separately and each displayed in a different colour to show the range of shapes encountered; the *yellow* crista is the most typical and shows a lamellar compartment with multiple crista junctions connecting it to the inner boundary membrane. (Reprinted with modification to caption from Frey TG, Renken CW, Perkins GA. Insight into mitochondrial structure and function from electron tomography. *Biochim Biophys Acta.* 2002;1555.196–203. Copyright 2002 with permission from Elsevier.)

outer membrane
intermembranous space
inner boundary membrane
crista junction
proteins around crista junction membrane
matrix space
crista tubule
intracristal space

Fig. 2.17 Crista Junction. The crista junction arises at a circular, pore-like opening in the inner boundary membrane. Proteins of MICOS are located in this region. The intracristal space is continuous with, but distinct from, the intramembranous space. The crista tubule leads into the cristae.

◎ ADVANCED CONCEPT

Mitochondria are closely but reversibly linked to the ER in specialized regions termed **mitochondria-associated ER membranes (MAMs).** These regions of the ER have specific associated proteins and serve specialized functions, including regulating calcium transfer as part of cell signalling, mediating mitochondrial reproduction through fission and creating membrane for wrapping structures in the waste disposal process of autophagy. It is apparent that the intimate association of specialized ER regions with mitochondrial membrane serves to coordinate several essential cellular functions.

👥 CLINICAL EXAMPLE

Mitochondrial Cytopathy Syndromes

Mitochondrial DNA is not inherited in the same way as nuclear DNA, and in humans, the whole mitochondrial complement of a developing embryo is derived from mitochondria present in the ovum (i.e. maternally derived); there is no paternal contribution. Nuclear genes also contribute to mitochondrial structure and function such that most mitochondrial proteins are determined by nuclear genes.

Abnormal mitochondrial DNA can impair mitochondrial function and lead to defective cell functioning, which results mainly in structural abnormalities of muscle and the nervous system, and metabolic abnormalities derived from failure of oxidative metabolism. Affected individuals can be considered to have mosaics of genetically different mitochondria, a concept termed *heteroplasmy*. If many abnormal mitochondria are inherited, then it is likely that severe disease will develop. If only a proportion are abnormal, then the resulting disease may be less severe.

The most common patterns of clinical disease are as follows:

- Muscle weakness, particularly affecting the extraocular muscles
- Degenerative disease of the central nervous system (e.g. loss of the optic nerve fibres, loss of cerebellar tissue or degeneration of brain white matter)
- Metabolic disturbances, marked particularly by the development of abnormally high levels of lactic acid

Such diseases may be seen at any age from childhood into adult life, and the diagnosis can be assisted by muscle biopsy (Fig. 2.18), in which abnormal mitochondria can be seen in a proportion of cases. Mutational analysis of mitochondrial DNA is the main method used in clinical diagnosis.

Fig. 2.18 Mitochondrial Cytopathy. Electron micrograph of abnormal mitochondria in the muscle cell of a person with muscle weakness. Characteristic paracrystalline inclusions (PCIs) are present and are thought to be composed of excess mitochondrial protein, which accumulates as a result of the genetic abnormality (compare with Fig. 2.15b).

ENDOPLASMIC RETICULUM AND GOLGI

> **The ER and Golgi are involved in protein and lipid biosynthesis.**

The ER and Golgi are two distinct regions of an intercommunicating membrane-bound compartment involved in the biosynthesis and transport of cellular proteins and lipids (Fig. 2.19). In addition to its functions in biosynthesis, the ER has other important roles:

- Detoxification or activation of foreign compounds, including several drugs, by ER proteins termed *cytochrome P-450 proteins*
- Storage of intracellular calcium
- Interaction with mitochondria in the processes of mitogenesis and lipid transport
- Membrane wrapping to bring material into the autophagic system for 'waste disposal'

The ER and Golgi are arranged as deeply folded, flattened membrane sheets or as elongated tubular profiles, with their quantity depending on cellular metabolic requirements. Few ER sheets are present in most metabolically inactive cells, but cells that synthesize and secrete protein-containing molecules contain vast amounts. Most cells have only a relatively small quantity of smooth ER, except for cells that secrete or process lipids.

> **Protein synthesis occurs through the interaction of ribosomes, RNA and rough ER.**

Protein synthesis begins in the cytosol, where mRNA attaches to free ribosomes and translation produces the new peptide. The first portion of the RNA forms a signal sequence. Proteins destined to remain in the cytosol have a signal sequence that is different from those destined for entry into membranes or for secretion.

Ribosomes producing peptides with the signal sequence for a membrane or secreted protein become attached to the surface of the ER mediated by signal recognition particles, and the rest of the peptide is translated into this space (Fig. 2.20). The attachment of ribosomes to the ER gives it a studded appearance; hence this portion is called *rough ER*.

Protein synthesis by rough ER results in either the attachment of membrane proteins to the ER membrane or retention of proteins destined for secretion or retention within the ER lumen. These newly made proteins then enter the smooth ER for transport to the Golgi.

> **The smooth ER is the site of membrane lipid synthesis and protein processing.**

Smooth ER is a vital cell membrane system. In addition to processing synthesized proteins, it is the site of cell lipid synthesis, particularly membrane phospholipids. The lipid synthetic enzymes are located on its outer (cytosolic) face with ready access to lipid precursors.

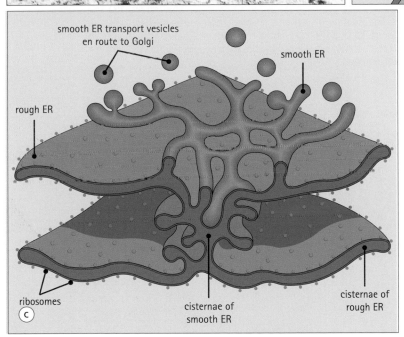

Fig. 2.19 Endoplasmic Reticulum. (a) Electron micrograph of rough ER composed of sheets of membrane with ribosomes on the cytosolic surfaces. **(b)** Relationship between ER and Golgi. The lumen of rough ER (RER) is continuous with the perinuclear space and with the lumen of smooth ER, whereas the Golgi forms a separate membrane system. Communication between ER and Golgi is mediated by small vesicles of ER, which break off, move through the cytosol and fuse with the Golgi membrane. The vesicles derived from RER are coated with a specific protein, COPII, which targets them for fusion with the Golgi. **(c)** The spatial relationship between rough ER and smooth ER. Smooth ER cisternae are tubular.

Once synthesized and incorporated into the outer part of the smooth ER membrane lipid bilayer, phospholipids are flipped over into the inner part by specific transport proteins colloquially termed *flipases*.

> **The Golgi is a membrane system involved in the sorting, packaging and transporting of cell products.**

From the smooth ER, further processing of synthesized macromolecules takes place in the Golgi. To reach the Golgi, vesicles bud from the smooth ER and travel in cytosol to fuse with its inner face. Membrane proteins are incorporated into the Golgi membrane, whereas luminal proteins enter the Golgi space (Fig. 2.21a).

The Golgi membrane system has three important roles:
- **Modification** of macromolecules by the addition of sugars to form oligosaccharides
- **Proteolysis** of peptides into active forms
- **Sorting** of different macromolecules into specific membrane-bound vesicles for subsequent incorporation into a membrane, transport into the lumen of a specific membrane-bound organelle or extracellular secretion

To facilitate the roles of modification, proteolysis and sorting, the Golgi is divided into three functional components (see Fig. 2.21b): the *cis* face, the **medial Golgi** and the *trans-Golgi network*.

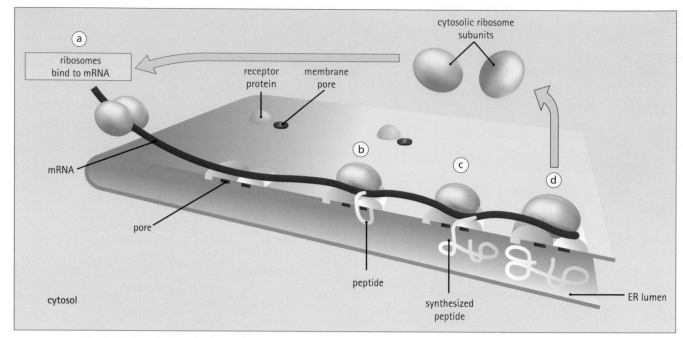

Fig. 2.20 Protein Synthesis on Rough Endoplasmic Reticulum. (a) Free cytosolic ribosomes attach to messenger RNA and begin to produce a peptide. **(b)** The ribosome attaches to a receptor on the ER membrane via a signal recognition particle, and the peptide is threaded into the ER lumen via a small protein-lined pore. At any one time, several ribosomes may be transcribing the same messenger RNA strand. **(c)** The original signal sequence that threads the peptide into the ER lumen is cleaved, and as the peptide is made, it forms in the lumen. Some proteins (i.e. those destined to be integral membrane proteins) can also form directly within the ER membrane. **(d)** After completion of peptide synthesis, the ribosome detaches from the receptor protein and returns to the cytosolic free pool.

Fig. 2.21 Golgi. (a) Ultrastructurally, the Golgi appears as parallel stacks of membrane (M) delineating Golgi lumen (L) from the cytosol (C). Transport vesicles (V) can be seen en route from the ER. **(b)** Golgi has three functional parts: the nuclear-facing *cis* face receives transport vesicles from smooth ER and phosphorylates certain proteins; the central medial Golgi adds sugar residues to both lipids and peptides to form complex oligosaccharides; the *trans*-Golgi network performs proteolytic steps, adds sugar residues and sorts different macromolecules into specific vesicles, which bud off the *trans* face. Golgi vesicles have a specific coat protein that targets vesicles to the correct compartment. Coat protein complexes (COPIs) coat vesicles moving between Golgi compartments. Sorting is performed by specific membrane receptor proteins, which recognize signal groups on macromolecules and direct them into correct vesicles. New membrane lipid synthesized in the smooth ER makes its way into the cell membrane via the Golgi.

VESICLES

> **Very small membrane-bound bodies are called vesicles and are derived from several compartments.**

Vesicles are small, spherical, membrane-bound organelles. They are formed by budding from existing areas of membrane and have two main functions:

- Transport or store material within their lumina
- Allow the exchange of cell membrane between different cell compartments

The main types of vesicles are:

- Cell surface–derived endocytotic (i.e. pinocytotic or phago-cytotic) vesicles
- Golgi-derived transport and secretory vesicles
- ER-derived transport vesicles
- Lysosomes
- Peroxisomes (see p. 33)

The cellular distribution of these vesicles can be determined by immunohistochemical staining for specific vesicle-associated proteins or specific vesicle contents (Fig. 2.22).

> **Lysosomes are part of the acid vesicle system, which is involved in the degradation of proteins.**

A lysosome is a membrane-bound organelle with a high content of hydrolytic enzymes operating in an acid pH. It functions as an intracellular digestion system, processing either material ingested by the cell or effete cellular components. This definition encompasses a variety of membrane-bound organelles derived from slightly different sources and with different functional roles.

Lysosomes are now considered to be only one part of the acid vesicle system, a group of vesicles so named because of their common membrane H^+-ATPase, termed the **vacuolar ATPase**, which can decrease their luminal pH to 5. This low pH activates powerful acid hydrolase enzymes, which are derived from vesicles that bud from the Golgi.

The membrane proteins required for lysosomal function (particularly the membrane pump, which increases H^+ concentration to maintain the acid pH), are not present in the initial Golgi hydrolase vesicles (also called *primary lysosomes*), which appear as membrane-bound vesicles with a dense core measuring 200–400 nm in diameter (Fig. 2.23a).

A functional lysosome, fulfilling the definition of an acid environment plus hydrolases, results from the fusion of hydrolase vesicles with endosomes that contain the correct membrane proteins to form an endolysosome (also termed a *secondary lysosome*). Endolysosomes are larger than Golgi hydrolase vesicles – 600–800 nm in diameter – and have an electron-dense core (see Fig. 2.23b). They can fuse with other endosomes derived from phagocytosis to form phagolysosomes. In this way, particulate matter brought into the cell is digested. Cells with a specific phagocytic function, such as certain white blood cells, have a well-developed acid vesicle system.

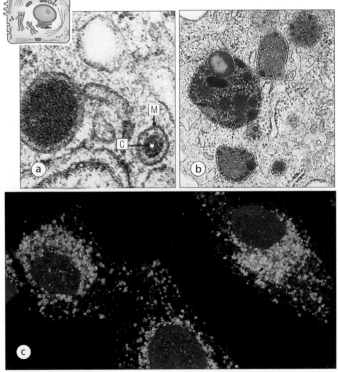

Fig. 2.23 Lysosomes. (a) Electron micrograph of Golgi hydrolase vesicles, which are bounded by membrane (M) and have an electron-dense core (C) composed of precursors of acid hydrolase enzymes. The membrane of this type of vesicle does not contain H^+-ATPase. **(b)** Electron micrograph showing several endolysosomes, which are produced by fusion of Golgi hydrolase vesicles with endosomes. Endolysosomes have a membrane containing H^+-ATPase, which can reduce pH to activate the hydrolases. **(c)** Cultured cells immunostained to show nuclei *(blue)* and lysosomes *(green)* (Image used under Creative Commons License https://creativecommons.org/licenses/by-sa/3.0/ from the Human Protein Atlas Antibody to TMEM106B HPA058342. https://www.proteinatlas.org/ENSG00000106460-TMEM106B/cell#img.)

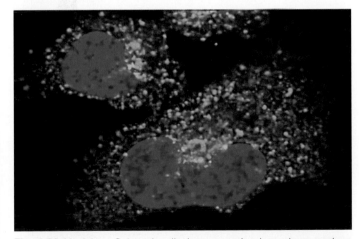

Fig. 2.22 Vesicles. Cultured cells immunostained to show nucleus *(blue)* and vesicles *(green)*. Vesicles are widely distributed in the cell cytoplasm. (Image used under Creative Commons License https://creativecommons.org/licenses/by-sa/3.0/ from the Human Protein Atlas https://www.proteinatlas.org/humancell/vesicles.)

It is possible to demonstrate the presence of lysosomes by histochemical staining for acid hydrolases, the most reliable being the demonstration of acid phosphatases. Immunohisto-chemical reagents can also be used to detect specific hydrolases: for example, cathepsin-B and β-glucuronidase (see Fig. 2.23c).

> **Autophagy is a process used to eliminate cellular constituents.**

All cells have a requirement to turn over proteins and organelles. Effete organelles are eliminated from cells by first becoming wrapped in membrane derived from the ER. These bodies subsequently fuse with an endolysosome to form an autophagolysosome; this enables old or damaged organelles to be recycled in a process termed **autophagy**.

Proteins in the cell membrane also need to be eliminated, and this happens by the formation of multivesicular bodies. In this process, a cell membrane containing the unwanted proteins is internalized into a body containing multiple bubble-like vesicles termed a *multivesicular body*. These bodies then fuse with vesicles containing lysosomal hydrolases, leading to protein degradation.

After digestion of material by acid hydrolases, indigestible amorphous and membranous debris may be seen in large membrane-bound vesicles called *residual bodies*. The relationships between members of the acid vesicle system are shown in Fig. 2.24.

Fig. 2.24 Acid Vesicle System. The relationships between the 'digestive' organelles of the acid vesicle system. Endosome forms from cell membrane and fuses with hydrolase-containing vesicles derived from the Golgi to form endolysosomes. The special Golgi membrane that forms the hydrolase vesicles is recycled back to the Golgi. Autophagy eliminates unwanted organelles. Unwanted cell membrane proteins are internalized for destruction by forming multivesicular bodies.

CLINICAL EXAMPLE

Lysosomal Storage Disorders

In the acid vesicle system, there are more than 30 defined and specific acid hydrolases, which not only degrade abnormal large molecules but also recycle or process normal cell constituents.

Genetic defects in the production of specific acid hydrolases lead to an inability to degrade specific classes of molecules, which then accumulate in the acid vesicle system. Most of these defects are inherited as single-gene autosomal recessive traits.

Lysosomal glycogen storage disease (acid maltase deficiency) leads to the accumulation of glycogen, which cannot be broken down (Fig. 2.25). Tay–Sachs disease results from a deficiency in an enzyme degrading one of the sphingo-lipids (hexosaminidase-A deficiency). Huge amounts of lipid accumulate in lysosomes and lead to severe neuronal degeneration.

Fig. 2.25 Acid Maltase Deficiency. Electron micrograph showing glycogen accumulation (G) in muscle cell cytoplasm and also within lysosomal bodies (L).

ADVANCED CONCEPT

Protein Degradation in Cells

There is a constant need for protein turnover in cells. Proteins in the cell membrane, unwanted organelles and proteins that enter cells from the extracellular space are degraded by the acid vesicle system, using lysosomal hydrolases.

In some cells, unwanted product in secretory vesicles is destroyed by the direct fusion of such secretory vesicles with lysosomes. This process is termed **crinophagy**. For example, when hormone-secreting cells in the pituitary gland no longer need to secrete their product, the secretory vesicles packed with hormone fuse with lysosomes, and the hormone is degraded.

Cytosolic proteins are mainly degraded by a distinct mechanism called the *ubiquitin–proteasome system*. In this system, unwanted proteins are recognized by specific enzymes and subsequently tagged by the protein ubiquitin. The resulting ubiquitinated protein is then recognized by large multicatalytic proteases termed *proteasomes* and degraded. In some cells this process of 'waste disposal' involves the reorganization of the cell to form a structure called an **aggresome**, centred around the centriole.

A highly efficient system for regulated elimination of proteins is essential for normal cell function. Certain proteins, such as those that control the cell cycle, those that activate transcription of genes or those that are intermediaries in intracellular signalling systems, are eliminated rapidly by the ubiquitin–proteasome system. If they were not eliminated, their activities would persist and lead to adverse effects in the cell.

Peroxisomes are membrane-bound vesicles important in the metabolism of long fatty acids.

Peroxisomes are small membrane-bound organelles containing enzymes involved in the oxidation of several substrates, particularly β-oxidation of very long-chain fatty acids (C18 and larger) and also involved in the synthesis of bile acids in addition to phospholipids.

Peroxisomes are small spherical bodies 0.5–1 μm in diameter with an electron-dense core. In some animals, but not in humans, there is a central paracrystalline core termed a *nucleoid*.

Peroxisomes are initially formed by budding of membrane from the ER together with required membrane-associated proteins. Once formed, further proteins are imported into the matrix core to form a mature peroxisome. The enzyme catalase is one of the more abundant matrix proteins (Fig. 2.26). Once mature, peroxisomes can replicate by fission.

CLINICAL EXAMPLE

Peroxisomal Disorders

There are around 20 rare inherited diseases that lead to defects in the peroxisomal enzymes responsible for processing very long-chain fatty acids. The main clinical features of such diseases are metabolic disturbances associated with acidosis or with the storage of abnormal lipids in susceptible cells, especially in the cells of the nervous system.

The most common example is **x-linked adrenoleukodystrophy**, caused by mutations in a lipid-transporter protein coded by the *ABCD1* gene and in which impaired β-oxidation of fatty acids results in abnormal lipid storage in the brain, spinal cord and adrenal glands, leading to intellectual deterioration (dementia) and adrenal failure. Other peroxisomal diseases are the result of gene mutations leading to defective peroxisomal biogenesis or causing a single enzyme deficiency.

Fig. 2.26 Peroxisomes. This image shows cultured human cells stained using immunofluorescence to show the enzyme catalase *(green)*, an abundant component of peroxisomes. For orientation, cell nuclei are stained *(blue)* and microtubules *(red)*. (Image used under Creative Commons License https://creativecommons.org/licenses/by-sa/3.0/ from the Human Protein Atlas Antibody to Catalase CAB001515. https://www.proteinatlas.org/ENSG00000121691-CAT/subcellular#img.)

CYTOSKELETON

The cytoskeletal proteins form filaments, which brace the internal structure of the cell.

Several functions of the cell are maintained by a set of filamentous cytosolic proteins, the cytoskeletal proteins, of which there are three main classes (depending on the size of their filaments):

- **Microfilaments** (5 nm in diameter), composed of the protein actin
- **Intermediate filaments** (10 nm in diameter), composed of six main proteins, which vary in different cell types
- **Microtubules** (25 nm in diameter), composed of two **tubulin** proteins

These filamentous proteins become attached to cell membranes and to each other by anchoring and joining proteins to form a dynamic three-dimensional internal scaffolding in the cell. This scaffolding is in a continual state of assembly and disassembly, but periods of stability serve specific functional roles, such as maintaining cellular architecture, facilitating cell motility, anchoring cells together, facilitating transport of material around the cytosol and dividing the cytosol into functionally separate areas.

Microfilaments are based on assemblies of the protein actin.

Actin accounts for about 5% of the total protein in most cell types. It is a globular protein (G-actin), which polymerizes to form filaments (F-actin), with all the actin subunits facing in one direction (polar filaments).

◎ ADVANCED CONCEPT

Actin

In association with other proteins, actin filaments form a layer (the cell cortex, Fig. 2.27) beneath the cell membrane. The actin is arranged into a stiff cross-linked meshwork by linking proteins, the most abundant being filamin. This meshwork resists sudden deformational forces but allows changes in cell shape by reforming, which is facilitated by actin-severing proteins.

Actin filament networks can provide mechanical support to the cell membrane by attachment to it via membrane-anchoring proteins; the best characterized of these are spectrin and ankyrin in red blood cells (see Fig. 7.3c), but similar proteins are present in most other cells. In addition, actin can become linked to transmembrane proteins in specialized areas of the plasma membrane, termed *adherent junctions* or *focal contacts* (see Fig. 3.5), which are externally attached to other cells or extracellular structures; thus the actin filament network of one cell can become linked to other cells or structures.

Actin filaments can form rigid bundles to stabilize protrusions of cell membrane termed *microvilli* (see Fig. 3.9). In these bundles, actin is associated with small linking proteins, the most abundant being fimbrin and fascin.

In all cells, actin filaments interact with a protein called *myosin* to generate motile forces. Myosin is an actin-activated ATPase composed of two heavy chains and four light chains arranged into a long tail and a globular head. These myosin heads can bind to actin and hydrolyse ATP to adenosine diphosphate (ADP). The interaction between actin and myosin to produce contractile forces is shown in Fig. 5.3.

Polymerization of actin filaments is responsible for the forces that drive local outgrowths of cell cytoplasm, such as spikes and ruffles, which are particularly evident in motile cells and cells undergoing migration in embryogenesis. Actin is also involved in bracing tunnelling nanotubules (see p. 21).

Fig. 2.27 Cell Cortex. (a) The cell cortex forms a layer that lines the cytosolic face of the cell membrane. It is composed of a stiff cross-linked meshwork of actin and actin-linking proteins, the most abundant being filamin but also including spectrin. Dynamic remodelling of this structure allows for membrane folding and cell motility. **(b)** This image is from cultured human cells stained using immunofluorescence for filamin. The green filaments can be seen at the cell margins at the location of the actin cortex. (Image used under Creative Commons License https://creativecommons.org/licenses/by-sa/3.0/ from the Human Protein Atlas Actin-binding protein Filamin A antibody HPA000368 https://www.proteinatlas.org/ENSG00000196924-FLNA/subcellular#img.)

There are several molecular variants (isoforms) of actin, which have specific distributions in different cell types: for example, isoforms restricted to smooth muscle or skeletal muscle.

> **Microtubules brace internal organelles and guide movement in intracellular transport.**

Microtubules are present in all cells except red blood cells. They are formed from two protein subunits, α and β **tubulin**, which polymerize in a head-to-tail pattern to form protofilaments. These are arranged into groups of 13 to form hollow tubes 25 nm in diameter (Fig. 2.28).

Other cellular elements, such as centrioles and cilia, are also made up of tubulin in the form of doublet or triplet tubules (see later).

Microtubules are constantly polymerizing and depolymerizing in the cell and grow out from the microtubule-organizing centre. They are stabilized by associating with other proteins (microtubule-associated proteins or MAPs, e.g. tau protein), which convert the unstable microtubular network into a relatively permanent framework. Microtubules are also stabilized by proteins that cap the growing end and prevent depolymerization.

Fig. 2.28 Microtubules. (a) Each microtubule is composed of 13 protofilaments of alternating α and β tubulin subunits. Microtubules are polar, with polymerization occurring at one end and depolymerization at the other. **(b)** In cross-section, each microtubule is 25 nm in diameter. **(c)** Electron micrograph showing the circular profiles of microtubules in cross-section. **(d)** Electron micrograph showing the faint parallel lines of microtubules in longitudinal section. **(e)** Cultured cell immunostained to show microtubules *(red)* and nucleus *(blue)*. (Image used under Creative Commons License https://creativecommons.org/licenses/by-sa/3.0/ from the Human Protein Atlas Antibody MAP7 HPA029712 https://www.proteinatlas.org/ENSG00000135525-MAP7/subcellular#img.)

Fig. 2.29 Centriole. (a) A centriole is composed of a cylindrical bundle measuring 200×400 nm composed of nine microtubule triplets arranged together by linking proteins. **(b)** In most cells, centrioles exist in pairs arranged at right angles to each other. **(c)** In electron microscopic preparations, one centriole is usually visible in cross-section, revealing the circular (C) arrangement of tubules, whereas its partner is cut either longitudinally or slightly obliquely (O). **(d)** Cultured human cells immunostained to show microtubules *(red)*, centriole *(green)* and nucleus *(blue)*. (Image used under Creative Commons License https://creativecommons.org/licenses/by-sa/3.0/ from the Human Protein Atlas. Antibody to centrosomal protein HPA030845 https://www.proteinatlas.org/ENSG00000135837-CEP350/subcellular#img.)

> **The centriole acts as a region which organizes the distribution of microtubules.**

Microtubules originate in the microtubule-organizing centre. This special region of the cell, known as the *centrosome*, is an organelle that contains a pair of centrioles (the centriole, Fig. 2.29).

The centrosome is composed of two centrioles. The first centriole (termed the **mother centriole**) forms in a cell at the time of completion of cell division, when it converts into a **basal body** to initiate development of a structure called a **primary cilium** in a process called *ciliogenesis* (see p. 37). In this process, a second centriole is formed called the **daughter centriole**. The mother centriole is associated with specific proteins that form appendages, which are responsible for anchoring the basal body and organizing microtubule structures.

Each centrosome, with its pair of centrioles surrounded by an amorphous electron-dense area of cytoplasm, acts as the nucleation centre for the polymerization of microtubules; these radiate from the centrosome in a star-like pattern called an *aster*. The protein forming the amorphous area is highly conserved in evolution and is present in both animal and plant cells. Each centrosome can act as the centre for about 250 microtubules.

The centriole has several roles in the cell:

- It organizes the cytoplasmic microtubular network in both normal and dividing cells.
- It organizes the development of specialized microtubules in motile cilia (see Fig. 3.11).

- It forms the basal body in the important signalling structures termed *primary cilia* (non-motile) (see p. 35 and Fig. 2.31).
- It organizes the spindle in cell division (see p. 40).
- It acts as the centre for cellular reorganization in the aggresomal response (see the Advanced Concepts box on p. 33).

◎ **ADVANCED CONCEPTS**

Microtubule Function

Microtubules form a network allowing transport around the cell, via the attachment protein dynein, which moves down a microtubule toward the cell centre, and kinesin, which moves up a microtubule toward the cell periphery. These attachment proteins are associated with the membranes of vesicles and organelles and facilitate their movement around the cell. This process is particularly important in the transport of organelles down the long cell processes of nerve cells (see Chapter 6).

Microtubules also form a network (cytoskeleton) for membrane-bound cell compartments (e.g. they maintain the extended tubular arrangement of the ER).

Chromosomes are organized in cell division along the microtubular cell spindle (see Fig. 2.35).

Specialized motile components of the cell, cilia (see Fig. 3.11), contain a core of microtubules bound together with other proteins.

Primary cilia, the ubiquitous sensing and signalling structure seen on all cells, are also centred on a core of microtubules (see Fig. 2.31).

Intermediate filament proteins vary between different functional classes of cells.

Intermediate filaments are a group of filamentous cytoskeletal proteins comprising six main types, which have a specific distribution in different cell types (Table 2.1). Ultrastructurally, they form relatively ill-defined bundles or masses in the cytosol of cells.

▶ **KEY FACTS**

Cytoskeleton
- Microfilaments are made of actin and have roles in movement and membrane stabilization.
- Microtubules are made of tubulin and have roles in intracellular transport and in the scaffolding of internal membranes.
- Intermediate filaments are made of proteins that vary between different cell types and function to link separate cells into structural units.

TABLE 2.1   Locations of Different Types of Intermediate Filaments

Intermediate Filament	Localization
cytokeratins	epithelial cells
desmin	muscle (smooth and striated)
glial fibrillary acidic protein (GFAP)	astrocytic glial cells
neurofilament protein	neurons
nuclear lamin	nucleus of all cells
vimentin	many mesenchymal cells

◎ **ADVANCED CONCEPTS**

Intermediate Filaments

Intermediate filaments are anchored to transmembrane proteins at special sites on the cell membrane (desmosomes and hemidesmosomes, see Figs 3.5, 3.6 and 3.8) and spread tensile forces evenly throughout a tissue so that single cells are not disrupted.

Although intermediate filaments have several defined roles in cells, as outlined later, detailed mechanisms of their function have not been elucidated, unlike those of the other cytoskeletal proteins.

In **epithelial cells of the skin,** keratin intermediate filaments become compacted with other link proteins to form a tough outer layer (see Fig. 18.3) and hence have an important structural role as an impermeable barrier, in addition to being the main constituent protein of hair and nail.

In **neurons,** neurofilaments have long side arms, which probably help maintain the cylindrical architecture of nerve cell processes when subjected to lateral tensile forces in bending. They also anchor membrane ion channel proteins via a link protein, 'ankyrin', to facilitate nerve conduction.

When cells are damaged, the intermediate filament network collapses around the centriole to form a perinuclear spherical mass associated with abnormal or damaged cellular proteins and elements of the ubiquitin–proteasome system used in protein degradation. This is termed the **aggresomal response.** It is possible that in this situation the intermediate filaments act to cocoon damaged cellular components in one spot for subsequent elimination by proteolysis and autophagy. After cell recovery, the intermediate filament network re-expands. This phenomenon occurs in liver cells in response to persistent alcohol excess, when collapsed bundles of cytokeratin intermediate filaments (Mallory's hyaline) accumulate. This is also believed to be a response that happens in neurons in the brain in Parkinson's disease, where the accumulations of material are termed *Lewy bodies.*

In the **nucleus,** the nuclear lamins form a square lattice on the inner side of the nuclear membrane, which probably acts with other link proteins in the organization of the nucleus (see Fig. 2.14).

The cell-specific restriction of distribution of intermediate filament proteins is used for the histological assessment of cell types, using immunohistochemical staining for the various filaments. This is particularly useful when small samples of malignant tumour are being assessed to determine their likely site of origin. The detection of cytokeratin argues strongly for an epithelial origin (Fig. 2.30), whereas the presence of desmin would suggest a muscle derivation, and glial fibrillary acidic protein (GFAP) is only seen in specialized central nervous system tumours.

Fig 2.30 Cytokeratin. This image is a section of salivary gland immunostained for one of the cytokeratins and counterstained with haematoxylin to stain nuclei blue. Epithelial cells are stained, but the background containing support cells, lymphoid cells, blood vessels and nerves remains unstained. Such tissue-restricted expression of cytokeratin is useful in identifying cells of epithelial origin. (Image used under Creative Commons License https://creativecommons.org/licenses/by-sa/3.0/ from the Human Protein Atlas. Cytokeratin antibody HPA012050 https://www.proteinatlas.org/ENSG00000108244-KRT23/tissue/salivary+gland#img.)

Primary cilia are found on most cells and act as a key structure for signalling pathways, for mechanical sensing and in the regulation of cell division.

The primary cilium is a hair-like extension of the cell membrane between 1 and 10 μm long and 0.2 and 0.3 μm in width and braced by a core of microtubules and associated proteins. Although this form of cilial structure is less well known compared with motile cilia (see p. 55), it plays vital roles in cell function, illustrated by the diseases now linked to the proteins in primary cilia, termed **ciliopathies**. It is becoming clear that the primary cilium is a highly distinct cell compartment that is essential for cell signalling. These structures are seen on most cells, including white blood cells, and have been likened to an 'antenna and control unit' for the cell, with several functions:

- Acts as a structural checkpoint involved in cell cycle progression: disassembly is required to form the mitotic spindle

- As an essential mediator for some forms of cell signalling, especially developmental signalling involving hedgehog (HH) and Wnt (wingless-related integration site) pathways
- Acts as a site for location of receptors responsible for sensing environmental information, including light (photoreceptor), movement (mechanoreceptors, including sensory cells in the ear), smell (olfactory sensing) and fluid flow in epithelial cells, including tubules of the kidney

The structure of a primary cilium includes a specialized covering cilial membrane, characterized by receptors, protein and lipid content different from the rest of the cell membrane; a transport system based on microtubules termed the *axoneme*; a gateway transition zone that functionally separates the cilium from the rest of the cell; and a zone within the cell termed the *basal body* and *bbsome* (a protein complex in the basal body), which are responsible for maintaining and organizing its structure (Fig. 2.31).

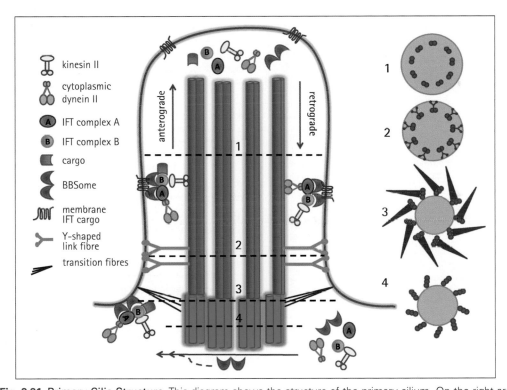

Fig. 2.31 Primary Cilia Structure. This diagram shows the structure of the primary cilium. On the right are drawings of cross-sections of the cilium at different levels indicated with *dashed lines:* ciliary axoneme **(1),** transition zone **(2),** distal end of the basal body with transition fibres **(3)** and basal body **(4).** At the core of this structure is a ring of nine microtubule doublets (in a 9+0 arrangement), termed the **axoneme,** that runs along its length. In contrast, motile cilia contain an additional central pair of microtubules and have a 9+2 axoneme structure (see Fig. 3.11). The axoneme grows out from the basal body. Proteins are linked to this microtubule core, where they function as molecular motors as part of the **intraflagellar transport (IFT) system**. These motors involve the proteins dynein and kinesin and bind to cargoes through structures called **IFT particles,** composed of multiprotein complexes. This transport system is vital to conducting signal molecules into the cell. The cell membrane of the primary cilium is the site of concentration of specialized receptor and channel proteins involved in signalling. At the base of the organelle is a structure called the **bbsome,** a concentration of proteins with a role in organizing transfer of material into the structure of the primary cilium and maintaining its structure. The proximal end of the cilium above the basal body is called the transition zone, characterized by the presence of Y-shaped link fibres that connect the axoneme with the ciliary membrane. The transition zone forms a functional ciliary gate that regulates the trafficking of ciliary components. The ciliary gate, IFT, and bbsome, by actively controlling ciliary trafficking, establish and maintain the cilium as a compartment with constituents distinct from the rest of the cell. (Reprinted and adapted from Yong HY, Young-Goo H. Primary cilia in brain development and diseases. *Am J Pathol.* 2018;188[1]:11–22. https://doi.org/10.1016/j.ajpath.2017.08.031. Copyright 2018, with permission from Elsevier.)

A Large Group of Inherited Diseases Affecting Brain, Eye, Kidney, Liver, Heart or Bone Is Caused by Defects in the Primary Cilium

The **ciliopathies** are a large group of disorders linked to mutations in genes coding for protein found in the structures of the primary cilium. These include proteins in the basal body, transition fibres, transition zone, intraflagellar transport and bbsome, which, when abnormal, disrupt ciliary function.

Given the ubiquitous presence of primary cilia in most cell types, clinical disease includes syndromes of neurological disorders, retinal degeneration, cardiac disease, cystic disease in the kidney and liver, and skeletal abnormalities.

Among the most common of the ciliopathies is the condition called **adult polycystic kidney disease,** which affects around 1:1000 persons worldwide. This is an autosomal dominant condition in which kidney failure develops in adult life, associated with destruction of the kidneys because of the formation of huge cysts derived from the normal renal tubule cells. Other associated features can include liver cysts, aneurysms (swellings) on arteries around the brain, and hypertension. There are two genes linked to the disease coding for proteins called *polycystin-1* (PC1) and *polycystin-2* (PC2, also called *TRPP1*). These two proteins together form a complex located in the membrane of the primary cilium of renal tubular epithelial, facing the lumen of the tubule. It has been proposed that PC1 acts as a mechanosensitive receptor that modulates calcium signals via PC2, which acts as a channel protein for calcium signalling. In experimental systems, disruption of primary cilia slows down the cyst growth caused by loss of polycystins, suggesting that signalling from the intact primary cilium is needed to develop cysts and develop disease. It is believed that the lack of polycystin leads to the inability of the primary cilium to sense shear stress (mechanosensation) of fluid flow in the tubule. With a lack of signal indicating the true level of fluid flow, the intact primary cilium signals instead to cause excessive secretion of fluid by the tubular epithelial cell. Over many years, this excessive fluid secretion in renal tubules leads to cyst formation.

Hypertension in this condition has been linked to failure of the primary cilia on vascular endothelial cells to sense shear stress and flow in blood vessels.

An Internet search for the term ciliopathy will produce the names of established and suspected diseases linked to functional abnormality of the primary cilium.

CELL INCLUSIONS AND STORAGE PRODUCTS

Accumulations of products within certain cells may occur in the form of cytoplasmic inclusions.

> **Lipofuscin pigment is mainly composed of phospholipids and is the result of 'wear and tear'.**

Lipofuscin appears as membrane-bound, orange-brown, granular material within the cytoplasm. Derived from residual bodies containing a mixture of phospholipids from cell degradation, lipofuscin is commonly referred to as a 'wear and tear' pigment, as it becomes more prominent in old cells. It is particularly common in tissues from elderly persons, and is most evident in nerve, heart muscle (Fig. 2.32) and liver cells.

Fig. 2.32 Lipofuscin. In this H&E section of cardiac muscle, lipofuscin pigment can be seen as brown-staining granules within the cardiac muscle cells.

> **Lipid is stored in cells as non–membrane-bound vacuoles.**

Lipids may accumulate as non–membrane-bound vacuoles, which appear as large clear spaces in the cytoplasm because paraffin wax processing dissolves out the fat. If the tissues are frozen and cut in a freezing microtome, the fat can be stained with certain dyes. Large fat vacuoles are a special feature of fat storage cells called *adipocytes* (see Fig. 4.24).

> **Glycogen may impart a pale, vacuolated appearance to cells.**

Glycogen forms as granules in the cell cytoplasm and can be seen by electron microscopy. Demands for energy are met by conversion of glycogen to glucose.

In certain cells, the presence of large amounts of glycogen causes pale staining or apparent vacuolation of cell cytoplasm. Glycogen can be stained by the periodic acid–Schiff (PAS) method.

Pathological accumulations of proteins can develop in certain disease states, where they form inclusion bodies, some of which have come to define certain diseases. The most common examples are seen in the brain in the group of neurodegenerative diseases. In Alzheimer's disease, inclusions called **neurofibrillary tangles** develop in nerve cells composed of tau protein (a microtubule binding protein). In Parkinson's disease, spherical inclusions called *Lewy bodies* form in nerve cells of the substantia nigra composed of the protein α-synuclein.

CELL DIVISION

> **Cell division for growth and renewal is achieved by the process of mitosis.**

An essential feature of development is the ability of cells to divide and reproduce. In addition, death of mature cells in the adult needs to be compensated for by the production of new cells.

Cells reproduce by duplicating their contents and dividing into two daughter cells. The phases involved in cell replication can be regarded as a cell cycle (Fig. 2.33). The phases of cell division are visible histologically, involving duplication of DNA, separation of cellular DNA into two separate areas of the cell (mitosis, Figs 2.34 and 2.35) and finally cell division (cytokinesis).

> **Different cell populations can be defined according to their pattern of growth.**

In adults, not all cells are capable of division. Several different populations of cells can be defined based on their capacity to replicate:

- Static cell populations are cells that do not divide in the developed tissue.
- Stable cell populations do not normally divide.
- Renewing cell populations normally divide constantly.

Nerve cells and cardiac muscle cells, for example, divide and form tissues during embryogenesis, but once tissues are formed, the cells do not divide again in postnatal life, and cells cannot be replaced if lost through disease. Stable cell populations, for example, liver cells, do not normally divide in postnatal life but can proliferate to replace cells lost through disease. Skin and gut-lining cells are renewing cell populations that divide continually in postnatal life to replace shed cells. In a similar way, blood cell populations have a short lifespan and are constantly renewed.

Tissues that are regarded as being composed of static cell populations (e.g. brain) have recently been shown to have a very low level of cell proliferation in postnatal life. However, this is currently not thought to contribute to functional renewal in postnatal life, and for practical purposes, once cells have been lost from such tissues through disease, they are not replaced in adult life. Clinical trials are taking place to see if the stimulation of local stem cells can be used in therapy for some diseases. Trials are also being done to see if injecting stem cells grown in vitro can be used for therapeutic purposes.

> **Stem cells are partly committed cells that function as a dividing population to produce a range of specialized cells.**

All cells in an adult must have originated from the single fertilized cell that originates from the fusion of the ovum and the sperm. Such a cell is regarded as being **totipotential**, as not only does it form the cells in the resulting adult but it also can form the extraembryonic tissues of the placenta.

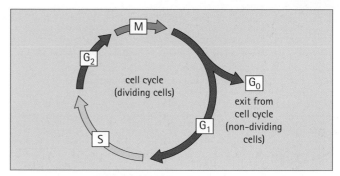

Fig. 2.33 Phases of Cell Cycle. Cells that leave the cycle are said to be 'in the G_0 phase'. Cells can enter a phase of proliferation in which they divide. Stages are detailed in Fig 2.34.

Fig. 2.34 The Cell Cycle. The DNA of cells is replicated only during certain phases of a cell's growth pattern, which takes place in several stages. The cell cycle is divided into two main periods: mitosis and interphase, which includes the G_1, S and G_2 phases. Cells which are not dividing are non-cycling, or G_0 cells, whereas G_1 cells have just entered a phase of cellular growth. S-phase cells actively synthesize DNA, G_2 cells have a double complement of cellular DNA and are resting before cell division, and M-phase cells are in mitosis, which comprises five stages. In most tissues, only a small proportion of cells will be in the cell cycle, the majority being differentiated cells in a G_0 phase. Stem cells may be in a G_0 phase and only come to re-enter the cell cycle if there is a demand, for example, after cell death. Progression through the cell cycle is carefully regulated by proteins such as cyclins that act at a series of checkpoints.

Prophase The duplicated chromatin becomes condensed into parallel sister chromosomes imparting a coarse stippling to the nuclear region, which is associated with loss of the nucleolus. The centriole replicates to form two microtubule organizing centres at opposite poles of the cell (the mitotic spindle), which is not visible by light microscopy.

nuclear membrane
centromere
centriole centre of spindle
two sister chromosomes held together at centromere
microtubules of spindle

Prometaphase The nuclear membrane breaks down to form small vesicles, allowing the microtubules of the spindle to interact with the chromosomes. Each chromosome pair has an attachment site (kinetochore), which binds to spindle microtubules from each pole of the spindle (kinetochore tubules). The chromosome pairs move toward the centre of the spindle.

spindle pole
kinetochore microtubule
nuclear membrane vesicle
polar microtubule

Metaphase Movement of chromosomes along the microtubules leads to alignment of the chromosomes at the equator of the cell between the poles of the spindle.

cell equator

Anaphase The kinetochore attachments to the paired chromosomes separate and the chromosomes move to opposite poles of the spindle. In late anaphase the spindle microtubules elongate, causing elongation of the cell and further separation of the spindle poles.

nuclear envelope vesicles migrate toward poles
elongation of polar microtubule
chromatids pulled towards pole of spindle
shortened kinetochrome microtubule

Telophase The separated chromatids become separated from the kinetochore microtubules and the nuclear membrane reforms around each group of chromosomes. The cell elongates further by elongation of the spindle microtubules. This phase signals the end of mitosis.

chromosomes decondense and lose microtubular attachment
nuclear envelope reforms

Cytokinesis Cleavage into two separate cells is produced by aggregation of an actin–myosin belt immediately beneath the equator of the telophase cell. The connecting region eventually separates with fusion of cell membranes to form two daughter cells. At this stage a nucleolus appears in the dense chromatin mass in the newly formed nucleus. The cell now enters the G_1 phase of the cell cycle.

centriole
actin–myosin belt
nuclear membrane

Fig. 2.35 Mitosis.

In a developing embryo, there is a population of cells termed **embryonic stem cells** (ES cells), which are **pluripotential** and have the capacity to develop into any functional cell type. These cells have been isolated from either the inner cell mass of the developing blastocyst phase of an embryo or from fetal gonads, and cell lines have been established in tissue culture that retain the capacity for differentiation into any cell type.

It is the identification and characterization of ES cells that has suggested that they might be used therapeutically, by transplantation, to treat a whole variety of diseases where there has been loss of permanent cells: for example, nerve cells. However, because they originate and must be harvested from an embryo, such work has led to ethical and moral debate, with some countries restricting or not allowing the development of therapeutic applications.

In postnatal life there are populations of cells that can develop into a restricted set of different cell types and are regarded as **multipotential**. They then act as a pool of dividing cells to replenish more specialized cell populations. Such partly committed cells are called **multipotential stem cells**, and it is now known that they are the basis for continued renewal of many constantly dividing cell types.

Several types of renewing cell populations are thought to originate from multipotential stem cells; for example, the different cells of the blood originate from a common haemopoietic stem cell, and enterocyte stem cells probably give rise to the different cell types in the epithelial lining of the gut.

In some tissues, cells exist that serve to generate only one cell type, termed **committed progenitor cells**. An example of this type of cell is the 'epidermal stem cell', which can form new epithelial cells in skin. Such cells have also been classed as **unipotential stem cells**.

A stem cell must reproduce itself each time it divides to maintain a stem cell population. After stem cell division, two types of cells may result: new stem cells to maintain the stem cell population, and committed cells, which differentiate along one cell line but may still divide in what are termed amplification divisions. Whereas stem cells typically have a low frequency of division, high rates of amplification divisions in committed cells are responsible for maintaining dynamic cell populations.

Multipotential stem cells typically represent a very small proportion of all cells in a tissue, and on microscopy, they are generally very hard to see, as they lack differentiated features and appear as inconspicuous small cells. Their morphological anonymity belies their importance. Single-cell RNA sequencing (scRNA-seq) technology coupled with histological methods using labelling antibodies and confocal microscopy have identified many types of stem cells, and this has allowed their isolation and study. It appears that the local environment of a stem cell and its attachments to the extracellular matrix influence its ability to divide and influence the formation of specific committed cell types. The concept that the local microenvironment controls stem cell differentiation is acknowledged by describing each type of stem cell as being in a **stem cell niche** – a local microenvironment that defines growth and differentiation.

Finally, investigation of the fate of bone marrow stem cell transplants in humans and rodents has recently challenged the dogma that multipotential stem cells can give rise to only a limited set of cell types. It is evident that cells from bone marrow transplants have differentiated into liver cells and neuronal cells in the brain. Such findings are not fully explained but raise the possibility that, given the correct environment, certain multipotential stem cells can become pluripotential again. This concept is termed **adult stem cell plasticity**. The pathways that allow such adult plasticity, by characterizing the stimuli in specific niches that switch differentiation of resulting cells, are under intense investigation.

> **The control and establishment of cell polarity are essential for the assembly of tissues.**

Within tissues, cells are arranged into ordered structures and are oriented with respect to each other and to the extracellular matrix. Many cells have a clear top (apical), bottom (basal) and side (lateral) polarity, with different structures associated with the different surface membranes. Specific mechanisms are used within cells to allow them to develop such individual cell polarity and, from cell polarity, to develop wider tissue polarity.

Many tissues are polarized within the horizontal plane of a sheet of cells such that cells are regularly arranged in relation to each other. This process is called *planar cell polarity* (PCP), which has been characterized in insect model systems that are now being extended to vertebrates.

A set of so-called core PCP genes have been identified, and the resultant proteins come to be located asymmetrically within the individual cells in a cellular sheet as the structural basis of cellular polarity. These core PCP elements affect the orientation of the mitotic spindle, layout of the internal cytoskeleton, cell adhesion and direction of cell movement. The primary cilia structure is an important signalling component in planar cell polarity. In vertebrate systems there is good evidence for PCP core genes being involved in the orientation of motile cilia (see p. 55), in the development of the central nervous system in the embryo and in the formation of specialized sensing elements in the inner ear.

However, although fundamental systems such as those controlling PCP have been discovered, the molecular basis of how individual cells that are widely dispersed within the three dimensions of a tissue are controlled to take up a specific orientation is still not fully understood.

> **Cell division to produce gametes for reproduction is achieved through the process of meiosis.**

Normal cells have two sets of complementary (homologous) chromosomes derived from the maternal and paternal germ cells at fertilization and are therefore called **diploid**, or **2n,** cells.

The germ cells (ova and spermatozoa), which are destined to fuse in fertilization to produce an embryo, have half the normal complement of chromosomes (i.e. are **haploid – n –** cells). They are the product of a modified form of cell division, **meiosis**. In preparation for cell division, a cell must form a structure called the *spindle*. This is formed from the disassembly of its primary cilium (see p. 37) from which the basal body is converted into the centriole in the centrosome that organizes the mitotic spindle.

In meiosis (Fig. 2.36), complementary chromosomes become paired on the mitotic spindle after the S phase of the cell cycle (see Fig. 2.33), with the maternal set attached to one pole and the paternal set attached to the opposite pole; the pole to which maternal- and paternal-derived chromosomes become attached is random for each chromosome. This is in contrast to mitosis, where complementary chromosomes do not align across the spindle.

Thus in meiosis, maternal and paternal complementary chromosomes are separated, migrating to opposite ends of the spindle by a first meiotic division. Once they are segregated in this way, a second division (virtually identical to a mitotic division, see Fig. 2.36) separates replicated chromosomes. The result of meiosis is four daughter nuclei, each containing one set of chromosomes.

CELL DEATH

> **Programmed cell death is a normal means of controlling dividing cell populations.**

In many replicating tissues, and particularly during embryogenesis, control of the cell population is achieved by controlling the rate of cell death. Normal cells require a balance of signals that maintain their viability. In the absence of a correct pattern of signals, certain genes are switched on, which bring about carefully controlled dissolution of the cell. Because of the genetic control of this process, it is referred to as *programmed cell death* and contrasts with cell death that occurs in many diseases or is brought about by deleterious stimuli.

The most important form of programmed cell death is **apoptosis**. In this process, the cell shrinks, becomes fragmented and is ingested by adjacent cells (Fig. 2.37).

Chromosome replication

replicated paternal chromosome

replicated maternal chromosome

First meiotic division

homologous chromosomes aligned on spindle

first meiotic division separates homologues

Second meiotic division

second meiotic division in two daughter cells

replicated chromosomes separate

Gametes

four haploid daughter cells

Fig. 2.36 Meiosis. Meiosis results in the formation of four daughter cells, each with half of the normal chromosomal complement (i.e. n, haploid).

Normal cells are arranged in close contact with each other and are united by cell junctions. Early in the process of apoptosis there is synthesis of enzymes needed to cause cell dissolution, but this is not associated with structural changes. This is termed **priming.** In development many cells are primed for apoptosis and survive only if rescued by a specific trophic factor.

The apoptotic cells lose surface specializations and junctions, shrinking in size. The nuclear chromatin condenses beneath the nuclear membrane. In contrast to necrosis, cell organelles remain normal. Endonuclease enzymes cleave chromosomes into individual nucleosome fragments.

loss of microvilli and junctions

nuclear changes

There is splitting of the cell into several fragments known as **apoptotic bodies.** Nuclear fragmentation also occurs. Each fragment contains viable mitochondria and intact organelles. The process takes a few minutes only.

apoptotic body

fragmentation

Apoptotic fragments are recognized by adjacent cells, which ingest them by phagocytosis for destruction. Some fragments degenerate extracellularly, while others are ingested by local phagocytic cells, not shown on this diagram.

Although apoptosis is a physiological process, it can also be induced by pathological conditions.

apoptotic body

phagocytosis

Fig. 2.37 Apoptosis. Apoptosis of cells is a programmed and energy-dependent process designed specifically to eliminate them. This controlled pattern of cell death, termed *programmed cell death*, is very different from that which occurs as a direct result of a severe damaging stimulus to cells (termed *necrosis*).

⊚ ADVANCED CONCEPT

Practical Histology

General principles can be usefully applied when looking at cells either in cytological preparations or in tissue sections to assess their activity, as outlined next.

Nucleus

A metabolically inactive cell has a compact round nucleus, which typically stains intensely, as little chromatin is being transcribed. No nucleoli are visible, as ribosome production is minimal.

A protein-synthesizing cell has a large, pale-staining nucleus with large or multiple nucleoli, reflecting active transcription of chromatin. Similar nuclear changes are evident in cells in an active phase of multiplication.

A dead cell has a shrunken nucleus, which appears as an amorphous compact mass of intensely staining material. This later fragments into separate particles and is completely lysed, leaving the cell devoid of any discernible nucleus.

Cytoplasm

Examination of cell cytoplasm should concentrate on the intensity and distribution of acidophilic *(pink)* and basophilic *(blue)* elements.

A granular, intensely pink-staining cytoplasm contains accumulations of organelles that take up acidic dye, which are usually mitochondria or secretory granules (e.g. neurosecretory granules, or specialized granules such as those seen in white blood cells).

A diffuse blue tint to the cytoplasm indicates the presence of cytoplasmic RNA in the form of ribosomes, and thus active protein production.

Large non-staining areas are generally large secretory vacuoles, such as those seen in the mucin-secreting cells. In some cell types, they may represent fat.

🐾 CLINICAL EXAMPLE

Nuclear Changes in Cancer

A cell containing a very large nucleus relative to the amount of cytoplasm is generally in a phase of cell division. Cells with inappropriately large nuclei raise the suspicion of cancerous change. For example, cells on the surface of the uterine cervix should have small nuclei unless there is abnormal cell growth, such as that associated with the development of a malignancy.

In any specialized cell type, all the nuclei in adjacent cells should be roughly the same size and have the same staining characteristics. In cancer, however, nuclei vary in size and shape (**nuclear pleomorphism**) and commonly show dense-staining chromatin in a coarse, clumped pattern (**nuclear hyperchromatism,** Fig. 2.38).

Fig. 2.38 Nuclear Changes In Cancer. Image of a malignant tumour showing variation in the size of nuclei (nuclear pleomorphism) and very dark staining of many nuclei (nuclear hyperchromatism).

CLINICAL EXAMPLE

Diagnostic Cytology

Cytology is the study of cellular form and refers to an important specialty in laboratory medicine, which concentrates on establishing the diagnosis of disease by examining small numbers of cells.

Cells for examination are obtained from patients either by scraping the surface of epithelia (e.g. the uterine cervix or gastric lining); by aspirating solid tissues with a needle (fine needle aspiration cytology); or by collecting cells from body fluids such as ascites, pleural effusion, cerebrospinal fluid (CSF), sputum or urine.

The aim is to detect abnormalities in the cell structure that point to the presence of disease. In clinical medicine, the most important aspect is the recognition of changes that herald the development of cancer (neoplastic changes) (Fig. 2.39).

Fig. 2.39 Fine Needle Aspiration Cytology. A patient presented with a lump in the neck, and an ultrasound examination revealed an enlarged lymph node. Under ultrasound guidance, cells were aspirated from the lymph node using a fine needle. The aspirate was smeared onto a glass slide, fixed and stained for microscopic examination. **(a)** Clumps of cells with dark-staining nuclei are seen. The nuclei show pleomorphism and were diagnosed as carcinoma. The pale, rounded profiles in the background are aspirated red blood cells. **(b)** After cytological diagnosis, further imaging was performed which did not reveal a primary site for the origin of the carcinoma. The lymph node was operatively removed, and histology showed a poorly differentiated carcinoma. Immunohistochemistry was used to refine the diagnosis and likely site of origin (see Chapter 3).

For online review questions, please visit https://studentconsult.inkling.com.

3

Epithelial Cells

INTRODUCTION

Epithelial cells are sheets of specialized cells that cover and line the interior and exterior surfaces of the body, for example, the outer layers of the skin and the inner luminal surface of the gastrointestinal tract. They have diverse functions such as secretion, absorption and protection (as a barrier), made possible by many specialized surface and internal modifications, with cells attached to each other by several types of cell junctions. Cells can be adapted to manufacture and secrete a product, and secretion of large amounts of product is facilitated by the folding and invagination of sheets of epithelium to form glands. Certain solid organs are composed of an intricate arrangement of epithelial cells, for example, the pancreas, kidney and liver.

> **Epithelial cells are specialized for absorption, secretion or to act as a barrier.**

Epithelial cells form very cohesive sheets of cells, called *epithelia*, which function mainly as:
- A covering or lining for body surfaces, for example, skin, gut, respiratory and genitourinary tracts; blood vessels; body cavities; and ducts
- The functional units of secretory glands and solid organs, for example, salivary tissue and liver

Epithelial cells are firmly joined together by adhesion specializations. These special structures serve to anchor the cytoskeleton of each epithelial cell to its neighbours and to anchor the epithelium to extracellular matrix materials. Epithelia are separated from their support tissues by a layer of extracellular matrix, the **basement membrane.** Epithelia do not have blood vessels, obtaining their nutrition via diffusion from capillaries running in the support tissue to which they are attached.

> **The classification of epithelial cells is based on their shape and how they are stacked together.**

Early microscopists described the cells simply by their observed shape, as function was not yet understood. This nomenclature persists to this day.

Traditionally, cells are classified into three main cell groups according to their shape. These groups are **squamous** (flat plate-like, Figs 3.1a and 3.1b); **cuboidal** (height and width similar, see Figs 3.1c and 3.1d); and **columnar** (height 2–5 times greater than width, see Figs 3.1e and 3.1f).

Epithelial cells form either a single layer, in which all of the cells contact underlying extracellular matrix (**simple epithelium**), or several layers, where only the bottom layer of cells is in contact with the extracellular matrix (**stratified epithelium**, Figs 3.2a and 3.2b). Stratified epithelia are described by the shape of the upper layers of cells, so that a multilayered epithelium with flat, plate-like cells at the surface is named **stratified squamous**.

A **transitional epithelium** is a further special type of stratified epithelium, which is restricted mainly to the lining of the urinary tract (see Figs 3.2c and 3.2d) and varies between cuboidal and squamous depending on the degree of stretching. **Pseudostratified epithelium** (see Figs 3.1g and 3.1h) contains epithelial cells that appear to be arranged in layers, but which are all in contact with the extracellular matrix.

Epithelia are also grouped according to whether they occur as a surface or glandular component.

The traditional morphological classification has limitations. Although two epithelia may be described as cuboidal, their function and biology may be so different that it is misleading to equate them. However, the use of a morphological classification of epithelia is still descriptively valuable and gives some potentially useful information about function. For example, simple squamous epithelia tend to be found in areas where transport via diffusion occurs such as lining the lung gas exchange areas (alveoli) or lining capillaries, whereas the multiple layers of stratified squamous epithelium tend to be found in areas of wear and tear such as the skin and the lining of the oesophagus, anal canal and vagina. Columnar epithelial cells, with their abundant cytoplasm, tend to be associated with absorption and secretion, as both require a large complement of organelles.

The traditional terms used to describe epithelia are found throughout this book but are always qualified to give insight into their function.

Fig. 3.1 Simple Epithelium. **Simple squamous epithelium. (a)** This type of epithelium is composed of a single layer of cells, which are flat and plate-like. **(b)** In histological sections, the nuclei (N) appear flattened and the cytoplasm is indistinct. Although 'squamous' refers to any flat epithelium, its use is restricted, as many flat epithelia are given more specific names, with the flat epithelium lining blood vessels being called *endothelium* and that lining the abdominal and pleural cavities *mesothelium*.

Simple cuboidal epithelium. (c) A simple cuboidal epithelium is composed of a single layer of cells whose height, width and depth are the same. Note that they are not strictly cuboidal. **(d)** In histological section, such cells usually have a centrally placed nucleus (N).

Simple columnar epithelium. (e) A simple columnar epithelium is composed of cells whose height is two to three times greater than their width. **(f)** The nuclei (N) of columnar cells are basal and arranged in an ordered layer.

Pseudostratified columnar epithelium. (g) Several layers of nuclei suggest several layers of cells, but in fact, all cells are in contact with the underlying extracellular matrix. **(h)** Routine histological preparations show several layers of nuclei.

Fig. 3.2 Stratified Epithelium. **(a) Stratified squamous epithelium.** This is composed of several layers, such that cells high up in the epithelium are not in contact with the underlying extracellular matrix. **(b)** Stratified squamous epithelium derives its name from the flattened (squamous) appearance of cells in the superficial part of the epithelium (S). Cells in the basal (B) and middle (M) layers of this type of epithelium are in fact pyramidal or polygonal and are not flattened. **(c) Transitional epithelium.** A transitional epithelium is also multilayered with cuboidal/polyhedral basal and middle layers and a surface layer that is unique to the lower urinary tract and bladder (see p. 324). This epithelium is named after the surface layer, which transitions from domed to squamous, depending on the distention of the bladder. The surface layer of cells is domed and almost columnar in appearance in the undistended state, becoming more flattened and squamous in appearance as the bladder distends. **(d)** Undistended transitional epithelium showing basal (B), middle (M) and surface (S) layers. The apical membrane is highly folded and specialized, giving it a fuzzy appearance in histological sections.

EPITHELIAL CELL JUNCTIONS

Specialized structures are present in epithelia that join individual cells into a functional unit.

The structural integrity of epithelium is maintained by adhesion of epithelial cells, both to each other and to the extracellular matrix (see Chapter 4). These adhesions are mediated by two main systems:

- Cell membrane proteins acting as specialized cell adhesion molecules
- Specialized areas of cell membrane incorporated into cell junctions

There are three types of cell junctions: **occluding junctions** link cells to form an impermeable barrier, **anchoring junctions** link cells to provide mechanical strength, and **communicating junctions** allow movement of molecules between cells.

> **Occluding junctions bind cells together and maintain the integrity of epithelial cells as a barrier.**

Occluding junctions have two main functions:

- Prevention of diffusion of molecules between adjacent cells, thereby contributing to the barrier function of the epithelial cells in which they are present
- Prevention of lateral migration of specialized cell membrane proteins, thereby delineating and maintaining specialized cell membrane domains

The occluding function is performed by intramembranous proteins (Fig. 3.3), which mediate the adhesion of adjacent cells.

Fig. 3.3 Occluding Junction (Tight Junction). **(a)** Occluding junctions are particularly evident between epithelial cells that have secretory or absorptive roles. A collar of occluding junction is present between each cell, sealing individual cells into a tight barrier to prevent back-diffusion of a secreted product. The intramembranous proteins that form these junctions are arranged as serpiginous intertwining lines (sealing strands), which stitch the membrane of adjacent cells together. Around 20 proteins are involved, including occludin and claudin, that span the cell membrane and bind cells together in addition to cytoplasmic proteins such as tight junction protein 1, which forms a plaque that anchors to cytoskeletal filaments. **(b)** Occluding (tight) junction function. Cells that transport molecules against a concentration gradient have occluding junctions to prevent back-diffusion of the transported substance. The protein claudin is mainly responsible for this diffusion barrier. In addition, it is desirable to concentrate specialized cell membrane components into certain areas of the cell, for example, a transport protein in the apical cell membrane. Cells use occluding junctions to prevent lateral migration of specialized membrane proteins, thus establishing specialized membrane domains. **(c)** Immunohistochemical staining for tight junction protein 1 (ZO-1) *(brown)*, which is part of the tight junction complex. The kidney tubular epithelial cells show sealing strands close to the apex of cells, which prevent back-diffusion of material from the lumen of renal tubules. (Image (c) used under Creative Commons License https://creativecommons.org/licenses/by-sa/3.0/ from the Human Protein Atlas Antibody to TJP1 (ZO-1) CAB010822 https://www.proteinatlas.org/ENSG00000104067-TJP1/tissue/kidney#img.)

Ultrastructurally, an occluding junction is seen as a focal area of close apposition of adjacent cell membrane corresponding to the site of membrane attachment proteins. This has led to its alternative name of **tight junction**.

Occluding junctions are particularly well-developed in the epithelial cells lining the small bowel, where they:
- Prevent digested macromolecules from passing between the cells
- Confine specialized areas of the cell membrane involved in absorption or secretion to the luminal side of the cell

Occluding junctions are also important in cells that actively transport a substance, for example, the active transport of an ion against a concentration gradient. In this situation, occluding junctions prevent back-diffusion of the transported substance (see Figs 3.3b and 3.3c).

> **Anchoring junctions link the cytoskeleton of cells both to each other and to underlying tissues.**

Anchoring junctions (Fig. 3.4) provide mechanical stability to groups of epithelial cells so that they can function as a cohesive unit in addition to being involved in cell:cell signalling.

The actin network interacts with two separate types of junctions:
- Adherent junctions link the actin filament network between adjacent cells (Figs 3.5a and 3.5b). In this type of junction, F-actin filaments in adjacent cells are linked by actin-binding proteins, including α and β catenins, vinculin and α actinin, to a transmembrane protein, which is one of a group of the cadherin family of cell surface glycoproteins (E-cadherin), which links cells in the presence of Ca^{2+}. In adherens-type cell–cell connections, β-catenin is located adjacent to the cell membrane (see Fig. 3.5b). β-Catenin also functions as a signalling factor, and dysregulation of this protein, involving separation of cadherin from its cell membrane location, is implicated in the pathogenesis of colon cancer.

Adherent junctions are seen towards the apex of adjacent columnar and cuboidal epithelial cells, where they link submembranous actin bundles into a so-called **adhesion belt.** They are prominent in the cells lining the small intestine, where they form a zone visible by light microscopy as an eosinophilic band (the **terminal bar**).

In embryogenesis, adherent-type junctions transmit motile forces generated by the actin filaments across whole sheets of cells. They are thus essential in mediating the folding of epithelial sheets to form early organs in the embryo.
- Focal contacts link the actin filament network of a cell to the extracellular matrix (see Fig. 3.5c). Bundles of actin

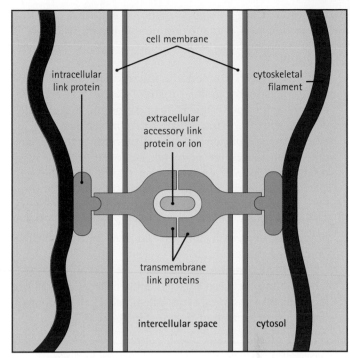

Fig. 3.4 Anchoring Junction (General Structure). Cytoskeletal filaments of adjacent cells are joined through intracellular link proteins, which attach the filaments to transmembrane link proteins. These can then interact with similar proteins on adjacent cells. The extracellular interaction may be mediated by additional extracellular proteins or ions, such as Ca^{2+}. Different (or multiple) link proteins and transmembrane proteins operate for the different classes of junction. An important class of proteins in this group are the cadherins, which link between adjacent cells using Ca^{2+}.

filaments interact with actin-binding proteins (α actinin, vinculin and talin) to link with a transmembrane link protein, which is one of a class of cell adhesion molecules termed an *integrin* (see also Fig. 4.10).

The intermediate filament network interacts with two separate types of junctions:
- Desmosomes connect the intermediate filament networks of adjacent cells (see Fig. 3.5d). Each desmosome consists of an intracellular plaque composed of several link proteins, the main type being desmoplakin associated with plakoglobin and plakophilin, into which cytokeratin intermediate filaments (tonofilaments in skin) are inserted. The cell adhesion is mediated by transmembrane proteins, desmoglein and desmocollin, which are members of the cadherin family of cell adhesion proteins. **Desmosomes** provide mechanical stability in epithelial cells that are subject to tensile and shearing stresses and are particularly well-developed in stratified squamous epithelium covering the skin.

Desmosomes are so characteristic of epithelial cells that their detection in malignant tumours of uncertain nature is indicative of an epithelial as opposed to a lymphoid or support cell origin.

- Hemidesmosomes connect the intermediate filament network of cells to extracellular matrix (see Figs 3.5e and 3.8). A hemidesmosome is similar to a desmosome, except that it interacts with the extracellular matrix rather than with an adjacent desmosome on another cell. In contrast to a desmosome, the cytokeratin filaments (tonofilaments in skin) commonly terminate end-on rather than looping through. The proteins in the hemidesmosome differ from those in desmosomes. The intracellular plaque contains the proteins plectin and BPAG1e. The transmembrane anchoring proteins comprise β_4 integrin, α_6 integrin and BPAG2 (BPAG, bullous pemphigoid antigen).

A **junctional complex** is the close association of several types of junctions between adjacent epithelial cells and reflects the requirement for several types of epithelial cell attachment to maintain structural and functional integrity (Fig. 3.6).

Communication junctions allow direct cell–cell communication.

Communication junctions (gap junctions) allow selective diffusion of molecules between adjacent cells and facilitate direct cell–cell communication (Fig. 3.7). The protein units that form this type of junction are called *connexins*. There are around 20 different coding genes, and mutations in several are linked to different disorders affecting a range of tissues, including the lens, skin, peripheral nerve and inner ear.

Gap junctions are usually present at relatively low density in most adult epithelia, but are found in large numbers during embryogenesis, when they probably have a role in the spatial organization of developing cells. Gap junctions are also important in cardiac and smooth muscle cells, where they pass signals involved in contraction from one cell to another.

The basement membrane anchors epithelial cells to underlying tissues.

The attachment of epithelial cells to underlying support tissues at hemidesmosome and focal contacts is mediated by a specialized layer of extracellular matrix materials: the basement membrane (Fig. 3.8 and see Fig. 4.11). The basement membrane contains a special form of matrix protein called *type IV collagen* and glycoproteins such as laminin, which are synthesized by the epithelial cells. It also contains elements (e.g. fibronectin) produced by the underlying connective tissue layer; the detailed structure and function of the basement membrane are fully discussed in Chapter 4. Using light microscopy, basement membrane is just visible as a linear structure at the base of epithelia. It can be stained with the periodic acid–Schiff (PAS) technique (see Fig. 4.13a) but is visible in electron micrographs (see Fig. 3.8). The function of the basement membrane is to attach the epithelium to the underlying tissue, to act as a barrier, and to organize the polarity of epithelial cells so specialized cell surfaces for absorption or secretion are orientated in the correct direction.

CLINICAL EXAMPLE

Disease of Cell Junctions: Pemphigus and Pemphigoid

In pemphigus, the body produces abnormal antibodies to the proteins forming desmosome junctions in the skin (desmoglein 1 and 3); this prevents normal adhesion between the desmosomes (autoimmune disease). Affected people develop widespread skin and mucous membrane blistering as the desmosomal junctions between adjacent squamous cells of the skin fall apart. Immunohistochemical staining can be used to demonstrate the abnormal antibodies adhering to the intercellular space between the diseased epidermal cells. Blisters develop within the cell layers of the epidermis (intraepidermal blisters) as the junctions affected are the desmosomes (see Fig. 18.5).

Bullous pemphigoid is a blistering disease in which autoantibodies form and are directed against proteins associated with hemidesmosome (bp180 and bp230; also called BPAG1 and BPAG2). The hemidesmosome links cytokeratin intermediate filaments in the basal layer of skin via integrin proteins that bind the cell to the basal lamina. In bullous pemphigoid, binding of antibody to these normal proteins leads to inflammation and separation of the epithelium from the basal lamina, causing skin blistering. The plane of separation leads to subepidermal blisters, as the problem lies with hemidesmosomes which anchor epidermis to basal lamina.

CLINICAL EXAMPLE

Epithelial Basement Membrane in Disease

The basement membrane is affected in many disease processes:

- Epidermolysis bullosa is a rare genetic condition with several causes. One type is called *junctional epidermolysis bullosa* in which affected children have very fragile skin and mucous membranes such that minimal trauma causes blisters and painful, raw areas of skin loss. This is caused by mutation of the genes encoding laminin-5 chains, which are normally found in basement membrane and which link to integrins expressed in skin epithelial cells, firmly anchoring the epidermis to the dermis. Lack of laminin-5 anchorage leads to skin fragility.
- Goodpasture's syndrome is a rare autoimmune condition where autoantibodies are directed against the α-3 domain of type IV collagen located in the basement membrane in lungs and kidneys. Patients develop renal failure because of damage to glomeruli in the kidneys and bleeding into the lungs because of damage to alveoli.

Fig. 3.5 Types of Anchoring Junctions. Four types of anchoring junctions provide mechanical stability in epithelial layers. Adherens junctions (a) and focal contacts (b) interact with the actin network; desmosomes (c) and hemidesmosomes (d) interact with the intermediate filament network. **(a) Adherent junctions** link actin filaments through a chain of proteins to E-cadherin that sits in the cell membrane. **(b)** Kidney tubular epithelium immunostained for β-catenin *(brown)*, which is located around lateral and basal cell membranes of adjacent epithelial cells as part of cell adhesion. **(c) Focal contacts** link actin filaments via actin-binding proteins to an integrin that sits in the cell membrane. **(d) Desmosomes** link intermediate filaments through a plaque composed of link proteins, which is attached to cadherin proteins that span the cell membrane and extend to the intercellular space. **(e) Hemidesmosomes** link intermediate filaments to the extracellular matrix through a plaque composed of link proteins, which is attached to integrin proteins that span the cell membrane and extend to the extracellular matrix. The proteins in the hemidesmosome differ from those in desmosomes. The linking proteins include some involved in the autoimmune disease bullous pemphigoid (BPAG, bullous pemphigoid antigen). (Image (b) used under Creative Commons License https://creativecommons.org/licenses/by-sa/3.0/ from the Human Protein Atlas Antibody to CTNNB1 HPA029159 https://www.proteinatlas.org/ENSG00000168036-CTNNB1/tissue/kidney#img.)

Fig. 3.6 Junctional Complex. **(a)** A junctional complex is commonly seen towards the apex of cuboidal and columnar cells. Immediately below the cell apex, an occluding junction (O) is followed by an adherent junction (A), and below this, by desmosomes (D). This example is obtained from cells lining the small bowel, where such complexes are well-developed. In other epithelia, particularly those in which occluding junctions are not required, such fully developed complexes are uncommon. **(b)** The disc-shaped adhesion plaques (P) in adjacent cells are seen as electron-dense areas into which cytokeratin filaments (CF) are inserted. The cell membranes (CM) between adhesion plaques are about 30 nm apart, and there may be an electron-dense band between cells in some desmosomes (X).

Fig. 3.7 Gap (Communication) Junction. **(a)** A small part of a gap junction. Each junction is a circular patch studded with several hundred pores, each formed by six protein subunits traversing the cell membranes and termed a *connexon*. Pores on adjacent cells are aligned, allowing small molecules to move between cells. **(b)** Ultrastructurally, a cross-section of a gap junction is seen as a flat area of closely apposing cell membranes, between which the connexons (C) can just be seen as dot-like granules.

Fig. 3.8 Basement Membrane. (a) An electron micrograph of a basement membrane between a basal epithelial cell in skin and the underlying support tissue. A hemidesmosome (Hd) can be seen, consisting of a dense plaque composed of intracellular link proteins into which the cell's cytokeratin intermediate filaments (IF) are inserted. Ultrastructurally, the basement membrane consists of two layers: lamina lucida (L) and lamina densa (D), with an external, ill-defined fibroreticular lamina. Fine anchoring fibrils (F), composed of type VII collagen, anchor the lamina densa to external collagen fibres (C).

EPITHELIAL CELL SURFACE SPECIALIZATIONS

> **The surface of epithelial cells is often adapted to allow a specialized function.**

The surface of epithelial cells is highly developed to fulfil specialized functions:

- The main adaptation requirement is for increased surface area, which in different cell types is achieved by microvilli, basolateral folds and membrane plaques.
- The need to move substances over their surface is met by motile cell projections termed *cilia*.

> **Microvilli are surface specializations to increase the surface area of cells.**

Microvilli are finger-like projections of the apical cell surface (Fig. 3.9). Small microvilli are found on the surface of most epithelial cells but are most developed in absorptive cells, such as kidney tubule cells and small bowel epithelium.

The shape of microvilli is maintained by a bundle of actin filaments, which form a core running through each villus; it is anchored to the actin cortex of the cell. In epithelial cells of the small bowel, the actin core is also linked to the actin network of adherent junctions between adjacent cells.

Fig. 3.9 Microvilli. (a) Each microvillus is a finger-like extension of cell membrane, which is stabilized by a bundle of actin filaments held rigidly 10 nm apart by actin-binding proteins. The actin bundle is bound to the lateral surface of the microvillus by a helical arrangement of myosin molecules, which bind on one side to the actin and on the other to the inner surface of the cell membrane. The bundle is also adherent to the apex of the microvillus in an amorphous area of anchoring proteins, which may represent capping proteins for the actin filaments to prevent their depolymerization. At the base of the microvillus, the entering actin bundle is stabilized by the actin/spectrin cell cortex, under which are cytokeratin intermediate filaments. **(b)** Electron micrograph showing the surface of a cell lining the small bowel. Microvilli (M) form finger-like projections, each having an actin filament (AF) core that enters the cell and merges with the actin cortex (AC), which is also known as the *terminal web*.

The cell membrane that covers microvilli bears specific cell surface glycoproteins and enzymes involved in the absorptive process. This cell surface specialization is just about visible ultrastructurally as a fuzzy coating but is much more evident when enzyme histochemistry or immunohistochemistry is used to detect specific proteins, such as lactase and alkaline phosphatase (see also Fig. 3.13).

Stereocilia are extremely long forms of microvilli and, despite their name, have nothing to do with true cilia. They are found on epithelial cells lining the epididymis and can also be seen in the inner ear, where they are sensors of cochlear hair cells (see Chapter 19).

Basolateral folds increase cell surface area.

Basolateral folds are deep invaginations of the basal or lateral surface of cells (Fig. 3.10). They are particularly evident in cells involved in fluid or ion transport and are commonly associated with high concentrations of mitochondria, which provide the energy for ion and fluid transport. The presence of basal folds and mitochondria imparts a striped appearance to the basal cytoplasm of such cells, giving rise to the descriptive term *striated epithelial cells*.

Basal folds are seen in renal tubular cells (see Figs 3.10a and 15.22) and in the ducts of many secretory glands.

Cell surface area can be similarly increased by folding of the lateral cell membrane, which can be seen in some epithelial cells, particularly absorptive cells lining the gut.

Membrane plaques are a specialized structure seen in the urothelium.

Membrane plaques are rigid areas of the apical cell membrane found only in the epithelium lining the urinary tract. They can fold down into the cell when the bladder is empty and unfold to increase the luminal area of the cell when the bladder is full (see Fig. 15.39).

Cilia are motile surface projections of cells involved in transport.

Cilia are hair-like projections, 0.2 μm in diameter, which arise from the surface of certain specialized cells and have a role in moving fluid over the surface of the cell or to confer cell motility. This type is termed **motile cilia** to distinguish them from the structure of the primary cilium, which is expressed on most cells and is involved in a range of cell-signalling functions (see p. 37). However, the unqualified use of the term *cilia* always refers to motile cilia.

Each cilium is a highly specialized extension of the cytoskeleton arising from a derivative of the centriole termed a *basal body* and composed of an organized core of parallel microtubules (the axoneme). These microtubules are bound together with other proteins to produce energy-dependent movement of the filaments, which results in side-to-side beating (Fig. 3.11).

Fig. 3.10 Basal Folds. (a) Electron micrograph showing a cuboidal epithelial cell in the proximal convoluted tubule of the kidney. A central nucleus (N) and abundant microvilli (M) can be seen projecting into the lumen (L). At the base of the cell the basement membrane (BM) is evident, as are membrane folds in the lateral and basal (BF) membranes. A capillary (C) can be seen in the underlying support tissue. **(b)** Electron micrograph showing deep infolding of basal cell membrane (BF) of a distal tubule kidney cell. This facilitates cell membrane transport of ions by greatly increasing the cell surface area.

Fig. 3.11 Motile Cilia. (a) Cross section of a motile cilium. The nine outer doublet tubules are made of tubulin, whereas arms composed of the protein dynein occur every 24 nm down the length of the cilium and interact with adjacent doublets as a 'molecular motor' to produce bending. Links composed of another protein, nexin, are more widely spaced (every 86 nm) and hold the microtubules in position. Radial spokes extend from each of the nine outer doublets towards a central pair of tubules at 29-nm intervals, and the central sheath projections are present every 14 nm. **(b)** Ultrastructural appearance of a cilium in cross-section. Because the different constituent proteins are periodically spaced at different intervals along the length of the axoneme, not all are visible in any one plane of section. **(c)** In longitudinal section, the base of each cilium (C) is seen to arise as a specialized derivative of the centriole (the basal body, BB). Here, the outer doublets of the cilium arise directly from the outer triplet of the centriole *(CM,* cell membrane; *Cy,* cytoplasm). **(d)** Micrograph of a ciliated epithelium. Cilia (C) form a hair-like layer at the apical cell surface. As they are quite fragile, they may not be well preserved in poorly fixed or processed tissue.

Cilia are particularly evident in:

- Epithelium lining the respiratory tract, where they move mucus over the cell surfaces (see Fig. 10.2).
- Epithelium lining the fallopian tube, where they convey released ova to the uterine cavity (see Fig. 17.12).
- Epithelium cells lining the ventricles of the brain called *ependymal cells* (see Fig. 6.22).
- An axonemal structure similar to that of cilia is found in the flagellum of spermatozoa (see Fig. 16.8).

👥 CLINICAL EXAMPLE

Cilial Defects and Disease

Genetic defects in genes coding for ciliary proteins give rise to poor ciliary beating (**primary ciliary dyskinesia**).

Ultrastructurally, elements of the cilia may be absent or abnormal (Fig. 3.12):

- In embryogenesis, defective cilia do not to move cell layers, and major organs do not assume normal anatomical positions (e.g. right-sided heart).
- Development of air sinuses in the skull is impaired.
- Failure of mucus removal from the lung results in recurrent and severe chest infections, leading to permanent dilation of the large air passages (bronchiectasis).
- Infertility is common because ovum transport along the fallopian tube depends on normal ciliary function, and ciliary proteins make up the motile tail of spermatozoa.

Fig. 3.12 Primary Ciliary Dyskinesia. Electron micrograph of cilia from a person with recurrent chest infections since childhood. The outer dynein arms are absent, and there are abnormal single microtubules (M), which prevent normal motility. Compare with Fig. 3.11b.

> **The cell surface is the location of enzymes, adhesion and cell recognition molecules.**

The external surface of epithelia is invested with a layer of proteins, sugar residues, glycoproteins, proteoglycans and glycolipids which, in many cells, can be resolved ultrastructurally as an amorphous fuzzy coating to the cell membrane. Because of the sugar content, it is stainable by techniques, such as the PAS method (see p. 7). This coating is termed the **glycocalyx.**

Fig. 3.13 Small Bowel Enzyme Activity in the Brush Border. The localization of cell membrane–associated maltase-glucoamylase on the surface of epithelial cells lining the small bowel is shown. Note that the enzyme activity (demonstrated as a brown stain deposit) is confined to the apical surface of the cells, as it is located in the membrane of the brush border. This enzyme is the final step in the breakdown of linear regions of starch to glucose. (Image used under Creative Commons License https://creativecommons.org/licenses/by-sa/3.0/ from the Human Protein Atlas Antibody to Maltase-glucoamylase HPA002270 https://www.proteinatlas.org/ENSG00000257335-MGAM/tissue/small+intestine#img.)

This layer has several functions, including:

- Barrier to infective pathogens
- Electrical charge barrier to limit the passage of charged proteins in renal glomeruli
- Coupling to mechanosensors to detect flow in blood vessel endothelium and renal tubules
- Cell adhesion and cell recognition in endothelium

Enzyme histochemical and immunohistochemical methods can be used to detect specific enzymes in this surface coating (Fig. 3.13), and it is apparent that epithelial cells at different sites have different functional attributes in terms of enzyme activity, despite similarities in their morphology.

Surface proteins are also used in a variety of cell recognition and adherence mechanisms, often of great importance to the function of the immune system (see discussion on CD molecules in Chapter 8).

SECRETORY ADAPTATIONS

> **Some organelles in epithelial cells develop to adapt a cell for secretion of macromolecules.**

Certain epithelial cells have structural specializations related to their role in the production and secretion of macromolecules, such as enzymes, mucins and steroids. In addition, epithelial cells can be adapted for the secretion and transport of ions. Such cells are characterized by an expansion of the specific organelle systems involved in the elaboration and secretion of the respective macromolecules (see pp. 28).

> **Protein-secreting epithelial cells have large nuclei and abundant rough endoplasmic reticulum (ER).**

Although all cells contain the apparatus to produce structural proteins, certain cells are specialized to secrete a protein product and have the following characteristics:

- A well-developed rough ER, which often results in blue colouration of the cytoplasm in haematoxylin and eosin (H&E)–stained sections (see discussion on plasma cells in Chapter 8)
- Distinct polarity with basal rough ER, a supranuclear Golgi just visible as an ill-defined lucent area of the cytoplasm and an apical zone containing granules filled with packaged protein ready for secretion by exocytosis

The staining characteristics of the apical portion of the cells depend on the nature of this protein (Fig. 3.14a).

> **Mucin-secreting epithelial cells have a greatly expanded Golgi system.**

Mucins (mixtures of glycoproteins and proteoglycans) have important functions in body cavities, for example, as a lubricant in the mouth and as a barrier in the stomach.

Cells that produce and secrete mucin (see Figs 3.14b and 3.17a) are characterized by the following features:

- A well-developed basal rough ER makes the protein core of mucins and imparts a faint blue colour to the basal cytoplasm.
- A well-developed supranuclear Golgi is the main site of protein glycosylation, but is not clearly visible by light microscopy.
- Large secretory vesicles of mucin at the cell apex impart an unstained vacuolated appearance to the apical cell cytoplasm.

Mucin-secreting cells may be part of a surface epithelium, when they are termed *goblet cells,* for example, in epithelia lining the gut (see Fig. 11.44) and respiratory tract. In addition, mucin-secreting cells can be aggregated into specialized glands, for example, in the genital tract, respiratory tract and intestinal tract.

Fig. 3.14 Appearance of Secretory Cells. **(a) Protein-secreting epithelial cells.** The cells shown in this micrograph are from the pancreas and are producing pancreatic enzymes. Cells show strong basophilia at the periphery of each acinus (P) caused by the abundant rough endoplasmic reticulum required in protein synthesis, whereas the apical cytoplasm towards the centre of each acinus (C) is eosinophilic because of the presence of the secretory protein product stored within vesicles. **(b) Mucin-secreting epithelial cells.** Micrograph of mucin-secreting epithelial cells aggregated into a gland showing the blue basal nuclei and the rest of the cells showing a vacuolated appearance of the apical cytoplasm because of extensive vesicles containing mucin (MV). **(c) Steroid-secreting epithelial cells.** According to their cytoplasmic composition, steroid-secreting cells vary in appearance in H&E-stained sections from granular pink-staining cells, which contain many mitochondria and little lipid, to pale pink-staining and vacuolated cells, which contain abundant lipid and dilated smooth endoplasmic reticulum. The cells shown here are from the adrenal gland and have a pale and finely vacuolated appearance. **(d) Ion-pumping epithelial cells.** Micrograph of striated duct epithelial cells from the salivary gland. Folding of the cell membrane (F) containing the active membrane protein produces a fine, striped appearance, whereas the large numbers of mitochondria impart a granular pink-staining appearance to the basal part of the cell. Tight junctions are visible ultrastructurally or by immunohistochemistry (see Fig 3.3c) (Micrograph (a) from digital pathology whole slide image provided by the University of Leeds Virtual Pathology Project https://www.virtualpathology.leeds.ac.uk. Reproduced with permission.)

Cells producing steroid hormones (see Fig. 3.14c) are found mainly in the adrenal gland, ovary and testis and have the following characteristics:

- A well-developed smooth ER, which gives the cytoplasm a granular pink appearance.
- Free lipid (lipids are the precursors of the steroid hormones) in vacuoles in the cell cytoplasm, which imparts a fine vacuolated appearance to the cells.
- Prominent mitochondria with tubular rather than flattened cristae. Mitochondria are involved in the biosynthesis of steroids from lipid, but the functional significance of the tubular shape of their cristae is not clear.

Cells in the kidney tubules and in the ducts of some secretory glands transport ions and water, whereas acid-producing cells of the stomach transport H^+ ions (see Fig. 11.29). Ion transport is mediated by membrane ion pumps; these use adenosine triphosphate (ATP) as a source of energy for the exchange of ions between cytosol and extracellular space.

The structural specializations of ion-pumping epithelial cells (see Fig. 3.14d) are as follows:

- The cell membrane is folded to increase the active surface area of membrane containing the membrane protein that acts as the ion pump.
- Large numbers of mitochondria are closely apposed to the membrane folds to supply ATP.
- Tight junctions between the cells prevent back-diffusion of pumped ions.

In cells of the intestine, gallbladder and kidney, the ion pumps move sodium and water from the apical surface to be absorbed, whereas in secretory glands, the cells move ions and fluid out of the apex of the cell, resulting in secretion of watery fluid (e.g. sweat).

There are four mechanisms of secretion of cell products by epithelial cells: merocrine, apocrine, holocrine and endocrine (Fig. 3.15).

Secretions from the apex of the cell onto a surface or into a lumen are termed *exocrine,* whereas secretions from the side or base of the cell, which enter the bloodstream directly, are termed *endocrine.*

A gland is an organized collection of secretory epithelial cells. In many epithelia, secretion is performed only by occasional specialized cells (e.g. mucin-secreting goblet cells) scattered among other, non-secretory cells (Figs 3.16 and 3.17).

Fig. 3.15 Types of Cell Secretion. Secretion of cell products may occur by exocytosis from the cell apex into a lumen (merocrine secretion), by pinching off apical cell cytoplasm containing cell products (apocrine secretion), by shedding of the whole cell containing the cell product (holocrine secretion) or by endocytosis from the cell base into the bloodstream (endocrine secretion, see also Fig. 14.1).

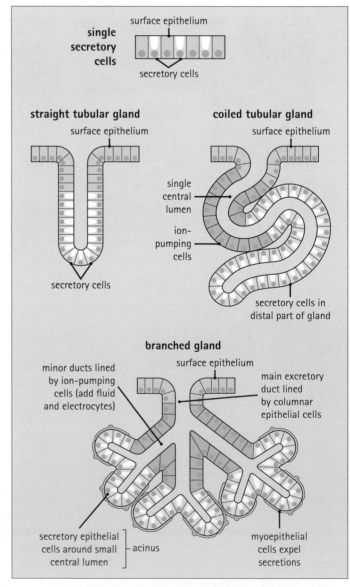

Fig. 3.16 Secretory Cells and Glands.

Fig. 3.17 Secretory Cells, Glands and Ducts. (a) Single cells in a surface epithelium secreting mucin. These are called *goblet cells* (G). **(b)** H&E-stained section showing a straight tubular colonic gland, which is typical of glands in the gut. Secretory cells (S) line straight tubules and discharge their mucin secretions on to the surface. **(c)** H&E-stained section of a sweat gland from the skin showing the arrangement of a coiled tubular gland. Secretory cells are present in the distal part, and there is zoning of secretory function, with an area of protein-secreting cells (P) being followed by an area of ion-pumping cells (I), which add fluid to the secretion in the lumen. The distal part of the gland (D) has no secretory function but is specialized for transporting secretions, having tight junctions to prevent back-diffusion of ions; such tubules are termed *ducts*. **(d)** H&E section of a branched gland showing the arrangement of secretory epithelial cells into acini (A) and main excretory duct (MD). Myoepithelial cells (see Fig. 5.16) are not readily visible at this low magnification but will be a component of acini and ducts. **(e)** Gland ducts carry exocrine secretion from a gland and discharge it onto an epithelial surface or into a body cavity. Ducts are lined by a tall columnar epithelium (E) and contain no specialized secretory cells. This duct has a clear bilayer lining; the luminal (inner) cells are epithelial in type, and the outer cells are myoepithelial in type. Note pale-stained secretion (S) in the lumen. (Micrograph (d) from digital pathology whole slide image provided by the University of Leeds Virtual Pathology Project https://www.virtualpathology.leeds.ac.uk. Reproduced with permission.)

When more secretions are required, the surface area of secretory epithelium can be increased by invagination of the surface to form straight tubular glands or by the formation of more complex coiled or branched glands, which may be divided into specialized zones for the secretion of different products.

The most structurally refined glands are those that have a branched architecture with secretory cells arranged in islands termed *acini*. Transport of secretion from this type of exocrine gland is via a series of ducts lined by columnar epithelium, with apical junctional complexes to prevent escape of the secretions (see Fig. 3.17e). In most complex glands myoepithelial cells form an outer layer to acini and ducts and have a contractile function in propelling secretions out of the gland (see Figs 3.17e and 18.20).

Whereas most glands form part of other tissues (e.g. mucous glands in the respiratory tract), many are anatomically distinct (e.g. salivary glands, pancreas, liver).

Gland secretions are under hormonal and innervatory control, and all glands have a rich vascular supply to provide the necessary metabolites.

BARRIER FUNCTION OF EPITHELIUM

Many epithelia function as a barrier, and this role is associated with certain specializations:

- Occluding junctions prevent diffusion of molecules between cells and therefore prevent diffusion of substances from one side of an epithelium to the other and ensure the controlled passage of substances through the epithelial layer.
- The apical cell membrane of epithelial cells lining the urinary tract (i.e. urothelial transitional epithelium) contains a high proportion of sphingolipids. These not only form membrane plaques (see p. 324) but are also believed to resist fluid and electrolyte movements out of the cells in response to the osmotic effect of concentrated urine.

- Desmosomal and hemidesmosomal junctions provide a tight mechanical linkage between cells and extracellular matrix to resist shearing forces and allow an epithelium to function as a mechanical barrier.
- Stratified squamous epithelial cells may undergo keratinization, a process in which the cytoskeleton of superficial cells of the epithelium becomes tightly condensed with other specialized proteins into a resilient mass. This results in cell death and the formation of a tough, impervious and protective layer (keratin) from the remaining cell membranes and cytoplasmic contents (see Fig. 18.3).

Keratinization ultimately transforms the cells into nonliving proteinaceous material, which remains attached by existing anchoring junctions. The surface keratin layer is mechanically strong but flexible; it is relatively inert and acts as a physical barrier, particularly preventing ingress of microorganisms. The intercellular phospholipid renders the epithelium impermeable to water. These features make it ideal for the epithelium of skin (see Fig. 18.3).

CLINICAL EXAMPLE

Tumours of Epithelial Cells

Cells may lose their normal growth control mechanisms and give rise to a tumour (neoplasm). Many such abnormal growths remain localized (benign neoplasms), but some invade adjacent tissues and metastasize to other parts of the body (malignant neoplasms).

A malignant neoplasm arising from squamous epithelial cells is termed a *squamous carcinoma*, whereas carcinoma derived from glandular epithelium is called an *adenocarcinoma* (Fig. 3.18). Note: The term *carcinoma* is a specific term meaning a malignant tumour derived from epithelium. The term *cancer* is non-specific and may refer to any type of malignant tumour.

In most cases, cells of a carcinoma resemble those of their tissue of origin. The diagnosis of malignancy is based on the presence of abnormal cytology and by locating cells that have invaded other tissues (Fig. 3.19).

In some cases, a carcinoma bears little resemblance to its cell of origin (undifferentiated carcinoma); such tumours commonly present with metastases, and their site of origin may not be clear. In this situation, histological knowledge of the pattern of expression of cell proteins can be explored using immunohistochemistry, and staining results, using a panel of antibodies to markers, can help to confirm a diagnosis. (See clinical example panel on Immunohistochemistry of Epithelia (page 62)).

Fig. 3.18 Adenocarcinoma. H&E section of colonic epithelium showing crypts lined by normal glandular epithelium (N) and carcinoma (T) forming gland-like structures (i.e. adenocarcinoma). The neoplastic epithelium is characterised by dark-staining, larger nuclei and fewer mucin-secreting cells than normal. (Micrograph (a) from digital pathology whole slide image provided by the University of Leeds Virtual Pathology Project https://www.virtualpathology.leeds.ac.uk. Reproduced with permission.)

Tumours of Epithelial Cells

Fig. 3.19 Histological Features of Epithelial Tumours. (a) Normal colonic epithelium. **(b)** Benign neoplasm of colon. **(c)** Well-differentiated malignant neoplasm of colon. **(d)** Poorly differentiated malignant neoplasm of colon. **(e)** Anaplastic malignant neoplasm of colon. Neoplastic change in an epithelium is associated with changes in the cytology and architecture of cells. The cells of a benign epithelial neoplasm of the colon (an adenoma) **(b)** resemble those of the normal epithelium **(a)**, in that they are columnar and have an orderly arrangement. Loss of some degree of differentiation is evident in that the neoplastic cells do not show mucin vacuolation. Cells of the well-differentiated malignant neoplasm (an adenocarcinoma) **(c)** have a haphazard arrangement, and although gland lumina are formed, they are architecturally abnormal and irregular. Nuclei vary in shape and size. Cells in the poorly differentiated adenocarcinoma **(d)** have an even more haphazard arrangement, with very poor formation of gland lumina. Nuclei show greater variation in shape and size than in **(c)**. Cells in anaplastic malignant neoplasm **(e)** bear no relation to the normal, with no attempt at gland formation. There is tremendous variation in the size of cells and of nuclei, with very intense staining (nuclear hyperchromatism) of the latter. Without knowing the site of its origin, it would be impossible to tell what sort of tumour this was by histology without special investigations.

CLINICAL EXAMPLE

Immunochemistry of Epithelia

Immunohistochemical techniques can identify epithelial cells and are useful in biopsy diagnosis of cancer.

In diagnostic histopathology, biopsy samples are looked at by a pathologist to diagnose disease. A common clinical problem is the evaluation of a biopsy of an abnormal growth, the most common type of which is malignant growth of epithelial cells as a carcinoma. The pathologist has to try and answer the following questions:

1. Is the tissue normal or abnormal?
2. If the tissue is abnormal, does it represent an abnormal growth of cells, a tumour?
3. If the abnormality is a tumour, what is the cell of origin? Is it epithelial?
4. If the abnormality is an epithelial tumour, is it one that would be predicted to grow only locally (benign – termed *adenoma* or *papilloma*), or is it one that would be predicted to spread by invasion or metastasis (malignant – termed *carcinoma*).

To answer these questions about a tumour of epithelial cells, the pathologist first uses conventional staining, usually H&E, and evaluates the tissue architecture. This will often give the diagnosis of the type of epithelial tumour and usually predicts behaviour.

- Benign growths closely resemble normal tissues, have few mitoses and cells have a uniform morphology.
- Malignant growths do not resemble normal tissues closely, have increased numbers of mitoses and cells vary in morphology – usually showing variation in size, with variation in the size and density of staining of nuclei.

In some instances, a carcinoma shows few distinguishing features when standard histological techniques are used. The pathologist then faces a problem in diagnosis. Different types of carcinoma require different types of treatment, as clinical trials have shown that certain types of epithelial tumour respond better to certain types of therapy. This is most important in situations where a tumour first presents by spread, for example, as a mass in a bone or a lymph node, and where imaging shows no clear origin. Histology shows a carcinoma, but there is no known primary site. In this case, the clinical team will ask the pathologist to try to state the likely primary site of origin of the tumour to help direct the further investigations and treatment.

The use of immunohistochemistry, applying a panel of antibodies that detect specific cellular components, is routinely used in clinical diagnosis (see p. 7). Depending on the pattern of expression of different antigens, it is possible to predict the cell type of a tumour and predict a likely primary site for a carcinoma.

For very poorly differentiated malignant tumours, it may first be necessary to discriminate between cells of different histogenesis using a broad panel of antibodies:

- Leucocyte common antigen (CD45) detects if the tumour is lymphoid in origin.
- Muscle-specific actin detects a tumour of muscle.
- MelanA detects tumours of melanocytes.

Epithelial cells have the following characteristics, detectable by immunohistochemical techniques:

- Expression of the cytokeratin class of intermediate filament proteins. This is not a feature of other classes of cells, for example, support cells or lymphoid cells.
- Expression of a class of cell surface glycoproteins (epithelial membrane antigen, EMA).

Once a broad panel of antibodies has established that a malignant tumour is of epithelial origin and is a carcinoma, further panels of antibodies may be employed to predict the likely primary site of origin of the tumour. Examples include:

- Possession of a specialized stainable epithelial product by some epithelia, for example, prostate-specific antigen and prostate-specific acid phosphatase in the ducts and acini of the prostate gland; thyroglobulin in cells of the thyroid gland.
- Cytokeratin 7 and cytokeratin 20 are differentially expressed in epithelia of different types and are commonly used in predicting the site of origin of carcinomas of glandular tissue, termed *adenocarcinomas*.
- Carcinoembryonic antigen (CEA) is strongly expressed in many tumours derived from glandular epithelium of the gastrointestinal tract.
- Thyroid transcription factor 1 (TTF-1) is a protein located in the nucleus of epithelial cells in lung tissue. TTF-1 has been shown to be present in a variety of lung and thyroid tumours and is not present in most other carcinomas.
- Tumours derived from mesothelial cells show a high frequency of staining for cytokeratins 5/6, thrombomodulin and calretinin.
- Tumours of hepatic epithelial cells show a high frequency of staining for Hep Par 1 (hepatocyte paraffin 1 monoclonal antibody), α-fetoprotein and CD10 antigen.
- Carcinoma of the breast may show immunoreactivity for oestrogen receptor, and this may direct therapy with anti-oestrogenic agents.

After evaluation of a panel of antibodies covering a variety of possible tumour sites, a pathologist can usually give a diagnosis and opinion that are clinically useful in directing further investigation and patient management.

For online review questions, please visit https://studentconsult.inkling.com.

Support Cells and the Extracellular Matrix

INTRODUCTION

The cells that form tissues can be divided into two types: **parenchymal cells**, which provide the main function of a tissue, and **support cells**, which provide the structural scaffolding of a tissue. Support cells comprise a set of highly developed cell types with complex metabolic functions and produce an extracellular matrix, which largely defines the physical characteristics of a tissue.

Support cells and their associated extracellular matrix are commonly termed **connective tissue**. However, this term does not emphasize the highly specialized nature of this class of tissues. The extracellular matrix is not merely a structural anchoring substance, it has essential roles in development, growth, homeostasis, and in response to disease.

This chapter covers the general characteristics and types of support cells and describes the main components of the extra-cellular matrix materials that are so vital to the structure and function of tissues and which define several types of what are termed *connective tissues*.

> **Support cells have common characteristics that distinguish them from other classes of cells.**

Support cells are vital in providing mechanical stability to tissues in addition to roles in growth, tissue remodelling and homeostasis. These are included in the class of connective tissue cells and have the following common characteristics:

- Embryological derivation from mesenchyme (Fig. 4.1)
- Production of a variety of extracellular matrix materials
- When mature, formation of sparsely cellular tissues in which the matrix is the main component
- Cell adhesion mechanisms that interact with extracellular matrix materials rather than other cells

> **There are five main classes of support cells.**

The support cells are as follows:

- **Fibroblasts** secrete the extracellular matrix components in most tissues, usually collagen and elastin.
- **Chondrocytes** secrete the extracellular matrix components of cartilage.
- **Osteoblasts** secrete the extracellular matrix components of bone.
- **Myofibroblasts** secrete extracellular matrix components and also have a contractile function.
- **Adipocytes** are specially adapted lipid-storing support cells, which not only act as an energy store but have an endocrine function and act as physical cushioning and padding in some anatomic regions.

Fig. 4.1 Embryonic Mesenchyme. Mesenchyme is an embryonic tissue. It is characterized by spindle-shaped cells with large nuclei (N), which develop into a variety of cell types in embryonic life, thus forming the family of support cells.

EXTRACELLULAR MATRIX

> **The extracellular matrix is the bioscaffold of tissues and is composed mainly of fibrillar proteins surrounded by glycosaminoglycans.**

The extracellular matrix can be considered as a bioscaffold, which provides both mechanical structural support and biological support (nutrition, growth factors) to the cells within any tissue. Some tissue types are characterized by only a relatively small volume fraction of extracellular matrix, for example, muscle, whereas others are almost entirely charac-terised by the extracellular matrix component, for example, in tendons and cartilage.

Extracellular matrix is produced by most support cells and is composed of two major materials: glycosaminoglycans (GAGs) and fibrillar proteins. In addition, smaller amounts of struc-tural glycoprotein are present in the extracellular matrix with important roles in cell adhesion.

The general structure of support tissue is a scattered net-work of support cells producing an organised extracellular network of fibrillar proteins arranged in a hydrated gel of GAG. Other cells (e.g. epithelial cells, contractile cells) are anchored to this tissue by cell matrix–anchoring junctions (see p. 50).

⊚ ADVANCED CONCEPT

GAGs Have the Following Properties

A high negative charge, because in all GAGs, one of the repeating units is an amino sugar (N-acetylglucosamine or N-acetylgalactosamine), which is commonly sulphated (SO_3^-), and in most GAGs, the second sugar is uronic acid with a carboxyl group (COO^-).

Strongly hydrophilic behaviour because they cannot fold into compact structures and therefore have a large, permanently open coil conformation.

Retention of positive ions (e.g. Na^+) together with water, thereby maintaining tissue architecture by an inherent turgor, which tends to prevent deformation by compressive forces.

Except for hyaluronic acid, **covalent attachment to proteins to form proteoglycans,** which are huge molecules capable of maintaining a large hydration space in the extracellular matrix. The spatial organization and charge of proteoglycans facilitate selective diffusion of different molecules, probably by allowing variation in pore size of the matrix gel. This is particularly important in the basement membranes of the kidney glomerulus (see Fig. 15.8).

They can be divided into four groups according to their structure: hyaluronic acid, chondroitin sulphate and dermatan sulphate, heparan sulphate and heparin and keratan sulphate (Fig. 4.2). They form the hydrated gel matrix of support tissues, the properties of which are determined by their charge and spatial arrangement. There is great variability in GAG distribution in different tissues, reflecting local requirements for specific pore sizes and charges in the extracellular matrix.

Glycosaminoglycan	Sulphation	Protein-linked	Distribution
Hyaluronic acid	no	no	cartilage, synovial fluid, skin, support tissue
Chondroitin sulphate	yes	yes	cartilage, bone, skin, support tissue
Dermatan sulphate	yes	yes	skin, blood vessels, heart
Heparan sulphate	yes	yes	basement membrane, lung arteries
Heparin	yes	yes	lung, liver, skin, mast cell granules
Keratan sulphate	yes	yes	cartilage, cornea, vertebral disc

Fig. 4.2 Glycosaminoglycans. There are four main groups of glycosaminoglycans, which have different tissue distributions. Sulphation causes the molecules to be highly negatively charged and contributes to their ability to retain Na^+ ions and water. With the exception of hyaluronic acid, the glycosaminoglycans become linked to proteins to form proteoglycans. The presence of specific types of glycosaminoglycan in different tissues confers special attributes to the extracellular matrix, particularly with regard to diffusion or binding of other extracellular substances.

GAGs are large polysaccharides that help provide turgor and determine the diffusion of substances through extracellular matrix. These polysaccharides link to backbone proteins to form proteoglycans. Many of the proteins that form the backbone of proteoglycans have been isolated and characterized.

GAGs are large, unbranched, polysaccharide chains composed of repeating disaccharide units (70–200 residues).

Fibrillar proteins determine the tensile properties and inherent strength of support tissues.

There are four major proteins that form fibrils in the extracellular matrix:
- Collagen
- Fibrillin
- Elastin
- Fibronectin

The role of these fibrillar proteins is to provide different tensile properties to support tissues and to provide anchorage for other cellular elements in tissues.

The collagens are a large family of proteins and comprise the most important fibrillar extracellular matrix components.

The collagens are a family of closely-related proteins, which can aggregate to produce filaments, fibrils or meshwork, which then interact with other proteins to provide support in the extracellular matrix. There are at least 28 types of collagen polypeptide chains (α chains) produced from different genes, which combine to produce different morphological forms (Fig. 4.3). The collagens can be divided into several families according to the types of structures they form:

- **Fibrillar collagens:** types I, II, III, V, XI
- **Non-fibrillar collagens**
  - **Facit collagens** (fibril-associated collagen with interrupted triple helix): types IX, XII and XIV
  - **Short-chain collagens:** types VIII and X
  - **Multiplexin collagens** (multiple triple-helix domains with interruptions): types XV and XVIII
  - **Basement membrane collagens:** type IV
  - **MACIT collagens** (membrane-associated collagens with interrupted triple helices) (types XIII and XVII)
- **Other collagens:** types VI and VII

Type	I	II	III	IV	V	VI	VII	VIII	IX	X	XI
Morphology	large banded collagen fibre	small banded collagen fibre	small banded collagen fibre	sheet-like layers	thin fibrils	thin fibrils	short striated fibrils	chains and lattices	fibril	short chain	fibril
Distribution	skin dermis, tendon, bone, ligaments, fascia, fibrous cartilage, cornea, loose fibrous tissue	hyaline and elastic cartilage, vertebral discs, vitreous of eye	blood vessels, parenchymal organs, bone marrow, lymphoid tissues, smooth muscle, nerves, lung, fetal skin	basement membranes, external laminae, lens capsule	basement membrane of placenta, smooth and skeletal muscle	ubiquitous	anchoring fibrils in basement membrane of skin and amnion	Descemet's membrane (cornea)	cartilage	mineralizing cartilage	cartilage

Fig. 4.3 Important Molecular Forms of Collagen.

Fig. 4.4 Collagen Fibres. In H&E-stained preparations, collagen fibres appear as pink-stained material, which is often difficult to delineate from other structures that stain equally pink (e.g. cytoplasms of support cells, walls of blood vessels). Special stains can be used to stain collagen (see also Fig. 4.16). Immunohistochemical staining can also be performed for different molecular types of collagen but is seldom used in the routine examination of tissues.

Collagen types I, II and III are arranged as rope-like fibrils and are the main forms of fibrillar collagen.

Collagen fibres (type I collagen) resist tensile stresses in tissues; thus their orientation and cross-linking vary according to the local environment. In histological preparations, collagen fibres appear as pink-staining material and have a dominant role in providing tensile strength to tissues (Fig. 4.4). Reticular fibres (also called *reticulin*) are thin fibrils (about 20 nm in diameter) of type III collagen (Fig. 4.5). They form a loose mesh in many support tissues and are particularly evident in a zone beneath basement membranes, where they are thought to have a support function as part of the fibroreticular lamina (see Fig. 4.13c).

Fig. 4.5 Reticular Fibres. Reticular fibres cannot be seen in H&E sections but can be stained by silver impregnation methods. **(a)** H&E of liver showing plates of cells separated by sinuses which contain blood cells. **(b)** A similar area stained using a silver method for reticulin. The black-stained network of reticulin fibres outlines the sinusoidal spaces and is the structural scaffold supporting the liver cells in columns and plates.

Fig. 4.6 Fibrillar Collagen. (a) Fibrillar collagen is formed from three polypeptide chains, which are initially secreted with both amino and carboxyl terminal extensions to prevent collagen forming inside cells. Initial assembly of these chains is into a triple helix (procollagen). **(b)** Cleavage of the amino and carboxyl extensions to leave the functional mid-domains (tropocollagen) allows the molecules to align themselves into linear arrays to form long filaments. The individual collagen molecules are 300 nm long and are arranged with a 67-nm overlap between adjacent molecules. This gives rise to a periodicity of 67 nm. **(c)** Electron micrograph of collagen showing the periodicity of 67 nm. **(d)** Electron micrograph of collagen in transverse section. **(e)** The initial filaments (collagen microfibrils) become arranged into fibres, and the fibres into larger bundles by tight cross-linking between adjacent molecules via lysine residues; this contributes to the mechanical strength of collagen fibres in tissues.

Reticular fibres can be considered a fine scaffolding, supporting specialised extracellular matrix components. In lymph nodes, spleen and bone marrow, reticular fibres form the main extracellular matrix fibres supporting the haemopoietic and lymphoid tissues. In parenchymal organs, such as the liver (see Fig. 4.5) and kidney, reticular fibres form a network supporting specialized epithelial cells.

Type IV collagen assembles into a meshwork rather than fibrils and is restricted to basement membrane formation (see p. 71).

Type V collagen is associated with type I collagen and is located in the skin at the dermoepidermal junction and in the placenta.

Type VI collagen forms microfilaments within extracellular matrix and has a very wide expression in many tissues. It is a useful marker of the mesangium in the renal glomerulus (see Chapter 15).

Type VII collagen forms the anchoring fibrils of some basement membranes.

Type VIII collagen forms a hexagonal lattice in Descemet's membrane in the cornea of the eye.

Although collagen is produced mainly by fibroblasts (see p. 73), it can be produced by other mesenchyme-derived cells of the support cell family and by a variety of epithelial and endothelial cells that produce the type IV collagen of basement membranes. Collagen fibres are constructed of precursor proteins (α chains) wound together to form rigid linear triple-helix structures, which are then secreted by fibroblasts. After proteolytic cleavage, the triple-helical portions of fibrillar collagen are assembled into long filaments and incorporated into cross-linked fibres and bundles (Fig. 4.6).

CLINICAL EXAMPLE

Diseases Caused by Disorders of Collagen

There are several inherited diseases caused by mutations in the genes coding for collagen. The main effect is reduced tensile strength in support tissues, leading to abnormal tissue laxity or susceptibility to injury.

Ehlers–Danlos syndromes are characterised by abnormal skin laxity and hypermobility of joints, which can predispose to recurrent joint dislocations. There are several genetic subtypes of disease, and six main forms have been described, characterized by distinct clinical associations. In some individuals, disease is caused by mutation in a collagen gene or in an enzyme related to collagen metabolism. Fig. 4.7 shows a patient with Ehlers–Danlos syndrome who kindly demonstrated the remarkable joint laxity characteristic of the condition by bending the hand backward.

In the condition called *osteogenesis imperfecta*, affected children have brittle bones that fracture with minimal force. This is caused by mutations in type I collagen.

Fig. 4.7 Hyperextensibility of Finger Joint in Ehlers–Danlos Syndrome.

Fig. 4.8 Elastin. (a) In the relaxed state, elastin has a random coil structure that can stretch but which reforms as a different random coil on relaxation. (b) Elastin molecules are covalently linked into arrays, which can reversibly stretch and recoil and may be arranged as fibres or sheets.

> **Elastin is a protein that assembles into stretchable and resilient fibres and sheets.**

Elastin is a hydrophobic protein that assembles into filaments and sheets by cross-linking (Fig. 4.8) and is the main component of elastic fibres. Like collagen, elastin is produced by fibroblasts.

Elastic fibres are formed by the interaction of elastin and fibrillin. The fibrillin microfibrils appear to organize secreted elastin so that it is deposited between the microfibrils to form distinct elastic fibres (Fig. 4.9). As their name implies, they confer elasticity to tissues and allow them to recoil after stretching. Elastic fibres are important constituents of many support tissues.

> **Microfibrils contain fibrillin and are important components of elastic fibres.**

Fibrillin is a fibril-forming glycoprotein and the main component of extracellular microfibrils. Microfibrils, 8–12 nm in diameter, are one constituent of elastic fibres (see Fig. 4.9). They are also found in the extracellular matrix of renal glomeruli (mesangium) and the suspensory fibres of the lens.

Microfibrils are prominent in elastic-containing extracellular matrix, particularly in lung, skin and blood vessel walls. The microfibrils are believed to mediate adhesion between different components of the extracellular matrix.

CLINICAL EXAMPLE

Mutations in Genes for Fibrillin Cause Marfan's Syndrome

People who have Marfan's syndrome are unusually tall, have a very wide arm span, are prone to developing subluxation of the lens and are also prone to developing rupture of the aorta. It is believed that the composer Sergei Rachmaninov had Marfan's syndrome.

The abnormality in this condition has been associated with the absence of fibrillin, which interacts with elastin in tissues. It is easy to understand why the lens dislocates, as its suspensory fibres normally contain fibrillin. It is also easy to understand how a lack of elastic recoil in the aorta would weaken the wall and predispose to rupture. It is assumed that the growth of long bones is somehow constrained by the presence of fibrillin, and hence bones grow longer in its absence.

Fig. 4.9 Elastic Fibre. (a) Elastic fibres are composed of glycoprotein microfibrils (fibrillin) associated with elastin microfibril interfacer proteins which surround and organize a core region of cross-linked elastin. **(b)** Ultrastructurally, the elastin core appears as an electron-dense area (E) with microfibrils (M) arranged peripherally. The microfibrils are prominent in early formed elastic tissue and decrease in number with ageing. **(c)** In H&E-stained tissues, elastic fibres (E) stand out as glassy, bright pink–stained structures, taking up acidic dyes such as eosin with much greater avidity than collagen fibres (F, fibroblast). **(d)** Elastic fibres can be stained by special techniques, including immunohistochemistry. This image shows brown-staining elastin fibres within the stroma of the uterine cervix using an antibody for elastin. **(e)** In this thin acrylic resin section, elastic fibres (E) in the dermis of the skin are stained darker blue by toluidine blue and contrast with the pale-staining collagen (C). [Image (d) used under Creative Commons License https://creativecommons.org/licenses/by-sa/3.0/ from the Human Protein Atlas Antibody to elastin https://www.proteinatlas.org/ENSG00000049540-ELN/tissue/cervix#img].

⊚ ADVANCED CONCEPT

Vesicles Are Present Within the Extracellular Matrix

It is recognized that cells can communicate by the formation of vesicles that are shed into the extracellular space (exosomes, see p. 19), some of which can then become part of the extracellular matrix as matrix-bound nanovesicles (MBNVs). The content of these membrane-bound structures includes proteins, lipids and nucleic acids (DNA, and microRNA). Increasing attention is being turned to understanding how MBNVs can interact with the immune system and with cells in control of cell growth and cell death.

Extracellular structural glycoproteins link cells and extracellular matrix.

Several non-filamentous proteins mediate interaction between cells and extracellular matrix and interact with specific receptors on the surface of cells. The best characterised of these proteins are fibronectins, the laminins, perlecan and the nidogens. A specialized structure termed **the basement membrane** is present in many tissues, and this sheet-like structure is formed from such specialized extracellular proteins (more about this later). In other tissues, adhesion of cells to the extracellular matrix is not mediated by a defined membrane structure.

> **Fibronectin mediates adhesion between a wide range of cells and extracellular matrix components.**

Fibronectin is a multifunctional glycoprotein and exists in three main forms. These are:

- A circulating plasma protein
- A protein that transiently attaches to the surface of many cells
- Insoluble fibrils forming part of the extracellular matrix, when fibronectin dimers cross-link to each other

The functional importance of fibronectin stems from its ability to adhere to several different tissue components because it possesses sites that bind collagen and heparin, in addition to cell adhesion molecules.

⊚ ADVANCED CONCEPT

Fibronectin is recognized by fibronectin receptor proteins in cell membranes, allowing cell adhesion to extracellular matrix. Such a fibronectin receptor is one of the class of cell surface receptors called *integrins* (Fig. 4.10). When tissues grow, fibronectin binds to cell surfaces via integrins, and through this interaction the fibronectin polymerizes to form a solid fibrillar matrix. This now-solid structural scaffold is thought to have an important role in organizing the subsequent deposition and orientation of early collagen fibrils through collagen attachment sites on the formed fibronectin fibrils.

Because fibronectin receptors are linked to intracellular actin, the orientation of the internal cytoskeleton of a cell influences the orientation of the extracellular matrix.

In disease, after tissue injury, fibronectin in the extracellular matrix is important in tissue repair, including mediating growth of new blood vessels (angiogenesis).

Fig. 4.10 Integrins. Integrins are a class of cell adhesion molecule, each comprising two protein subunits. An α subunit is composed of two protein chains and has a globular head. The β subunit extends through the membrane and binds via link proteins to the actin cytoskeleton. The fibronectin receptor shown in the diagram is the best characterized of the integrin family, possessing a cytosolic domain binding to actin (via talin), a transmembrane domain and extracellular domains binding to fibronectin. Thus this molecule links the intracellular actin network with extracellular matrix at focal contacts (see also Fig. 3.5b). The laminin receptor also belongs to the integrin family. Integrins may bind to other cell surface proteins, thus acting as intercellular adhesion molecules. In addition, some integrins bind to extracellular matrix components and allow cell–matrix adhesion, with the main extracellular matrix ligands being fibronectin, laminin and collagens.

BASEMENT MEMBRANE AND EXTERNAL LAMINA

> **Basement membranes and external lamina are specialized sheets of extracellular matrix that lie between parenchymal cells and support tissues.**

Basement membranes and external lamina are specialised sheet-like arrangements of extracellular matrix proteins and GAGs and act as an interface between parenchymal cells and support tissues.

Basement membrane refers to the structure which is associated with a surface epithelium, and *external lamina* refers to the structure which surrounds certain non-epithelial cell types such as muscle or Schwann cells. An external lamina also forms a limiting membrane around the central nervous system. They all have a similar structure (Fig. 4.11). The term *basement membrane* refers to the structure seen by light microscopy. Using electron microscopy, the basement membrane can be resolved into three layers termed the *lamina lucida*, the *basal lamina* and the *reticular lamina*.

Basement membranes have four major components: type IV collagen (Fig. 4.12), laminins, perlecan, and nidogens (entactins), which are synthesized by parenchymal cells within the tissue. In addition, there are numerous, less abundant protein and GAG components.

⊚ ADVANCED CONCEPT
Important Components of Basement Membrane

Type IV collagen is composed of six different alpha chains which can assemble into three heterotrimers, and these have different distributions in the basement membrane of different tissues. This form of collagen forms a planar, sheet-like network and gives mechanical stability to the basement membrane structure.

Laminins are a family of around 16 different sulphated glycoproteins and are a major component of basement membranes, in which they also form a planar, sheet-like network. They are produced by most epithelial and endothelial cells and have a cross-shaped structure with binding sites for specific cell receptors (integrins) (see Fig. 4.10). The pattern of binding ligands for laminins makes them a major extracellular link molecule between cells and extracellular matrix. There are several forms of laminin specific to different tissues and expressed at different stages of embryonic development.

Nidogens (nidogen-1 and -2) function as a link protein that bind laminins to type IV collagen and are important in stabilizing the sheet structure of basement membrane, especially in tissue growth. Nidogens are glycoproteins that also bind with integrins as part of adhesion systems.

Perlecan is a proteoglycan which also bridges and stabilizes the type IV collagen and laminin networks in basement membrane. It is also recognized to bind to growth factors and mediates control of cell proliferation in many tissues. During the tissue response to damage, in which new blood vessels are formed, perlecan is involved with binding of growth factors involved in angiogenesis.

Fibronectin is a component of the reticular lamina of the basement membrane. This part of the basement membrane is synthesized by support cells.

Other proteins. Cell biological studies show many more basement membrane–associated proteins with roles in cell adhesion, cell signalling, growth regulation and tissue remodelling.

Fig. 4.11 A Basement Membrane or External Lamina is Composed of Three Layers. Adjacent to the cell is a sheet mainly composed of laminin termed the lamina lucida. Next, there is a sheet composed mainly of type IV collagen termed the lamina densa (basal lamina). These two lamina are produced by the cell. Outside these two layers is the fibroreticular lamina which is produced by support cells of the extracellular matrix. Within these three layers many other proteins and glycoproteins perform linking and adhesion functions. On the left of this figure is a column showing the ultrastructural appearance of each layer, shown further in Fig. 4.13b.

Fig. 4.12 Basement Membrane. The basement membrane can be demonstrated by immunostaining for constituent proteins such as **(a)** laminin and **(b)** type IV collagen.

The basement membrane seen by light microscopy has been well characterized by electron microscopy (Fig. 4.13). Superimposed on this general structure, minor protein and carbohydrate components are specific to certain tissues, giving rise to the concept that basement membranes in different tissues are different from each other and have localised specialised functions. The basement membrane in the glomerulus of the kidney is different from that seen around the glands of the intestine. The interaction of stem cells with the local microenvironment (stem cell niche) is also believed to involve specific structural components in the associated basement membrane (see p. 41).

In some tissues, one epithelial cell layer is anchored directly to another epithelial cell layer by basement membrane in the absence of other extracellular matrix components, forming a **fusion basement membrane** (Fig. 4.14).

> **The main functions of basement membrane are cell adhesion, diffusion barrier and regulation of cell growth.**

Basement membrane has three main functions:

First, it forms an adhesion interface between parenchymal cells and underlying extracellular matrix, the cells having adhesion mechanisms to anchor them to basement membrane, and the basement membrane being in turn tightly anchored to the wider extracellular matrix. Where such an interface occurs in non-epithelial tissues, for example, around muscle cells or Schwann cells, it is referred to as an **external lamina**.

Fig. 4.13 Basement Membrane. (a) Basement membrane is only around 0.05 mm thick and stains poorly with H&E; however, a high content of glycoprotein renders it stainable with periodic acid–Schiff (PAS), when it appears as a magenta-stained line. This image shows basement membrane surrounding tubules in the kidney. Epithelial cells adhere to the basement membrane and in turn are anchored within the renal interstitium. In this site, anchorage is via reticulin fibres composed of type III collagen. **(b)** On electron microscopy, basement membrane resolves into several layers (laminae). The lamina densa (D) is a dark-staining band 30–100 nm thick and corresponds to the location of type IV collagen. Between this and the attached cell (C) is a lucent zone, the lamina lucida (L), which is usually 60 nm wide and corresponds to the location of laminin. On the other side of the lamina densa is a rarefied layer of variable thickness, the fibroreticular lamina (FR), which merges with fibrous proteins of the extracellular matrix and corresponds to the location of fibronectin and other structural proteins synthesized by support cells. **(c)** The fibroreticular lamina anchors the basement membrane to adjacent extracellular matrix by three main mechanisms, which vary according to site and are illustrated in this figure.

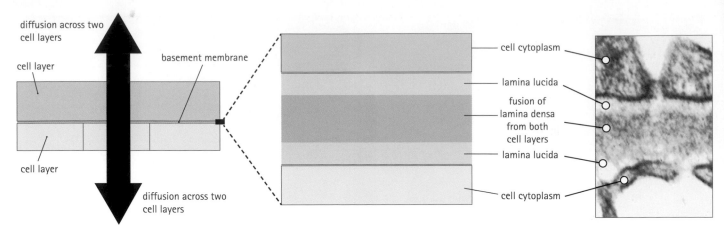

Fig. 4.14 Fusion Basement Membrane. In some locations there is a need for one cell layer to be structurally anchored to another cell layer by attachment of their basement membranes. This is especially seen in the alveoli of the lung and in the glomeruli of the kidney, where diffusion is required across a cellular barrier. In these circumstances, the lamina densa of each basement membrane fuses into one layer and a so-called fusion basement membrane is formed. In this situation there is no associated fibroreticular lamina. The functional significance is to minimize the thickness of the diffusion barrier between the two sides of a double-cell layer. On the right of this diagram is an electron microscopic image of the fusion basement membrane from the kidney (see also Fig. 15.9).

Second, the basement membrane acts as a molecular sieve (permeability barrier), with pore size depending on the charge and spatial arrangement of its component GAG. Thus the basement membrane of blood vessels prevents large proteins from leaking into the tissues, that of the kidney prevents protein loss from filtered blood during urine production and that of the lung permits gaseous diffusion.

Third, basement membrane is involved with control of cell organization and differentiation by the mutual interaction of cell surface receptors and molecules in the extracellular matrix. The involvement of basement membrane in cell interactions includes cell proliferation, differentiation and migration in development. The basement membrane is also important in cancer biology and is the subject of wider research, particularly in the investigation of mechanisms that might prevent the spread and proliferation of cancer cells throughout the body.

CELL ADHESION TO EXTRACELLULAR MATRIX

> **Adhesion of cells to the extracellular matrix is mediated by four main types of junctions.**

The organization of cells into functional tissues and organs depends on the support functions of the extracellular matrix and the cells that produce it. Although various types of intercellular junctions tie cells together (see p. 48), the junctions between cells and the extracellular matrix are equally important in maintaining structural integrity.

CLINICAL EXAMPLE

Basement Membrane in Disease

There are several inherited disorders of basement membrane or external lamina of muscle caused by mutation in genes coding for structural components. Examples include:

Laminin-α2–related congenital muscular dystrophy is an inherited disorder caused by mutations in the gene coding for one of the laminin proteins which normally binds skeletal muscle fibres to the external lamina. The condition typically presents in neonatal life as a so-called *floppy baby* and progresses in childhood with muscle weakness and joint rigidity. Spinal deformity with scoliosis is common, with most requiring use of mobility aids. In a diagnostic muscle biopsy no laminin-α2 can be detected on immunostaining.

Alport syndrome and thin basement membrane disease are conditions that affect the renal glomeruli and are caused by mutations in genes coding for type IV collagen. Mutations in genes coding for α3(IV), α4(IV) or α5(IV) chains cause Alport's syndrome, characterized by renal failure, deafness and retinal degeneration in affected persons.

Goodpasture's syndrome is an autoimmune conditions in which abnormal antibodies, termed *anti–glomerular basement membrane (anti-GBM) antibodies*, are directed against components of the basement membrane of kidney glomeruli and lung alveoli causing immune-mediated damage. The most common autoantibody is directed at a domain of the α3 chain of type IV collagen. Patients develop abnormal renal function with blood and protein in the urine (the basement membrane is no longer intact) together with bleeding into the lungs caused by disrupted alveolar walls. As part of the diagnosis, a renal biopsy can be examined, which shows antibodies binding to the basement membrane.

The basement membrane of renal glomeruli is also the site of pathology in several immune-mediated disorders (see Fig. 15.10) in addition to being the target of damage in **diabetes mellitus** leading to leaking of protein into the urine (proteinuria).

Junctions between cells and extracellular matrix include the following:

- Hemidesmosomes (see Fig. 3.5) anchor the intermediate filament cytoskeleton of cells to basement membrane.
- Focal contacts (see Fig. 3.5) anchor the actin cytoskeleton to basement membrane. The interaction is mediated through proteins that bind fibronectin (see Fig. 4.10).
- Laminin receptors (see Fig. 4.10) anchor cells to the major laminin component in basement membrane.
- Non-integrin glycoproteins (possessed by many cells) bind to collagen and other cell matrix components.

SUPPORT CELL FAMILY

Support cells derive from embryonic mesenchyme.

During embryogenesis, a proportion of developing mesenchymal spindle-shaped cells differentiate into the following types of support cells: fibroblasts, myofibroblasts, lipoblasts, osteoblasts and chondroblasts.

The addition of 'blast' to the root name of a support cell indicates that the cell is actively growing or secreting extracellular matrix material. Support cells in a quiescent phase in tissues are indicated using the suffix '-cyte' (e.g. osteocyte, chondrocyte).

CLINICAL EXAMPLE

Tumours of the Support Cell Family

Tumours may arise from support cells and may be either benign or malignant.

Cell Type	Benign	Malignant
Fibroblast	Fibroma	Fibrosarcoma
Chondrocyte	Chondroma	Chondrosarcoma
Adipocyte	Lipoma	Liposarcoma
Osteocyte	Osteoma	Osteogenic sarcoma

Fibroblasts populate fibrocollagenous tissue, which is the most important of the support tissues.

Fibroblasts (Fig. 4.15) produce fibrocollagenous (fibrous) tissue, which is composed mainly of collagen fibres associated with GAG, elastic fibres and reticular fibres (Fig. 4.16). Fibrocollagenous tissue is described as **loose connective tissue** when collagen fibres are thin, haphazardly arranged and widely spaced, or **dense connective tissue** when collagen fibres are broad and virtually confluent. The degree of organization and collagen orientation varies from site to site according to local tissue stresses. Highly organized dense fibrocollagenous tissue forms tendons and ligaments.

Fibrocollagenous tissue is the major support tissue in most organs and has the following specific functions:

- Support of nerves, blood vessels and lymphatics; vessels and nerves are a conspicuous feature, particularly in loose fibrocollagenous support tissue.

- Separation of functional layers in organs and tissues (e.g. separation of mucosa from underlying tissues). Its loose arrangement and variable elastic content allow mobility and stretching.
- Support for transient and resident immune cell populations (i.e. macrophages, lymphocytes, plasma cells, mast cells).
- Formation of fibrous capsule, which surrounds most parenchymal organs, such as the liver, spleen and kidneys.
- Formation of fibroadipose tissue, which is a component of most tissues, by enclosing and blending with adipocytes.

Fibroblasts are extremely robust and resist the damaging stimuli that kill most other cell types, such as nerves, epithelial cells or muscle. They are important in tissue repair (see p. 76).

ADVANCED CONCEPT

In adult tissues, fibroblasts adopt a quiescent functional profile when they are termed **quiescent fibroblasts (QFs)**.

There is evidence that QFs in different anatomical locations have different profiles in terms of protein expression.

The main functional role of QFs is in maintaining local tissue homeostasis by remodelling the local extracellular matrix (synthesis and degradation). Other functions include secretion of growth factors, roles in the innate immune response and acting as a progenitor cell for a range of mesenchymal cell types in response to tissue injury.

Functional subsets of fibroblasts are present in different tissue locations. The ability to perform single-cell analysis on fibroblasts in different locations has led to deeper understanding of such tissue-specific functions. Fibroblasts in lung differ from those in heart or those in skin.

In response to tissue injury, fibroblasts can proliferate and accumulate in affected areas. These fibroblasts can be derived from QFs but also from endothelial cells, bone marrow–derived fibroblasts or stellate cells. In an activated state, such fibroblasts may differentiate to form other mesenchymal cell types, including myofibroblasts. They are one of the most important cell types involved in repair and healing.

Mesenchymal stem cells/stromal cells are pluripotent cells found in support tissues.

Mesenchymal stem/stromal cells (MSCs) are derived in embryogenesis from mesoderm and take part in developmental growth. In adult tissues they can be seen in small numbers. In routine light microscopy, they are inconspicuous, with barely defined cytoplasm and a round nucleus; however, immunohistochemistry can be used to distinguish this cell type.

This cell type is pluripotent, and after local immune activation or tissue damage they can proliferate and differentiate into other cell types, including fibroblasts, osteoblasts, chondroblasts and myofibroblasts. Subtypes of MSCs are found in adipose tissue, bone marrow and umbilical cord, and small numbers can be harvested from circulating blood. There is currently great interest in harvesting MSCs and using them in a range of therapeutic applications.

Such cells are grown in tissue culture systems for therapeutic or experimental applications (Fig 4.17).

Fig. 4.15 Fibroblasts. (a) In the embryo, collagen-secreting cells develop from mesenchyme and appear as plump, spindle-shaped cells separated by extracellular matrix (pale blue) and early secreted collagen (C), which stains pink in H&E preparations. **(b)** In the adult, active collagen-secreting cells are called *fibroblasts* and are characterized by a large oval nucleus and large nucleolus, a tapering spindle-shaped morphology with small additional cell processes and basophilic cytoplasm reflecting active collagen synthesis. The collagen (C) is seen as pink-stained fibrillar material between fibroblasts. **(c)** Once collagen secretion has stopped, the fibroblasts lose their voluminous basophilic cytoplasm and the nucleus shrinks, reflecting non-transcription of DNA. The cells are termed quiescent fibroblasts (fibrocytes) to indicate this inactivity. The collagen appears more compact, and is aligned in parallel bundles. **(d)** Ultrastructurally, fibroblasts have a well-developed rough endoplasmic reticulum (RER), Golgi and secretory vesicles, reflecting active collagen secretion. Mitochondria (M) are numerous. Collagen fibres (C) are visible adjacent to the cells. Fibroblasts can also secrete elastic and reticular fibres, and when they form reticular fibres in lymphoid tissue and bone marrow, they have a highly branched stellate shape and are called *fibroblastic reticular cells*.

> **Myofibroblasts have features that overlap between fibroblasts and smooth muscle cells.**

Myofibroblasts resemble fibroblasts on light microscopy, but ultrastructurally contain aggregates of actin fibres associated with myosin to subserve a contractile function similar to that seen in smooth muscle (see p. 89). They are not typically prominent in normal support tissues, being found only in small numbers, and are identifiable by immunohistochemical or ultrastructural methods.

⊚ ADVANCED CONCEPT

Myofibroblasts

Myofibroblasts develop during repair after tissue damage and may originate from local quiescent fibroblasts or MSCs stimulated by factors released by immune cells, including macrophages at the site of tissue injury. They can also originate from epithelial cells, through the process of epithelial-to-mesenchymal transition.

Myofibroblasts express smooth muscle α-actin and vimentin, they produce collagen and their contractile properties contribute to wound retraction and shrinkage of early fibrocollagenous scar tissue.

Fig. 4.16 Fibrocollagenous (Fibrous) Tissue. (a) Fibrocollagenous tissue contains many extracellular matrix components, with collagen fibres being predominant. Only collagen (C) is evident in H&E sections, staining light pink. Fibroblasts (F) are widely scattered and inconspicuous. Immune cells (i.e. lymphocytes [L], plasma cells, macrophages, mast cells) are occasionally found. **(b)** The collagen fibres (C) in loose fibrocollagenous tissue can be stained by dyes with affinity for collagen (e.g. van Gieson's, shown here). The bundles are haphazardly arranged and of varying thickness. **(c)** In most loose fibrocollagenous tissues, elastic fibres are present, but are usually inconspicuous in H&E preparations. They are revealed by special stains (elastic stain) as wavy, black-staining fibres (E), which contrast with the orange-stained collagen. Elastic fibres form a minor and variable component of most fibrocollagenous tissues. **(d)** Stains for the GAG component of fibrocollagenous tissue reveal that the unstained areas of the H&E preparations are rich in this extracellular material (seen here stained *blue* with Alcian blue stain) (C, collagen). In contrast with loose fibrocollagenous tissue, dense irregular fibrocollagenous tissue has little space for GAG and appears uniformly pink with few architectural features. Collagen-secreting fibroblasts are widely spaced and inconspicuous.

Fig. 4.17 Mesenchymal Stem Cells. Cells are inconspicuous in adult tissues and can only be identified using immunohistochemical methods. This image shows mesenchymal stem cells grown in cell culture and stained with haematoxylin and eosin, where they have a spindle-cell appearance. (Image from Jin-Xiang F, et al. Homing efficiency and hematopoietic reconstitution of bone marrow-derived stroma cells expanded by recombinant human macrophage-colony stimulating factor in vitro. *Exp Hematol.* 2004;32[12]:1204–1211 with permission.)

> **Chondroblasts and chondrocytes form cartilage.**

Chondroblasts elaborate a special support tissue called *cartilage*, which is composed mainly of GAG associated with collagen fibres. Developing from embryonic mesenchyme, chondroblasts first appear as clusters of vacuolated cells with a rounded morphology. These contrast with the spindle-shaped cells of surrounding undifferentiated mesenchyme, which develop into fibroblasts and form a confining sheet of cells termed the **perichondrium**.

Chondroblasts contain abundant glycogen and lipid, and their active synthesis of extracellular matrix proteins is indicated by their basophilic cytoplasm, which is the result of a high content of rough endoplasmic reticulum (Fig. 4.19a).

Growth of cartilage results from proliferation of chondroblasts within established matrix (interstitial growth) and also by the development of new chondroblasts from the perichondrium (appositional growth). After depositing cartilage matrix, chondroblasts become less metabolically active and have small nuclei with pale, indistinct cytoplasm (i.e. they become chondrocytes; see Fig. 4.19b).

CLINICAL EXAMPLE

Tissue Damage is Repaired by Proliferation of Support Cells and Secretion of Matrix to Form Scar Tissue

After tissue damage (e.g. by infection), the loss of specialized cells can be rectified by regrowth only if the architecture of the support tissues (particularly basement membrane) is preserved; for example, epithelial cells lining the lung can regrow after some types of pneumonia (e.g. lobar pneumonia caused by *Streptococcus pneumoniae*).

If damage has been severe and the specialized support tissue architecture is destroyed, such regrowth is usually not possible, and the area of dead tissue is repaired by means of the growth of non-specialized support tissue, which forms a fibrous scar.

Chemical mediators produced by damaged tissue attract phagocytic cells, such as neutrophils and monocytes (see Chapter 7) from the blood into the tissue. These cells ingest the dead cells, whereas inactive support cells, including fibroblasts and MSCs, are stimulated to proliferate by the secretion of growth factors (e.g. platelet-derived growth factors and fibroblast growth factor).

The stimulated support cells have characteristics of MSCs; are multipotential; and can differentiate into endothelial cells, myofibroblasts and fibroblasts, the damaged area being replaced by a mixture of these cell types, which form new blood vessels and lay down collagen. The resulting fibrocollagenous tissue is termed a **fibrous scar** (Fig. 4.18).

During this process of healing by fibrous repair, which is one of the basic responses to cell death in most body tissues, stromal cells adopt a multipotential role and behave in a manner similar to that of primitive mesenchyme from which they were derived, by differentiating into a variety of cell types.

This ability to transform into a variety of cell types in adult life to facilitate healing and repair is an important attribute of the support cell family.

Fig 4.18 Scar in Myocardium. After death of cardiac muscle caused by myocardial infarction, the cardiac muscle (M) has been replaced by collagenous scar tissue (S). Healing by scarring replaces the specialized and functional parenchymal tissue with non-specialised fibrous scar.

Fig. 4.19 Chondroblasts and Chondrocytes. (a) Chondroblasts are metabolically active and have large vesicular nuclei with prominent nucleoli. Their cytoplasm is pale and vacuolated because of a high lipid and glycogen content and tends to draw away from the extracellular matrix when fixed and embedded in paraffin, forming an artefactual space called a *lacuna* (L). **(b)** Chondrocytes are smaller than chondroblasts, with densely staining nuclei and less cytoplasm, reflecting their low level of metabolic activity.

⊚ ADVANCED CONCEPT

Cartilage has two main extracellular components:
- Fibrous proteins (predominantly type II collagen), which confer mechanical stability
- Abundant GAG, which resist deformation by compressive forces

The collagen fibres are thin and arranged in an interwoven lattice, which merges into the extracellular matrix of adjacent support tissues. The major GAGs are hyaluronic acid, chondroitin sulphate and keratan sulphate, which are bound to a core protein called *aggrecan* to form a large proteoglycan. These are attached to the collagen lattice by so-called *link protein*.

Because of its high content of sulphated GAG, cartilage stains with basic dyes such as haematoxylin, which gives it a slightly blue colour in haematoxylin and eosin (H&E) preparations; this is particularly evident around the chondrocytes.

The arrangement of extracellular matrix in cartilage confers important properties:
- The tightly bound proteoglycans form a hydrated matrix with an inherent turgor that resists deformation by compressive forces.
- Small molecules can diffuse freely through the extracellular matrix.

Different types of cartilage contain different fibrous proteins.

The three types of cartilage – hyaline, fibrocartilage and elastic – are distinguished by their fibrous protein content. **Hyaline cartilage** contains type II collagen only (Fig. 4.20). In fetal development, it forms the temporary skeleton until it is replaced by bone; it forms the growing point in long bones in childhood, the articular surface in joints (see Chapter 13), and is present in the respiratory passages where it acts as a support tissue (see Fig. 4.20c and Fig. 10.10).

Fibrocartilage contains both type II and type I collagen (Fig. 4.21) and is a component of intervertebral discs, tendon attachments to bones and the junctions between the flat bones of the pelvis. **Elastic cartilage** contains elastic fibres in addition to type II collagen (Fig. 4.22). It is located in the auricle of the ear, the walls of the external auditory canal and eustachian tubes (see Chapter 19) and in the epiglottis of the larynx (see Fig. 10.8).

Osteoblasts and osteocytes form bone, which contains an extracellular matrix material termed osteoid.

Osteoblasts elaborate the support matrix of bone – osteoid – which subsequently calcifies to form bone.

Osteoid is composed mainly of type I collagen, which is associated with the extracellular GAGs chondroitin sulphate and keratan sulphate. Two glycoproteins, sialoprotein and osteocalcin, are found mainly in the bone matrix and bind calcium; hence they may have a role in bone mineralization. The cytology and structure of bone and its matrix are discussed in Chapter 13.

Adipose tissue stores fat and has a role in heat regulation in the young.

Adipocytes are characterized by their intracellular storage of fat. There are two types of fat-storing tissue: unilocular and multilocular.

Fig. 4.20 Hyaline Cartilage (H&E). (a) This hyaline cartilage is from a child and therefore in a state of growth. The perichondrium (P) is a layer of spindle-shaped fibroblasts with associated type I collagen, which merges with the outer layer of the pink-staining extracellular matrix of the hyaline cartilage. New chondroblasts develop from the perichondrium and allow appositional growth. The chondroblasts show artefactual vacuolation, forming the characteristic lacunae around the cell bodies. In actively growing cartilage, many appear in small clusters (C), which will eventually move apart as the cells secrete extracellular matrix material during interstitial growth. Hyaline cartilage is associated with perichondrium in most sites except where it lines synovial joints. **(b)** This section of hyaline cartilage is from the joint of an adult and so is not in an active phase of growth. Chondrocytes are more widely dispersed, mostly as single cells (C) within the pink-staining extracellular matrix. **(c)** This micrograph shows hyaline cartilage from the wall of the trachea. A perichondrium (P) is seen. The chondrocytes (C) are present in small groups in lacunae separated by the extracellular chondroid matrix.

Unilocular adipose tissue ('white fat') develops from embryonic mesenchyme with the formation of spindle-shaped cells (lipoblasts) containing small fat vacuoles (Fig. 4.23). These mature into adipocytes, storing fat which is used as a source of energy by other body tissues (Fig. 4.24).

Ultrastructurally, adipocytes have prominent smooth endoplasmic reticulum and numerous pinocytotic vesicles, these being involved in lipid biosynthesis and transport.

Each cell is surrounded by an external lamina, and there is an extracellular matrix composed of reticular fibres (type III collagen).

Multilocular adipose tissue ('brown fat') is most prominent in the newborn, its development in the fetus being separate from that of unilocular adipose tissue. Its function is to metabolize fat to produce heat in the neonatal period (Fig. 4.25).

Ultrastructurally, multilocular adipose cells contain huge numbers of mitochondria in addition to lipid vacuoles; this correlates with their function of heat generation through mitochondrial metabolism of fatty acids.

Fig. 4.21 Fibrocartilage. (a) In this H&E section of fibrocartilage, small inactive chondrocytes are dispersed in a pink-stained extracellular matrix, in which coarse collagen fibres (C) are visible. These are type I collagen fibres and merge with the type I collagen fibres in surrounding fibrocollagenous support tissue. **(b)** The presence of type I collagen is highlighted in this van Gieson–stained section of fibrocartilage, in which it stains red.

Fig. 4.22 Elastic Cartilage (H&E). (a) The structural arrangement of elastic cartilage is similar to that of hyaline cartilage, with a perichondrial layer (P) and chondrocytes set in an extracellular matrix, but differs because it contains elastic fibres. These appear as bright pink–staining linear bundles running in the matrix between cells and confer great resilience and elastic recoil in the cartilage. **(b)** At a slightly higher magnification, the bundles of elastic fibres are seen more clearly as linear bright pink–stained material. The inset image is from a van Gieson–stained section and shows the elastic fibres as dark-stained linear bundles within the extracellular matrix.

Fig. 4.23 Lipoblasts. (a) In the fetus, the first indication of differentiation into a fat-storing cell is when the spindle-shaped mesenchymal cells (M) accumulate fat in their cytoplasm in multiple small vacuoles (V). **(b)** The vacuoles fuse to form a larger perinuclear vacuole, and the cell is recognized as a maturing lipoblast (L), losing its spindle shape. With increased fat storage, the cytoplasm becomes attenuated around a single huge lipid vacuole and the nucleus is displaced to one side. Each developing lipoblast produces extracellular matrix material, and a basement membrane forms around each cell.

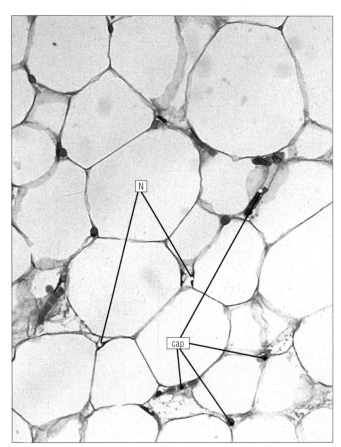

Fig. 4.24 Unilocular Adipose Tissue. Unilocular *(white)* adipose tissue cells (adipocytes) are 50–150 μm in size and polyhedral in shape. In H&E-stained preparations, as here, they appear as stringy wisps of cytoplasm surrounding an empty vacuole because embedding in wax involves immersion in lipid solvents, which remove all the fat. Close examination reveals inconspicuous flattened nuclei (N) to one side of the cells. Numerous fine arborizing capillary vessels (cap) transfer metabolites to and from the cells.

Fig. 4.25 Multilocular Adipose Tissue. Multilocular adipose tissue is so-called because cells contain multiple small lipid droplets. It develops as a cluster of plump eosinophilic cells differentiating from fetal mesenchyme and has a restricted distribution, being concentrated in support tissues in the neck, shoulders, back, perirenal and para-aortic regions. As shown in this micrograph, two populations of cells can be seen: lipid-rich cells (L) with a central nucleus and multiple small unstained vacuoles and polyhedral-shaped cells (P) with a granular, pink-stained cytoplasm, a central nucleus and only occasional lipid vacuoles. A capillary vascular supply, together with thin fibrocollagenous septa, divides the tissue into small lobules.

The high mitochondrial density is responsible for both the eosinophilia seen histologically and the brown colour seen macroscopically, which gives this tissue its alternative name of 'brown fat'. Multilocular adipose tissue does not usually persist in adult life: it becomes lost during childhood, although small amounts may remain in certain sites (Fig. 4.26).

Fig. 4.26 Mixture of Unilocular and Multilocular Adipose Tissue. Certain adipose tissue, particularly in the subcutaneous tissue over the back and shoulders, contains a mixture of both unilocular (U) and multilocular (M) adipose tissue.

> **Adipose tissue has a secretory and endocrine function.**

In addition to their energy-storage role, it is evident that adipocytes have an important secretory role. In this way, adipocytes modulate energy metabolism and influence general metabolism in coordination with hormones, such as insulin, to regulate body mass.

Adipose tissue is also responsible for the secretion of several proteins into the blood, collectively known as **adipokines**, that regulate general metabolism. There are over 100 cell-signalling and regulatory factors associated with adipocytes, which include leptin, adiponectin, adipsin, chemerin, resistin, tumour necrosis factor alpha (TNF-α), and interleukin-6. Adipose tissue also contains a population of macrophages, the **adipose tissue macrophages**, which become abnormally activated in obesity and are then involved in wider tissue dysfunction (see Chapter 8). It is evident that there is cross-talk between adipose tissue and the immune system, and this subject area is being studied extensively in understanding the system-wide effects of obesity on health.

> **KEY FACTS**
>
> Unilocular adipose tissue is the main form of fat-storing cell in the adult and is adapted as a support tissue and as an energy store by means of:
> - Receptors for growth hormone, insulin, glucocorticoids, thyroid hormones and norepinephrine (noradrenaline) that modulate the uptake and release of fat.
> - A rich capillary blood supply and innervation by the autonomic nervous system. Local release of noradrenaline stimulates the release of stored fat into the blood.
> - Organization into pads by sheets of fibrocollagenous tissue at certain sites to act as deformable shock-absorbing support tissues, particularly in the soles of the feet, the buttocks, around the kidneys and in the orbit around the eye.

For online review questions, please visit https://studentconsult. inkling.com.

Contractile Cells

INTRODUCTION

Several cell types are specialized to generate motile forces through contraction. This chapter presents an overview of the main types of contractile cells. The general structure of each type of cell is described, together with details of their fine structure and how this relates to the molecular basis of contraction.

> **There are four main groups of contractile cells.**

Contractile cells are specially adapted to generate motile forces by the interaction of the proteins actin and myosin (contractile proteins).

There are four groups of contractile cells: muscle cells, myofibroblasts, pericytes and myoepithelial calls. Muscle cells are the main type and comprise striated (voluntary) muscle, cardiac muscle and smooth (involuntary) muscle. Myofibroblasts have a contractile role in addition to being able to secrete collagen. Pericytes are smooth, muscle-like cells that surround blood vessels. Myoepithelial cells are an important component of certain secretory glands.

Different arrangements of actin and myosin in each type of contractile cell, together with important structural adaptations, modulate and control contraction.

SKELETAL MUSCLE

Skeletal muscle cells form the structural basis of muscles (see Chapter 13), which are responsible for voluntary movement under the influence of the nervous system and for maintenance of posture. This section presents the characteristics of muscle cells related to contraction. The innervation, specialisations and attachment of muscle to the skeletal system are discussed in Chapter 13.

> **Each skeletal muscle fibre is a multinucleate syncytium formed by the fusion of individual cells in development.**

In embryogenesis, each skeletal muscle cell forms from the fusion of many hundreds of precursor cells (myoblasts), so in the adult each is a syncytium containing hundreds of nuclei, which are located just beneath the cell membrane. Each skeletal muscle cell is a long, thin, cylindrical structure, typically 50–60 μm in diameter in an adult and up to 10 cm long, depending on its location (Fig. 5.1).

In adult muscle, there is a resident population of muscle precursor cells (satellite cells), which can divide to form new muscle cells after tissue damage.

In addition to contractile proteins, skeletal muscle cell cytoplasm contains numerous mitochondria, along with abundant glycogen to provide energy. Each muscle cell is surrounded by an external lamina (see p. 69).

Because of long usage, special terms are often used to describe skeletal muscle cell components. These are *sarcolemma* (cell membrane), *sarcoplasm* (cell cytoplasm) and *sarcoplasmic reticulum* (endoplasmic reticulum).

> **Skeletal muscle contracts as a result of organized assemblies of actin and myosin.**

The contractile elements of skeletal muscle cells (myofibrils) are thin, cylindrical structures 1–2 μm in diameter. They are composed of overlapping, repeating assemblies of thick (mainly myosin) and thin (mainly actin) filaments.

Any one muscle fibre has hundreds of myofibrils running parallel along its length, the alternating zones of thick and thin filaments giving rise to the descriptive term *striated muscle* (Fig. 5.2a).

Ultrastructurally, the thick and thin filaments are held in place by plates of accessory proteins, visible as lines, which

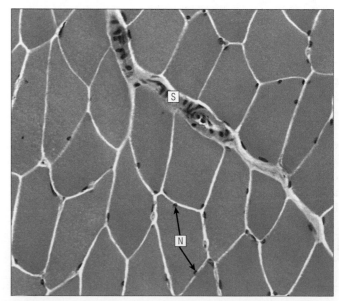

Fig. 5.1 Skeletal Muscle. In cross-section, skeletal muscle cells have a roughly pentagonal profile with individual cells moulded together. Nuclei (N) are arranged beneath the cell membrane. Fibrocollagenous septa (S) contain blood vessels.

Fig. 5.2 Myofibrils. (a) Individual skeletal muscle cells appear to have cross-striations in longitudinal section owing to the presence of stacks of myofibrils composed of alternating overlapping zones of thick (dark-stained) and thin (light-stained) filaments. (b) Ultrastructurally, several zones of staining can be discerned along myofibrils. The A (dark) band refers to the thick filament band and includes a zone where the thin filaments overlap the thick filaments. The H zone is a pale-staining area in the centre of the A band and indicates where no thin filaments overlap the thick filaments. The I (light) band is the zone of thin filaments that does not overlap the thick filaments, the Z line is a dark band in the centre of the I band and the M line runs down the centre of the H band. The unit delineated between two Z discs is termed a *sarcomere*. (c) The arrangement of filaments in a sarcomere. The thin filaments are composed mainly of actin, the thick filaments mainly of myosin. (d) When viewed in cross-section at the level of overlap between the A and I bands, as in (b), each myofibril is seen to have a regular spaced arrangement of thick and thin filaments, such that each thick filament is surrounded by six thin filaments arranged in an approximately hexagonal lattice.

divide the myofibrils into functional units called *sarcomeres* (see Fig. 5.2b). Sarcoplasm, mitochondria and other cellular elements are packed between the myofibrils.

There is a regular arrangement of contractile proteins within each sarcomere, with each thick filament being surrounded by six thin filaments (see Fig. 5.2c and d). Contraction of muscle occurs as thick and thin filaments slide past each other (Fig. 5.3) and is therefore accompanied by a decrease in the width of the light bands. The width of the dark bands remains unchanged.

> **Accessory proteins maintain the alignment of actin and myosin filaments.**

Skeletal muscle function depends on a precise alignment of actin and myosin filaments within each myofibril. This is achieved by accessory proteins, which link the different components and hold them in register with each other. These proteins can only be visualized using immunohistochemical techniques.

Fig. 5.3 Muscle Contraction. During muscle contraction, the thin filaments of the myofibrils slide over the thick filaments. This is reversed on muscle relaxation.

◉ ADVANCED CONCEPT

Myofibrils

Thin Filaments are Mainly Formed from Actin

Thin filaments are 8 nm in diameter and composed mainly of the protein actin. Each thin filament (F-actin) is formed by the polymerization of many single molecules of globular actin (G-actin). These actin filaments are polar, with all G-actin molecules pointing in the same direction.

To form a complete thin filament, two actin filaments become attached by their tail ends to α actinin in the Z line so that they face in opposite directions (i.e. away from the Z line).

Thick Filaments are Mainly Formed from Myosin

Thick filaments are composed mainly of the protein myosin. Like the actin filament, the myosin filament is polar. To form a complete heavy filament, two myosin filaments become attached by their tail ends so that they face in opposite directions (i.e. away from the M line) (Fig. 5.4). Different molecular types (isoforms) of myosin are present in different types of skeletal muscle fibre.

Fig. 5.4 Myosin Molecule. Each myosin molecule is composed of two tadpole-shaped heavy chains, the tails of which coil around each other, with four small light chains attached to the head portions. The coiled, rod-like tail portions of many myosin molecules aggregate and pack together in a regular staggered array to form the filament, and the head portions project out in a regular helical pattern.

◉ ADVANCED CONCEPT

Accessory Proteins of Muscle

Actinin holds actin filaments in a lattice arrangement in the Z disc. Other Z disc proteins include filamin, amorphin and Z protein.

Nebulin is associated with actin-containing thin filaments.

Myomesin holds myosin filaments in a lattice arrangement in the region of the M line, associated with creatine kinase and M protein.

Titin (connectin) is an extremely long elastic protein, which runs from the Z disc parallel to the filament array and links the ends of the thick filaments to the M line, maintaining their ends in register with the lattice of thin filaments.

Desmin filaments (one of the class of intermediate filament proteins) link adjacent myofibrils to each other and maintain their register. In addition, they link myofibrils to the cell membrane.

Myosin-binding protein C1 is a myosin-binding protein localized in stripes running parallel to the M band in the first half of the A band.

Mutations may develop in genes coding for proteins involved with myofibril organization, leading to diseases called *muscular dystrophies*.

Contraction of skeletal muscle is mediated by a cycle of binding and release between actin and myosin.

In muscle contraction, the actin filaments slide along the myosin filaments. This is driven by the heads of the myosin molecules, which bind to actin and, in a sequence of binding and release movements, 'walk' along the actin filament. This repetitive binding and release is powered by the hydrolysis of adenosine triphosphate (ATP) (Fig. 5.5), and myosin can be regarded as an ATPase that is activated by the binding of actin.

Control of muscle contraction is achieved by proteins that bind to actin and prevent muscle contraction by blocking the myosin–actin interaction (Fig. 5.6). This is reversed by high concentrations of Ca^{2+} ions in the cell cytoplasm (Fig. 5.7).

◉ ADVANCED CONCEPT

The Force of Muscle Contraction is Transmitted to the Extracellular Matrix by a Series of Link Proteins

The cytoskeleton of each skeletal muscle fibre is linked to the external lamina by a series of link molecules. Actin filaments inside the cell are linked to the protein dystrophin. Dystrophin then links with a complex composed of several glycoproteins that bridge through the muscle cell membrane to the cell surface. On the outer surface of the muscle cell, the glycoprotein complex links to the protein merosin, which is a laminin component of the basement membrane. In this way, forces generated inside the muscle are transferred to the extracellular matrix in the external lamina.

If there is a genetic absence of one of the linking proteins, then muscle fibres are prone to undergo tearing on contraction, and the affected person develops one of the many forms of muscular dystrophy.

It is being increasingly recognized that the different forms of muscular dystrophy can be related to defects in structural proteins in the muscle fibres. Duchenne muscular dystrophy is described on page 249.

Special internal membrane systems called *triads* control muscle contraction by regulating calcium release.

There is a specialized internal membrane system in skeletal muscle called the *T-tubular system*. This extends from the surface membrane as thin tubules, which extend deep through the muscle fibre running along the region of the AI junction

Fig. 5.5 Use of ATP by Myosin Binding to Actin. A myosin molecule uses the energy of ATP to move along an actin filament. **(a)** ATP bound to myosin is hydrolysed to ADP and phosphate (Pi). **(b)** This causes myosin to bind loosely to actin. **(c)** Pi is released, and myosin binds tightly to actin. **(d)** This binding initiates molecular folding of the myosin molecule to cause the movement of the molecule relative to the actin filament. ADP is released, fresh ATP binds and the myosin returns to its non-attached state. The cycle repeats, and the myosin head 'walks' along the actin filament.

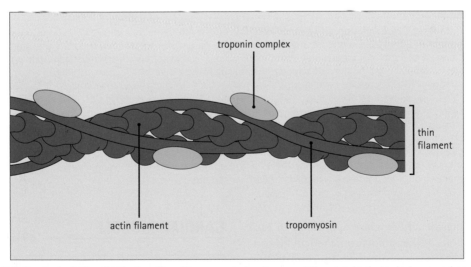

Fig. 5.6 Control of Muscle Contraction. Tropomyosin is a long, rod-like protein that winds around an actin filament to stabilize and stiffen it. The troponin complex, which regulates the binding of actin to myosin, is attached to tropomyosin and composed of three separate polypeptides termed *troponins T, I* and *C*. Troponin T binds the complex to tropomyosin and positions the complex on the actin filament at the site where actin would bind to myosin. Troponin I physically prevents myosin from binding to actin. Troponin C binds Ca^{2+} ions, which causes a conformational change in the troponin complex, allowing myosin access to the actin filament.

AI junction   AI junction

T-tubular system

sarcoplasmic reticulum

myofibrils

mitochondria

external lamina

Fig. 5.7 Muscle Cell Excitation and Intracellular Ca²⁺ Ions. After a nerve signal, excitation of the muscle cell membrane is conveyed to the interior of the cell via a series of membranous channels (the transverse tubular system of T tubules) that extend from the muscle surface to surround each myofibril. Running alongside each T tubule are two portions of sarcoplasmic reticulum, called *terminal cisternae,* which contain a high concentration of Ca²⁺ ions and have electrically sensitive Ca²⁺ ion channels in their wall. Membrane excitation of the T-tubular system causes these Ca²⁺ ion channels to open, thus allowing Ca²⁺ ions to flood into the sarcoplasm. In the resting state, muscle cells have few intracellular free Ca²⁺ ions, and a sudden increase in free cytosolic Ca²⁺ ions initiates muscle contraction. Membrane pumps (Ca²⁺-ATPase) in the sarcoplasmic reticulum pump the Ca²⁺ ions back into the sarcoplasmic reticulum rapidly (within about 30 ms) and stop contraction. The close association of T tubules and sarcoplasmic reticulum forms three tubules in cross-section (a membrane triad). In human muscle, there is a membrane triad surrounding every myofibril in the AI junction region; thus there are two triads to each sarcomere.

(Fig. 5.8). Running alongside and in close apposition to each T tubule are two extensions of the sarcoplasmic reticulum containing a very high calcium concentration. In cross-section these three tubes form a triad (Fig. 5.9). In response to membrane depolarization in the T-tubular system, calcium channels in the membrane of the sarcoplasmic reticulum release calcium into the cytosol of the muscle fibre, causing contraction.

▶▶ KEY FACTS

Skeletal Muscle

- Each muscle fibre is surrounded by an external lamina.
- Actin is arranged as thin filaments anchored to the Z line.
- Myosin is arranged as thick filaments anchored to the M line.
- Cytosolic calcium regulates contraction at membrane triads.

CARDIAC MUSCLE

Cardiac muscle is a form of striated muscle but differs significantly from skeletal muscle.

Like skeletal muscle, cardiac muscle is a type of striated muscle and is characterized by a similar arrangement of actin and myosin filaments to mediate contraction. The important differences between cardiac muscle and skeletal muscle are as follows:

- Cardiac muscle cells have a central nucleus and are much shorter than those of skeletal muscle (Fig. 5.10).
- Long cardiac muscle fibres are produced by linking numerous cardiac muscle cells end to end via anchoring-type cell junctions.

Fig. 5.8 Electron Micrograph of a Skeletal Muscle Triad. The T tubule is seen as a small open tube (T) and on each side are extensions of the sarcoplasmic reticulum. In humans, the sarcoplasmic reticulum contains electron-dense material, making these relatively indistinct structures in comparison to illustrations taken from animal material. A single triad is shown at higher magnification in the inset.

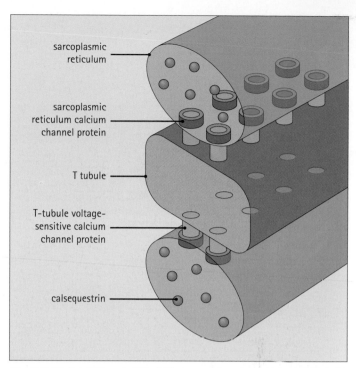

Fig. 5.9 Skeletal Muscle Triad. The sarcoplasmic reticulum (SR) Ca^{2+} channel protein lines up with the Ca^{2+} channel protein in the T-tubular system. Depolarization of the T-tubular system causes opening of the SR calcium channels. Calcium, which is held in the SR lumen by calsequestrin, can then be released into the muscle cytoplasm.

Fig. 5.10 Cardiac Muscle. Cardiac muscle cells appear as elliptical or lobulated structures in transverse section. Their nuclei are centrally placed and have irregular shapes, and thin fibrocollagenous septa containing small blood vessels run between fibres. Between individual cardiac muscle cells, there is a rich capillary blood supply. The eosinophilic cytoplasm has a granular appearance related to myofilaments cut in cross-section. Cardiac muscle is a type of striated muscle (see Fig. 5.11).

There is no resident stem cell population in cardiac muscle analogous to the satellite cells of skeletal muscle (see p. 249). Damage to cardiac muscle in disease leads to replacement of dead cells by collagenous scar.

> **Individual cardiac muscle cells are linked into long chains by specialized cell junctional systems.**

Instead of fusing to form syncytia as for skeletal muscle (see p. 247), cardiac muscle cells align into long chains and have anchoring cell junctions (Fig. 5.11).

In the adult, a cardiac muscle cell is about 15 μm in diameter and about 130 μm in length, with a central nucleus; approximately 50% of human heart myocytes have two nuclei. Intercellular junctions, which can be seen by light microscopy as faint lines running transversely across fibres, are termed **intercalated discs**. These contain three types of cell junctions:

- Desmosomal junctions tightly link adjacent cells via the intermediate filaments (see Fig. 3.5).
- Adherent-type junctions anchor the actin fibres of the sarcomeres to each end of the cell (see Fig. 3.5).
- Communicating gap junctions (see Fig. 3.7) facilitate passage of membrane excitation and synchronization of contraction.

Fig. 5.11 Cardiac Muscle. (a) In longitudinal section, cardiac muscle appears as a series of anastomosing cords of cells, which branch and join with adjacent fibres at cell junctions (intercalated discs, ID), seen as dark lines by the immunocytochemical method for α-B crystallin. Note the striations within each fibre. **(b)** Micrograph immunostained for desmoglein 2, one of the proteins in the intercalated disc. **(c)** Ultrastructurally, cardiac muscle cells contain myofibrils with thick and thin filament systems virtually identical to those in skeletal muscle but composed of different structural isoforms. Mitochondria are prominent and make up a much larger proportion of cell volume than in skeletal muscle. Several regions of the intercalated disc structure can be resolved, showing desmosome-like junctions (D), adherent-type junctions (A) and, in the lateral portions of the intercalated disc, prominent communicating gap junctions (G). **(d)** The structural arrangement of adjacent cardiac muscle cells. Cells are bound together by desmosomal junctions at interdigitating areas at the ends of adjacent cells to form the intercalated disc. Gap junctions facilitate transmission of the contractile stimulus between cells. [Image (b) used under Creative Commons License https://creativecommons. org/licenses/by-sa/3.0/ from the Human Protein Atlas Antibody to desmoglein 2 HPA004896 https://www. proteinatlas.org/ENSG00000046604-DSG2/tissue/heart+muscle#img.]

The molecular basis of contraction of cardiac muscle is similar to that of skeletal muscle.

Contraction of cardiac muscle cells is regulated by cytosolic Ca^{2+} ion concentration similar to skeletal muscle (see Figs 5.5 and 5.6), but:

- The cardiac transverse (T) tubular system consists of much wider invaginations of the cell surface.
- Sarcoplasmic reticulum associated with T tubules is not as regular or as well organized as in skeletal muscle.
- The association of sarcoplasmic reticulum with T tubules is as dyads rather than triads and is at the Z lines rather than the AI junction.

CLINICAL EXAMPLE

Cardiac Muscle and Disease

The cardiac muscle is the most hard-worked muscle in the body; it contracts and relaxes 60–100 times per minute from intrauterine life until death, often 80–90 years later, without rest. Stress and physical activity can increase the number of beats per minute to well above 120, often for long periods. The cardiac muscle in the wall of the left ventricle has a particularly heavy workload, having to force oxygenated arterial blood all around the body. It is not surprising that any factor affecting the function of the cardiac muscle has a major impact on the left ventricle and its function. The most important factor affecting the function of the cardiac muscle is inadequate oxygenation, usually the result of an inadequate coronary artery supply. Once a cardiac muscle cell dies, other cells must increase their size and work output to compensate (these cells undergo hypertrophy).

- Other causes of cardiac muscle hypertrophy are given in the Clinical Example box on page 92.
- The structural and functional consequences of failure of oxygenation of cardiac muscle cells are given in the Clinical Example box on page 175.
- Genetic disorders which affect the structure and function of cardiac muscle (primarily myosin heavy chains) are termed *cardiomyopathies*.

The adult heart does not contain stem cells for myocytes, and there is no population of cells able to grow into new muscle cells after damage caused by disease. Experimental techniques are being investigated to grow stem cells ex vivo and inject them back into damaged hearts. These trials show promise but are very early in their development.

SMOOTH MUSCLE

Smooth muscle is the main contractile cell in the walls of viscera and in blood vessels.

Smooth muscle cells have a much less organized system of contractile proteins than striated skeletal and cardiac muscle cells. Forming the contractile portions of the wall of most hollow viscera (e.g. gut, urinary bladder and uterus), in addition to the contractile elements in blood vessel walls and secretory gland ducts, smooth muscle cells are found in situations requiring sustained slow or rhythmic contractions not under voluntary control.

Individual smooth muscle cells are anchored together into functional units by basement membrane material.

Smooth muscle cells are typically spindle-shaped and, depending on site, vary in size from 20 μm (small blood vessels) to 400–500 μm (uterus). Each cell has a single, centrally located nucleus, which is elongated or elliptical in shape (Fig. 5.12).

Fig. 5.12 Smooth Muscle (Light Microscopy). (a) In longitudinal section, smooth muscle cells occur in linear bundles. The cells have abundant pink-staining cytoplasm and central elongated nuclei. **(b)** In transverse section, the smooth muscle cells have polygonal profiles. **(c)** This special stain demonstrates *(in black)* the external laminae that surround each smooth muscle cell and to which the cell membranes adhere. The laminae are composed of type IV collagen and glycoproteins and bind individual cells into a functional mass.

In cross-section, smooth muscle cells have polygonal profiles, but in longitudinal section they appear as linear bundles.

Each smooth muscle cell is surrounded by an external lamina to which cell membranes adhere; small groups of cells are organized into bundles by fine collagenous tissue containing blood vessels and nerves.

Fig. 5.13 Motor Innervation of Smooth Muscle. Smooth muscle is arranged in bundles of many thousands of small, individual, electrically coupled cells. In most organs the bundles are connected by smaller bands of muscle. Muscle bundles are functionally innervated by around 20 or more axons (4 are shown here). Different numbers of these axons can be active, thus grading the effects of the nervous system on the muscle. Each axon forms a terminal arbour, consisting of varicose branches. Every time an action potential passes into the terminal arbour, there is release of transmitter from a minority of varicosities. Connected smooth muscle bundles, which themselves are also innervated *(shown in grey)*, are influenced through the connecting bands of smooth muscle cells. (Reprinted from Di Natale MR, Stebbing MJ, Furness JB. Autonomic neuromuscular junctions. *Auton Neurosci.* 2021;234:102816 with permission from Elsevier.)

> **The initiation and modulation of smooth muscle contraction is controlled by pacemaker cells and neuronal and paracrine factors.**

Smooth muscle contraction can be initiated or modulated by several factors:
- Smooth muscle cells may act as 'pacemaker' cells and initiate contraction. Gap junctions between individual cells propagate signalling.
- Autonomic innervation modulates smooth muscle contraction. Whereas in skeletal muscle, a motor endplate is a discrete structural and functional unit that initiates contraction (see Fig. 13.8), in contrast, the innervation of smooth muscle by autonomic nerves (see Chapter 6) is delivered through varicosities located along a network of axons (Fig. 5.13). Each varicosity contains neurosecretory vesicles which are released upon stimulation of the nerve.
- The smooth muscle of the bowel is associated with interstitial cells of Cajal that serve to modulate contraction (see p. 217).

> **Contraction of smooth muscle cells is mediated by a dispersed arrangement of actin and myosin, which is quite different from that of striated muscle.**

Ultrastructurally, smooth muscle does not show the highly organized system of contractile proteins (i.e. myofilaments) seen in striated muscle, but has an arrangement whereby bundles of contractile proteins crisscross the cell and are inserted into anchoring points (focal densities). Focal densities are similar to adherent junctions and are studded around the cell membrane (Fig. 5.14).

Tension generated by contraction is transmitted through the focal densities to the surrounding network of external laminae, thus allowing a mass of smooth muscle cells to function as one unit. The abundant intermediate filaments of smooth muscle, desmin, are also inserted into the focal densities.

Energy is supplied by numerous mitochondria, which tend to be located, along with endoplasmic reticulum and other organelles, around the nucleus, in an area devoid of contractile filaments.

Although each smooth muscle cell is surrounded by an external lamina, this is deficient where the cells communicate with each other via gap junctions. These junctions, which are also termed *nexus junctions* in smooth muscle, are widespread and allow the spread of membrane excitation between cells.

A characteristic feature of smooth muscle cells is the presence of numerous invaginations of cell membrane–forming structures that resemble caveolae. It is thought that these invaginations function in a similar way to the specialized transverse (T)-tubular system of striated muscle by controlling the entry of Ca^{2+} ions into the cell after membrane excitation. Terminal sacs of Ca^{2+} ion–containing endoplasmic reticulum terminate beneath the cell membrane close to these vesicles.

> **The molecular basis of contraction in smooth muscle differs from that in skeletal muscle.**

The contraction mechanism of smooth muscle differs from that for striated muscle. Because the contractile proteins are arranged in a crisscross lattice inserted circumferentially into the cell membrane, contraction results in shortening of the cell, which assumes a globular shape in contrast to its elongated shape in the relaxed state (see Fig. 5.14f).

Fig. 5.14 Smooth Muscle (Ultrastructure). (a) Low-power electron micrograph of a smooth muscle cell showing scattered focal densities (D) around the cell membrane. **(b)** High-power electron micrograph of one of the focal densities in **(a)**, showing the insertion of large numbers of very fine contractile filaments into it. **(c)** Very low-power electron micrograph of smooth muscle fibres in transverse section showing a central nucleus (N), distinct surrounding external laminae (EL), the bulk of the cytoplasm occupied by tightly packed contractile protein filaments (CP) and a perinuclear lucent zone (PLZ) in which most of the mitochondria and non-contractile organelles reside. **(d)** Gap junctions (G) connect adjacent cells at defects in the external lamina. **(e)** A terminal sac of the endoplasmic reticulum (ER) lies close to caveolae-like endocytotic vesicles (V) on the surface. External lamina material (EL) lies between two adjacent smooth muscle cells. **(f)** Contractile protein filaments are inserted into focal densities around the cell membrane. With contraction of the tethered filaments, each cell assumes a short, rounded shape.

ADVANCED CONCEPT

Smooth Muscle Contraction

Thin filaments of actin (an isoform specific to smooth muscle) are associated with tropomyosin (see Fig. 5.6), but in contrast to striated muscle, there is no troponin.

The thick filaments are composed of myosin, but of a type different from that in skeletal muscle and will only bind to actin if its light chain is phosphorylated; this phenomenon does not occur in skeletal muscle.

Although Ca^{2+} ions in smooth muscle cells cause contraction as in striated muscle, the control of Ca^{2+} ion movements is different. In relaxed smooth muscle, free Ca^{2+} ions are normally sequestered in sarcoplasmic reticulum throughout the cell. On membrane excitation, free Ca^{2+} ions are released into the cytoplasm and bind to a protein called *calmodulin* (a calcium-binding protein). The calcium–calmodulin complex then activates an enzyme called *myosin light-chain kinase,* which phosphorylates the myosin light chain and permits it to bind to actin. Actin and myosin subsequently interact by filament sliding to produce contraction in a manner similar to that for skeletal muscle.

In the cell membrane of smooth muscle cells are calcium channels, which can open and let calcium into the cell. Some of these channels are activated by hormones (ligand-gated channels), whereas others are activated by membrane depolarization (voltage-gated channels). These channels provide another mechanism for initiation or modulation of contraction.

Contraction of smooth muscle can be modulated by surface receptors activating internal secondary messenger systems. Expression of different receptors allows smooth muscle in different sites to respond to several different hormones.

Compared with skeletal muscle, smooth muscle can maintain a high force of contraction for very little ATP use.

Smooth muscle can be arranged into two functional types, termed *unitary* and *multiunit*.

Most smooth muscle is present in the walls of hollow viscera (e.g. gut, ureter, fallopian tube) where it is arranged in sheets with cells aligned circumferentially or longitudinally, with contraction resulting in reduction of the luminal diameter. In these so-called *unitary smooth muscles*, cells tend to generate their own low level of rhythmic contraction, which may also be stimulated by stretch, and is transmitted from cell to cell via the gap junctions. Such smooth muscle is richly innervated by the autonomic nervous system (see Chapter 6), which increases or decreases levels of spontaneous contraction rather than initiating it. Physiologically, this is termed *tonic smooth muscle* and is characterized by slow contraction, no action potentials and a low content of fast myosin.

A second arrangement of smooth muscle is typified by that in the iris of the eye. Here, rather than simply modulating spontaneous activity, autonomic innervation controls contraction precisely, resulting in opening and closing of the pupil. Similar neurally controlled or multiunit smooth muscle is found in the vas deferens and some large arteries. Physiologically, this is termed *phasic smooth muscle* and is characterized by rapid contraction associated with a distinct action potential and a high cell content of fast myosin.

 ADVANCED CONCEPT

Support Cell Function of Smooth Muscle

Smooth Muscle Cells Have to Secrete Elements of Their Extracellular Matrix
Depending on the site, smooth muscle cells produce collagen, elastin and other components of the extracellular matrix. Thus they have a support cell function and a contractile cell function. In most situations, this support cell function is limited to manufacturing extracellular matrix to anchor the smooth muscle.

▶ **KEY FACTS**

Smooth Muscle

- Spindle-shaped cells surrounded by external lamina
- Main contractile cell of hollow viscera, blood vessels and airways
- Contractile proteins inserted into focal densities around cell periphery
- Contraction modulated by local cells and neuronal and endocrine factors
- Innervation is served by varicosities along a web of autonomic axons
- Two main smooth muscle types (tonic and phasic) characterized by arrangement and speed of contraction

▣ **CLINICAL EXAMPLE**

Muscle Hypertrophy, Hyperplasia and Atrophy

Cells, including muscle cells of all types, can adapt to handle a heavier workload. They can do this by either increasing the size of the cell, and hence its work output, or by increasing the number of cells doing the job. Increasing a cell's capacity for work by increasing its size is called **hypertrophy,** and by increasing the number of cells is called **hyperplasia.** For hyperplasia to occur, the mature functioning cells must be capable of cell division, and neither skeletal muscle nor cardiac muscle cells are capable of cell division, so the cells can only increase their output by hypertrophy. Smooth muscle cells are capable of cell division and can therefore increase their work output by both hypertrophy and hyperplasia.

Similarly, muscle that has to deal with greatly reduced workload can adapt by each cell becoming smaller **(atrophy).**

Here are some examples:

Skeletal muscle undergoes hypertrophy in increased physical exercise, for example, in athletes, but undergoes atrophy when the muscles are underused, for example, in someone who is immobilized by paralysis or limb injury.

Cardiac muscle can undergo hypertrophy in many circumstances, both as a result of increased physiological demand (again in athletes) and as a result of some disease processes. For example, if the aortic outflow lumen in the heart is reduced by valve disease (see Chapter 9), the cardiac muscle fibres of the left ventricle will undergo hypertrophy to increase the force with which blood can be pushed through the partially obstructed outflow. Hypertrophy of cardiac muscle cells makes the heart abnormally large.

Smooth muscle can undergo both hypertrophy and hyperplasia and usually responds to increased demands by doing both, although hypertrophy is usually the major component. A good example is the smooth muscle of the uterus (myometrium), which increases enormously in both bulk and power during the 9 months of pregnancy in preparation for the immense contractile effort required at childbirth. Atrophy of uterine smooth muscle occurs after menopause, indicating that the status of uterine smooth muscle is under hormonal control.

MYOFIBROBLASTS

> **Myofibroblasts are important in tissue responses to injury.**

Myofibroblasts are spindle-shaped cells that secrete collagen (i.e. fibroblast-like) but also have well-defined contractile properties similar to those of smooth muscle.

In conventional histological sections, myofibroblasts cannot be readily distinguished from fibroblasts, but immunohistochemical detection of their content of smooth muscle actin and desmin (not seen in fibroblasts) and ultrastructural demonstration of contractile proteins show that they are distinct. Myofibroblasts lack an external lamina, in contrast to true smooth muscle cells.

In normal tissues, myofibroblasts are inconspicuous and form populations of cells within mesenchymal tissues, for example, in the alveolar septa of the lung and around the crypts of glands in the gut (Fig. 5.15). They also form a sparse population in loose collagenous support tissue.

Fig 5.15 Myofibroblastic Cells. Micrograph of colonic mucosa stained to show alpha smooth muscle actin *(brown)*. The smooth muscle of the muscularis mucosae is seen (MM). Two gland crypts (C) are seen surrounded by spindle-shaped cells (colonic pericryptal sheath myofibroblasts) (P) that contain alpha smooth muscle actin. This type of myofibroblastic cell has a role in homeostasis, healing and repair in the gut mucosa. (Image used under Creative Commons License https://creativecommons.org/licenses/by-sa/3.0/ from the Human Protein Atlas. Antibody to smooth muscle actin CAB000045 https://www.proteinatlas.org/ENSG00000143632-ACTA1/tissue/colon#img.)

CLINICAL EXAMPLE

Myofibroblasts in Disease

In addition to being prominent in wound healing and in the normal processes of repair, myofibroblasts are found in several diseases characterized by fibrosis of tissues, for example, fibrosis of the lung after damage by immune-mediated diseases, atheroma in the lining of arteries (see Fig. 9.6) and cirrhosis of the liver (see Fig. 12.9). In these diseases, the stimuli that cause myofibroblast proliferation are uncertain, but include local production of growth factors.

During wound healing, however, myofibroblasts become active and proliferate, and their role appears to be to repair defects resulting from tissue damage. They secrete collagen to provide a firm scaffold to consolidate a damaged area (fibrous scar). As healing proceeds, myofibroblasts contract and pull the extracellular matrix together to reduce the physical size of the damaged area.

PERICYTES

> **Pericytes are found around vessels and can act as mesenchymal stem cells.**

Pericytes are spindle-shaped cells that are found circumferentially arranged around capillaries and venules (see Fig. 9.11). They are surrounded by external lamina and, in normal tissues, show little cytoplasmic differentiation ultrastructurally, but contain actin and myosin immunohistochemically, suggesting a contractile function.

After tissue injury, pericytes proliferate and assume the role of primitive mesenchymal cells, able to differentiate into myofibroblasts, in addition to mesenchymal tissue, which develops into collagenous support tissue and new blood vessels.

MYOEPITHELIAL CELLS

> **Secretions from glands are expelled by the contractile function of myoepithelial cells.**

Myoepithelial cells are found in exocrine glands, including highly developed glands, such as the breast, where they form a major population surrounding glandular acini and ducts and squeeze secretions from the glandular lumina.

Myoepithelial cells are generally inconspicuous in routine haematoxylin and eosin (H&E) sections, appearing as a layer of flat cells running around acini and ducts. They have dark-staining, rounded nuclei and clear or vacuolated cytoplasm.

Around acini, myoepithelial cells have a stellate, multiprocessed morphology in three dimensions and form a contractile meshwork, which encloses secretory units of glands. Around ducts they are fusiform in shape and surround the periphery of ducts in a way analogous to barrel hoops.

Ultrastructurally, myoepithelial cells contain contractile proteins arranged in a manner similar to that in smooth muscle and have numerous desmosomal connections with adjacent cells.

Immunohistochemically, they can be detected by their content of the muscle-specific intermediate filament desmin (Fig. 5.16).

Myoepithelial cells are controlled by the autonomic nervous system and on stimulation contract and expel glandular secretions.

For online review questions, please visit https://studentconsult. inkling.com.

Fig. 5.16 Myoepithelial Cells. Myoepithelial cells in this section from a salivary gland can be shown by an immunoperoxidase technique that demonstrates desmin, which is the muscle-specific intermediate filament and stains brown.

Nervous Tissue

INTRODUCTION

The nervous system allows rapid and specific communication between widely spaced areas of the body by the action of specialized nerve cells (neurons), which gather and process information and generate appropriate response signals.

The nervous system is divided into two main parts:
- The **central nervous system** (CNS), comprising the brain and spinal cord.
- The **peripheral nervous system** (PNS), comprising the nerves which run between the CNS and other tissues, together with nerve 'relay stations' termed *ganglia*.

NERVE CELLS (NEURONS)

> **Nerve cells are responsible for direct communications between different groups of cells.**

Neurons form a network of highly specific connections between different groups of cells to:
- Gather information from sensory receptors.
- Process information and provide a memory.
- Generate appropriate signals to effector cells.

> **A neuron is divided into several regions, each with a different function.**

Neurons (Fig. 6.1) are characterized by:
- A cell body containing the nucleus and most of the organelles responsible for maintaining the cell.
- A long cell process (**axon**) stretching from the cell, often over a long distance, which is responsible for transmitting signals from the neuron to other cells.
- Numerous short cell processes (**dendrites**) that increase the surface area available for connecting with axons of other neurons (dendrites can run in many directions from the neuronal cell body).
- Specialized cell junctions (**synapses**) between its axon and other neurons to allow direct cell communication.

The functional attributes of the nervous system are determined mainly by the network of connections between neurons rather than by specific structural features of individual neurons.

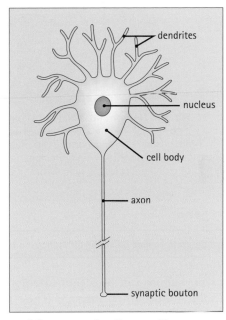

Fig. 6.1 General Structure of a Neuron. Neurons consist of a cell body, axon and dendrites, the axon carrying impulses to its terminal, the synaptic bouton, which makes contact with another cell. The dendrites connect with synaptic boutons from other neurons.

> **Neurons have a characteristic cytology reflecting a high metabolic activity.**

Neurons are highly metabolically active, as they not only maintain a massive surface area of cell membrane but also constantly require energy to develop electrochemical gradients. This activity is reflected in their histological appearance (Fig. 6.2), in which the nucleus is typically large and rounded, with a large central nucleolus, reflecting a high degree of transcriptional activity. There is abundant rough endoplasmic reticulum, which synthesizes the necessary proteins and is visible in the cytoplasm in haematoxylin and eosin (H&E) sections as blue-stained granules, the so-called **Nissl substance**. This is present in the cell body (perikaryon) and dendrites but not the axon. There is also a well-developed Golgi to produce secretory products and large numbers of mitochondria to supply the high energy requirements. Lysosomes are numerous because of a high turnover of cell membrane and other cell components, and residual bodies containing lipofuscin are often prominent, particularly in the elderly.

Fig. 6.2 Neuron. (a) Electron micrograph of a neuron showing the axon (A) containing mitochondria and cytoskeletal filaments and the cell body containing a nucleus (N), dark-staining lysosomal bodies (L) and abundant rough endoplasmic reticulum (Nissl substance; NS). **(b)** Micrograph showing a neuron with a large nucleus (N) containing a prominent nucleolus. Within the cell body, blue-staining NS can be seen, composed of rough endoplasmic reticulum. The axon (A) stretches away from the cell body.

Neurons have different shapes reflecting differences in function.

Several types of neurons can be identified according to the pattern of axons and dendrites (Fig. 6.3). These appearances are only apparent when special staining methods are used to highlight cellular anatomy.

Motor neurons have a large cell body to provide metabolic support for the large axon. They also have many dendritic processes and are therefore classed as multipolar neurons. Examples of motor neurons include the Betz cells of the cerebral motor cortex and the anterior horn cells in the spinal cord (Fig. 6.4).

Sensory neurons are commonly unipolar cells, which are characterized by the possession of one major process. This divides into two branches, one running to the CNS and one to a sensory area of the body.

Interneurons are generally small, simple cells with short processes that provide local connections within the CNS. Many such cells are bipolar, having two main processes of equivalent size, one dendritic and one axonal. Other types of interneurons have multiple cell processes and wrap around the cell body of a target nerve cell to create multiple connections; they are termed *basket cells*.

Many of the nerve cells in the cerebral cortex are called **pyramidal cells** because they have a roughly triangular shape (Fig. 6.5).

In addition to these general types of neurons, there are many types of neurons that are unique to a particular part of the brain; for example, **motor neurons** are found in the anterior horn of the spinal cord (see Fig. 6.4). They are very large cells compared with other types of neurons, given that the cell body

has to maintain an axon that might, for example, need to extend from the cervical spine to a muscle in the hand, a distance of around 100 cm. **Purkinje cells** are very large, multipolar neurons seen in the cerebellar cortex (Fig. 6.6). Granule cells are small multiprocessed neurons seen in the cerebellum (see Fig. 6.6) and hippocampus.

◎ ADVANCED CONCEPT

The Cytoskeleton of the Neuron Is Vital for Axonal Transport

The cytoskeleton of neurons is highly organized to maintain the unique shape of these cells, particularly axons, which may be up to 1-m long.

Neurofilament protein, the intermediate filament of nerve cells, is thought to act as an internal scaffold to maintain the shape of the axon and cell body. In the axon, certain membrane proteins are anchored in place in an organized pattern by attachment to cellular neurofilaments.

There is also a highly organized network of microtubules, which transport substances and organelles up and down the axon.

The metabolic maintenance of the long cell process of the axon requires a transport system for organelles, enzymes and metabolites from the cell body, which is largely directed by the microtubular cytoskeleton. Enzymes and elements of the cytoskeleton are transported down the axon at a speed of 1–5 mm/day by a stop–go system (**slow axonal transport**). Membrane-bound organelles, such as neurosecretory vesicles, are transported at speeds of 400 mm/day (**anterograde fast axonal transport**). This method is mediated by microtubular transport mechanisms using the molecule kinesin as a molecular motor.

The return of effete organelles and recycled membrane from the synaptic ending back to the neuronal cell body for processing occurs at a rate of 300 mm/day (**retrograde fast transport**). This is mediated by microtubular transport mechanisms using the molecule dynein as a molecular motor.

Fig. 6.3 Types of Neurons. (a) There are many different types of neurons, which are shaped according to their function. Bipolar cells are commonly interneurons, whereas unipolar cells tend to be sensory neurons. The majority of neurons are multipolar, including motor neurons and pyramidal neurons in the cerebral cortex. **(b)** 3D image of a pyramidal neuron of the human temporal cortex made from reconstruction of high-resolution confocal stacks of images. **(c)** 3D reconstruction showing just the dendrites of the same cell. **(d)** The neuronal processes running in different directions have been coloured. The apical dendrite is in *red* and four reconstructed basal dendrites are in *blue, green, orange* and *purple*. Scale bar [in **(c)**]: 50 μm. (Images b–d reproduced under https://creativecommons.org/licenses/by/4.0 from Anton-Sanchez L, Larranaga P, Benavides-Piccione R, et al. Three dimensional spatial modelling of spines along dendritic networks in human cortical pyramidal neurons. *PLOS One.* 2017;12(6):e0180400. https://doi.org/10.1371/journal.pone.0180400.)

Fig 6.4 Motor Neuron. This image shows one of the motor neurons located in the spinal cord. A large nucleus is seen in the cell body. Around the periphery of the cell body, the Nissl substance is clearly seen as purple-stained speckles in the neuronal cytoplasm. There are many nuclei in the surrounding neuropil, which are different types of glial cells (see Fig. 6.17).

Fig. 6.5 Pyramidal Neurons in the Cerebral Cortex. High-magnification H&E micrograph of cerebral cortex. Most of the cerebral cortex has six distinct layers of different neuronal types. Neurons (N) vary in size and have a triangular shape representing pyramidal cells in layers II and V. In routine histological sections such as this, it is not possible to see details of cell processes, and only the cell body is evident. Special staining methods are needed to show the cell processes of neurons. Many of the other nuclei (G) seen in the image are support cells termed *glial cells* (see Fig. 6.17). The pink-stained background is a mat of neuronal and glial cell processes termed neuropil. The thin structure (C) is a small blood vessel.

Fig. 6.6 Cerebellum. (a) Micrograph of the cerebellum, which is a distinct part of the brain and is characterized by complex folding of cerebellar cortex, generating a pattern of pleats (cerebellar folia). The folia contain the nuclei of nerve cells, which produce a blue-staining ribbon at this low magnification. The centre of the cerebellum is composed of white matter (W), in which a serpiginous aggregate of nerve cells, termed a nucleus (N), can be seen. **(b)** Higher-power micrograph of cerebellum showing that the outer part of the cerebellar cortex is composed of a mat of pink-stained nerve cell processes with scanty glial cells (the molecular layer, M), whereas the bulk of the blue-staining ribbon is formed by a band of small nerve cells with dark-staining rounded nuclei (the granular layer, G). Below the granular layer is the white matter (W), which contains axons. At the junction of the molecular layer with the granular layer is a row of large nerve cells (Purkinje cells, P) characterized by a vast branching pattern of dendrites in the molecular layer, but this is only visible by special staining methods.

CLINICAL EXAMPLE

Motor Neuron Disease

Motor neuron disease is a progressive disease, seen mainly in old age, in which symptoms include weakness of voluntary muscles caused by the death of motor neurons. The disease progresses to severe paralysis, leading to death in 2–3 years. Although mutations in several genes have been found to cause this type of disease, the reason for the peculiar susceptibility of motor neurons (rather than other neuronal types) to spontaneous death is not fully understood. All motor neurons are vulnerable, and the symptoms in each case depend on which groups of motor neurons are most severely involved. Death of motor neurons in the brain stem produces the symptom complex called **progressive bulbar palsy;** that of the lower motor neurons of the spinal cord produces **progressive muscular atrophy**. The most common pattern is called **amyotrophic lateral sclerosis** and is the result of death of motor neurons in the cerebral cortex, brain stem and spinal cord.

Neurons transmit signals by changes in the electrical polarity of the cell membrane.

Neuron signalling is controlled by an electrical (ionic) gradient across the cell membrane. Firing is associated with depolarization of the cell membrane which, in a resting axon, has a negative membrane potential (−70 mV). This depolarization is propagated along the axon of the cell at up to 100 m/s.

The cell membrane of neurons is divided into several regions, each containing highly specialized membrane proteins. **Membrane ion pumps** maintain the baseline electrical gradient between the outside and inside of the cell and are widely distributed in the cell membrane. **Ion channel proteins** modify the electrochemical gradient across the neuron cell membrane by forming pores or gates, which can switch their permeability to ions in response to specific signals (gated channels):

- **Ligand-gated channels** close or open in response to binding to chemical transmitter substances and are located mainly in synapses.
- **Voltage-gated channels** are involved mainly in the explosive and rapid depolarization that occurs as nerve cells fire and are widely distributed in the cell membrane.

If an area of the axon membrane is locally depolarized and the current is small, then no gated channels will open. The current flows down the axon by passive local spread for a small distance before dissipating because of leakage from the membrane. In this situation, the axon behaves like an electrical cable, simply conducting a current along its surface, with the speed of conduction related to the resistance and capacitance of the axon.

If an area of axon membrane is depolarized and the current is large, Na$^+$- and K$^+$-gated channels open and lead to an explosive change in the membrane potential, termed an **action potential.**

The opening of voltage-gated channels to produce an action potential can be considered a local amplification system for membrane depolarization; the current does not now dissipate over a small length of the axon, but propagates to the end of the axon by causing a chain reaction triggering of gated ion channels along the way.

Action potentials propagate along an axon at the speed of passive local spread, which is determined by the resistance and capacitance of the axon: the larger the diameter of the axon, the greater the speed of propagation.

> **Nerve cells signal to each other through structures called synapses.**

A *synapse,* also termed a *chemical synapse,* is a special type of cell junction that allows direct communication between cells; a transmitter substance is secreted in a highly localized fashion by one cell and received uniquely by the other.

> **Each synapse has vesicles containing neurotransmitter substances.**

The terminal end of an axon is swollen to form a synaptic bouton, which is closely applied to the surface of a target cell, leaving a small gap 20-nm wide (the synaptic cleft). The cell membrane on each side of the synaptic cleft contains special membrane proteins and receptors involved in neurotransmission.

Ultrastructurally, the cell membrane on each side of the synaptic cleft is slightly thickened, and the synaptic bouton contains mitochondria, microtubules and neurofilaments, in addition to membrane-bound vesicles 40–65 nm in diameter (neurosecretory vesicles; Fig. 6.7). The appearance of these vesicles is variable; most are small and round with a clear centre; others are elliptical. Certain neurosecretory granules (dense-core granules) have an electron-dense core with a pale 'halo' beneath the membrane.

In tissue sections, it is possible to detect transmitter substances in neurons and their terminals by immunochemistry, using antibodies specific for the transmitter.

Neurosecretory granules also contain unique non-transmitter proteins, which are vital to their function. Again, these may be detected by immunochemistry; for example, synaptophysin, which is a glycoprotein in the membrane of neurosecretory granules, and chromogranins, proteins involved in the packaging of transmitter into dense-core vesicles.

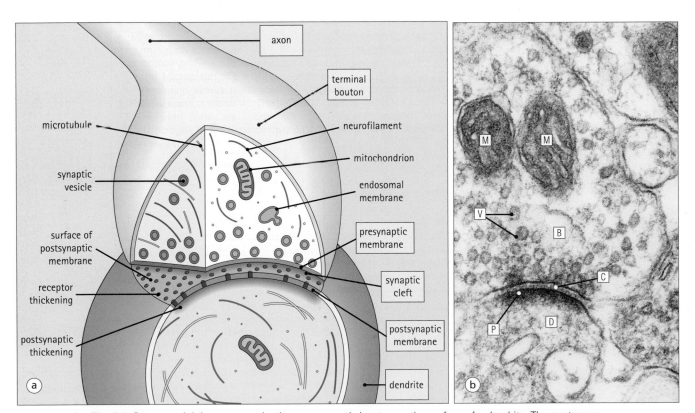

Fig. 6.7 Synapse. (a) An axon terminating as a synaptic bouton on the surface of a dendrite. The postsynaptic membrane bears arrays of receptors for the neurotransmitter contained in the synaptic vesicles. Vesicles are released into the synaptic cleft by exocytosis. **(b)** Electron micrograph showing the synaptic bouton (B) making contact with the dendrite (D). The bouton contains small vesicles (V), mitochondria (M) and cytoskeletal filaments. The synaptic cleft (C) contains faint granular material above the thickened postsynaptic membrane (P).

Neurosecretory vesicles release transmitter by fusion with the presynaptic membrane.

When a wave of depolarization reaches the synaptic bouton, it triggers the release of a transmitter substance from the neurosecretory granules by exocytosis (Fig. 6.8). The transmitter substance then diffuses across the synaptic cleft and can interact with receptors in the postsynaptic membrane of the target neuron. The membrane of the synaptic vesicle is recovered as a coated pit and recycles back to an endosome compartment in the nerve terminal. There is thus a constant recycling of membrane in the nerve terminal. Neurosecretory vesicles also arrive in the axon terminal by transport from the cell body, but others are formed locally by budding off from the endosome compartment in the synapse. Neurotransmitter substances can be imported into vesicles formed from the endosome compartment of the nerve terminal by reuptake systems.

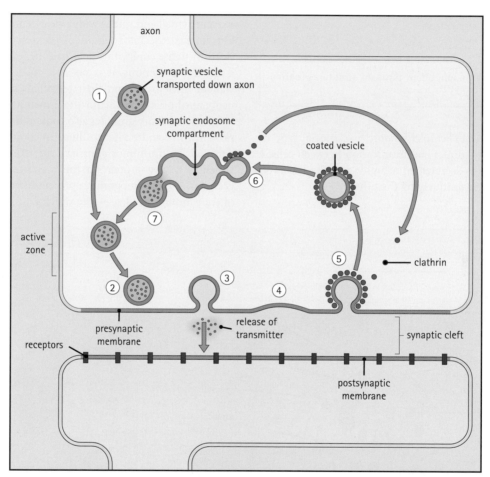

Fig. 6.8 Turnover of Synaptic Vesicles. Synaptic vesicles (NSVs) are formed in the neuronal cell body and are transported down the axon (1). Once in the terminal bouton, proteins in the NSV membrane direct vesicles to an area just above the presynaptic membrane, termed the active zone. Vesicles from the active zone bind to special docking proteins in the presynaptic membrane and become primed for exocytosis (2). Exocytosis is associated with the release of the transmitter substance into the synaptic cleft (3) and integration of the membrane of the vesicle with the presynaptic membrane (4). The protein clathrin associates with vesicle membrane and forms coated vesicles, which recycle the vesicle membrane back into the nerve terminal (5). Recycled vesicle membrane fuses with an endosome membrane compartment in the nerve terminal (6), and clathrin is released. New synaptic vesicles can bud off from the endosome compartment (7). Transmitter substances that are free in the nerve terminal can be imported into these recycled vesicles via special membrane pumps. Astrocytes around the synapse can also take up transmitter substance from the cleft. The terminal bouton also has a full complement of organelles to locally synthesise proteins, making each a separate domain within the neuron.

Neurosecretion Is Mediated by Proteins in the Synaptic Vesicle and Presynaptic Membrane

Many of the proteins involved in neurosecretion have now been characterized (Fig. 6.9).

The membrane of the synaptic vesicle contains an anchoring protein (synaptobrevin), which ties the vesicle to a docking protein in the presynaptic membrane (syntaxin) by a group of linking proteins called the *SNARE complex*. In the resting state, a calcium-sensitive trigger protein on the synaptic membrane (synaptotagmin) prevents the linking complex from allowing membrane fusion. If an action potential reaches the terminal bouton, voltage-sensitive calcium channels open and increase the concentration of calcium in the nerve terminal. Calcium then binds to synaptotagmin, and a conformational change mediated by proteins in the SNARE complex brings the membrane of the synaptic vesicle and the adjacent presynaptic membrane into close contact, and there is fusion of the lipid bilayers leading to pore formation and exocytosis of neurotransmitter within the vesicle.

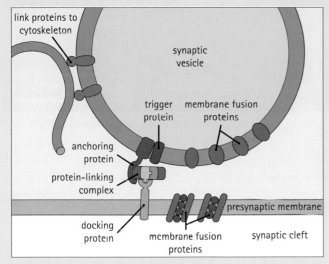

Fig. 6.9 Synaptic Docking and Exocytosis. Many of the proteins involved in the exocytosis of synaptic vesicles are characterized. Fusion of vesicle to presynaptic membrane takes place only when an increase in calcium causes an alteration in the configuration of proteins involved in docking.

Three possible effects of transmitter release are depolarization, hyperpolarization or altered cell sensitivity.

When a released transmitter binds to receptors on the postsynaptic cells, there are three possible effects: depolarization, hyperpolarization or altered cell sensitivity.

The target cell **depolarizes** if the transmitter substance binds to a ligand-gated receptor (i.e. Na^+ ion channel protein) and causes it to open, allowing ions to diffuse into the neuron. If many receptors are activated at the same time, the alteration in membrane potential causes activation of voltage-gated ion channels, leading to an action potential.

Only a small group of transmitter substances act in this way, which generally results in rapid neural transmission. These include acetylcholine, which is the major transmitter in this group, and glutamate.

The target cell **hyperpolarizes** if the transmitter substance binds to a ligand-gated receptor that admits small negative ions into the cell. Hyperpolarization inhibits depolarization.

The main transmitter substances causing hyperpolarization are γ-aminobutyric acid and glycine.

The overall **sensitivity of a cell** to stimulation is altered if the transmitter substance binds to one of the class of non–channel-linked receptors. These receptors generate secondary messengers (e.g. cyclic adenosine monophosphate [cAMP]) within the target neuron to modify the overall sensitivity of the cell to depolarization mediated by the ligand-gated receptors. Such behaviour is called *neuromodulation*.

Many of the transmitters causing altered cell sensitivity are monoamines (e.g. dopamine, serotonin), but some are small neuropeptides.

In any given nerve terminal, more than one transmitter substance may operate.

Synapses form different patterns of connection between neurons.

Within the CNS, synapses form in a diversity of combinations between axons and dendrites, axons and cell bodies, and axons and other axons (Fig. 6.10).

Fig. 6.10 Patterns of Synapse. (a) The combination of synapses. Synapses can form between axons and dendrites (most common), axons and cell bodies, and axons and other axons. **(b)** Electron micrograph showing two axodendritic synapses (S) onto the same dendrite (A). Firing of (A) will depend on the integration of these separate inputs.

Fig. 6.11 Dendritic Spines. (a) Confocal microscopy image of an intracellular injected layer III pyramidal neuron of the human cerebral cortex. DAPI staining shows nuclei in *blue*. **(b)** High-magnification image showing a horizontally projecting basal dendrite. There is a virtual lack of dendritic spines in the proximal dendritic segment and more distally on the right. **(c)** High-magnification image of an apical dendritic segment 100 μm away from the cell body. **(d)** Three-dimensional reconstruction of the complete morphology of each dendritic spine shown in **(c)** with spines coloured *red*. **(e)** Estimation of the spine volume values shown in **(d)** by colour codes (*blue-white*: 0.0–1.345 μm^3). Scale bar [in **(b)**]: 40 μm. (Reprinted from Benavides-Piccione R, Fernaud-Espinosa I, Robles V, et al. Age-based comparison of human dendritic spine structure using complete three-dimensional reconstructions. *Cereb Cortex*. 2013;23[8]:1798–1810. https://doi.org/10.1093/cercor/bhs154. Copyright 2013, with permission.)

Because axons may be excitatory, inhibitory or modulatory, certain synapses are formed from the coincidence of many axons from different neurons onto one part of a target neuron. The target neuron can then integrate the overall input into an appropriate output. Such functional clusters of synapses are commonly isolated from the adjacent nervous system by support cells of the brain, such as astrocytes.

The neuromuscular junction or motor endplate (see Chapter 13) is a specialized form of synapse between a motor nerve axon and skeletal muscle.

> **Synapses are formed mainly on the dendrites of neurons at structures called dendritic spines.**

The most common target for synapse formation is onto the dendrites of a target neuron. Such dendritic synapses form on buds of membrane which push out from the dendrite termed **dendritic spines,** with an individual dendrite containing hundreds to thousands of spines. Spines vary in size, and it has only recently become possible to quantitate spatial patterns using confocal microscopy and three-dimensional (3D) reconstruction of individual neurons (Fig. 6.11).

Dendritic spines are thought to be the anatomical location for memory storage and are dynamic structures which change shape and functional sensitivity (synaptic strength) in response to the activity of their synaptic connections.

Fig. 6.12 The Basic Types of Dendritic Spines. Dendritic spines have been classified into four basic types termed (A) stubby, (B) thin, (C) mushroom and (D) ramified.

Fig. 6.13 Detailed Morphology of Dendritic Spines. Dendritic spines show a continuum between the four basic types, which can be seen in the three-dimensional reconstruction of spines. The red areas are the site of a synapse. **(a)** Spines showing the four named types: stubby (1), thin (2), mushroom (9–11) and ramified (15). Most spines have shapes that are intermediate between these four types (3–8, 12–14). **(b)** Spines appear different depending on the angle of observation. 16–18 illustrate two spines from three points of view after 90 degrees rotation. Scale bar is 0.5 μm. (Koepsell Kilian, Wang Xin, Hirsch Judith, Sommer Friedrich, Exploring the function of neural oscillations in early sensory systems, Frontiers in Neuroscience, 3, 2010. https://www.frontiersin.org/articles/10.3389/neuro.01.010.2010.)

> **Dendritic spines change in structure in response to synaptic inputs.**

Dendritic spines show a range of shapes, and four basic types have been defined ranging from low and broad-based through to tall structures that appear as a globular head on a stalk (neck) attached to the shaft of the dendrite (Fig. 6.12). Three-dimensional reconstruction from ultrastructural studies shows a continuum of morphologies (Fig. 6.13). Within each dendritic spine there is an actin-based cytoskeleton associated with systems that can remodel the shape of the spine. In a manner similar to the terminal bouton, larger spines contain mitochondria and rough endoplasmic reticulum such that local protein synthesis can take place.

More than one synapse can be found on each dendritic spine, and although most synapses are excitatory, inhibitory synapses also terminate on spines. It is believed that spines that are elongated correlate with synapses with a higher strength, whereas low dome-shaped spines are a feature of synapses with low strength. The neck region of elongated spines has been shown to be able to modulate signalling and depolarization, thereby allowing for selective modulation of synaptic inputs to the target neuron.

Remodelling of spines can take place over a matter of hours in response to synaptic activity. Shrinkage of spines back to the low dome-shaped form is believed to relate to a reduction in synaptic strength, correlating to a reduction of function; for example, memory. In experimental systems, environmental enrichment, increased sensory stimulation and training are associated with development and stabilization of large dendritic spines. It has been proposed that creation of long-term memory is mediated through enlargement of specific dendritic spines.

MYELIN

> **Myelin wraps around axons and increases the speed of conduction.**

The speed of conduction along nerves is limited by the electrical capacitance and resistance of the axon.

Because wide axons have a lower capacitance than narrow ones, increasing their diameter is a useful means of increasing the speed of nerve conduction. This is inefficient, however, as giant axons require high metabolic upkeep.

The speed of conduction along axons can also be increased if leakage of current from the membrane is minimized by insulation.

The two functions of insulation and reduction of electrical capacitance are performed by a substance called **myelin,** which is produced by specialized support cells. These cells, which wrap layers of membrane containing the lipid-rich insulating layer around axons, are called **oligodendrocytes** in the CNS and **Schwann cells** in the PNS.

A Schwann cell myelinates only one axon, but an oligodendrocyte may myelinate several adjacent axons. Although largely identical in structure, there are significant differences in the composition of myelin formed by these two cell types.

Myelin can be stained by histological methods with affinity for the lipid or protein components of the myelin sheath, and such methods highlight the structural difference in the CNS between neuron-rich areas lower in myelin (grey matter) and tracts of axons with abundant myelin (white matter).

> **Myelin is a spiral layer of closely apposed cell membranes.**

The myelin sheath is formed by the oligodendrocytes or Schwann cells wrapping spiral layers of cell membrane around the axon. Each layer of cell membrane is linked to its neighbour by specialized cell adhesion proteins.

Myelination begins with the invagination of a single axon into the support cell, which brings its outer cell membranes into close apposition and seals them together to form a sheet of internal membrane (the mesaxon; Fig. 6.14). The line of fusion is mediated by proteins in the outer surfaces of the cell membrane and ultrastructurally forms a line (the intraperiod line). Myelination then proceeds as the support cell wraps numerous layers of the mesaxon around the axon. A tight spiral composed of double-thickness cell membrane fused together forms because the cytoplasm of the support cell is excluded from most of the space between the membrane layers.

The inner surfaces of the cell membranes also fuse together and form a dense line, the **major dense line.**

The thickness of the myelin sheath depends on the number of layers (lamellae) wrapped around the axon.

In addition to the specialized cell adhesion proteins, the cell membrane of the support cells that forms myelin also contains special lipids; for example, the glycolipid galactocerebroside, which is abundant in myelin.

The myelin insulation is not continuous along axons, being limited by the size of the myelinating cell. The small bare areas of axon between myelin sheaths are termed the **nodes of Ranvier** and are physiologically important.

Fig. 6.14 Myelin. (a) Myelin formation. First, an axon invaginates a myelin-forming cell, and the outer leaflets of the myelin-forming cell's membrane fuse to form the mesaxon. The myelin-forming cell then wraps layers of the mesaxon around the axon; the inner cytoplasm is lost when the inner leaflet of the cell membrane fuses to form the major dense line. Myelin forms into numerous lamellae of fused membrane, the lamellae being separated by alternating major dense lines and mesaxon (intraperiod line). **(b)** Low-power electron micrograph showing an axon (A) surrounded by myelin (M) and the nucleus (N) of a Schwann cell. **(c)** Medium-power electron micrograph showing the fine structure of myelin. The axon (A) is surrounded by myelin lamellae (M). Note the outer mesaxon (OM). The areas of cytoplasm in the myelin represent Schmidt–Lanterman incisures (S) (see Fig. 6.15) and the inner collar of cytoplasm (IC). **(d)** High-power electron micrograph showing the fine detail of myelin lamellae; the dark lines are the major dense lines, whereas the intraperiod lines are barely visible in between.

◎ ADVANCED CONCEPT

Cell Membranes in Myelin Are Linked Together by Specialized Proteins

The layers of cell membrane which are wrapped to form myelin are tightly bound together by special proteins. The proteins involved are different for CNS myelin and PNS myelin.

In the myelin of the CNS, proteolipid protein (PLP) links the exoplasmic surfaces of myelin membranes together. The cytoplasmic surfaces are linked through interactions with another protein called *myelin basic protein* (MBP).

In the PNS, P0 protein associates with myelin basic protein to form the major dense line. P0 protein accounts for about 50% of protein in PNS myelin.

Myelin-associated glycoprotein (MAG) is expressed on the surface of oligodendrocytes and is a member of the family of immunoglobulin-like proteins, acting as a cell-surface ligand-binding protein.

Peripheral myelin protein-22, like P0, is also involved in the formation and maintenance of myelin in the PNS.

👥 CLINICAL EXAMPLE

Abnormalities in Myelin Proteins Cause Disease of the Nervous System

Several inherited diseases of the nervous system are now recognized to be caused by abnormalities in the genes coding for myelin-related proteins.

Dominantly inherited hereditary motor and sensory neuropathy type 1 (HMSN-1) is caused by mutations in peripheral myelin protein-22 (PMP-22) in 90% of affected families. Patients develop weakness and impaired sensation caused by degeneration of the myelin in peripheral nerves.

Deletion of the gene for PMP-22 gives rise to hereditary neuropathy, with liability to pressure palsies. Patients are unusually susceptible to nerve damage after relatively trivial pressure to nerves.

Mutations in the *PLP* gene can cause two disorders. In Pelizaeus–Merzbacher disease, affected children develop degeneration of their CNS myelin and develop progressively severe mental disability. Other mutations can cause degeneration of myelin in the spinal cord, leading to spastic paraparesis. The gene for PLP is on the X chromosome, and so these diseases are seen in males.

> **Myelin is maintained by extensions of cytoplasm from the parent myelin-forming cell.**

The cell membranes forming myelin are a dynamic structure. The cytoplasm of the myelin-forming support cell remains in the myelin sheath at four sites to maintain the cell membrane. These sites are located:
- Adjacent to the axon (inner collar)
- Between the internodal myelin lamellae of PNS myelin formed by Schwann cells (Schmidt–Lanterman incisures)
- At each end of the myelin segment adjacent to the nodes of Ranvier (paranodal area, see later)
- Adjacent to the cell body on the outer aspect of the myelin (outer collar)

The cytoplasm in all these areas is in continuity with that of the cell body of the support cells so that the membrane forming the myelin can be maintained (Fig. 6.15).

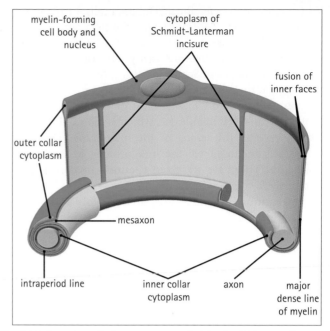

Fig. 6.15 Cytoplasmic Compartments in Myelin. If the myelin around an axon is theoretically unwrapped, the relationships between the cytoplasmic compartments become evident. The inner collar and outer collar run along and parallel to the axon, whereas the cytoplasm of the Schmidt–Lanterman incisures is wrapped around the axon in between myelin lamellae. These zones of cytoplasm are continuous with the cell body of the myelin-forming cell and serve to maintain the membrane forming the myelin.

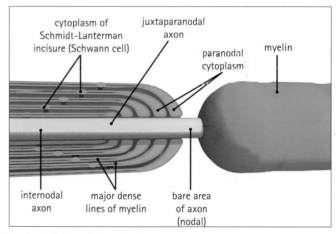

Fig. 6.16 Node of Ranvier. A node of Ranvier in longitudinal section. At the end of a myelin segment, the myelin lamellae give way to a series of paranodal loops containing cytoplasm. The adjacent bare area of axon is generally slightly wider than the internodal axon and is the region containing the voltage-gated Na⁺ channels, which are necessary for the formation of an action potential. Compare the Schmidt–Lanterman incisures in this plane with those in Fig. 6.15.

> **The nodes of Ranvier contain bare areas of axon devoid of myelin.**

Myelination of an axon is not continuous along its length but occurs in small units 1–2-mm long, each unit being formed by an individual support cell. The small space between each unit of myelin is the node of Ranvier and has an important physiological role in increasing the efficiency of nerve conduction (Fig. 6.16).

At the node of Ranvier, the myelinating cells form paranodal loops of cytoplasm in continuity with the cell body.

In the CNS, the axons in the nodes of Ranvier are bare, whereas those in the PNS are partly covered by tongues of cytoplasm from adjacent Schwann cells.

The axon at the node of Ranvier is slightly thicker than in the internodal regions and contains most of the Na$^+$-gated channels of the axonal cell membrane, which is reflected ultrastructurally as a fuzzy thickening of the membrane. These gated channels are anchored via the link protein, ankyrin, to the cytoskeleton. There are no gated channels in the internodal region beneath the myelin sheath.

Depolarization at a node of Ranvier is followed by rapid passive spread of the depolarization current along the axon beneath the myelin to the next node because leakage of current is minimized by the insulation. As the membrane capacitance is low, which is also the result of the myelin, only a small change is required to cause a significant voltage difference.

When such passively spread conduction encounters the zone of highly concentrated gated channels in the next node of Ranvier along the axon, there is further local depolarization. Thus the depolarization progresses in a series of jumps, with passive spread of charge in between.

Depolarization in a myelinated nerve is much more efficient metabolically than in a non-myelinated nerve because the restricted entry of Na$^+$ ions to small areas, instead of to the whole axonal surface, reduces the demand for energy to pump the ions back out again.

◎ ADVANCED CONCEPT

Molecular Organization Around the Node of Ranvier

Myelin-producing cells (Schwann cells or oligodendrocytes) organize the cell membrane of the axon into four specific functional areas.

The node of Ranvier: The axonal membrane in this region is enriched in Na$^+$ channels held in a molecular complex with ankyrin G and cell adhesion molecules NrCAM and neurofascin.

The paranodal region: This part of the axon lies beneath the paranodal loops of cytoplasm derived from the myelinating cell. This area is characterized by membrane-associated cell junctional proteins, such as caspr/paranodin and contactin, that bind the paranodal loops of the myelinating cell to the axon. These junctions are known as the *paranodal septate junctions*. In addition to anchoring myelin loops to the axon, these specialized junctions form a diffusion barrier into the periaxonal space and help to maintain the specialized axonal domains by preventing cell membrane diffusion.

The juxtaparanodal region: This part of the axon lies just beyond the paranodal region, with overlying compact myelin. This region has a high concentration of the delayed-rectifier K$^+$ channels, Kv1.1 and Kv1.2, held in place by contactin-associated protein-like 2 (caspr2) and mediate repolarization

The internodal region: This region of the axon is not specifically enriched in specialized proteins. Some proteins concentrated in the paranode and juxtaparanode, such as caspr, contactin, Kv1.1 and Kv1.2, extend into the internodal axon membrane as a narrow spiral aligned with the inner mesaxon of the myelinating cell.

⟫ KEY FACTS
Myelin

- Is formed by Schwann cells in the PNS and oligodendrocytes in the CNS
- Ultrastructurally is a spiral of membrane wrapped around an axon
- Contains special cell adhesion proteins and lipids which differ between the CNS and PNS
- Functions to increase the speed of conduction along axons
- Occurs in small units with a space between termed the *node of Ranvier*

CENTRAL NERVOUS SYSTEM

The CNS comprises the brain and spinal cord, which contain nerve cells and their processes, together with a series of specialized support cells.

> **The specialized support cells of the CNS are collectively called glia.**

The CNS contains numerous non-neural support cells. These are astrocytes, oligodendrocytes, ependyma and microglial cells (Fig. 6.17), which are collectively called the **glia.**

> **Astrocytes are stellate cells with roles in embryogenesis, fluid transport and structural support.**

Astrocytes are large, multiprocessed cells with several functions:
- In embryological development, forming a structural framework to guide the migration of developing nerve cells.
- Transporting fluid and ions from the extracellular space around neurons to blood vessels, regulating extracellular volume.
- Developing and eliminating synapses in addition to modulating synaptic activity and clearance of neurotransmitters.
- Propagating Ca^{2+} signals and contributing to electrical depolarization events in brain.
- They are intimately associated with synapses and can themselves release glutamate, which acts as a neurotransmitter in a process termed *gliotransmission*. These excitatory phenomena are being investigated in relation to certain forms of epilepsy.

In light microscopy, astrocytes are characterized by oval or slightly irregular nuclei with an open chromatin pattern and a typically stellate morphology, with numerous fine processes radiating in all directions. These processes contain a specific form of cytoskeletal intermediate filament called **glial fibrillary acidic protein** (GFAP).

The stellate morphology is not evident in conventional H&E sections because the processes merge with the processes of other cells, but it is seen with special staining methods (Fig. 6.18).

Four types of astrocytes have been identified in the human brain (Fig. 6.19).

Interlaminar astrocytes are seen in layer I of the cerebral cortex and have tangential processes orientated radially in addition to longer processes that run vertically down into layer III and processes that extend up to the pia to form the glia limitans (see p. 111).

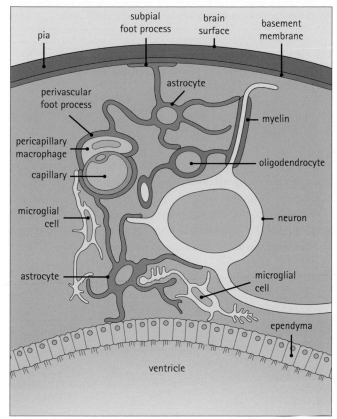

Fig. 6.17 Support Cells of the CNS. The support cells of the CNS are called glia and have several roles. Astrocytes not only support neurons and their synapses but also extend foot processes around capillaries to maintain a blood–brain barrier. At the surface of the brain, astrocytes line a basement membrane and form the glia limitans, which surrounds the whole CNS. Oligodendrocytes myelinate the axons of the nerve cells, and a vast network of antigen-sensing microglial cells is present throughout the CNS. Phagocytic macrophages, which also have an immune defence role, reside in the perivascular space, outside the CNS substance. The ependymal cells form an epithelial sheet which, unlike other epithelia, does not lie on a basement membrane. This sheet lines the fluid-filled ventricular cavities of the brain and the central canal of the spinal cord.

Fig. 6.18 Astrocytes. Micrograph stained by an immunoperoxidase method to show glial fibrillary acidic protein (GFAP), the intermediate filament of astrocytes. This example of a fibrous astrocyte is stained *brown* and shows the characteristic stellate morphology.

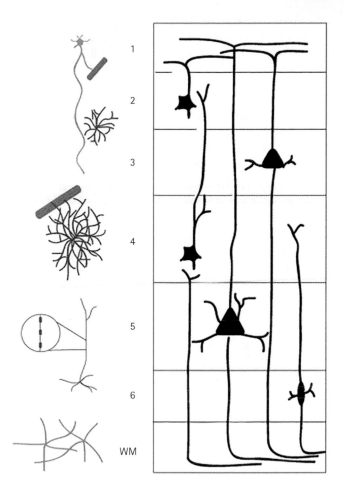

Fig. 6.19 Four Main Types of Astrocytes. Distinct classes of human astrocytes *(left)* are located within different layers of the cortex *(right)*. Interlaminar astrocytes *(light blue)* are in layer I and send long fibres that extend throughout the cortex, terminating in layers III and IV. Protoplasmic astrocytes *(dark blue)* characteristically inhabit layers II–VI and vary in size (shown here only in layers II and IV). Protoplasmic astrocytes are associated with neurons and blood vessels *(red)*. Astrocytes with varicose projections *(pink)* also extend long processes but are found in layers V and VI rather than near the pia and have varicosities along their processes *(inset)*. Fibrous astrocytes *(green)* reside in the white matter (WM). Scale bar, 100 μm. (Reprinted from Oberheim NA, Wang X, Goldman S, et al. Astrocytic complexity distinguishes the human brain. *Trends Neurosci.* 2006;29: 547–553. doi: 10.1016/j.tins.2006.08.004. Copyright 2006, with permission.)

Fibrous astrocytes are most evident in the white matter and have long cell processes, which are rich in bundles of GFAP. They contact blood vessels with foot processes, forming part of the blood–brain barrier (see p. 112) and provide metabolic support to axons and associated myelin.

Protoplasmic astrocytes are the most numerous astrocyte type and are typically seen in layers II–VI of the cerebral cortex. They have around 40 long thin processes that radiate in all directions, containing bundles of GFAP. These astrocytes are involved in formation of the blood–brain barrier (see p. 111) and also surround groups of synapses, where they have a support and modulating function.

Astrocytes with varicose projections are seen in layers V and VI of the cerebral cortex. They have poorly branched cell processes associated with multiple varicosities around 10 μm apart.

As noted earlier, one important structural adaptation of astrocytes is seen in their interaction with the blood vessels of the brain, which they surround by forming flat plates termed *end feet* (see Fig. 6.17 and p. 112). The interaction, together with changes in the associated basement membranes, induces changes in the structure of the cerebral vascular endothelium, rendering it highly impermeable, so that it acts as a barrier to diffusion between the blood and the brain. The clinical significance of this is that certain drugs cannot cross from the bloodstream to enter the brain.

CLINICAL EXAMPLE

Gliosis

When neurons die, the dead cells are removed by macrophages, by phagocytosis. The damaged area is then repaired by proliferation of astrocytic cells, which fill the defect and form an astrocytic scar in a process termed **gliosis.**

Oligodendrocytes are the myelin-forming cells of the CNS.

Oligodendrocytes produce myelin within the CNS, each cell sending out several cell processes and myelinating several nearby axons (Fig. 6.20).

In routine histological preparations of oligodendrocytes, their branching morphology is not seen, but they do show a rounded nucleus with moderately dense-staining chromatin and, in most preparations, a cytoplasm containing a clear 'halo' around the nucleus. Such a halo is an artefact of preparation because oligodendrocytes are fragile and contain few cytoskeletal elements.

Immunohistochemical staining for myelin-related proteins – for example, MBP – can be used specifically to identify oligodendrocytes (see Figs 6.20c and 6.20d).

Fig. 6.20 Oligodendrocytes. (a) Oligodendrocytes myelinate several adjacent axons within the CNS. **(b)** Ultrastructurally, the oligodendrocyte (O) has abundant mitochondria and Golgi but few cytoskeletal elements. Note processes (P) myelinating nearby axons (A). **(c)** Oligodendrocytes can be identified by immunochemical staining for specific proteins: in this instance highlighting oligodendrocytes *(brown)*, but not other cells such as microglia or astrocytes. **(d)** This section has been stained using an antibody to myelin basic protein *(brown)*. Several oligodendrocytes are seen *(arrows)*, and in the background myelin surrounding individual axons is stained. The long linear profiles are myelin sheaths around axons cut in the plane of the section. (Image used under Creative Commons License https://creativecommons.org/licenses/by-sa/3.0/ from the Human Protein Atlas Antibody to myelin basic protein CAB002300 https://www.proteinatlas.org/ENSG00000197971-MBP/brain/cerebral+cortex#img.)

Disease Affecting Myelin

Multiple Sclerosis

The myelin of the CNS is the target for attack by the immune system in multiple sclerosis (Fig. 6.21), which is of unknown cause.

Myelin is vital for the CNS to function effectively, and its destruction in multiple sclerosis results in severe functional deficits, such as paralysis, loss of sensation and/or loss of coordination. The nature of the deficit depends on the area of the CNS affected.

Fig. 6.21 Multiple Sclerosis. Low-power micrograph of cerebral cortex from a patient with multiple sclerosis (MS). Tissue is stained with *Luxol fast blue* to demonstrate myelin in the white matter (W), whereas the grey matter (G) contains far less myelin. Two pale non-staining areas, called MS plaques (P), demonstrate focal areas of myelin loss caused by immune-mediated damage to myelin.

Fig. 6.22 Ependyma. (a) Micrograph showing ependymal cells (E) lining the lateral ventricle (V) of the brain. They are cuboidal epithelial cells and rest on underlying glial processes in the brain (B). **(b)** Scanning electron micrograph showing that many of the ependymal cells bear tufts of surface cilia.

Ependymal cells are epithelial-like and have cilia.

Ependymal cells are epithelial in type and line the cavities in the brain (ventricles) and the central canal of the spinal cord, forming a sheet of cuboidal cells in contact with the cerebrospinal fluid.

Each ependymal cell has a small oval basal nucleus with dense chromatin, and many are ciliated (Fig. 6.22).

Ultrastructurally, the cells are bound to each other by prominent desmosomal junctions and have apical microvilli in addition to cilia.

Unlike other epithelial cells, the ependymal cells do not lie on a basement membrane but have tapering processes, which merge with the processes of underlying astrocytic cells.

Microglia are specialized immune cells in the CNS.

The CNS has its own unique set of immune cells, the main type being the microglial cells, which are similar to specialized macrophages.

In conventional H&E preparations, microglial cells are not easily seen, appearing only as rod-shaped nuclei, with no discernible cytoplasmic borders. Immunohistochemical staining (Fig. 6.23), however, shows that they have extensive fine ramifying processes and form a widespread network of cells throughout the brain.

Fig. 6.23 Microglia Showing a Range of Morphology in Resting and Activated States. (a) Ramified microglia exhibit highly branched processes with which they are in contact with the surrounding microenvironment. **(b)** Activated microglia retract processes and become enlarged because of organelle build-up and increased metabolic activity. **(c)** Phagocytic microglia often appear as rounded brain macrophages. **(d)** Dystrophic microglia most characteristically display beaded, twisted or fragmented processes. Human cerebral cortex stained with Iba1 antibody. (Reprinted from Streit WJ, Xue QS, Tischer J, et al. Microglial pathology. *Acta Neuropathol Commun.* 2014;2:142. http://doi.org/10.1186/s40478-014-0142-6. Copyright 2014, with permission.)

In the normal resting state microglia are ramified and have a stellate appearance of multiple radiating cell processes. In response to disease, microglia become larger and the cell processes become thicker. If microglia are activated to remove dead cells from damaged areas of the brain, they adopt a less ramified structure in which they phagocytose material from the brain for degradation and elimination. It has been found that in the aged brain, microglia develop fragmented and distorted cell processes, termed *dystrophic microglia* (see Fig. 6.23d).

Microglia have several roles in the CNS. The phenotype of microglia suggests that they are similar to dendritic antigen-presenting cells, having a low level of phagocytic activity and expressing class II major histocompatibility molecules. They are involved in remodelling neuronal networks by promoting programmed cell death and removing dead cells through phagocytosis. They are involved in synapse formation and remodelling through removal of dendritic spines. Similar to other immune mediators, microglia express receptors that recognize pathogens and can release cytokines to recruit inflammatory defence mechanisms. In such disease states, microglial cells become activated and increase in size and number. Under these circumstances, they are usually supplemented by monocytes, which enter the brain from the blood and form macrophagic cells.

In addition to the microglial cells, which are intrinsic to the brain, there are macrophages in the perivascular spaces outside the brain substance, and these cells can also act as immune effector cells.

The brain appears to have only a small traffic of lymphoid cells in the normal state.

> **The meninges are membrane systems covering and supporting the CNS.**

The CNS is invested by three protective coats, the meninges, which are composed of fibrocollagenous support tissue and epithelial cells (Fig. 6.24). There are three meningeal layers: the dura, the arachnoid and the pia.

The **dura** is a tough fibrocollagenous layer, which forms the outer coat of the CNS. It blends with the periosteum of the skull and is attached to the periosteum of the vertebral canal by the dentate ligaments. It is covered on its internal surface by an incomplete layer of flat epithelial cells.

Fig. 6.24 Meninges and Glia Limitans. (a) The meninges cover the CNS and are divided into three layers: the dura, arachnoid and pia. Below the pia, there is a basement membrane that gives rise to a set of astrocytic cells, which form a barrier around the CNS, termed the *glia limitans*. The subarachnoid space contains the cerebrospinal fluid. **(b)** Micrograph showing the arachnoid (A), subarachnoid space (SAS) and underlying brain (B). Blood vessels (BV) run in the subarachnoid space. **(c)** Meningothelial cells are normally flat, inconspicuous cells that line the dura, arachnoid and pia, but with age, some of these cells become histologically prominent; in this micrograph from the arachnoid of a 60-year-old man, the meningothelial cells (M) form a small aggregate (A). **(d)** Electron micrograph showing the glia limitans (GL), which forms an outer barrier investing the whole of the CNS. It is composed of a basement membrane, which is seen just beneath the pia collagen (P) and is produced by a sheet of closely adherent foot processes from astrocytic cells in the underlying brain.

The dura is reflected down from the skull to form sheets of tissue, the tentorium cerebelli and the falx cerebri, which separate the structures of the brain. The venous sinuses of the brain run at the base of these sheets of dura.

The **arachnoid** is a layer of fibrocollagenous tissue covered by inconspicuous flat epithelial-type cells called **meningothelial cells** and is located beneath, but not anchored to, the dura. Web-like strands of fibrocollagenous tissue extend down from the arachnoid into the subarachnoid space, which contains the cerebrospinal fluid. The main arteries and veins to and from the brain run in the subarachnoid space.

The **pia** is a delicate layer of epithelial cells associated with loose fibrocollagenous delicate tissue. It lies external to a basement membrane, which completely invests the CNS. This basement membrane is formed by a special set of astrocytes, termed the **limiting glia** (**glia limitans**).

👥 CLINICAL EXAMPLE

Meningeal Spaces in Disease

Several spaces defined by the meninges are of clinical importance. These are the subdural space, the subarachnoid space and the extradural space.

Extradural Haematoma

Fracture of the skull can cause an accumulation of blood outside the dura in the extradural space.

Subdural Haematoma

After trauma, bleeding may occur from venous channels into the space between the dura and the arachnoid (subdural space).

Subarachnoid Haemorrhage

Rupture of arteries running on the surface of the brain causes bleeding into the subarachnoid space between the arachnoid and the pia.

Meningitis

The cerebrospinal fluid in the subarachnoid space is the site of bacterial and occasionally viral infection causing meningitis.

The choroid plexus is responsible for production of cerebrospinal fluid.

The choroid plexuses are in the ventricular system of the brain and produce cerebrospinal fluid. Each choroid plexus consists of a vascular stroma covered by columnar epithelial cells, which form large frond-like masses (Fig. 6.25). The epithelial cells are anchored by junctional complexes, rest on a basement membrane, have apical microvilli and are adapted for secretion.

The cerebrospinal fluid produced in the ventricles flows out through exit foramina at the base of the brain and circulates in the subarachnoid space. It is reabsorbed by the venous sinuses in the dura.

Fig. 6.25 Choroid Plexus. **(a)** Micrograph showing a portion of choroid plexus covered with a columnar epithelium (E), which is arranged as papillae over vascular stromal cores (C). **(b)** Scanning electron micrograph showing the convoluted surface of the choroid plexus, which is thrown into deep folds, and the fine microvilli on the apical surface of the covering epithelium.

👥 CLINICAL EXAMPLE

Tumours of the Nervous System

Gliomas

Primary brain tumours are most commonly derived from the glial cells and are collectively termed **gliomas.**

The most common glioma is derived from astrocytes (**astrocytoma**) and varies from a slow-growing lesion, which diffusely infiltrates the brain over many years, to a rapidly growing lesion, termed **glioblastoma,** that soon compresses vital structures.

Ependymomas commonly arise in childhood in the region of the ventricles and are recognized histologically by their epithelial characteristics. **Oligodendrogliomas** are most common in the temporal lobe, where they may be a cause of temporal lobe epilepsy.

Certain tumours of the CNS resemble the primitive embryonic cells of the developing brain and are grouped together as **primitive neuroectodermal tumours** (PNETs). These are most common in childhood and may show differentiation toward neuronal, astrocytic or ependymal cells.

Meningiomas

The epithelial cells of the meninges (meningothelial cells) may form tumours termed *meningiomas*. These tumours appear macroscopically as rounded nodules, typically 3–4 cm in size, but can be much larger. Histologically, meningiomas are made up of sheets of meningothelial cells which characteristically form spherical whorls.

Confirming the Diagnosis

The diagnosis of CNS tumours must be confirmed by histology of tumour biopsies, and immunohistochemistry is used routinely to identify cell types within a tumour. Finding GFAP is a strong indication that a tumour is of glial origin,

Blood vessels entering the CNS are surrounded by a perivascular space.

A blood–brain barrier prevents diffusion of materials into the CNS from the blood.

The brain is supplied with blood from major arteries that form an anastomotic link around the base of the brain. From this region, the arteries run in the subarachnoid space before turning and dipping down into the brain.

Around the large vessels within the brain is a perivascular space, called, eponymously, the **Virchow–Robin space.** In humans, this space is sealed from the subarachnoid space by reflections of the pia on to the blood vessels as they enter the brain (Fig. 6.26) and is therefore continuous with the potential subpial space.

The perivascular space is bounded externally by the basement membrane of the glia limitans (see Fig. 6.24d) and extends as far as the capillaries, where the vascular and glial basement membranes fuse.

The microvascular system in the nervous system is highly specialized. The endothelial cells of brain capillaries are joined by occluding junctions and are not fenestrated; hence they form a barrier to the diffusion of substances from the blood to the brain. The brain endothelial cells have systems for active transport of substances, such as glucose, into the brain.

External to the capillary endothelium is a basement membrane, and external to this is a layer composed of the foot processes of astrocytes (see Fig. 6.17).

These three layers (endothelium, basal lamina, astrocyte foot processes) form a functional **blood–brain barrier,** which is important in the physiology of CNS function. There is considerable evidence that, in embryogenesis, it is the interaction of astrocyte foot processes that is responsible for induction of the special properties of the cerebral capillary endothelial cells.

Fig. 6.26 Vascular Arrangement in the Brain. (a) Arteries running in the subarachnoid space penetrate the pia, which is reflected up onto the wall of the vessel, thus isolating the perivascular space from the subarachnoid space. The layer of pia reflected onto the vessel is composed of a single layer of flat meningothelial cells anchored by junctional complexes. The perivascular space is continuous with the potential subpial space. **(b)** Micrograph showing vessels (V) penetrating the surface of the brain (B) from the subarachnoid space (SAS). The pia (P) is reflected onto the vessel wall and separates the subarachnoid space from the perivascular space (PVS). **(c)** Scanning electron micrograph showing the subarachnoid space (SAS) with an artery (A) becoming invested by pia (P). Note the underlying subpial space (SPS) and brain (B).

PERIPHERAL NERVOUS SYSTEM

> **The PNS is made up of nerve cells and support cells.**

The PNS is described in terms of nerves and ganglia.

A **peripheral nerve** is a collection of axons, linked together by support tissue into an anatomically defined trunk. The axons may be either motor or sensory, myelinated or non-myelinated.

A **ganglion** is a peripheral collection of nerve cell bodies together with efferent and afferent axons and support cells. Ganglia may be sensory (e.g. spinal sensory ganglia) or contain the cell bodies of autonomic nerves (i.e. sympathetic or parasympathetic ganglia).

> **Peripheral nerves are bundles of axons associated with support tissues.**

A peripheral nerve is composed of:
- Axons
- Schwann cells, which make myelin
- Spindle-shaped fibroblast support cells, which produce fibrocollagenous tissue
- Blood vessels

> **The endoneurium, perineurium and epineurium are composed of support tissues.**

There are three types of support tissue in a nerve trunk: the endoneurium, perineurium and epineurium (Figs 6.27–6.29).

Endoneurium is composed of longitudinally orientated collagen fibres, extracellular matrix material rich in glycosaminoglycans and sparse fibroblasts. It surrounds the individual axons and their associated Schwann cells, in addition to capillary blood vessels.

Perineurium surrounds groups of axons and endoneurium to form small bundles (fascicles). It is composed of 7–10 concentric layers of epithelium-like flattened cells separated by layers of collagen (see Fig. 6.29). The cells are joined by junctional complexes, and each layer of cells is surrounded by an external lamina.

Epineurium is an outer sheath of loose fibrocollagenous tissue that binds individual nerve fascicles into a nerve trunk. The epineurium may also include adipose tissue and a main muscular artery supplying the nerve trunk.

Fig. 6.27 Support Tissue of Peripheral Nerve. (a) The arrangement of support tissue in a peripheral nerve. Individual axons and their associated Schwann cells are surrounded by endoneurium and bound into fascicles by the epithelial-like perineurium. The epineurium binds individual fascicles into a nerve trunk and contains the main muscular artery supplying the nerve trunk. **(b)** Resin-embedded section of a sural nerve stained with *toluidine blue*. The epineurium (E), which binds eight nerve fascicles (F) into a nerve trunk, contains intraneural blood vessels (BV) and grey-stained adipose tissue and pale-blue collagen. A thin layer of perineurium (P) can be identified around each fascicle. At this low magnification, not much detail can be seen within each fascicle – *toluidine blue* stains myelin, and this is the reason for the dense staining within each fascicle. **(c)** Micrograph from a wax-embedded H&E section showing nerve fascicles (F) surrounded by perineurium (P) and grouped into a nerve trunk by epineurium (E). Note blood vessels (BV). (Micrograph (b) from digital pathology whole slide image provided by the University of Leeds Virtual Pathology Project https://www.virtualpathology.leeds.ac.uk. Reproduced with permission.)

Fig. 6.28 Peripheral Nerve Longitudinal Section. This H&E micrograph shows the appearance of a peripheral nerve sectioned along its length. The axons and myelin are pale-stained. It is possible to see linear structures, but little detail can be appreciated of the fine structure in such routine sections. Myelin becomes vacuolated in wax-embedded tissue, as shown here. The numerous elongated nuclei seen within the fascicle are Schwann cell nuclei. The perineurium (P) is also seen. (Micrograph from digital pathology whole slide image provided by the University of Leeds Virtual Pathology Project https://www.virtualpathology. leeds.ac.uk. Reproduced with permission.)

Fig 6.29 Perineurium. The perineurium (P) is composed of several layers of flattened cells. Ultrastructurally, these are ramified, surrounded by an external lamina and anchored together by tight junctions. The perineurial layer has between 8 and 20 layers of perineurial cells, with a thicker layer in larger nerves. On the *left* of this figure is part of a nerve fascicle stained by H&E and on the *right* stained using immunohistochemistry with an antibody to epithelial membrane antigen (EMA), which strongly stains perineurial cells. These cells are of epithelial type and are understood to have a barrier function in establishing the endoneurial space within the nerve bundle. (Micrograph from digital pathology whole slide image provided by the University of Leeds Virtual Pathology Project https://www.virtualpathology.leeds.ac.uk. Reproduced with permission.)

> **Schwann cells support both myelinated and non-myelinated axons in the PNS.**

Within a peripheral nerve, there are both myelinated and non-myelinated axons, which are both supported by Schwann cells. Each Schwann cell has a well-defined external lamina, which separates the cell from the endoneurium.

The myelin of a peripheral nerve differs from that in the CNS, as it has a different set of myelin-related proteins. Each Schwann cell produces myelin for one axon, and this contrasts with oligodendrocytes in the CNS (p. 108).

In addition to producing myelin, Schwann cells support non-myelinated axons, which bury themselves into the Schwann cell cytoplasm (Figs 6.30 and 6.31).

Nerves vary in their relative composition of myelinated and non-myelinated fibres from one anatomical site to another. Myelinated fibres in a typical peripheral nerve in the lower limb of an adult vary in diameter from 2 to 17 μm (including myelin), there being a bimodal distribution with peaks around 5 μm and 13 μm.

> **Ganglia are neuronal relay centres in the PNS.**

There are two locations of ganglia: sensory (e.g. spinal sensory ganglia, trigeminal ganglia) and autonomic (i.e. sympathetic or parasympathetic ganglia).

A ganglion is composed of:
- Neuron cell bodies
- Support cells (satellite cells and Schwann cells)
- Axons
- Loose fibrocollagenous support tissue, including a capsule (Fig. 6.32)

The neuron cell bodies are large; they have abundant cytoplasm containing Nissl substance and large nuclei with prominent nucleoli.

Satellite cells are small support cells resembling Schwann cells that surround the neuron cell bodies.

Myelinated and non-myelinated axons run to and from the ganglion and are also present within the capsule.

Fig. 6.30 Peripheral Nerve. (a) Micrograph of the edge of a single fascicle from a peripheral nerve stained with osmium, which stains myelin *black*. The perineurium (P) surrounds the fascicle. The myelinated axons appear as circular profiles with the central non-staining area occupied by axon. Non-myelinated fibres are not visible. **(b)** Micrograph of a small nerve fascicle embedded in resin and stained with *toluidine blue*. The increased resolution allows myelinated axons (M) to be seen with associated Schwann cell nuclei (S) and endoneurial support tissue (E). The perineurium (P) is visible as two to three thin cell and collagen layers. **(c)** Non-myelinated fibres are buried into and thereby supported by the cytoplasm of Schwann cells. **(d)** Electron micrograph showing non-myelinated axons (A) of a peripheral nerve embedded in the cytoplasm of Schwann cells (S).

Fig 6.31 Axon Ultrastructure. This electron micrograph shows axons (A) in cross-section. Some are myelinated axons and surrounded by myelin (M), and others are non-myelinated and simply surrounded by Schwann cell cytoplasm. The axons contain small, dark, dot-like structures, which are transversely sectioned microtubules. Also within the axon are less well-defined grey-coloured filaments, which are intermediate filaments composed of neurofilament protein. Within some axons, large, rounded bodies are seen, which are cargo in transit along the axon.

Fig. 6.32 Ganglion. Micrograph showing a peripheral autonomic ganglion containing neurons (N) with large nuclei and prominent nucleoli surrounded by small satellite support cells with darkly stained rounded nuclei. Axons running to and from the ganglion are supported by Schwann cells, and a loose fibrocollagenous stroma is seen surrounding the ganglion cells. A perineurial capsule surrounds the ganglion.

CLINICAL EXAMPLE

Repair in the PNS

The axons of neurons can regenerate after damage if the cell body remains alive.

After section of a nerve supplying a muscle, the axons and myelin beyond the area of damage degenerate and are removed by Schwann cell lysosomes and by macrophages, which migrate into the nerve. This is called *Wallerian degeneration*. The neuron cell body accumulates large amounts of neurofilaments, and the Nissl substance and nucleus migrate peripherally, so that it appears pale and swollen with an eccentric nucleus (chromatolysis).

The Schwann cells proliferate and form longitudinal columns of cells in the distal damaged nerve. At the proximal end the damaged axons regrow by sprouting, with the sprouts growing down the cords of Schwann cells at 2–5 mm/day. One fibre may eventually connect with the muscle, become remyelinated and re-establish innervation (Fig. 6.33). The cell body then resumes a normal appearance.

Fig. 6.33 Repair in the PNS. After damage to a myelinated neuron innervating a muscle fibre, the distal axon and myelin are phagocytosed by proliferating Schwann cells. The muscle fibre, devoid of innervation, undergoes wasting, while the cell body of the neuron undergoes chromatolysis, with swelling, lateral migration of the nucleus and loss of Nissl substance. Axons then sprout from the damaged end of the nerve and grow down the column of Schwann cells, eventually restoring innervation of the muscle. The Schwann cells remyelinate the axon, but the myelin segments are much shorter than before the damage.

For online review questions, please visit https://studentconsult.inkling.com.

Blood Cells

INTRODUCTION

> The blood is a mixture of cellular elements, fluid, proteins and metabolites.

Blood has four major elements:

- **Red blood cells** (erythrocytes) transport oxygen from the lungs to the peripheral tissues.
- **White blood cells** (leukocytes) have a defensive role, destroying infecting organisms, such as bacteria and viruses, and assisting in the removal of dead or damaged tissues.
- **Platelets** (thrombocytes) are the first line of defence against damage to blood vessels, adhering to defects and participating in the blood clotting system.
- **Plasma** is the proteinaceous solution in which the previously mentioned cells circulate and carries nutrients, metabolites, antibodies, hormones, proteins of the blood clotting system and other molecules throughout the body.

In postnatal life, under normal circumstances, the formation of the cellular elements of the blood (**haematopoiesis**) occurs in the **bone marrow** in various bones (see p. 131). Most of the proteins in the plasma are made by the liver.

BONE MARROW–DERIVED STEM CELLS

> The bone marrow contains at least two kinds of stem cells.

One population, called *haematopoietic stem cells,* can form all the types of blood cells in the body. These are the cells useful clinically for bone marrow transplants.

A second population is called *bone marrow stromal stem cells* or *mesenchymal stem cells.* These non-haematopoietic stem cells make up a small proportion of the stromal cell population in the bone marrow and can generate bone, cartilage, fat, cells that support the formation of blood and fibrous connective tissue (see Fig. 4.17). These cells are under study as sources of different cell types for regenerative medicine.

METHODS OF STUDYING THE BLOOD CELLS

In haematoxylin and eosin (H&E)–stained histological sections blood is usually encountered within the blood vessels, and it is important to be able to identify blood when encountered in histological sections (Fig. 7.1). However, in clinical work, morphological examination is usually performed on a blood sample taken with a needle and syringe. The name for the two main types of cells in blood derives from what is seen if blood is prevented from clotting and left to stand in a tube. Blood settles into several layers: a thick layer of clear plasma is seen at the top of the tube, beneath which is a very thin layer of white material ("buffy coat") on top of a thick layer of red material. The cells in the white material are called *white cells,* and the cells in the red material are called *red cells.*

The usual way to look at blood is to make a very thin smear on a glass slide. The names applied to the white cells are largely derived from the stains used to examine blood smears. The main staining method used (Romanowsky stain) involves applying several dyes that have an affinity for different cellular constituents (Fig. 7.2).

Under the microscope it is possible to count the proportion of different cell types in blood, and as it has been found that this reflects disease processes, a blood count is a valuable diagnostic tool. In modern laboratory practice, routine counting of cells in blood is done electronically on preparations of cells in suspension. Smears of blood are still examined for morphological abnormalities of cells.

Fig. 7.1 Micrography of Blood Inside a Blood Vessel (V). In H&E sections red cells (R) are brightly eosinophilic. Plasma proteins form pink-staining material (P). White blood cells can be identified proportional to their numbers in the blood; hence neutrophils (N) and lymphocytes (L) may be often seen but eosinophils, basophils or monocytes are less commonly encountered. The quality of morphology is not as good as can be obtained by a smear preparation, as shown in Fig. 7.2.

Fig. 7.2 Blood Film. A blood film is made by smearing a sample of peripheral blood, previously mixed with an anticoagulant, on a slide and staining it with a mixture of dyes. Four types of white blood cells (nucleated) are seen against a background of numerous smaller anucleate red blood cells. Very small, purple-stained structures are platelets.

RED BLOOD CELLS

Red blood cells are highly deformable and are specialized for carrying oxygen.

The red blood cells are responsible for oxygen transport. Red cells in peripheral blood smears (Figs 7.3a and 7.3b) appear as rounded, bright pink–stained cells. They are 6.5–8.5 μm in diameter and have a biconcave shape, appearing paler in the centre and darker at the periphery. The biconcave shape maximizes their surface area–to–volume ratio and thereby maximizes oxygen exchange. The bright pink colour (acidophilia) is a result of the content of oxygen-carrying haemoglobin, which binds the acidic eosin dye used in staining. Red cells do not have a nucleus, as this is lost during formation. In paraffin-processed tissue sections, red cells appear smaller and the biconcave shape is generally not discernible.

Ultrastructurally, red cells have a cell membrane, which surrounds an electron-dense cytoplasm that contains haemoglobin. There are no discernible organelles, as these have been lost during differentiation. Despite a lack of organelles, red cells are metabolically active and derive energy from anaerobic metabolism of glucose and through adenosine triphosphate (ATP) generation by the hexose monophosphate shunt.

Functionally, red cells are highly deformable and can squeeze through small blood vessels down to 3–4 μm in diameter. The cell membrane is braced by an actin/spectrin-containing cytoskeletal meshwork, which is largely responsible for maintaining the distinctive biconcave shape (see Figs 7.3c and 7.3d).

Fig. 7.3 Mature Red Cell. (a) Typical appearance of a mature red cell in a stained smear of the peripheral blood. It is a biconcave disc 1.8 μm thick and ranges from 6.5 to 8.5 μm in diameter, the size decreasing slightly with age. Its main cytoplasmic constituent is the protein complex haemoglobin, which results in its characteristic acidophilic-staining property. Because of its biconcave shape, which facilitates oxygen exchange, the centre of the cell appears pale. **(b)** Scanning electron micrograph showing the typical biconcave structure of a mature red cell. **(c)** The red cell cytoskeleton maintains its distinct shape. A filamentous skeleton of the protein spectrin is anchored to the cell membrane by three main proteins (band 3 protein, ankyrin and band 4 protein), with short actin pieces, about 15 actin monomers long, linking spectrin to the band 4 protein. Other proteins are also involved but have been omitted for clarity. **(d)** Micrograph immunostained for spectrin *(brown)* showing red cells in a blood vessel. The cells show staining of their membranes corresponding to the location of cytoskeletal proteins bracing the red cell membrane. (Image **(d)** used under Creative Commons License https://creativecommons.org/licenses/by-sa/3.0/ from the Human Protein Atlas Antibody to erythrocytic spectrin B HPA003394 https://www.proteinatlas.org/ENSG00000070182-SPTB/tissue/bone+marrow#img.)

Red cells have a limited lifespan and are eventually destroyed in the spleen.

Red cells have a lifespan of 100–120 days in the circulation. The mature red blood cell is unable to synthesize new enzymes to replace those lost during normal metabolic processes. Diminishing efficiency of ion pumping mechanisms is probably the main factor in red cell ageing, the cell becoming progressively less deformable until it is unable to negotiate the splenic microcirculation and is removed by phagocytosis. The spleen, liver and bone marrow all dispose of aged and defective red cells, but their relative contributions under normal conditions are uncertain; the spleen appears to be the most active.

 CLINICAL EXAMPLE

Hereditary Spherocytosis

Hereditary spherocytosis is caused by an abnormal arrangement of the internal cytoskeleton of red cells. Normally the internal surface of the cell membrane is braced by cytoskeletal proteins via interactions between ankyrin and spectrin (see Fig. 7.3c). In hereditary spherocytosis, a defect in spectrin or the ankyrin binding of spectrin is the main underlying abnormality. As a result, the red cell membrane is not braced and is easily deformed.

In hereditary spherocytosis, red cells do not form their normal biconcave disc shape, but rather appear round and convex (Fig. 7.4). They are abnormally brittle and less deformable than normal red cells, and so do not pass easily through the splenic microcirculation (see Fig. 8.21). They are trapped there and rapidly destroyed in large numbers; this excessive breakdown of red blood cells is called **haemolysis**.

Fig. 7.4 Hereditary Spherocytosis. Micrograph showing the abnormal round convex blood cell of hereditary spherocytosis. Many of the cells do not have the normal pale-stained central area as is seen in a normal concave-shaped red cell (compare with Fig. 7.3a) and are called spherocytes.

⟫ **KEY FACTS**

Red Cells

- Biconcave shape for high surface area–to–volume ratio
- Main function is oxygen and carbon dioxide transport
- Contain haemoglobin
- Have no cell organelles
- Cell membrane is braced by an actin/spectrin-containing cytoskeleton which maintains shape

CLINICAL EXAMPLE

Anaemia

The most common blood disorder is anaemia, in which an inadequate haemoglobin supply reduces oxygen-carrying capacity in blood and causes tiredness, weakness, pallor and, sometimes, breathlessness. It may be the result of either impaired red cell formation or excessive red cell destruction.

The most common cause is **deficiency of iron,** which is essential for the formation of haemoglobin. Red cells are released into the circulation containing much less haemoglobin than normal and are therefore pale staining (hypochromic) and small (microcytic) (Fig. 7.5).

Excessive red cell destruction usually occurs because the red cells are structurally abnormal and therefore more liable to damage while circulating. Such cells are removed prematurely and in excess by the spleen, causing **haemolytic anaemia.** This can be the result of a genetic abnormality of red cell structure and occurs in hereditary spherocytosis (see Fig. 7.4). Point mutations in the haemoglobin gene may cause abnormal red cells. Sickle cell anaemia is caused by such a mutation, leading to precipitation of haemoglobin in red cells subject to hypoxia, which causes a sickle shape instead of the biconcave disc. Sickled cells become disrupted and can also block blood vessels.

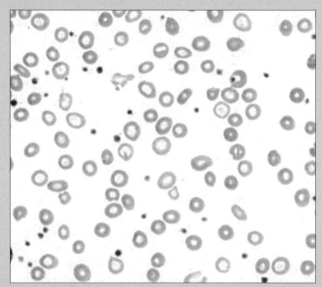

Fig. 7.5 Hypochromic, Microcytic Anaemia. Micrograph of blood smear showing that most red cells are very pale, especially in the concave central part (hypochromic), and many are also very small (microcytic). This is the result of iron deficiency. The pale appearance is because of a very low concentration of haemoglobin pigment in each cell. The blue dot-like structures in the film are platelets. A feature of many patients with iron deficiency is an increased platelet count (thrombocytosis). Compare density of red cell staining with Fig. 7.2 and 7.3a.

WHITE BLOOD CELLS

There are five main types of white blood cells.

White cells use the blood for transport from the bone marrow to their major sites of activity. Most functions of white blood cells take place when they leave the circulation to enter tissues. The total number of white cells in peripheral blood is normally $4.0–11.0 \times 10^9/L$.

There are five types of white cells, and their names and relative proportions in the circulation are as follows:

- Neutrophils: 40%–75%
- Eosinophils: 5%
- Basophils: 0.5%
- Lymphocytes: 20%–50%
- Monocytes: 1%–5%

If there is a requirement for increased activity of any one cell type in the peripheral tissues, the number and proportion of that cell type rise accordingly.

Neutrophils, eosinophils and basophils are known as **granulocytes** because their cytoplasm contains prominent granules, and they may also be referred to as *myeloid cells* because of their origin from bone marrow. Neutrophils are also commonly called *polymorphonuclear leukocytes* or *polymorphs* because of their multilobed nucleus.

Lymphocytes and monocytes are classed as white blood cells because they are a constituent of the blood and ultimately originate from bone marrow. They are found mainly in tissues such as lymph nodes and spleen. In the tissues, monocytes transform into macrophages.

> **Neutrophils are the most common type of white blood cell.**

Neutrophils (Fig. 7.6) are the most abundant of the circulating white cells. They circulate in a resting state but, with appropriate activation, leave the blood and enter tissues, where they become highly motile, phagocytic cells. Their primary function is as part of the innate immune system (see Chapter 8) to ingest and destroy invading micro-organisms in tissues. They play a central role in the early stages of the acute inflammatory response to tissue injury and are the major constituents of purulent exudate ('pus').

There are normally $1.5–10 \times 10^9$/L neutrophils in peripheral blood; a rise to above 10×10^9/L is called **neutrophilia** and is usually an indication of bacterial infection or tissue necrosis (e.g. myocardial infarction). A reduction in numbers of circulating neutrophils below 1.5×10^9/L is called **neutropenia** or agranulocytosis; this reduction in numbers can be the result of decreased production in the bone marrow or increased destruction in the tissues. The danger of persistent neutropenia is that the patient becomes highly vulnerable to severe bacterial infections.

> **The neutrophil nucleus has several lobes.**

The characteristic neutrophil nucleus is composed of two to five distinct lobes, joined to one another by fine strands of nuclear material, with the lobulation developing with cellular maturity. The chromatin is highly condensed, reflecting a low degree of protein synthesis.

In females, about 3% of nuclei exhibit a small, condensed nuclear appendage (drumstick chromosome), which represents the quiescent X chromosome (Barr body).

Fig. 7.6 Neutrophil. **(a)** A mature neutrophil is 12–14 μm in diameter and has a characteristic multilobed nucleus (N) and pale-staining cytoplasm, in which only a few of the many granules it contains can be seen with routine stain. **(b)** Electron micrograph of a neutrophil from the blood, showing its characteristic multilobed nucleus (N), cytoplasmic processes (CP) and a mixture of granule types within its cytoplasm. At this magnification, individual granule types cannot be identified.

⊚ ADVANCED CONCEPT

White Cell Traffic From Blood Vessels Is Mediated by Cell Adhesion Molecules

Normally, white cells circulate in the blood in an inactive state. To leave a capillary vessel and enter tissues, white cells have first to stick to the endothelium lining the capillaries and then pass into the tissues by traversing the vessel wall. The adhesion to endothelium is mediated by complementary cell adhesion molecules expressed on the white cell surface and the surface of the endothelium. In the healthy state, such molecules are not strongly expressed, and so there is little traffic. In disease states, cytokines cause activation of both white cells and endothelium, there is high expression of adhesion molecules and cells stick firmly to the endothelium. Further cell signals then cause white cells to become motile and gain the ability to actively migrate into the tissues.

> **Neutrophils contain three types of granules.**

Neutrophil cytoplasm contains three types (i.e. primary, secondary and tertiary, related to the sequential phases of neutrophil maturation at which they appear) of membrane-bound vesicles (granules) and secretory vesicles (Fig. 7.7).

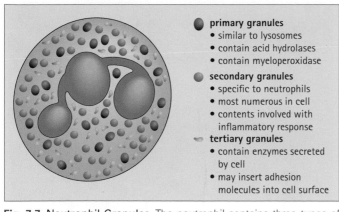

Fig. 7.7 Neutrophil Granules. The neutrophil contains three types of granules.

- **primary granules**
  - similar to lysosomes
  - contain acid hydrolases
  - contain myeloperoxidase
- **secondary granules**
  - specific to neutrophils
  - most numerous in cell
  - contents involved with inflammatory response
- **tertiary granules**
  - contain enzymes secreted by cell
  - may insert adhesion molecules into cell surface

◎ ADVANCED CONCEPT

Neutrophils Are Adapted for Anaerobic Metabolism

The neutrophil cytoplasm contains few organelles apart from granules. There are only a few scattered profiles of rough endoplasmic reticulum and free ribosomes, with the remnants of the Golgi complex involved in granule packaging earlier in development. Although mitochondria are also few, they provide about 50% of energy needs.

Once activated, neutrophils need to be able to operate in devascularized tissue, where oxygen and glucose may be in short supply. They therefore contain abundant glycogen for anaerobic metabolism, which occurs mainly via the glycolytic pathway. Energy production may also take place via the hexose monophosphate shunt, but this is used to generate microbicidal oxidants rather than for general cellular upkeep.

Once neutrophils have become activated in tissues, they do not live for long, only a day or two. The neutrophil cytoplasm also contains various antioxidants to destroy potentially toxic peroxides that may be generated during lysosomal activity.

Primary or azurophilic granules are the first granules to appear at the promyelocytic stage during neutrophil formation, but as the cell matures, their number falls with respect to secondary granules (see below), making them more difficult to see with light microscopy. With electron microscopy, they are large and electron-dense. Primary granules contain antibacterial substances linked to the innate immune system, including elastase, myeloperoxidase, cathepsins and defensins. Myeloperoxidase, which can be detected by the peroxidase stain, is therefore a useful light microscopic marker not only for these granules but also in establishing cell lineage in the diagnosis of leukaemias (see p. 126).

Secondary or specific granules develop during the myelocyte stage of neutrophil maturation and are twice as numerous as primary granules. With a diameter of 0.2–0.8 μm (i.e. smaller than primary granules), they are barely visible on light microscopy.

Ultrastructural studies have shown secondary granules to be variable in size, shape and density; are myeloperoxidase-negative; and contain lactoferrin and proteolytic enzymes. These substances are secreted into the extracellular environment.

Tertiary or gelatinase granules are formed during the metamyelocyte stage and contain proteolytic enzymes (e.g. matrix metalloprotease 9 [gelatinase] and collagenase) that are secreted into the extracellular environment. These enzymes degrade structural components of the extracellular matrix, helping to facilitate neutrophil extravasation and migration during inflammation.

Neutrophils also contain secretory vesicles which contain integrins and other factors thought to promote apoptosis and help to mediate inflammatory reactions.

> **Neutrophils migrate into areas of tissue damage, where they have a defensive role.**

Phagocytosis (Fig. 7.8) is the process whereby cells ingest extracellular particles for destruction. Neutrophils have a role in the phagocytosis of bacteria and dead cells.

Fig. 7.8 Neutrophil Phagocytosis. (a) Neutrophils have membrane receptors, mainly for the Fc portion of antibodies, complement factors bound to foreign particles and bacterial polysaccharides. Neutrophils do not phagocytose material to which they do not bind. **(b)** As the first step in phagocytosis, the neutrophil binds to the abnormal particle by its specific receptors. The cell pushes out pseudopodia to surround the particle, driven by assembly and disassembly of actin filaments. **(c)** The pseudopodia fuse to enclose completely the abnormal particle and form an endocytotic vesicle. Special proteins probably allow final sealing of the membrane. **(d)** The internalized particle in the endocytotic vesicle is called a phagosome. **(e)** The phagosome fuses with neutrophil granules, particularly primary granules, which discharge their contents, exposing the particle to a potent mixture of lysosomal enzymes. If the particle is a bacterium, killing is enhanced by hydrogen peroxide and superoxide generated by the enzymatic reduction of oxygen by respiratory burst oxidase (RBO), a membrane enzyme. **(f)** Foreign particle destruction is associated with the formation of a residual body containing degraded material.

To reach an area of infection or tissue damage, neutrophils leave the circulation by adhering to endothelial cells using adhesion molecules expressed in response to local secretion of cytokines and move through the endothelium and basement membrane.

Once in the extravascular tissue, neutrophils respond to chemicals (chemotaxins), moving towards the highest concentration. Chemotaxins include degradation products of complement, products leaking from dead cells and bacterially derived polysaccharides in the extracellular space. Neutrophil motility is derived from the assembly and disassembly of cellular actin filaments.

Activation of membrane receptors, some linked to phagocytosis, signals the neutrophil to release the contents of its granules by exocytosis in a process termed **neutrophil degranulation**. The activation of neutrophils can also release an extracellular meshwork composed of chromatin and proteases called **neutrophil extracellular traps (NETs)**, which immobilize and can kill bacteria.

Neutrophils typically die soon after phagocytosis and degranulation, as this highly energy-dependent process uses up their glycogen reserve. The granule contents, which have been released into the extracellular space, contribute to liquefaction of adjacent tissue and are directly toxic to many types of bacteria. They also cause activation of local macrophages (p. 140) and local dendritic cells responsible for antigen presentation (p. 141).

The collection of dead neutrophils, tissue fluid and debris is described as purulent exudate, or *pus*.

Fig. 7.9 Eosinophil. (a) The eosinophil is 12–17 μm in diameter in blood films and is easily recognizable by its large granules, which stain bright red. Most have a bilobed nucleus, but nuclear detail is often obscured by the numerous overlying, densely packed granules. **(b)** Electron micrograph of an eosinophil from blood showing its characteristic bilobed nucleus (N), scattered mitochondria (M) and cytoplasmic glycogen. The characteristic granules (LG) are large and ovoid in shape (0.15–1.5 μm long and 0.3–1.0 μm wide) and contain a central electron-dense crystalloid (C), surrounded by a less dense matrix. In humans, the crystalloid has a cubic lattice structure and consists of an extremely alkaline (basic) protein called *major basic protein,* in addition to other basic proteins, hydrolytic lysosomal enzymes and eosinophil peroxidase, which has a different substrate specificity to the neutrophil myeloperoxidase. Smaller granules (G) 0.1–1.5 μm in diameter are also present in mature eosinophils and contain acid phosphatase and aryl sulphatase, which is eight times more concentrated than in other white cells and appears to be secreted in the absence of phagocytosis and degranulation.

> ▶▶ **KEY FACTS**
>
> *Neutrophils*
>
> - One of the myeloid series of white blood cells
> - One of the granulocyte type of white blood cells
> - Main role as part of innate defences in phagocytosis and bacterial killing
> - Contain granules in cytoplasm
> - Cells marked by myeloperoxidase
> - Increased numbers in blood during bacterial infections and inflammation ('neutrophilia')

Eosinophils have a bilobed nucleus and acidophilic granules.

Eosinophils have a bilobed nucleus and contain strongly eosinophilic granules (Fig. 7.9). They are phagocytic, with an affinity for antigen–antibody complexes but have less microbicidal activity than neutrophils.

After production in the bone marrow, eosinophils are stored for approximately 8 days before release into the circulation, where they remain for 6–12 hours before preferentially migrating to the skin, lungs and gastrointestinal tract, where they reside for 1–2 weeks. They may enter lung and gut secretions via lymphatics or by direct migration. A population is resident in the thymus gland (see Chapter 8).

Circulating eosinophil numbers show a marked diurnal variation, being maximal in the morning and minimal in the afternoon. Eosinophils are an important component of innate defences and in modulating adaptive immune responses (see Chapter 8). In disease, they are involved in asthma, a range of allergic disorders and in the responses to parasitic diseases. Tissue (and sometimes blood) eosinophil numbers are increased in certain allergic states; for example, in the nasal and bronchial mucosae in hay fever and asthma and in adverse reactions to drugs. Eosinophils do not usually re-enter the circulation after tissue migration.

Basophils and mast cells have similar functions.

Basophils are the least common white cell in the blood. They are characterized by large, intensely basophilic, cytoplasmic granules (Fig. 7.10a). Mast cells are tissue-resident cells and have large basophilic granules (see Fig. 7.10b). Although it was thought that mast cells were derived from basophils, studies have shown that mast cells are derived from a separate haematopoietic progenitor cell.

Mast cells reside in support tissues, especially those beneath epithelia, around blood vessels and lining serous cavities. They are long-lived (weeks to months) and can proliferate in the tissues.

Eosinophil Phagocytosis and Degranulation

Like neutrophils, eosinophils move chemotactically in response to signalling systems. The cytokine interleukin-5 (IL-5), mainly produced by T-helper lymphocytes (see Chapter 8), is most important. Eosinophils respond to a group of eosinophil-specific chemokines termed **eotaxins**.

All eosinophils have surface receptors for IgE (not found on neutrophils), which may be involved in the destruction of parasites. Only a few eosinophils have IgG-Fc receptors, but these increase in eosinophilia. Eosinophils can act as part of the innate immunity system through expression of receptors for pathogen- and damage-associated molecular patterns (PAMPs/DAMPs) (see Chapter 8).

In response to activation signals, eosinophils release granule contents into the external environment (**eosinophil degranulation**). This may be by simple exocytosis, but in some circumstances, granules fuse inside the cell to form a giant granule, which then fuses at a single pore in the cell membrane, something seen in the response to large parasites.

The granule contents such as eosinophil cationic proteins (ECPs), major basic protein (MBP) and eosinophil peroxidase (EPX) have cytotoxic properties. When degranulated, cells can also form eosinophil extracellular DNA traps (EETs), composed of a net of mitochondrial DNA and granule proteins, which together can trap bacteria and facilitate bacterial killing. Eosinophils can also recruit helper T cells, forming a link between innate defences and the adaptive immune response (see Chapter 8).

Mast cells and eosinophils are seen together in several allergic conditions. The activation of eosinophils is supported by the activation of mast cells which produce IL-5. In return, eosinophil MBP activates mast cells, causing them to release histamine, tumour necrosis factor α (TNF-α) and other cytokines.

In mucosae, but not in other sites, proliferation appears to depend on interaction with T lymphocytes.

The granules of basophils and mast cells contain the sulphated proteoglycans heparin and chondroitin sulphate, together with histamine and interleukin-4 (IL-4).

Both basophils and mast cells have highly specific membrane receptors for the Fc segment of IgE produced in response to allergens (see Chapter 8). Exposure to allergens results in rapid exocytosis of their granules, thereby releasing histamine and other vasoactive mediators and resulting in **an immediate hypersensitivity (anaphylactoid)** reaction. Such a reaction causes allergic rhinitis (hay fever), some forms of asthma, urticaria and anaphylaxis.

Mast cell granules contain mast cell tryptase, which is released upon degranulation. Levels of this protein can be detected in the blood as a way of detecting mast cell activity, for example, in diagnosing severe allergic reactions.

Monocytes are part of a cell network: the monocyte–macrophage system.

Monocytes that circulate in blood and their bone marrow–located precursors (monoblasts and promonocytes) are an important component of the innate immune system (see Chapter 8). These cells have a close interplay and functional

Fig. 7.10 Basophil and Mast Cell. (a) The basophil is 14–16 μm in diameter. Its nucleus (N) is bilobed, with the two lobes exhibiting marked chromatin condensation. The cytoplasmic granules are large, dark-blue staining and often obscure the nucleus. **(b)** Mast cells in tissues are ovoid or elongated spindle cells with a non-segmented nucleus. Their granule content imparts a diffuse purplish colour to the cytoplasm in haematoxylin and eosin (H&E) paraffin sections unless special stains are used to demonstrate individual granules (as here). In thin resin H&E sections, the granules can be resolved by light microscopy. **(c)** Ultrastructurally, mast cell granules (BG) are round or oval, membrane bound and contain dense particles and less dense matrix. There is also a small population of smaller uniform granules found near the nucleus. Mast cell cytoplasm also contains free ribosomes, mitochondria and glycogen, and the cell membrane exhibits blunt, irregularly spaced surface projections.

overlap with tissue-resident cells called **macrophages** to form the **monocyte–macrophage system** (mononuclear phagocyte system). At one time it was understood that bone marrow–derived monocytes were the precursor cells that gave rise to tissue-resident macrophages. Studies have shown that although tissue-resident macrophages are derived from a common monocyte/macrophage and dendritic cell precursor (MDP), they do so independently of monocytes or bone marrow. However, in disease states, monocytes can enter damaged tissues and form a new population of macrophagic cells, but this is a distinct process from that which originally populates tissues with their resting tissue-resident macrophage populations.

Included in the system of tissue-resident macrophages are the following:
- Küpffer cells of the liver
- Sinus lining cells of the spleen and lymph nodes (see Chapter 8)
- Pulmonary alveolar macrophages (Chapter 10)
- Synovial lining cells (Chapter 13)
- Dendritic antigen-presenting cells (see Chapter 8)
- Microglia in the brain (Chapter 6)
- Adipose macrophages found in fatty tissues (Chapter 4)

The monocyte–macrophage system has three main functions: phagocytosis of cells and material for further processing, antigen presentation as part of mounting an immune response and cytokine production stimulated by recognition of pathogens.

> **Monocytes have structural features related to their phagocytic role.**

Monocytes are large, motile, phagocytic cells. In blood films, they often have vacuolated cytoplasm (Fig. 7.11).

Ultrastructurally, monocyte cytoplasm contains numerous small lysosomal granules and cytoplasmic vacuoles. The granules are electron dense, homogeneous and membrane bound and are of two types. One type represents primary lysosomes; they contain acid phosphatase, aryl sulphatase and peroxidase and are analogous to the primary granules of neutrophils. Numerous small pseudopodia extend from the monocyte,

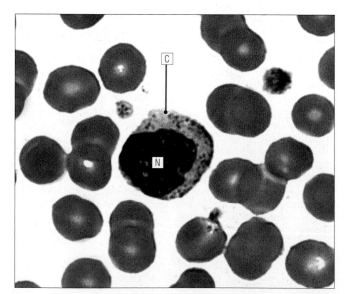

Fig. 7.11 Monocyte. This monocyte is a large cell, up to 15–20 μm in diameter, with a pale-staining cytoplasm (C), which often contains granules. The nucleus is often reniform with a distinct indentation, or it can be irregular in shape as in this case, with this monocyte and an irregular nucleus (N), often with a deep indentation on one side.

reflecting its phagocytic ability and amoeboid movement. Cells express the major histocompatibility (MHC) class II molecule as part of their role in participating in immune responses in collaboration with lymphocytes (see Chapter 8).

Monocytes respond chemotactically to the presence of bacteria, necrotic material and cytokines secreted in the process of inflammation. They leave the blood to enter the tissues, where they take on protective roles, forming histiocytes and macrophages.

◉ ADVANCED CONCEPT

Monocytes play an important role in innate immunity (see Chapter 8) and can be divided into three functionally distinct subsets detected by expression levels of CD14 (a receptor for bacterial lipopolysaccharide involved in innate immunity) and CD16 (an Fc receptor involved in antibody recognition involved in adaptive immunity):
- Classical monocyte with high expression of CD14 and no expression of CD16 (CD14^{++}CD16^{-})
- Non-classical monocyte with low expression of CD14 and high expression of CD16 (CD14^{dim}CD16^{++})
- Intermediate monocyte with high expression of CD14 and low expression of CD16 (CD14^{++}CD16^{+})

It is understood that each type may have slightly different roles in ability to produce proinflammatory factors after activation and differentiation into macrophages.

> **Lymphocytes are responsible for generating specific immune responses.**

In adults and older children, lymphocytes are the second most numerous white cell in the blood, their numbers increasing in response to viral infections; they are the most numerous white cell in young children. Most circulating lymphocytes are small (Fig. 7.12), but about 3% are large, with a diameter of 9–15 μm. Their nuclei are ovoid or kidney-shaped, with the dense chromatin typical of cells with little biosynthetic activity. There are two main types of lymphocytes, termed *B and T cells,* which perform different but linked roles in the generation of specific immune responses (see Chapter 8).

The small mature lymphocytes circulating in the blood emigrate into tissues and into special organs of the immune system. They are responsible for immune surveillance, constantly sampling their environment for foreign material. Lymphocytes then transform into active cells, mediating the immune responses, particularly in specialized lymphoid tissues (see Chapter 8). Large lymphocytes may be seen in the blood, representing such activated lymphocytes en route to the tissues.

> **Plasma cells are formed from B lymphocytes and secrete immunoglobulin.**

Plasma cells are a differentiated form of B lymphocytes (see Chapter 8) and actively synthesize immunoglobulin.

Plasma cells form a small population in normal marrow and are usually seen in support tissues and specialized lymphoid organs. In health, they are not found in the blood.

Fig. 7.12 Lymphocyte. (a) In small lymphocytes, which have a diameter of 6–9 μm, the nucleus occupies about 90% of the cell. The cytoplasm appears only as a narrow rim and is slightly basophilic, owing to the presence of free ribosomes (RNA); rough endoplasmic reticulum is minimal. **(b)** Ultrastructurally, the lymphocyte cell membrane shows small cytoplasmic projections (CP), which appear as short microvilli with the scanning electron microscope and are most numerous on B lymphocytes. Cytoplasm is sparse and contains only a few mitochondria (M) and occasional aggregates of glycogen.

Plasma cells are large and have an eccentrically located, round or oval nucleus with the chromatin coarsely clumped in a characteristic cartwheel or clock-face pattern, reflecting active transcription.

Their cytoplasm is moderately basophilic, owing to its large content of ribosomal RNA in abundant rough endoplasmic reticulum, required to manufacture the immunoglobulin protein. A well-developed Golgi complex displaces the nucleus and is visible as a paranuclear halo or pale zone (Fig. 7.13).

Fig. 7.13 Plasma Cell. Plasma cells have a rounded nucleus, with a speckled chromatin pattern and a central nucleolus, which is often likened to a clock face. The cytoplasm stains a deep purple, reflecting the RNA content. Note the clear, pale-stained area next to the nucleus, which is the area occupied by the Golgi complex (G).

CLINICAL EXAMPLE

White Blood Cell Abnormalities

Analysis of the peripheral blood is an important part of diagnosing disease. Part of a full blood count lists the numbers of white cells in the peripheral blood. The number of circulating white blood cells is altered in many disease processes, and changes in different cell types are associated with different diseases.

For example, although in these cases the white cells are qualitatively normal, there is:

- A considerable and sustained increase of circulating neutrophils in bacterial infections (neutrophilia)
- An increase of circulating eosinophils in parasitic infestations and some allergies (eosinophilia)
- An increase in circulating lymphocytes in certain viral infections (lymphocytosis)

Reduction in the number of white blood cells can also be detected in certain conditions. Reduction in the number of circulating neutrophils (neutropenia or agranulocytosis) can be caused by:

- Damage to the bone marrow: for example, after infiltration and replacement by tumour or after treatment for malignancy using chemotherapy

- Increased destruction of neutrophils seen in several conditions; for example, in association with some autoimmune diseases and in diseases where the spleen is enlarged causing hypersplenism

Reduction in the number of lymphocytes (lymphopenia) can be seen in association with some autoimmune diseases, such as systemic lupus erythematosus; in some infections, such as typhoid and brucellosis; and in association with rare inherited diseases.

The most important disorders of white cells are the leukaemias, in which there is a malignant proliferation of the white cell precursors in bone marrow. This produces vast numbers of white cells, which spill over into the blood.

Leukaemias are classified according to the cell line involved (i.e. granulocytic, monocytic, lymphocytic) and according to their degree of malignancy.

In chronic leukaemias (Fig. 7.14a), the proliferating cells are relatively well differentiated and resemble the normal cell precursors. Disease is slowly progressive, and residual bone marrow still produces some normal elements.

In acute leukaemias (Fig. 7.14b), the proliferating cells are primitive precursor (blast cells). Acute leukaemias are rapidly progressive with failure of bone marrow and reduction of normal cells, and the presentation is often dramatic.

Continued

White Blood Cell Abnormalities

Fig. 7.14 Leukaemia. (a) In this blood film from a patient with chronic myeloid leukaemia (CML), there are increased numbers of mature white cells, mainly neutrophils (N), in addition to precursor cells, mainly myelocytes (Mc) and metamyelocytes (Mm). **(b)** In this blood film from a patient with an acute myeloid leukaemia (AML), the malignant cells are immature granulocyte precursors, mainly myeloblasts (Mb). Very few mature neutrophils (N) are being formed.

PLATELETS

> **Platelets are small cell fragments derived from megakaryocytes and are important in haemostasis.**

Platelets (also called *thrombocytes*) are an essential component of the blood coagulation system. They are small, disc-shaped anuclear structures (Fig. 7.15) that are formed by the cytoplasmic fragmentation of huge precursor cells (megakaryocytes) (see p. 134). Platelets contain mitochondria, microtubules, glycogen granules, occasional Golgi elements and ribosomes, in addition to enzyme systems for aerobic and anaerobic respiration. Many functions of platelets rely on their ability to rapidly secrete mediators and adhesion molecules. This is achieved by having preformed factors stored, ready for use in secretory granules of which there are three types:

- α Granules are variable in size and shape and are believed to be heterogeneous in content and function. Various α granules contain the following: adhesive proteins such as P-selectin, fibrinogen and von Willebrand factor (vWF), platelet factor 4 (PF4), platelet-derived growth factors, insulin-like growth factor 1, and proteins involved in blood clotting (fibronectin, thrombospondin).
- Dense granules (δ granules) are electron dense and contain small molecules such as adenosine diphosphate (ADP), serotonin and calcium. These components are critical for platelet activation and vasoconstriction.
- Lysosomal granules contain lysosomal enzymes (e.g. glycosidases, acid hydrolases and cationic proteins).

Some of the most important functional components of platelets are surface receptors and adhesion molecules expressed on the surface membrane. These surface molecules are essential for platelet interaction with endothelium, white blood cells and elements of the coagulation system. Among these receptors is an ADP receptor involved in aggregation of platelets and glycoprotein IIb/IIIa (GPIIb/IIIa), which is a receptor for fibrinogen and vWF, both involved in platelet activation. Certain antiplatelet drugs prescribed to reduce the risk of pathological blood clotting inhibit these receptors.

> **Platelets aggregate together and degranulate in haemostasis.**

Platelets are essential to normal haemostasis, undergoing aggregation in the process (Fig. 7.16).

Haemostasis is achieved by the following steps:

After loss of the lining endothelium of blood vessels, platelets adhere to vWF bound to exposed collagen through a platelet glycoprotein (GP) receptor complex on the platelet membrane.

Platelet actin, myosin and microtubules cause reversible platelet moulding and adhesion along a broad surface. They then irreversibly release the contents of their granules through the canalicular system in a secretion reaction and synthesize thromboxane.

Thromboxane, ADP and Ca^{2+} ions mediate adhesion of other platelets. Platelet phospholipids (with Ca^{2+} ions) activate the blood clotting cascade, leading to the formation of fibrin.

CLINICAL EXAMPLE

Platelet Disorders

A severe reduction in the number of platelets well below 150×10^9/L in circulating blood is called *thrombocytopenia*. It causes spontaneous bleeding because of the failure of platelets to plug microscopic breaches in vessel walls, resulting from minor trauma.

In the skin, this manifests as a reddish-purple blotchy rash, either small blotches (purpura) or larger, bruise-like patches (ecchymoses).

Severe thrombocytopenia may be a stand-alone condition, for example, idiopathic thrombocytopenic purpura. It may also be part of a wider failure of haematopoietic bone marrow, when it is associated with a reduction in the number of circulating neutrophils (neutropenia) and red cells. This may arise, for example, when normal haematopoietic marrow is suppressed by tumour invasion in acute leukaemia (see Fig. 7.14b) or caused by drugs, such as the cytotoxic drugs used in cancer therapy.

The presence of excessive numbers of circulating platelets is called *thrombocytosis* and occurs frequently as a transient phenomenon when a general burst of bone marrow hyperactivity follows acute blood loss. A more persistent thrombocytosis occurs as a part of so-called *myeloproliferative disorder*, an uncontrolled clonal proliferation of the blood-forming cell colonies in the bone marrow. Thrombocytosis is an important predisposing factor in the development of pathological thrombosis.

Fig. 7.15 Platelets. (a) Platelets (P) are 1.5–3.5 μm in diameter in peripheral blood. **(b)** Scanning electron micrograph showing the smooth disc shape of an inactive platelet. The surface canalicular pores cannot be seen at this magnification. **(c)** Platelet structure. Platelet cell membrane, which has a prominent glycocalyx that includes cell adhesion molecules for platelet adhesion, contains many external pits which connect a system of interconnected canalicular membrane channels (open canalicular system) with the external environment. The cytoplasmic aspect of these membranes is associated with an actin cortex (see p. 34). This canalicular system secretes the contents of the α granule, whereas the contractile proteins in the actin cortex (previously called thrombosthenin) are involved in clot retraction and extrusion of granule contents. A well-developed cytoskeleton incorporates a marginal band of microtubules arranged beneath the cell periphery; these polymerize into component filaments at the onset of platelet aggregation. Deep to the marginal band of microtubules and also scattered throughout the cytoplasm is the dense tubular system (DTS), consisting of narrow membranous tubules containing a homogeneous electron-opaque substance This system is involved in calcium sequestration and releases stored calcium to the cytosol on activation. **(d)** Electron micrograph of a platelet. The circumferential band of microtubules (MT) and elements of the dense tubular system (DTS) and open canalicular system (CS) can be seen, as can a selection of granules, including α and δ granules and some lysosomes (L).

Fig. 7.16 Aggregating Platelets. (a) Scanning electron micrograph of platelets in the early stages of aggregation. They show extensive alteration in shape, becoming contracted. They also develop numerous long, thin cytoplasmic processes (CP). Compare with Fig. 7.15b. **(b)** Transmission electron micrograph of aggregating platelets. Note the interlinking of some cytoplasmic processes and the decrease in granule numbers in some platelets. Compare with Fig. 7.15d.

HAEMATOPOIESIS

> **Blood cells are made in the bone marrow in adult life.**

The site of blood cell formation (haematopoiesis) changes several times during fetal development, the earliest sites being the yolk sac, followed by the developing aorta and then the major expansion taking place in the fetal liver (Fig. 7.17).

Fig. 7.17 Haematopoiesis in Fetal Liver. Micrograph showing haematopoietic cells (H) in the sinusoidal spaces (S) between plates of liver cells (L) in a fetus.

At 5 months, the fetal bone marrow begins to produce white cells and platelets, whereas red cell production by bone marrow starts later, at around 7 months. Once the bone marrow is established, it becomes the main site of haematopoiesis.

⊚ ADVANCED CONCEPT
Haematopoietic Progenitor Cells

The different types of progenitor cells and their relationship to each other are shown in Figs 7.18–17.20. All of the cellular elements in blood are derived from a multipotential stem cell called the *hematopoietic stem cell (HSC)*, which originates in the yolk sac during fetal development. These stem cells have little cytological specialization that discriminates one from another, but they can be identified by their expression of CD markers $CD34^+$ and $CD90^+$. This HSC divides to produce further multipotential cells, finally producing two main branches of cellular differentiation. Different progenitor cells require the presence of specific growth factors in order to mature along different lines (see Figs 7.18– 7.20).

- Common lymphoid progenitor cells, which express CD10 give rise to the different types of lymphocytes (B and T cells, natural killer cells and a population of lymphoid cells involved in innate immunity) (see Chapter 8).
- Common myeloid progenitor cells, which express CD33, give rise to the main types of circulating blood cells through the formation of further progenitor cell groups:
  1. Megakaryocyte/erythroid progenitor cells lead to differentiation pathways producing red blood cells and the megakaryocytes that produce blood platelets.
  2. Granulocyte/monocyte progenitor cells give rise to granulocytes and macrophage by forming further subsets of specific lineage-restricted progenitor cells to form eosinophils, basophils and neutrophils.
  3. A distinct progenitor cell arising from the myeloid line gives rise to macrophage and dendritic cells, both classic dendritic cells and plasmacytoid dendritic cells (see Chapter 8).

At birth, the bone marrow is the main site of red cell production, and almost all bones in the body are involved.

Over the next few years, with the rapid increase in bone size, the haematopoietic capacity of the bone marrow expands far beyond even emergency requirements, and so the haematopoietic bone marrow occupies less of the marrow space available. By skeletal maturity, only the marrow of the vertebrae, ribs, skull, pelvis and proximal femurs is haematopoietic, the rest having been replaced by adipose tissue, although retaining its capacity to resume haematopoiesis should the need arise.

In adult life, cell formation from the bone marrow is sufficient to meet normal requirements. If there is disease of the bone marrow, such that it can no longer make adequate numbers of blood cells, then haematopoietic activity may develop once again in the liver and spleen; this is termed *extramedullary haematopoiesis*.

> **Pluripotential stem cells give rise to all the different types of blood cells.**

All cellular elements of the blood originate from a common progenitor stem cell (HSC; see Figs 7.18–7.20). These stem cells are found in very small numbers at sites of blood cell formation, and even smaller numbers can be found in the peripheral blood. Histologically, they resemble lymphocytes, but can be identified by immunohistochemical techniques, as they have distinctive cell-surface antigens. The stem cells divide and give rise to cells with a more restricted line of growth.

It is possible to divide blood-forming cells into four groups, depending on their capacity for self-renewal, cell division and ability to form different cell types (see Fig. 7.19).

The **haematopoietic stem cells** are capable of forming any type of blood cell; **multipotential progenitor** cells are capable of forming a wide range of blood cells; **lineage-restricted progenitor cells** are capable of forming only one or two types of blood cells; and **maturing cells** are undergoing structural differentiation to form one cell type, and so are incapable of division.

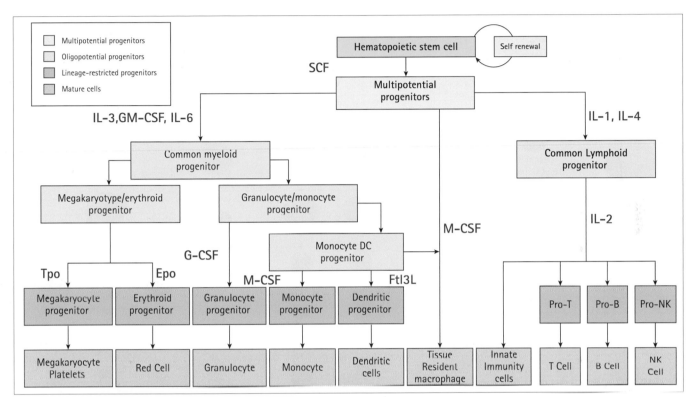

Fig. 7.18 Haematopoietic Stem Cells. All the cellular blood elements are formed from one multipotential stem cell (haematopoietic stem cell). This self-renewing stem cell gives rise to two main progenitor cell types (common myeloid progenitor and common lymphoid progenitor). The main growth factors are shown in red. *Epo,* erythropoietin; *Tpo,* thrombopoietin; *SCF,* stem cell factor; *IL,* interleukin; *CSF,* colony-stimulating factor.

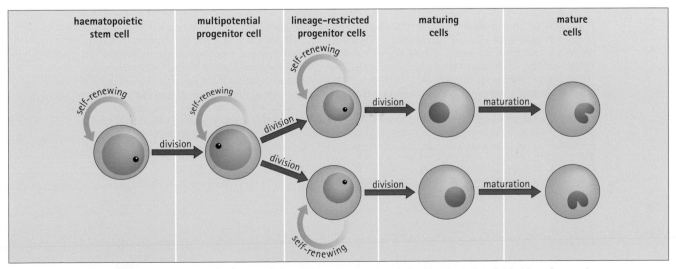

Fig. 7.19 Haematopoietic Precursor Cells. The precursor cells of the blood can be divided into four main classes according to their ability to differentiate into different cell types and their capacity for self-renewal.

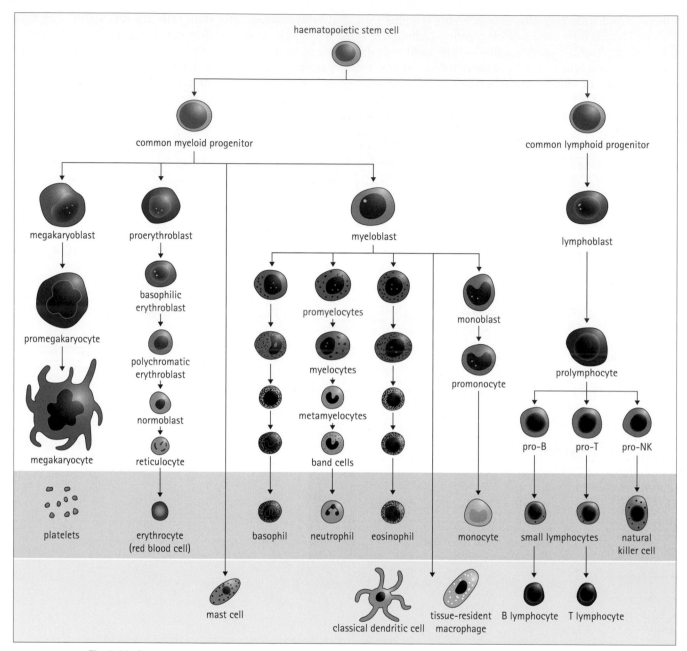

Fig. 7.20 Cell Lineages Formed From Haematopoietic Stem Cells. The relationship between the different progenitor cells seen in bone marrow and the mature cells that are found in blood and tissues is shown. There are two main branches derived from a common myeloid progenitor cell and a common lymphoid progenitor cell. Cell lineages are characterized by expression of specific cell surface markers (CD molecules), which can be used to isolate cells in clinical work. The artwork background is coloured to show which cells are in the bone marrow *(yellow)*, the peripheral blood *(pink)* and tissue *(green)*. Details of each differentiation pathway are described in more detail later in the chapter. For some mature cell types, a named precursor has not been ascribed using histological terminology, as cell markers, transcription factors and other methods have been used to show origin. For example, it was previously thought that tissue-resident macrophages and dendritic cells were derived from monocytes and mast cells were derived from basophils (compare with Fig. 7.18).

A bone marrow stem cell niche creates the microenvironment required for haematopoiesis.

The **haematopoietic stem cell niche** creates the local micro-environment needed for growth and differentiation of HSCs into mature cellular elements of the blood. The niche in bone marrow involves cell adhesion to extracellular matrix, cell-to-cell interactions and the presence of secreted growth factors.

The best-understood component is the action of growth factors. These substances are secreted systemically or locally and modulate three aspects of cell growth:
- Proliferation
- Differentiation
- Maturation

The main growth factors and points where they act are illustrated in Fig. 7.18. Stem cell factor is a cytokine that binds to CD117 (c-KIT receptor) and is important in maintaining HSC populations. Some growth factors, such as erythropoietin and certain colony-stimulating factors, are used in the treatment of diseases of the blood.

Less well understood is the nature of the cell-to-cell interactions involved in haematopoiesis. One niche is located adjacent to bone trabeculae and called the *endosteal niche*. In this site HSCs interact with osteoblasts, bone matrix and local growth factors. A second niche is located adjacent to blood vessels in the marrow cavity called the *perivascular niche*. At this site HSCs interact with mesenchymal stromal cells, endothelial cells and local growth factors.

BONE MARROW

The bone marrow is the main site of haematopoiesis.

Bone marrow occupies the spaces between the trabeculae of medullary bone (see Chapter 13) and consists of highly branched vascular sinuses and a reticulin scaffolding, with the interstices packed with haematopoietic cells (Fig. 7.21).

In addition to its haematopoietic function, the bone marrow, along with the spleen and liver, contains fixed macrophagic cells, which remove aged and defective red cells from the circulation by phagocytosis. It also plays a central role in the immune system, being the site of maturation of B lymphocytes, which produce antibodies (see Chapter 8).

Bone marrow has a highly developed set of vascular sinusoids.

Bone marrow is supplied by medullary branches derived from the nutrient artery of the bone, which pierces the cortical bone through a nutrient canal, giving off a series of small branches to the cortical and medullary bone. This is augmented by smaller vessels from the muscle and periosteum surrounding the bone, which similarly penetrate the cortical bone. A capillary network opens into a well-developed series of thin-walled sinusoids, which empty into a large central sinus. Blood leaves the bone via the nutrient canal.

Fig. 7.21 Bone Marrow. (a) Micrograph of decalcified vertebra showing haematopoietic bone marrow (H) in the spaces between the bony trabeculae (T) of the ilium. Some of the space is also occupied by adipocytes (A). **(b)** At a higher magnification the most eye-catching feature of marrow is large megakaryocytes (M). Careful inspection of nuclei and cytoplasm of bone marrow cells shows myeloid precursors, for example, forming neutrophils (N) and eosinophils (Eo). Erythroid precursors usually form small islands (E). Many larger cells with prominent nucleoli (B) represent blasts for the different marrow cell lineages. **(c)** An important method of examination of bone marrow involves aspiration of marrow and preparation of a smear. This micrograph is a marrow smear stained with Giemsa. The most prominent cell is a megakaryocyte (M). The background consists of red blood cells. The nucleated cells are precursors of erythroid and myeloid cell lines, described in other parts of this chapter. (Micrograph (b) and (c) from digital pathology whole slide image provided by the University of Leeds Virtual Pathology Project https://www.virtualpathology.leeds.ac.uk. Reproduced with permission.)

The bone marrow sinusoids are lined by flat cells (endothelial cells), which normally line blood vessels, and these lie on a discontinuous basement membrane. In places, the cytoplasm of endothelial cells is so thin that the endothelial barrier is little more than the inner and outer layers of endothelial cell membrane. Mature blood cells adhere to the marrow sinusoidal endothelium before being released into the circulation.

> **The bone marrow stromal cells have important roles in haematopoiesis.**

Outside the endothelium and basement membrane of the marrow sinusoids is a discontinuous layer of fibroblast-like support cells called *bone marrow stromal cells* (reticular cells) that synthesize collagenous reticulin fibres (see Fig. 4.5) and extracellular matrix materials and are responsible for producing growth factors. Bone marrow stromal cells have extensive branched cytoplasmic processes, which enclose well over 50% of the outer surface area of the sinusoid wall. The stromal cells also ramify throughout the haematopoietic spaces, forming a regular sponge-like matrix, a meshwork to support the haematopoietic cells.

By accumulating lipid, the stromal cells may transform into the adipocytes found in bone marrow.

The extracellular matrix in the haematopoietic compartment contains coarse collagen fibres, in addition to laminin and fibronectin, which facilitate adhesion of the haematopoietic cells to the marrow stroma. The associated proteoglycans, chondroitin sulphate, hyaluronic acid and heparan sulphate, may also bind growth factors, which control haematopoiesis.

There is an intimate contact between developing blood cells and stromal cells in the marrow. It is believed that such cell–cell contacts are important in the control of haematopoiesis as part of the stem cell niche.

> **Erythropoiesis is associated with the formation of distinct precursor cells termed *erythroblasts*.**

Red cells are the terminal differentiated progeny of one cell line derived from multipotential bone marrow stem cells which is committed to erythropoiesis only.

The common myeloid progenitor cell forms a more restricted progenitor cell, the megakaryocyte/erythroid progenitor, and under influence of the growth factor erythropoietin, this leads to a lineage-restricted erythroid progenitor cell line. The erythroid progenitor cells are few and cannot easily be identified on routine bone marrow histology. Immunochemical techniques have allowed their characterization, revealing cells with large nucleoli, many polyribosomes and large mitochondria. Differentiation of these progenitor cells into mature red cells is associated with:

- Decreasing cell size
- Haemoglobin production
- Gradual decrease and eventual loss of all cell organelles
- Changing cytoplasmic staining, from intense basophilia resulting from large numbers of polyribosomes to eosinophilia caused by haemoglobin
- Condensation and eventual extrusion of the nucleus

Along the path of red cell differentiation, certain morphological cell types can be distinguished in routine marrow smears: proerythroblast, basophilic erythroblast, polychromatic erythroblast, normoblast (orthochromatic erythroblast) and reticulocyte (Fig. 7.22).

> **Red cell formation occurs in small cellular islands in the marrow.**

Red cells are formed in small erythroblastic islands consisting of one or two specialized macrophages surrounded by erythroid progenitor cells. The macrophages have long cytoplasmic processes and deep invaginations to accommodate the

| Proerythroblast | Basophilic erythroblast (early normoblast) | Polychromatic erythroblast (intermediate normoblast) | Orthochromatic erythroblast (late normoblast) | Reticulocyte |

Fig. 7.22 Morphological Stages in Erythropoiesis. Red blood cells constantly develop from a dividing population of erythropoietic cells in the bone marrow. Differentiation into mature red cells is associated with distinctive morphological and functional changes. A proerythroblast divides to form 8–16 cells. As seen in the micrographs, as cells mature they decrease in size from 25 μm for a proerythroblast to 10 μm for a reticulocyte. Nuclei in the dividing blast cells are large, with prominent nucleoli. With differentiation, the nucleus becomes condensed and smaller and is eventually extruded. Stippled material in reticulocytes is not nuclear material. As a red cell matures, it accumulates haemoglobin in the cytoplasm, causing increasing eosinophilia. This contrasts with dividing cells that have basophilic cytoplasm, reflecting large amounts of RNA from the protein synthetic machinery of the cell. A pale-staining perinuclear halo is the result of a Golgi apparatus. Reticulocytes mature into red cells in 24–48 hours and leave the bone marrow via the sinusoids.

dividing erythroid cells, which migrate outward along the cytoplasmic process as they differentiate.

When mature, the red cell contacts nearby sinusoidal endothelium and passes out to enter the circulation.

Red cell production is controlled by erythropoietin.

The term **erythron** describes the whole mass of mature red cells and their progenitors. It functions as a dispersed organ, with the number of red cells in the circulating blood being regulated to meet oxygen-carrying needs and the rate of red cell production varying with changing rates of their removal from the circulation.

This behaviour is mediated by a number of factors, but particularly by the growth factor **erythropoietin,** which adjusts red cell production to match oxygen demand. Erythropoietin is secreted mainly by the kidneys in adults and by the liver in the fetus.

Erythropoietin (or EPO) production is stimulated by low tissue oxygen tension (e.g. hypoxia), whatever the cause; the most common stimulus is anaemia, but other causes of tissue hypoxia, such as heart or lung disease, can also increase the production of EPO. EPO increases the number and proliferative activity of erythroid progenitors. EPO deficiency is a common feature of chronic kidney disease, which can be corrected by treatment with synthetic human EPO.

Certain factors are required by the bone marrow for the formation of red cells, notably iron (as a component of haemoglobin), folic acid and vitamin B_{12}. Lack of any of these factors leads to defective red cell formation and the development of anaemia.

Neutrophil granulopoiesis occurs with the formation of five distinctive cell types.

The formation of granulated white cells is termed *granulopoiesis*. This takes place under the influence of growth factors (see Fig. 7.18). The first recognizable precursor of neutrophil formation is the myeloblast. The stages of subsequent maturation through promyelocyte, myelocyte, metamyelocyte and band cell are shown in Fig. 7.23.

Maturation from myeloblast to neutrophil takes about 7–8 days and involves five cell divisions between myeloblast and metamyelocyte stages, after which no further multiplication divisions take place and chemotactic ability, complement and Fc receptors are acquired.

Structurally mature neutrophils remain in the marrow for about 5 days and are then released into the blood. After circulating for about 6 hours they migrate into the peripheral tissues, where they survive for 2–5 days unless they become activated, when they may degranulate and die (p. 122).

Fig. 7.23 Morphological Stages in Neutrophil Granulopoiesis. Micrograph showing granulocyte precursors at various stages of maturation. The myeloblast (Mb) is a large cell largely occupied by a nucleus in which nucleoli are prominent; its scanty cytoplasm contains a few granules. The promyelocyte (Pm) contains more abundant cytoplasm and more primary granules; nucleoli are still present. The myelocyte (Mc) shows early flattening or invagination of one face of the nucleus, from which the nucleoli have disappeared. Its cytoplasm contains a mixture of a few primary granules and smaller secondary granules. The metamyelocyte (Mm) shows more advanced invagination of the nucleus to a reniform shape, and a later stage, the band or stab form (B), has a horseshoe-shaped nucleus. Increasing lobation of the nucleus produces the mature neutrophil (N), which features a multilobed nucleus and abundant cytoplasm containing small secondary granules.

Increase in numbers of circulating neutrophils may occur by two mechanisms.

A reserve pool of stored neutrophils is maintained, loosely adherent to the sinusoidal endothelium in the bone marrow. This pool can be mobilized rapidly when there is a disease process. Stimuli cause a sudden outpouring of granulocytes from the bone marrow, leading to an increase in the number of blood neutrophils (neutrophilia, see p. 120). This mechanism copes with a sudden demand for neutrophils.

If it is necessary to maintain a high blood neutrophil count, for example, during bacterial infection, there is increased proliferation of the granulocyte precursors in the marrow. This is regulated by systemic secretion of cytokines, especially interleukin-1 (IL-1), granulocyte-macrophage colony-stimulating factor (GM-CSF) and granulocyte colony-stimulating factor (G-CSF).

Eosinophil and basophil formation morphologically resembles neutrophil granulopoiesis.

Eosinophils are derived from granulocyte–monocyte progenitor cells under the influence of cytokines. Eosinophil myeloblasts resemble neutrophil myeloblasts, and there are comparable subsequent developmental stages. Eosinophils are readily distinguishable from neutrophils at the early myelocyte stage by the appearance of their larger granules, most of which are stained bright red (eosinophilic), but a few are initially basophilic.

Basophils are also derived from granulocyte–monocyte progenitor cells (see Fig. 7.20). Basophil myeloblasts resemble neutrophil myeloblasts; development then proceeds through analogous stages to those of neutrophils and eosinophils. Basophil granules are distinguishable at the early myelocyte stage.

Monocytes leave the marrow soon after formation, with no marrow pool.

Monocytes are derived from monocyte–dendritic progenitor cells (see Fig. 7.18) under the influence of cytokines, including M-CSF. Two morphological monocyte precursors are recognized: the monoblast and the pro-monocyte. At least three cell divisions occur before the mature monocyte stage is reached. Mature monocytes leave the bone marrow soon after their formation, and there is no reserve pool. They spend about 3 days in the blood before migrating into the tissues, where they are understood to patrol as part of innate immune defences (see Chapter 8); they are then unable to re-enter the circulation.

The relationship between monocytes, tissue-resident macrophages and dendritic cells is further discussed in Chapter 8.

Lymphoid precursors migrate to peripheral lymphoid tissues.

The bone marrow is the site of formation of primitive lymphocyte precursors derived from the common lymphoid progenitor, which subsequently give rise to both T and B lymphocytes, natural killer cells and other cells involved in innate immunity (see Fig. 7.20).
- B cells undergo initial maturation in the bone marrow and move on to colonize peripheral lymphoid tissues.
- T cells migrate to the thymus, where they undergo initial maturation before moving on to colonize peripheral lymphoid tissues (see Chapter 8).

Lymphoid cells are capable of division in adult life when expansion of selected clones is desirable to mount a specific immune response. **Lymphoblasts** are recognizable dividing lymphocytes, having a large open nucleus, a prominent nucleolus and a small amount of cytoplasm. Expansion of numbers of lymphocytes also takes place in the specialized peripheral lymphoid tissues, as discussed in Chapter 8.

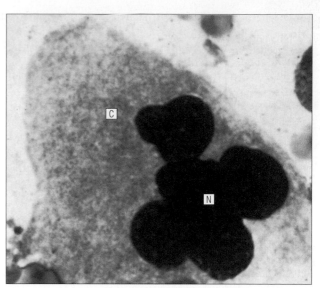

Fig. 7.24 Megakaryocyte. Megakaryocytes are huge polyploid cells 30–100 μm in diameter with a large irregular, multilobular nucleus (N), which contains dispersed chromatin and is devoid of nucleoli. Their extensive cytoplasm (C) is filled with fine basophilic granules, reflecting their profusion of cytoplasmic organelles. With light microscopy the cell margin is often difficult to define clearly owing to the presence of numerous disaggregating platelets, cytoplasmic processes, ruffles and blebs.

Megakaryocytes are large multinucleate cells which give rise to the platelets.

Megakaryocytes (Fig. 7.24) are the largest cells seen in bone marrow aspirates, and they produce platelets by cytoplasmic fragmentation.

The precursor of the megakaryocyte in bone marrow is the megakaryoblast, which duplicates its nuclear and cytoplasmic constituents up to seven times without cell division, each causing increased ploidy, nuclear lobulation and cell size.

Cytoplasmic maturation involves the elaboration of granules, vesicles and demarcation membranes (see below) and progressive loss of free ribosomes and rough endoplasmic reticulum.

Megakaryocyte cytoplasm is divided into three zones. First, the perinuclear zone contains the Golgi and associated vesicles, rough and smooth endoplasmic reticulum, developing granules, centrioles and spindle tubules. It remains attached to the nucleus after platelet shedding. Second, the intermediate zone contains an extensive system of interconnected vesicles and tubules (the demarcation membrane system [DMS]), which is in continuity with the cell membrane and has the function of delineating developing platelet fields (i.e. potential platelets) which, like platelets, are uneven in size. Finally, the marginal zone is filled with cytoskeletal filaments and traversed by membranes connecting with the DMS.

Megakaryocytes produce platelets in bone marrow, and there is also a population found in the lung.

For online review questions, please visit https://studentconsult.inkling.com.

Immune System

INTRODUCTION

> The immune system is part of an array of defence systems used to combat disease.

The body must constantly protect itself from invasion by a variety of pathogens, which may gain entry via the skin, gut, respiratory tract and other routes. This protection is provided by a range of cells which together form the immune system. The main cell types involved are white blood cells, especially **lymphocytes, granulocytes, macrophages** and **dendritic cells.**

The two primary organs of the immune system, responsible for the creation of lymphocytes, are the **bone marrow** and the **thymus gland.** The secondary organs of the immune system, responsible for developing specific immune responses, are **lymph nodes,** the **spleen,** and the lymphoid tissues present in epithelial surfaces collectively called **mucosa-associated lymphoid tissue (MALT).**

There are two basic mechanisms:

- Innate immunity
- Adaptive immune response

Systems involved in protection (barrier functions) at epithelial surfaces are considered part of general defence systems that guard against pathogens. These include the barrier provided by keratin in the skin, mucus in the respiratory and alimentary tracts and an acid environment in the stomach and vagina. If pathogens gain access to tissues, then a further general line of defence is activated.

Innate immunity is served by a range of cells capable of first detecting a danger signal, and secondly activating generic cellular defence systems. Receptors on immune cells can either identify elements that are generically expressed in broad groups of pathogens called **pathogen-associated molecular patterns (PAMPs)** or are able to recognize signal molecules that are expressed when cells become damaged called **damage-associated molecular patterns (DAMPs).** When the innate immune system is activated, pathogens are destroyed or neutralized by complement, interferon, cytokines, natural killer cells, neutrophil leukocytes and macrophages. Innate immunity is non-specific, with the understanding that the system is only responding to pathogens in a generic manner and is not providing long-lasting immunity. Its importance is in its immediate ability to respond to pathogens.

In contrast, the **adaptive immune response** is specific, with the understanding that each pathogen encountered is met with a unique programmed (adaptive) response that involves recognition of 'non-self'. In an adaptive response, immune effector cells (lymphocytes) are programmed to destroy or neutralize the pathogen based on recognition of these 'non-self' targets, which are termed **antigens.** Antigen-specific immune responses create a set of lymphocytes that 'remember' the pathogen, such that any repeated exposure is rapidly managed. A second exposure to a pathogen is dealt with before it can take hold because the adaptive immune response provides long-lasting immunity; however, this takes time to develop.

> The two main types of adaptive immune responses are termed cell-mediated and humoral.

The immune response is served by several types of cells acting synergistically. Exogenous agents (commonly micro-organisms) are first recognized by **antigen-presenting cells** (APCs), which constantly survey their local environment and are mainly dendritic cells and macrophages. The exogenous agents are broken down within the APCs into key fragments. These fragments act as antigens, which are then presented to specialized effector cells **(lymphocytes).** Lymphocytes bind to these foreign antigens, and this starts a process of creating an expanding pool of cells that can specifically destroy or neutralize the antigen. Lymphocytes capable of recognizing and binding to the antigen then proliferate and can mount an immune response, which may be one of two main types:

- **Cell-mediated immunity** – characterized by the joint action of lymphocytes and macrophages to destroy or neutralize the foreign agent.
- **Humoral immunity** – characterized by the secretion of proteins (antibodies) by one type of lymphocyte. Antibodies neutralize foreign agents by specifically binding to the antigen (see Key Facts box, p. 136).

These two systems usually work together in the elimination of a pathogen.

Whereas the immune response occurs in all body tissues, the growth, maintenance and programming of immune cells take place preferentially in the lymph nodes, spleen, thymus gland and bone marrow, which are the special organs of the immune system.

KEY FACTS

Antibodies

- Are synthesized by B lymphocytes (as plasma cells) and bind to specific antigens
- Are also known as immunoglobulins and fall into five different structural classes: IgG, IgA, IgD, IgM and IgE
- Have two main components: immunoglobulin light chain (κ or λ) and immunoglobulin heavy chains (γ, α, δ, μ or ε)
- Have heavy and light chains with highly variable regions (antigen-binding sites) and constant regions, which form the main part of the molecules
- May circulate in the blood and body fluids or remain bound to the B-lymphocyte surface, where they activate the B cell on meeting the appropriate antigen

---

Different cells of the immune system can be identified by characteristic markers.

Many of the different but highly specialized lymphocytes of the immune system were originally defined by morphology and only more recently by expression of surface marker.

To recognize different cell types, it is necessary to stain tissues to detect the presence of various markers of cells, most of which are cell-surface proteins. The many cytoplasmic and cell membrane proteins that characterize cells of the immune system have been given names according to an international system, which relates them to proteins expressed at different phases of cell maturation. These are called **cluster of differentiation** molecules (also known as **cluster of designation** or **classification determinant**) and abbreviated as **CD.** Antibodies to the different CD molecules can be used to identify specific subtypes of lymphoid cells using immunohistochemical staining. The nomenclature has the prefix CD, followed by numbers and letters. In this chapter, reference is made to CD markers (Fig. 8.1). The definition of cell types is being extended to include expression of growth and transcription factors; for full details, it is recommended that the reader refer to a specialized immunology or haematology textbook.

KEY FACTS

CD Molecules

CD molecules can be considered in three main groups:
- Markers which are expressed by a cell line throughout its life.
- Markers which are expressed transiently during one phase of differentiation.
- Markers which are expressed when cells are activated.

Cell types are specified by the suffix '+' or '−' to indicate expression or lack of expression of a CD molecule. For example, a CD4$^+$ CD8$^-$ cell is one that expresses CD4 but not CD8.

CD markers are membrane-associated proteins often representing receptors and ligands involved in cell-to-cell interactions to mediate cell adhesion or to cause cell signalling.

The precise typing of a cell and discrimination from another type may involve considering the expression of multiple CD molecules.

B lymphocyte	CD45$^+$ CD3-CD19$^+$ CD20$^+$ CD21$^+$ CD22$^+$ CD24$^+$ CD38$^+$ CD72$^+$ CD79a$^+$
T lymphocyte	CD45$^+$ CD3$^+$
Helper T cell	CD45$^+$ CD3$^+$ CD4$^+$
Regulatory T cell	CD45$^+$ CD3$^+$ CD4$^+$ CD25$^+$ CD39$^+$ CD73$^+$
Cytotoxic T cell	CD45$^+$ CD3$^+$ CD8$^+$
Natural killer cell	CD45$^+$ CD3-CD16$^+$ CD30$^+$ CD31$^+$ CD56$^+$

Fig. 8.1 Cluster of Differentiation Molecules. Common CD profiles for cells considered in this chapter.

LYMPHOCYTES

Lymphocytes are particularly important cells of the immune system. The three main types of lymphocytes are termed *B cells*, *T cells* and *natural killer* (NK) *cells*.

B cells turn into plasma cells and secrete antibodies.

B lymphocytes (B cells) are mainly concentrated within the specialized lymphoid organs. They also circulate in the peripheral blood – accounting for between 5% and 15% of blood lymphocytes – and migrate through body tissues (Fig. 8.2). The constant movement of this type of lymphoid cell means they are readily available for immune defence. When stimulated by an appropriate antigen, B cells undergo proliferation and convert into **plasma cells,** which then secrete specific proteins called *immunoglobulins*. B cells, plasma cells and antibodies in the blood and body fluids are the basis of the **humoral response.**

Fig. 8.2 Lymphocytes in Tissues. Haematoxylin and eosin (H&E) micrograph from the dermis of skin. Small blood vessels are surrounded by lymphocytes, which have dark-stained nuclei and no visible cytoplasm. There is adjacent, pink-stained collagenous tissue. Informally, microscopists use the size of lymphocyte nuclei, being roughly 10 μm, as a ruler against which to judge the size of other cells.

◎ ADVANCED CONCEPT

B-Cell Antigen Receptor Complex

B cells recognize antigen by expressing immunoglobulin, commonly IgM antibody, on their surface as part of a B-cell receptor complex. The other proteins that form the receptor complex are signal transduction proteins detected by antibodies to CD79a and CD79b.

All developing B cells have common genes encoding the production of immunoglobulins. At this stage they are called *germline* B-cell genes. During B-cell maturation, and before antigen stimulation, these genes undergo rearrangement to produce different unique immunoglobulin proteins, which can specifically interact with a particular antigen. In this way, the diversity of the humoral immune response is generated. Cells that produce an immunoglobulin recognizing a normal body (self) antigen are eliminated, and immune responses are regulated by subsets of T cells (discussed in detail later in the chapter). Some activated cells become dormant and remain as so-called *memory cells.* These can rapidly proliferate on repeated encounter with the same antigen.

B cells originate in haematopoietic tissues and later colonize lymphoid tissues.

B cells mature from small inactive cells to large immunoglobulin-secreting cells. Their cytological appearance varies according to their activity.

Originating in the haematopoietic tissues of the liver and bone marrow, B cells develop from lymphoid stem cells. This occurs in niches within the marrow and is stimulated by interleukin (IL)-7.

B cells leave their site of development and populate specialized lymphoid tissues (lymph nodes, spleen, tonsils and gut mucosa in particular). In birds, B cells develop in a structure called the *bursa of Fabricius,* hence the origin of the term *B (bursal) cell.*

Inactive B cells are small cells, 6–8 μm in diameter, with barely discernible cytoplasm. The nucleus is rounded with compact chromatin, reflecting a lack of DNA transcription (Fig. 8.3).

Fig. 8.4 Plasma Cells. In tissue sections plasma cells have rounded nuclei and basophilic cytoplasm. In some cells, a perinuclear pale-stained area can be seen *(arrows)* which is the location of the Golgi apparatus. Nuclei are said to resemble a clock face, having an open chromatin pattern with chromatin granules arranged at the periphery and a large central nucleolus.

When B cells become activated and proliferate, they develop large nuclei with prominent nucleoli and moderate amounts of cytoplasm. These cells are termed **lymphoblasts, centroblasts** and **immunoblasts.**

The fully differentiated immunoglobulin-secreting B cell is termed a **plasma cell** and has cytological features that reflect its function as a protein-secreting cell (Fig. 8.4 and see Fig. 7.12). The cytoplasm is basophilic because of a high content of rough endoplasmic reticulum, and there is a clear area near the nucleus corresponding to the Golgi complex.

ᴍ CLINICAL EXAMPLE

A malignant tumour of plasma cells is called a **myeloma.** In this condition, a single malignant clone of plasma cells develops and spreads through the bone marrow. Given that the function of plasma cells is to produce immunoglobulin, a blood test can be used to detect if there is a single dominant antibody in the plasma (monoclonal band). Myeloma is often associated with the development of lytic areas within bone, which can lead to fractures.

◎ ADVANCED CONCEPT

Markers of B Cells

- Pre–B cells express CD10; this is lost with maturation.
- B cells in blood express IgM and IgD on their surface in addition to major histocompatibility (MHC) class II antigens.
- CD19, CD20, CD22 and CD79a are the main markers used in identification.
- CD21 and CD35 (complement receptors) are expressed when cells are activated.
- CD40 is expressed and is involved in activation signalling with helper T (Th) cells.
- B cells in tissues may express IgM and IgD, IgG, IgA or IgE. The latter three are produced as a consequence of 'class switching', when activated B cells stop producing μ and δ heavy chains and start producing γ, α or ε heavy chains instead.

Fig. 8.3 Inactive Lymphocytes. H&E micrograph of wax-embedded tissue. Lymphocytes have no visible cytoplasm. The nuclei are rounded with dense, dark-stained chromatin.

T cells are specialized lymphocytes responsible for cell-mediated immunity.

T lymphocytes (T cells) originate from stem cells in the haematopoietic tissues of the liver and bone marrow and are so named because they undergo maturation in the thymus gland, hence the 'T' from the thymus gland. T cells leave to populate specialized lymphoid tissues (lymph nodes, spleen and gut mucosa, in particular). Although T cells are found concentrated within the specialized lymphoid organs, they also circulate in the peripheral blood and migrate through body tissues. T-cell receptors are located on the cell surface and bind to specific antigen in a manner similar to that of antibodies (although T cells bind only to peptide antigens held on the surface of APCs, whereas B cells can bind to many chemical varieties of antigens that are in solution or on the surface of microbes). When stimulated by binding to an appropriate antigen and receiving reciprocal stimulation from the cell presenting that antigen, T cells undergo proliferation and can direct and recruit other cells of the immune system and attack diseased cells directly.

Activated T cells also have an important secretory function and produce cytokines (lymphokines).

T cells, T-cell receptors and cytokines are the basis of the **cell-mediated immune response** and are also essential for organizing many aspects of the humoral response.

◎ ADVANCED CONCEPT

T-Cell Receptor Complex

The T-cell receptor proteins are assembled with proteins of CD3 to form a complex which sits on the T-cell surface (**T-cell receptor complex**). All developing T cells have common genes encoding T-cell receptor proteins. At this stage, they are called *germline T genes*. During maturation, genetic mechanisms (somatic mutation and T-cell receptor gene rearrangement) generate the diversity of T cells needed to respond to different antigens. Cells that recognize a normal body (self) antigen are eliminated during development (discussed in detail later in the chapter).

The T-cell receptors have variable regions which, like antibodies, can bind to different antigens. The receptors are assembled as pairs (dimers) of antigen-binding peptides:

- 95% of lymphocytes in blood express α and β chains together (αβ T-cell receptor) and are referred to as α:β (or αβ) T cells.
- 5% of lymphocytes in the blood express γ and δ chains together (γδ T-cell receptor) and are referred as γδ T cells.

T cells have a varied morphology.

The histological appearance of T cells depends on their activity.

Inactive T cells can be of two morphological types. The most common form in peripheral blood, accounting for between 60% and 90%, is called a **small lymphocyte.** This is 6–7 μm in diameter, with barely discernible cytoplasm and a rounded nucleus with compact chromatin (see Fig. 7.12a).

The second type of inactive T cell is called a **large granular lymphocyte** (Fig. 8.5). These cells are 7–10 μm in diameter; they have a moderate amount of cytoplasm, which contains small numbers of granules that stain with azure dyes (**azurophilic granules**).

Fig. 8.5 Large Granular Lymphocyte. Blood film showing a large granular lymphocyte. Note that the nucleus is larger than in a small lymphocyte and that there is a moderate amount of cytoplasm with small numbers of pink-staining (azurophilic) granules.

T cells that have been stimulated to divide as part of an immune response are larger than the inactive cells and have a moderate amount of basophilic cytoplasm. The nucleus is large, with a convoluted appearance (in contrast to that of B cells) and an open vesicular chromatin pattern and a visible nucleolus, reflecting gene transcription.

Lymphokine-secreting activated T cells have basophilic cytoplasm owing to their high content of rough endoplasmic reticulum (ER) and a large nucleus with a convoluted contour.

It is not possible to distinguish between different specialized types of T cells using routine histological methods, and it is necessary to use immunohistochemical staining to detect expression of specific markers which may be present in the cytoplasm, on the cell membrane or in the case of a transcription factor, in the nucleus.

There are several functional subsets of T lymphocytes.

There are several subtypes of T cells, which can be defined by their expression of specific surface markers, transcription factors, secreted products and their functional activity.

During processing and maturation in the thymus gland, T cells may differentiate into an **effector T cell** (cytotoxic, helper and regulatory types) or a **memory T cell,** responsible for providing long-lived protection through immunity (Fig. 8.6).

NK cells are activated to become cytotoxic lymphocytes.

NK cells are the third main type of lymphocyte and in the peripheral blood have the morphology of large granular lymphocytes (see Fig. 8.5). NK cells do not express T-cell receptors, including an absence of CD3. In addition to forming a population in the blood, they are also present in the spleen. NK cells are an important part of **innate immunity** and express several classes of receptors through which they can be activated, with the ability to kill other cells (**cell-mediated cytotoxicity**) by secreting perforin and granzymes. The main role of this type of cell is in the elimination of virus-infected cells and in the surveillance and elimination of cancer cells. Among other signals, NK cells may be activated by recognizing interleukins and cytokines produced by virally infected cells.

NK cells can produce IFN-γ to stimulate macrophages to engulf viral-infected cells and TNF-α that can mediate tumour cell killing.

◎ ADVANCED CONCEPT

T-Cell Subtypes

Naïve T cells express either **CD8** or **CD4** together with CD3 and the αβ T-cell receptor. These cells are present in lymph nodes and, by sensing antigens presented with molecules of the MHC on APCs, can respond to pathogens that the immune system has not previously encountered.

- CD4+ cells interact with MHC class II. If activated by binding to antigen and co-stimulated, they differentiate into helper or regulatory T lymphocytes. Some may also develop into memory T cells
- CD8+ cells interact with MHC class I. If activated by binding antigen and co-stimulated, they differentiate into cytotoxic T lymphocytes. Some may also develop into memory T cells.

Helper T cells (Th cells) express **CD4** together with **CD3** and the αβ T-cell receptor plus receptors for different cytokines and chemokines. There are several recognized sets within this subtype depending on the nature of secreted products and functions. The ability of Th cells to secrete cytokines – for example, different types of interleukin – allows them to promote immunity against different classes of pathogen (e.g. virus, bacterium, fungus, protozoan). In addition, a group of Th cells plays a vital part in humoral immunity through interaction with B cells to promote differentiation into plasma cells and formation of memory B cells.

Cytotoxic T cells (TC cells) express **CD8** and CD3 together with the αβ T-cell receptor. They can kill target cells by secreting perforin and granzyme. This subtype is especially involved in immune responses to viral infections within cells, in transplant rejection and in immune surveillance against the development of cancerous cells.

Regulatory T cells (TReg) express **CD4** together with CD3 and the αβ T-cell receptor. They have roles in promoting immune tolerance and suppressing the extent of an immune response. Several types of regulatory T cells have been characterized according to function and expression of marker proteins. They can secrete IL-10 and transforming growth factor (TGF)-β as part of suppressing a T-cell–mediated immune response.

Natural killer T cells (NKTs) (not to be confused with NK cells; see earlier) express the αβ T-cell receptor, but the α chain is usually restricted in its diversity. Cells may be either CD4 or CD8 positive. A small number of subgroups have been characterized. This subtype of T cell can respond to lipid antigens. NKT cells have been implicated in the immune response to mycobacteria, in autoimmune diseases, and when activated are responsible for secreting a range of cytokines that recruit other immune cells and modulate local cellular responses.

Gamma delta T cells (γδ T cells) express the γδ T-cell receptor together with CD3 and are a type of so-called *unconventional* T cell. This type of T cell forms a very small proportion of lymphocytes in the blood and is seen mainly in the bowel, where they are a major type of lymphocyte infiltrating between epithelial cells lining the gut (intraepithelial lymphocytes). In contrast to Th and TC cells, γδ T cells do not need to be presented with antigen together with MHC molecules but are able to recognize whole antigens: for example, as expressed on a bacterial surface. Subgroups of γδ T cells have been characterized and shown to have restricted forms of T-cell receptor functioning as a pattern recognition receptor and hence are linked more to innate immunity rather than adaptive immunity. The lymphocytosis seen in certain bacterial infections is believed to derive from this class of lymphocyte. When activated, they can produce cytokines (interferon [IFN]-γ, tumour necrosis factor [TNF]-α) and chemokines (RANTES, lymphotactin) and cause the death of target cells by secreting perforin and granzyme.

Memory T cells express the T-cell receptor, including CD3 and CD45RO (a receptor protein involved in later activation). On encountering a repeated antigen challenge, they can quickly combat a pathogen by producing effector cytokines and proliferating to create a new population of effector T cells. Their function as effector cells depends on whether they express CD4 (helper or regulatory) or CD8 (cytotoxic). Several populations of memory T cells have been characterized in different tissue locations.

Anergic T cells, exhausted T cells and senescent T cells: These three T-cell types are associated with a state of hyporesponsiveness and can be recognized using cell surface markers.

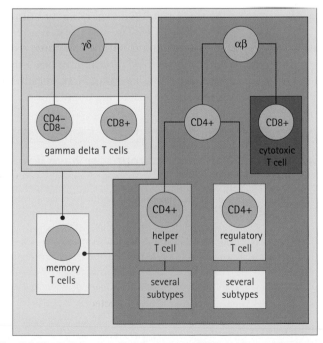

Fig. 8.6 T-cell Subtypes. T cells express different types of T-cell receptors. Cytotoxic cells, helper cells and regulatory cells are associated with the expression of other surface markers not illustrated in this diagram. There are subtypes of helper T cells and regulatory T cells defined by markers and function. Memory T cells can form from different T-cell types.

🕅 CLINICAL EXAMPLE

HIV Infection and the Immune System

The virus that causes acquired immunodeficiency syndrome (AIDS), HIV-1, gains entry to cells by using the CD4 surface protein as a receptor. One of the most important markers of progression in HIV infection is reduction in CD4+ T-cell numbers in the blood.

▶ KEY FACTS

Lymphocytes

- There are three main types: T cells, B cells and NK cells.
- There are two morphological types of inactive lymphocytes: small lymphocytes and large granular lymphocytes.
- The different types of lymphoid cells are identified using immunochemical techniques to detect specific markers.
- B cells mature into plasma cells and secrete immunoglobulin.
- T cells have several roles as cytotoxic cells, helper cells and regulatory cells.
- NK cells have a primary cytotoxic role as part of the innate immunity.

MACROPHAGES AND DENDRITIC CELLS

Macrophages are part of the mononuclear phagocytic system.

Monocytes (see Chapter 7), macrophages and dendritic cells (discussed in detail later in the chapter) are part of the mononuclear phagocyte system, a system of primarily phagocytic cells dispersed in all tissues, with some specialized forms present as **tissue-resident phagocytic cells.**

Macrophages and dendritic cells are derived from myeloid progenitor cells (see p. 129). Macrophages are important as an effector cell in innate immunity and in the removal of dead cells as part of normal tissue cell turnover, including in fetal development. In disease, after tissue damage, macrophages become activated and local populations are supplemented by monocyte-derived cells that come from the blood.

Macrophages can recognize pathogens by pattern-recognition receptors and Fc receptors, after which they can kill bacteria through phagocytosis and production of reactive oxygen species (ROS) with myeloperoxidase. They also recruit other effector cells by secreting inflammatory cytokines.

Macrophages may also serve as effector cells in adaptive immunity, becoming activated in response to cytokines produced by T cells.

Tissue-resident macrophages have a variety of morphological appearances, as they differentiate to serve specialized roles:
- They may form a population of cells adapted mainly for phagocytosis (tissue-resident macrophages or histiocytes).
- They may be stimulated by T cells to secrete cytokines that control local cellular immune responses.
- They may perform immune surveillance (antigen presentation).

The cells adapted mainly for phagocytosis remove or store material by assuming a rounded morphology with short, broad pseudopodia. They contain large numbers of lysosomes (see Fig. 2.23).

Secretory-type macrophages are large cells with voluminous pink-staining cytoplasm caused by expansion of the Golgi complex and smooth ER. They are seldom seen in normal tissues but are important in T-cell–mediated immune responses when they are termed **epithelioid cells** because of their superficial resemblance to epithelial cells (type IV hypersensitivity response).

Macrophagic cells are widely distributed in most tissues.

The morphology of macrophages is variable according to their site and function.

Macrophages are an important component of the specialized organs of the immune system, especially in the spleen. They are also particularly abundant in loose fibrocollagenous support tissue, which is found in most parts of the body (Fig. 8.7).

Fig. 8.7 Macrophages. Macrophages are particularly abundant in the loose fibrocollagenous support tissue found in most organs. In this site they are adapted for major phagocytic activity, which is reflected in their high lysosome content. **(a)** In H&E sections, normal macrophages are inconspicuous; **(b)** they may be detected by immunochemical staining for CD68, a heavily glycosylated type I transmembrane glycoprotein located in the endosomal/lysosomal compartment and strongly expressed in macrophages. In the micrograph, macrophages are stained brown. Comparing the morphology of cells in **(a)** it is apparent that some of the elongated cells adjacent to the vessels are likely macrophages.

Specialized tissue-resident macrophages are seen in the lung (alveolar macrophages, see p. 190), liver (Küpffer cells, see Fig. 12.3), brain (microglial cells, see Fig. 6.23), placenta (Hofbauer cells), spleen (sinusoidal lining cells) and adipose tissue (see Chapter 4). Most tissue-resident macrophages are established before birth from primitive haematopoietic cells originating in the yolk sac and are self-sustaining populations.

ADVANCED CONCEPT

Two Polarized Forms of Macrophages have been Characterized

- The M1 type of macrophage is adapted for promoting inflammatory responses and is nicknamed a 'killer macrophage'. This type is activated by bacterial wall lipopolysaccharide (LPS) and IFN-γ. As part of their phenotype they produce IL-12 (activates T cells) and low levels of IL-10 (anti-inflammatory cytokine). This functional state of macrophage is understood to be involved in the elimination of pathogens, killing virally infected cells and eliminating cancer cells as part of wider immune surveillance.
- The M2 type of macrophage is adapted for modulating and downregulating inflammatory responses and promoting healing and repair. As part of this phenotype they produce high levels of IL-10 and TGF-β (inhibits immune responses) and low levels of IL-12.

CLINICAL EXAMPLE

Macrophages and the Pathology of Obesity

A distinct subset of macrophages is found in adipose tissue – **adipose tissue macrophages.** Dysregulation of function linked to obesity has been associated with the development of wider immune dysfunction and correlated with production of proinflammatory molecules. In those with normal body mass, macrophages comprise about 5% of cells in adipose tissue. However, in the obese state, macrophages can comprise 50% of cells in adipose tissue. Inflammation originating in this way has been implicated in the development of insulin resistance and type 2 diabetes in obesity.

> **Most APCs are dendritic cells derived from a common bone marrow progenitor.**

APCs phagocytose antigenic material, process it through proteolytic systems and present the resulting fragments to lymphocytes at the cell surface in combination with molecules of the MHC. The main type is termed a **classical dendritic cell** (cDC). Such cells are present in all tissues and can account for around 5% of all cells. They are characterized by the following features:

- Elongated ramified cell processes and ruffles to present a large membrane surface area for antigen trapping
- Specialized proteolytic system that can cut out antigenic structures from larger proteins
- Motile and can migrate from tissues to carry any encountered antigen to T cells in lymph nodes
- Surface expression of MHC class II and the integrin CD11c and can present antigen to T cells
- Derived from a distinct progenitor cell and express markers of white cell lineage (leukocyte common antigen)

Cells that can be classified as dendritic APCs are:

- Langerhans' cells of the skin
- Dendritic cells of lymph nodes and spleen (Fig. 8.8)
- Interstitial dendritic cells, which form a population of dendritic cells in the support tissues of most organs
- Veiled cells of the blood, which are thought to be circulating forms of dendritic APCs in transit between tissues; three main types have been characterized by expression of surface markers using flow cytometry
- Microglia of the central nervous system (see Fig. 6.23)

In each of these sites, both in lymphoid and non-lymphoid tissues, dendritic cells can constantly sample the local environment and acquire and process antigens. Despite certain common attributes, each of these cell types is microenvironmentally specialized, and each has slightly different cell-surface receptors and proteins which adapt them to antigen presentation in different sites.

In addition to antigen presentation, this class of dendritic cells can play a role in innate immunity independent of T-cell activation and can also modulate local immune responses.

In contrast, some other cells which are also termed dendritic cells have a mesenchymal origin; for example, the **follicular dendritic cells** of lymph nodes. The follicular dendritic cells also differ, as they present antigen to B cells (not T cells) and lack MHC class II expression.

Fig. 8.8 Dendritic Antigen-Presenting Cells. Micrograph showing dendritic antigen-presenting cells from a lymph node. This section is immunostained for CD14, which is expressed on this type of cell as a pattern recognition receptor (PRR) as part of the innate immune response.

> **Plasmacytoid dendritic cells are a second main type of dendritic lineage cell.**

Plasmacytoid dendritic cells (pDCs) are found in blood and are also resident in lymphoid tissues. They are derived from the same common dendritic cell progenitor in bone marrow as cDCs (see Chapter 7) and play an important role in innate immunity. Although termed *plasmacytoid dendritic cells,* this is a name derived from cell lineage studies rather than morphology. Histologically they appear as rounded cells with a basophilic cytoplasm and abundant rough ER typical of a protein-producing cell. They are seen in low numbers in blood and are present in lymphoid organs and tissues. This class of dendritic cells carries pattern-recognition receptors and can detect viral and bacterial pathogens, after which they show a characteristic response of producing very high levels of type I interferons. The secreted interferon can then locally stimulate other immune cells to target virally infected cells or cancer cells. Although pDCs have low levels of MHC class II, once activated, they can also interact with T cells and present antigen as part of the adaptive immune response.

BONE MARROW

The bone marrow is the site of origin of B- and T-cell precursors and of macrophages and is discussed in detail in Chapter 7.

THYMUS

> **The thymus is the site of T-cell development.**

Immunologically naïve lymphocytes from bone marrow called **thymocytes** differentiate into mature T cells in the thymus. During this process, the immune system distinguishes self from foreign antigens and develops self-tolerance.

Fig. 8.9 Thymus. (a) In the child, the cortex (C) of the thymus is divided into lobules by fibrocollagenous septa (S) and is surrounded by adipose tissue of the mediastinum. The medulla (M) is less cellular. **(b)** In the adult, there is involution of the thymus, with replacement by adipose tissue (A). The division into a cellular cortex (C) and a less cellular medulla (M) is still apparent. **(c)** The dominant feature of the thymic cortex is its vast number of densely packed lymphocytes (thymocytes), which range in size from small to large, depending on their activity. Most, if not all, of the thymocytes are in direct contact with thymic epithelial cells (E), which permeate the whole gland and act as a supporting framework. They are difficult to identify in the sea of lymphoid cells but are visible where they surround blood vessels entering the gland. Numerous macrophages (Mc) are scattered throughout the cortex and contain the phagocytosed debris of eliminated lymphocytes. **(d)** The dominant feature of the thymic medulla is its epithelial component, the cells having large pale nuclei and abundant eosinophilic cytoplasm. Thymocytes are less densely packed than in the cortex; most are T cells en route to the general circulation. Hassall's corpuscles (H) are derived from thymic epithelial cells, which first appear during fetal development and form continuously thereafter. The process begins with the enlargement of a single medullary epithelial cell, which undergoes progressive degenerative changes characterized by nuclear disintegration and increasing cytoplasmic eosinophilia. Vacuoles appear in the cytoplasm, taking up the nuclear debris. This process is repeated in nearby epithelial cells, which form concentric lamellae around a central hyalinizing mass. Hassall's corpuscles may grow as large as 100 μm in diameter and undergo a variety of degenerative changes, becoming infiltrated by lymphocytes, macrophages and eosinophils; they may also show cystic change or calcification.

The thymus is also an endocrine organ, secreting hormones and other soluble factors, which not only control T-cell production, differentiation and maturation in the thymus but also regulate T-cell function and interactions in peripheral tissues.

The thymus is the first lymphoid organ to develop and is derived from the endoderm and a small ectodermal element of the ventral wing of the third pharyngeal pouch on each side.

> **The thymus is a soft lobulated organ located in the superior and anterior mediastinum.**

At birth, the thymus is pinkish-grey in colour and weighs 10–15 g, increasing to 30–40 g by puberty. Thereafter, it undergoes progressive involution and extensive fatty infiltration and assumes a yellowish colour.

In children, the thymic parenchyma is divided into an outer, highly cellular cortex and a pale-stained central medulla. The cortex is divided into irregular lobules 0.5–2.0 mm in diameter by fine septa extending in as far as the corticomedullary junction from a loose fibrocollagenous capsule. The less cellular medullary tissue forms a continuous central core. The main cell types in the thymus are thymic epithelial cells (TECs), thymocytes (lymphocytes), dendritic APCs and macrophages (Fig. 8.9).

> **The thymic epithelial cells have essential roles in regulating thymic function.**

Thymic epithelial cells promote T-cell differentiation, proliferation and subset maturation. In addition, they secrete hormones and other substances that regulate T-cell maturation and proliferation within the thymus and other lymphoid organs.

The thymic epithelial cells form the stromal meshwork of the thymus and have a variety of ultrastructural and immunohistochemical features. Three cell types are recognizable: cortical thymic epithelial cells (cTECs), medullary thymic epithelial cells (mTECs) and Hassall's corpuscle cells (see Fig. 8.9). These cells are all believed to derive from a common thymic epithelial cell precursor.

Beneath the capsule, the thymic epithelial cells form a continuous layer, which is carried deeply into the thymus to invest the septa and vessels entering and leaving the organ.

Within the cortex, **cTECs** form a sponge-like structure containing an extensive network of spaces which becomes colonized by thymocytes (see Fig. 8.9c).

In the medulla, sheets of **mTECs** converge to form a coarser, more solid structure of medullary cells with smaller interstices accommodating much smaller numbers of thymocytes.

Deep in the medulla, the thymic epithelial cells form bulky cords and whorls, some of which contain lamellated structures (**Hassall's corpuscles**; see Fig. 8.9d).

Thymic epithelial cells have pale-staining oval nuclei and eosinophilic cytoplasm and can be readily identified in the medulla. In the cortex, however, their fine cytoplasmic extensions make them difficult to identify within the mass of lymphocytes.

With the electron microscope, typical desmosomes (see Fig. 3.6b) are seen to bind the epithelial cells, which contain bundles of intermediate (cytokeratin) filaments.

> **Thymic epithelial cells in the cortex are in close contact with thymic lymphocytes and are called *nurse cells*.**

Once they enter the thymus gland, thymocytes first move to the cortex (Fig. 8.10). In the thymic cortex, individual cTECs are in intimate contact with multiple thymocytes and completely enclose them by deep infoldings of surface membrane. Described as thymic nurse cells, they are the environment in which thymocytes undergo genetic recombination to produce the diversity of T-cell receptors (α and β chains) needed for immune recognition. The developing thymocytes undergo a process called *positive selection,* which ensures that each unique T-cell receptor is effective in being able to bind to the major histocompatibility molecules, and hence that the developing T cell can function once fully mature. Thymocytes that have developed useless, non-functional T-cell receptors do not manage to achieve positive selection and undergo cell death by apoptosis because they do not receive survival signals from cTECs, so-called *death by neglect*. Thymocytes that pass positive selection move to the thymic medulla.

> **Medullary thymic epithelial cells can express most self-antigens, which is essential in developing immune self-tolerance.**

Medullary thymic epithelial cells ectopically express and present many self-antigens, including those which are otherwise highly specific tissue-restricted antigens (TRAs) in a process termed *promiscuous gene expression*. Each specific TRA is expressed by a very small proportion (<3%) of mTECs

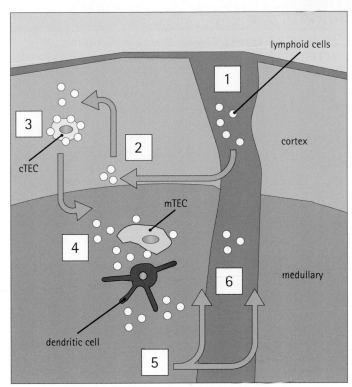

Fig. 8.10 Lymphocyte Development in the Thymus. 1. Lymphocytes enter the thymus from blood vessels in the stroma. 2. Now called thymocytes, they pass to the cortex. 3. Thymocytes interact with cortical thymic epithelial cells (cTECs) (positive selection for functional MHC binding). 4. Thymocytes that are positively selected pass to the medulla, where they interact with medullary epithelial cells (mTECs) and dendritic cells, which negatively select cells that bind to self-antigens. 5. T cells leave the medulla to enter blood vessels in the stroma. 6. T cells of different types now migrate to secondary lymphoid organs.

at any one time. The thymic medulla, by producing an environment in which many self-antigens can be encountered, is believed to be the site where self-tolerance is acquired by developing T cells.

Positively selected thymocytes migrate to the medulla from the cortex (see Fig. 8.10), where they are presented with all tissue-restricted self-antigens by both mTECs and classical dendritic APCs. If any T cell shows avid binding to these self-antigens, response signals lead to the death of the self-reacting thymocytes through apoptosis in a process termed *negative selection*. In this way, only T cells that recognize non–self-antigens can survive. Most developing thymocytes are killed in this process, and only a minority go on to form the naïve CD4⁻ or CD8⁻ positive T cells that then leave the thymus to populate peripheral tissues and lymphoid organs. Certain thymocytes which show less avid binding to self-antigens are signalled to develop into regulatory T cells, which will later be capable of modulating any immune reaction that might develop to self-antigens.

Any failure of negative selection and the subsequent deletion of self-reactive thymocytes would lead to the development of disease caused by autoimmunity.

CLINICAL EXAMPLE

Failure to Express Tissue-Specific Antigens on MTECs Leads to Autoimmune Disease

The ability of thymic epithelial cells to express many TRAs is linked to the action of a transcription factor called *autoimmune regulator* (AIRE), which is expressed in mTECs. The rare human autoimmune disease APECED is characterized by defective functional development of mTECs and is caused by mutations in the AIRE.

In this condition, mTECs fail to express TRAs, and so the process of negative selection of autoreactive T cells in the thymic medulla cannot take place. The thymus instead allows the production of T cells that recognize a wide range of self-antigens.

APECED is an acronym for autoimmune polyendocrinopathy candidiasis ectodermal dystrophy. The condition is also called *autoimmune polyendocrinopathy syndrome type 1* (APS1). Patients who have mutations in AIRE develop multiorgan autoimmune disease in childhood.

The *AIRE* gene codes for the AIRE transcriptional activator, acting on downstream transcription of a wide range of other genes. In the thymus lack of function of AIRE leads to the failure of mTECs to express tissue-specific genes coding for TRAs.

The presence of this rare inherited autoimmune disorder illustrates the importance of promiscuous TRA expression in mTECs in the development of T-cell immune tolerance.

The thymus has a rich vascular supply, which allows migration of lymphoid cells.

The thymus receives its arterial supply via many small branches of the internal thoracic and inferior thyroid arteries, which enter the thymus mainly via the interlobular septa.

In the region of the corticomedullary junction, the vessels give rise to small radially arranged arterioles and capillary loops to supply the cortex and medulla.

The cortical capillaries have continuous endothelium (see Chapter 9), whereas those of the medulla and septa may be fenestrated.

At the corticomedullary junction, the postcapillary venules have a taller endothelium with features of high endothelial venules.

Venous tributaries follow the course of the arterial vessels in the septa, with some forming a plexus within the thymic capsule before draining via the thymic veins into the left brachiocephalic, internal thoracic and inferior thyroid veins.

The thymus receives no afferent lymphatics, but the medulla and corticomedullary area give rise to efferent lymphatics, which follow the course of the arteries and veins.

The thymus undergoes involution after puberty.

The thymus reaches its maximum weight at puberty, declining thereafter, so that in old age, it may be so small as to be unrecognizable. Involution involves replacement of the gland by adipose tissue (fatty infiltration) and a decline in its lymphocyte content.

Fatty infiltration begins at birth but accelerates after puberty. Adipocytes increase in number in the perivascular compartment. Initially, this is most apparent in the septa; thus the cortex is involved first and then the process is extended into the medulla (see Fig. 8.9b).

Thymocyte depletion begins after 1 year of age and thereafter continues at a constant rate, independent of puberty. It results in progressive collapse of the sponge-like TEC framework, which nevertheless remains intact, so that cords of TECs can be seen histologically, even in the most atrophic thymic remnants. Such cells probably continue to secrete thymic hormones into old age.

Despite the progressive decrease in their number with involution, thymic lymphocytes continue to differentiate and proliferate, thus maintaining a supply of T cells throughout life.

CLINICAL EXAMPLE

An Inherited Form of Immunodeficiency is Linked to Failure of Thymic Epithelial Cell Function

Severe combined immunodeficiency (SCID) is characterized by defects in T-cell development and function with knock-on effects in the development of B cells and NK cells and a clinical presentation in early childhood with life-threatening infections. Although there are several different genetic causes, a rare form of SCID is caused by mutation of *FOXN1*. Forkhead box N1 protein (FOXN1) is a transcription factor found in TECs, hair follicles and the nail bed. FOXN1 is vital for the differentiation of TECs, and in its absence, thymocytes do not differentiate to form T cells.

Affected patients have an absent thymus (athymia) and associated severe immunodeficiency, a 'nude' phenotype with complete loss of body hair (alopecia universalis) and deformity of the nails.

Much of the understanding of immunology, transplantation biology and T-cell function has come from work done in animal models. Nude mice are congenitally hairless and have no thymus: hence they have no T cells and no cell-mediated immune responses. The phenotype is also caused by mutation of *FOXN1*.

LYMPH NODES

The lymph nodes are an important site for generation of immune responses.

Lymph nodes are small organs found in groups or chains at sites where lymphatic vessels draining an anatomical region converge to form larger lymphatic vessels; for example, in the neck, axillae, groins and para-aortic area. They have two main functions:

- Phagocytic cells within the nodes act as non-specific filters for particulate matter, such as micro-organisms and carbon, preventing them from reaching the general circulation.
- They provide an elegant mechanism whereby lymphocytes can interact with new antigens and APCs at an interface between lymph and the blood. Starting with only a small number of lymphocytes recognizing an antigen, lymph nodes facilitate proliferation of activated cells and consequently amplification of the immune response by forming clones of lymphocytes.

When relatively inactive, each lymph node is only a few millimetres in length, but they may become greatly enlarged when functional demands are increased.

The cells of the lymph node can be divided into three functional types: lymphoid cells, immunological accessory cells and non-immunologically active stromal cells.

Lymphoid cells in lymph nodes include lymphocytes of all types and their derivatives. Most of the lymphocytes enter the node via the blood, but a few enter via lymph draining from the tissues.

Immunological accessory cells comprise a variety of macrophages, including those with phagocytic antigen-processing, antigen-presenting and non-specific effector functions.

Non-immunologically active stromal cells comprise the lymphatic and vascular endothelial cells and fibroblasts, which elaborate the stromal reticular framework. Many of the endothelial cells are highly specialized for interaction with lymphoid cells.

Each lymph node is divided into several functional compartments.

The lymph node is a bean-shaped organ with a fibrocollagenous capsule from which fibrous trabeculae extend into the node to form a supporting framework (Fig. 8.11).

The convex surface of the gland is penetrated by a number of afferent lymphatic vessels, which drain into the node, whereas at the hilum there is an efferent lymphatic vessel that transports lymph toward larger collecting lymphatic vessels. In turn these vessels drain into more proximal nodes or chains of nodes before entering the blood via either the thoracic duct or the right lymphatic duct.

Lymph nodes contain three functional compartments (Fig. 8.12):

- A network of endothelial-lined **lymphatic sinuses** continuous with the lumina of the afferent and efferent lymphatic vessels
- A network of small blood vessels, where circulating lymphocytes enter the node
- A parenchymal compartment composed of superficial cortex, deep cortex (paracortex) and medulla

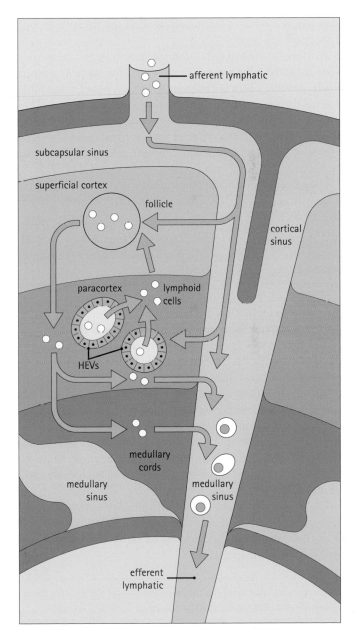

Fig. 8.12 Functional Compartments of the Lymph Node. Antigens, accessory cells and lymphocytes enter the lymph node via the afferent lymphatics, which drain into the subcapsular sinus and thence into the cortical sinuses. These antigens, accessory cells and lymphocytes may then enter the cortex or remain in the sinuses and leave the lymph node via the efferent lymphatic vessel. Most lymphocytes enter the node from the blood via the high endothelial venules (HEVs), which are lined by a special endothelium bearing lymphocyte-homing receptors.

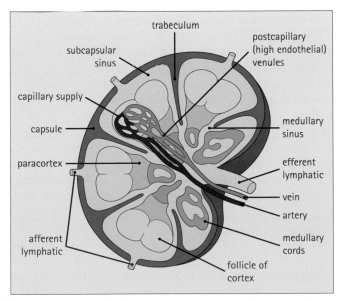

Fig. 8.11 Lymph Node Structure. The bean-shaped lymph node has a hilum into which blood vessels enter and from which efferent lymphatics emerge. It has an investing capsule. Afferent lymphatic vessels penetrate the convex surface of the gland and drain into the subcapsular and medullary sinus system. The lymphoid parenchyma is divided into cortex, paracortex and medulla. The most prominent structures in the cortex are the lymphoid follicles.

The structural integrity of the lymph node is provided by a framework of reticulin fibres (see p. 65), which are linked to the fibrous trabeculae. These fibres are most dense in the parenchymal compartment, although some do traverse the lymphatic compartment, where they are completely invested by endothelial cells.

> **Lymph node sinuses carry lymph throughout the nodal structure.**

Afferent lymphatics drain into a major subcapsular sinus running around the periphery of the lymph node. From this sinus, cortical sinuses pass down toward the medulla through the cortical cell mass.

Within the medulla, the dominant feature is a network of interconnected lymphatic channels called the *medullary sinuses,* which converge upon the efferent lymphatic vessel at the hilum.

Only the larger channels of the lymphatic compartment can be seen by light microscopy. The cortical sinuses are generally difficult to see because of their highly convoluted shape and numerous fine extensions, which penetrate the cellular mass of the cortex.

The extremely thin and pale-staining endothelial lining cells of the sinuses are almost impossible to identify with ordinary staining methods.

> **The blood supply of lymph nodes is the main route of entry of lymphocytes into the node.**

The blood supply also provides the metabolic needs of the lymph node. One or more small arterial vessels enter the node via the hilum and then divide in the medulla into branches, which ramify into a capillary network corresponding to the cortical follicles and deep cortex.

Within the deep cortex, the postcapillary venules (see Chapter 9) have cuboidal endothelium-bearing specialized cell receptors (lymphocyte-homing receptors), which are recognized by circulating lymphocytes and facilitate the passage of lymphocytes from the blood and into the lymph node. The postcapillary venules are often described as **high endothelial venules** (HEVs).

The blood vessels of the superficial cortex and medullary cords are thought to be non-specialized and do not appear to allow the exit of lymphocytes. Small veins draining the node leave via the hilum.

> **The superficial cortex of the lymph node contains the densely staining spheroidal aggregations of lymphocytes (lymphoid follicles).**

The superficial cortex of a lymph node is initially composed of **primary follicles** made up of naïve B cells in a network of follicular dendritic cells. The B cells in primary follicles are small lymphocytes with dark-staining, dense chromatin and barely visible cytoplasm (Fig. 8.13).

Fig. 8.13 Superficial Cortex Primary Follicles. In this micrograph, part of a lymph node is shown with the capsule (C). Two primary follicles (PF) are seen composed of closely packed lymphocytes with no visible cytoplasm. Below the primary follicles is the deep cortex (paracortex).

When lymph draining to the node brings a foreign antigen, this stimulates proliferation of B cells resulting in the formation of **germinal centres,** so forming **secondary follicles.** The proliferation of B cells is part of clonal expansion in response to antigen stimulation, which displaces the small lymphocytes of the primary follicle to the periphery of the secondary follicle, where they come to form the **mantle zone** around the germinal centre (Fig. 8.14).

The lymphocyte population of the germinal centres in secondary follicles consists predominantly of B cells, but there are smaller populations of Th cells, macrophages and accessory cells.

The **mantle zone** of a follicle is an outer ring of small lymphocytes surrounding a germinal centre. The mantle zone is composed of antigen-naïve B lymphocytes

A marginal zone composed of lymphocytes with moderate amounts of cytoplasm is described around secondary follicles in white pulp of the spleen and in some mesenteric lymph nodes but is not typically present elsewhere. Marginal zone lymphocytes have receptors that bind to microbial molecular patterns as part of innate immune responses and are understood to play an important role in defence against blood-borne capsulated bacteria such as pneumococci.

> **The main cells of the lymphoid follicles are B cells.**

B cells enter a lymph node via the HEV of the paracortex. Within a few hours, many have migrated to the superficial cortex. If activated, they proliferate and remain in the lymph node for an extended period as memory cells or plasma cells. In contrast, non-activated cells re-enter the general circulation within a matter of hours via the efferent lymph.

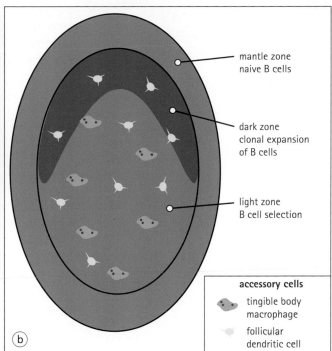

mantle zone
naive B cells

dark zone
clonal expansion
of B cells

light zone
B cell selection

accessory cells

tingible body
macrophage

follicular
dendritic cell

Fig. 8.14 Superficial Cortex Secondary Follicles. In micrograph **(a)**, part of a lymph node is shown with the capsule (C). Two secondary follicles (SF) are seen with a pale, oval centre called the germinal centre and a surrounding belt of small lymphocytes. Below the secondary follicles is the deep cortex (paracortex). **(b)** This diagram shows the different parts of the germinal centre of a secondary follicle. In addition to B cells the follicle contains accessory cells. **(c)** At a higher magnification, a capsule (C) is seen composed of collagen, beneath which is the subcapsular sinus (S). A secondary follicle containing a germinal centre (G) with a mantle zone (M) is present in the underlying cortex.

The primary follicles contain mainly naïve B cells and some memory cells. The secondary follicles, in contrast, contain small naïve B cells peripherally and activated B cells in their germinal centres.

It is possible to identify several stages in the maturation of B cells in the follicles (Fig. 8.15). Activated B cells proliferate and mature and thereby produce an expanded population of identical cells recognizing the same antigen. This takes place in the dark zone of the germinal centre. The light zone clonal selection takes place involving a subset of T cells and accessory cells.

The activated B cells in the germinal centre are collectively called **follicle centre cells.** They are characterized by open nuclei and have more cytoplasm and are less densely packed than the smaller, more peripheral follicular B cells; this explains the lighter staining intensity of the germinal centres. Immunohistochemical staining is able to highlight different aspects of the germinal centre and secondary follicle (Fig. 8.16).

The proliferation and differentiation of antibody-secreting plasma cells is thought to result from T cell–B cell interaction in the paracortex. The plasma cells then migrate directly to the medullary cords, where they are conveniently situated to secrete antibody into the efferent lymph.

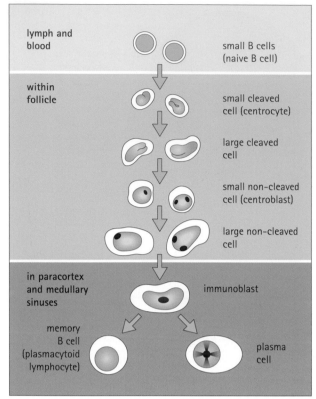

Fig 8.15 B-cell Development in the Lymph Node. The maturation of B cells from small naïve cells to dividing cells responding to a specific antigen is associated with a distinct series of morphological changes. From the small lymphocyte, the cell changes first into a centrocyte with a cleft nucleus and then into a centroblast. This cell enlarges, leaves the follicle and migrates to the paracortex and medullary sinuses as an immunoblast, ultimately transforming into a plasma cell or a memory B cell.

Accessory cells in the superficial cortex are involved in antigen processing.

A variety of immunological accessory cells are found in the superficial cortex. These are derived from bone marrow and reach the lymph node via the afferent lymph. These cells all appear to play some role in antigen processing; this also applies to the accessory cells of the paracortex and medulla. These immunological accessory cells cannot be readily distinguished in haematoxylin and eosin (H&E), sections but may be stained by immunochemical techniques for special macrophage markers.

The main accessory cell types in the superficial cortex are:

- **Sinus macrophages,** highly phagocytic cells of the subcapsular and cortical sinuses
- **Tingible body macrophages,** so named because they contain cellular debris and are found within the germinal centres with an abundance of lysosomal enzymes (see Fig 8.16e)
- **Marginal zone macrophages,** which constitute a morphologically diverse group of phagocytic cells located within the follicular interstitium immediately beneath the subcapsular sinus
- **Follicular dendritic cells** (see Fig. 8.16f) which have numerous fine branching surface projections covered by electron-dense material

Fig 8.16 Cells Populating the Germinal Centre. This panel shows germinal centres stained using a variety of methods to highlight different cell components. **(a)** H&E micrograph showing the dark zone (D) and light zone (L) and mantle (M) within a secondary follicle. **(b)** This follicle is immunostained using MiB-1, an antibody, to show nuclei of dividing cells in cycle. The cells of the germinal centre are actively proliferating. The dark zone (D) has a higher density of nuclei than the light zone (L). Few lymphocytes in the mantle (M) are in cycle. **(c)** Follicle stained using a B-cell marker, CD20. The germinal centre, mantle zone and many surrounding cells are B cells. **(d)** Follicle stained using a T-cell marker, CD3. A few T cells are seen in the germinal centre involved in clonal selection as helper T cells. T cells are also present outside the mantle zone. **(e)** Follicle stained using a macrophage marker, CD68, to show tingible body macrophages in the germinal centre. B cells that are not clonally selected undergo cell death and are removed by these macrophages. **(f)** Follicle stained to show a marker of follicular dendritic cells, which form a scaffold within the germinal centre and are involved in antigen processing and presentation. (Image used under Creative Commons License https://creativecommons.org/licenses/by-sa/3.0/ from the Human Protein Atlas Antibody to CD21 CR2 HPA060715 follicular dendritic cells https://www.proteinatlas.org/ENSG00000117322-CR2/tissue/lymph+node#img.)

Follicular dendritic cells retain antigen on their surface for many months. These cells present antigen directly to B cells and lack the MHC class II expression normally seen on other APCs.

The main cells of the lymph node deep cortex are T cells.

The cell population of the deep cortex (paracortex) consists of lymphocytes and accessory cells, which constantly move in and out of the region.

T cells dominate the deep cortex (Fig. 8.17), entering the node from the blood via the HEV and leaving 6–18 hours later via the efferent lymphatic.

When activated, T cells enlarge to form lymphoblasts. These then proliferate to produce an expanded clone of activated T cells. In a T-cell–dominated immunological response, the paracortex may expand into the medulla, producing a so-called **paracortical reaction**. Activated T cells are then disseminated via the circulation to peripheral sites, where much of their activity occurs.

Accessory cells of the deep cortex act as APCs.

Interdigitating cells are prominent in the deep cortex and are one form of 'dendritic APC', being so named because of their numerous cytoplasmic processes which interdigitate with those of other cells. These cytoplasmic processes also make numerous contacts with other cell types in the vicinity.

Macrophages are also found in the deep cortex. Their cytoplasm is often observed packed with lipid (possibly engulfed cell membrane) and nuclear debris.

Fig. 8.17 Lymph Node Deep Cortex (Paracortex). (a) Micrograph of lymph node paracortex showing sheets of T cells, which vary in morphology from small inactive cells to large cells representing activated proliferating T cells. The high endothelial venules (HEVs) are prominent, but accessory cells are inconspicuous even at high magnification. **(b)** Area immunostained with an antibody to CD34, which is a cell adhesion molecule expressed on the endothelium of HEVs and required for T cells to migrate through the walls of these vessels. Endothelial cells lining the HEV stain brown. Note the plump pericytes surrounding each vessel. The blue nuclei in the background are T lymphocytes of the paracortex. **(c)** Micrograph of lymph node stained by an antibody to CD3 that detects T cells. The deep cortex (paracortex) (D) stains darkly (i.e. is T cell in nature), whereas the middle of the germinal centre (G) is faintly stained, being mostly composed of B cells. A few T cells are seen in the germinal centre and represent helper T cells involved in the maturation of B-cells. See also Fig. 8.16c.

> **The lymph node medulla is composed of a series of sinuses separating cords of cells.**

The medulla of the lymph node contains mainly:
- Cell-rich medullary cords
- Wide medullary sinuses (separating the medullary cords) through which lymph percolates toward the hilum from the cortex
- Larger blood vessels and their supporting trabeculae

As in the cortex, the interstitial compartment of the medulla is supported by a framework of reticulin fibres, a small number of which traverse the sinuses.

> **The medulla contains plasma cells and macrophages.**

The most common cells in medullary cords are plasma cells and their precursors. Plasma cells synthesize antibody, which is carried from the node to the general circulation via the efferent lymph. In addition, some mature plasma cells probably migrate from the node.

Classic macrophages are the main accessory cell type in the medulla. They are located in the sinuses and derive support from the traversing reticulin fibres (Fig. 8.18).

> **Lymph entering the node is filtered, and antigens are presented to lymphoid cells.**

Lymph draining into a lymph node via afferent lymphatics first enters the subcapsular sinus and then percolates through the cortical sinusoidal maze to drain into the medullary sinuses before leaving the node via the efferent lymphatics.

Fig. 8.18 Macrophages in Lymph Node Medulla. This is a section stained with CD68 showing brown-stained macrophages populating the medulla of the node.

Some particulate matter is probably taken up from the lymph and disposed of by the phagocytic activity of the endothelial cells without evoking any immune response.

Antigens are phagocytosed and processed by various types of APCs exposed to the lymph. They are then transferred via the APC cytoplasmic extensions to sites where they may be encountered by lymphocytes.

Lymphocytes entering a lymph node in the afferent lymph constitute less than 10% of all the lymphocytes entering the node, except in the case of mesenteric nodes, where they may constitute up to 30%. The rest of the lymphocytes gain entry via the high endothelial venules.

Activated lymphocytes pass through the endothelium of the subcapsular sinus and enter the germinal centres of the cortical follicles.

CLINICAL EXAMPLE

Spread of Cancer to Lymph Nodes

Cancerous cells may break off from primary tumours and enter lymphatic vessels, from where they migrate to lymph nodes. Once in the node, they adhere to and proliferate in the sinuses (Fig. 8.19).

Fig. 8.19 Spread of Cancer to Lymph Nodes. Micrograph showing clumps of cancer cells from a carcinoma of the stomach in the subcapsular (S) and cortical (C) sinuses of a lymph node.

KEY FACTS

Lymph Nodes

- Function to allow interaction between antigen and lymphoid cells
- Main site for proliferation of lymphoid cells in an immune response
- Follicles are composed of B cells (follicle centre cells)
- Deep cortex (paracortex) is composed of T cells
- Medulla contains plasma cells and macrophages
- Most lymphocytes enter the node from specialized high endothelial venules
- Antigen from tissues enters the node in lymph, which circulates around a series of sinuses

SPLEEN

The spleen lies in the left upper abdomen and weighs around 150 g in the adult.

The two principal functions of the human spleen are:

- To mount a primary immune response to antigens in the blood
- To act as a filter to remove particulate matter and aged or abnormal red cells and platelets from the circulation

The following description is specific to **human** spleen. The spleen has a thin fibrocollagenous capsule containing elastic fibres, and its external surface is covered by peritoneal mesothelial cells. Arising from the capsule are short, radially arranged collagenous septa which extend into the organ. These support an extensive network of reticulin fibres that forms the scaffold for the splenic parenchyma.

Blood vessels enter the spleen at the hilum and branch within its structure, surrounded by collagenous tissue, which form vascular trabecula.

Most of the spleen is composed of a vast array of sinusoids and vascular sinuses filled with blood (**red pulp**). A branching array of arteries (central arteries) associated with aggregates of lymphoid tissue is called **white pulp** and accounts for 5%–20% of the total mass of the spleen (Fig. 8.20).

Fig. 8.20 Spleen Anatomy. H&E micrograph of spleen showing its fibrous capsule (C) and areas of white pulp (W) seen as dense-staining aggregates of lymphoid cells adjacent to central arteries The red pulp (R) is less densely stained, as it has fewer nuclei, and at this magnification it is not possible to distinguish between the various sinuses and parenchymal components. Within the parenchyma are collagenous trabeculae containing the trabecular arteries (T). No septa arising from the capsule are shown in this histological section.

> **The splenic red pulp is composed of cords of cells separated by sinusoids.**

The red pulp consists of loose support tissue supported by reticulin fibres with several functional areas:

- **Capillaries,** which terminate by draining into a fusiform shaped structures called the *ellipsoidal (sheathed) capillaries.*
- A **parenchyma** composed of stellate reticular support cells, which surrounds sponge-like cavities through which blood from sheathed capillaries slowly percolates. These are called the splenic cords.
- **Venous sinuses,** which run adjacent to columns of parenchymal tissue and drain blood that has filtered through the parenchyma, along with blood that has come directly from the sheathed capillaries.

The sinuses are lined by flattened endothelial cells resting on a discontinuous basement membrane, which is interrupted by numerous narrow slits through which red cells squeeze. Phagocytic cells are closely associated with the walls of these sinuses (Fig. 8.21 and see Fig. 8.23).

> **The splenic white pulp is composed of lymphoid cells and is divided into three zones.**

The white pulp of the spleen is related to the branching arterial tree, and is composed of lymphocytes and accessory cells supported by a reticulin scaffold. It is divided into three zones (Fig. 8.22).

Periarteriolar lymphoid sheath (PALS). This zone contains T cells and B cells and typically has a densely cellular area surrounded by a less densely cellular part. The area adjacent to the central artery is mostly composed of small T cells with the outer part also containing some B cells and a majority of T cells.

Follicles. The white pulp may include follicles composed of B cells which are usually located near an arteriole merging into the PALS. In young people, many of the follicles have germinal centres and a mantle zone similar to secondary follicles seen in lymph nodes; the proportion of such follicles diminishes with age.

Marginal zone. This zone surrounds the PALS and is the most peripheral part of the white pulp at the interface between the white pulp and the red pulp. It is composed of small lymphocytes, less densely packed larger lymphocytes and dendritic APCs which surround fine vascular channels with a reticulin scaffold (Fig. 8.23).

In addition to these lymphoid areas associated with the central arteries, a significant number of small B-cell, T-cell and plasma-cell aggregates are present in the splenic parenchyma.

> **The marginal zone of the white pulp defends against pathogens in the bloodstream.**

The marginal zone is composed of B cells in a sparse reticulin scaffold and anastomosing fine vascular channels surrounded by dendritic APCs and a specialized subset of macrophages.

About 10% of blood entering the spleen is believed to pass into the marginal zone parenchyma, from where it drains into the sinusoids or directly into the venous sinuses of the red pulp.

The marginal zone and its associated lymphocytes are arranged to maximize the interaction of APCs and marginal zone lymphocytes as part of the splenic lymphoid immune response against antigens that are blood-borne rather than tissue-based.

Fig. 8.21 Splenic Red Pulp. (a) H&E micrograph of red pulp, which is composed of parenchymal areas (P), termed splenic cords and sinusoids (S). The endothelial cells protrude into the sinuses. **(b)** This micrograph is stained with an antibody to NOS3 that detects endothelial cells and highlights the anatomy of the splenic sinuses. The cellular, blue-stained areas are the tissues of the cords of the red pulp. **(c)** Micrograph of splenic red pulp venous sinusoids, which have been immunostained for the lysosomal enzyme cathepsin-D *(brown)* and highlights the abundant phagocytic macrophages associated with the walls of the venous sinusoids (S). **(d)** H&E micrograph of an ellipsoidal sheathed capillary (C), seen here in cross-section. **(e)** Micrograph of splenic red pulp immunostained for CD271 *(brown)*, which is a marker for sheath cells and highlights the ellipsoidal sheathed capillaries. (Images (b) and (e) used under Creative Commons License https://creativecommons.org/licenses/by-sa/3.0/ from the Human Protein Atlas. (b) Antibody to NOS3 CAB002168 https://www.proteinatlas.org/ENSG00000164867-NOS3/tissue/spleen#img; (e) Antibody to Nerve Growth Factor Receptor CD271 CAB000143 https://www.proteinatlas.org/ENSG00000064300-NGFR/tissue/spleen#img.)

Fig. 8.22 Spleen White Pulp. The white pulp is composed of the periarterial lymphatic sheath seen as a densely cellular area (PD) surrounding the central arterioles (A) and merging with a less densely cellular outer area (PL). No follicle is seen in this image of the white pulp. The edge of the white pulp merges into the marginal zone (MZ), which forms an interface with the red pulp (R). Splenic sinusoids (S) of the red pulp can also be seen. The splenic white pulp is a key site responsible for provision of an immune response to blood-borne infections. The peripheral part of the PALS (PL) includes both T and B lymphocytes, as well as macrophages. This outer part of the PALS is an important site for development of plasma cells responsible for secretion of immunoglobulin following antigenic stimulation.

The following labels appear in the figure:

- reticulin 'hoop'
- endothelial cells and macrophages line sinuses
- slits in sinus wall
- Splenic venous sinus
- marginal zone perilymphoid sinuses
- sheathed capillaries
- penicillar arteries
- central artery
- splenic cords
- radial arterioles to perilymphoid sinuses
- venous sinuses
- follicle
- trabecular vein
- trabecular artery
- white pulp (mainly T lymphocytes)
- fibrocollagenous support tissue
- marginal zone network
- marginal sinus
- perimarginal cavernous sinus
- antigen-presenting cell (APC)
- (A), (B), (C)

Fig. 8.23 Vascular Anatomy of the Spleen. The spleen has two main functions: it removes aged and effete red cells from the circulation, and it mounts an immune response to antigens, particularly bacteria, circulating in the blood. Blood enters the spleen in the splenic artery; this branches to form the trabecular arteries, which give rise to a series of central arteries surrounded by T cells of the white pulp. For red cells to be removed, blood passes along the central arteries and then enters the red pulp through a series of specialized vessels (penicillar arteries and sheathed capillaries) to drain into the splenic parenchyma (splenic cords). The blood then percolates through spaces between the reticular cells forming the splenic cords and squeezes through narrow slit spaces to enter the splenic venous sinuses. Normal red cells are deformable and survive this passage, but aged red cells have rigid membranes and are lysed. Fragments of destroyed red cells are removed by phagocytic cells along the sinus walls. Red cells leave the system via trabecular veins and enter the splenic vein. This pathway is the open circulation (A). A proportion of the splenic circulation enters small arterioles to reach a series of marginal sinuses, which run around the lymphoid sheaths in the marginal zone. In this area, blood comes into contact with dendritic antigen-presenting cells, and foreign antigens can be trapped and presented to marginal zone lymphocytes. Most of the blood from the marginal sinuses around the lymphoid sheaths enters the red pulp and then drains into the venous sinuses (B), but a small proportion passes directly into the sinuses and forms what is termed the closed circulation (C).

Marginal zone lymphocytes are B cells with an unusual profile such that they are capable of recognizing and binding to conserved microbial determinants in a PAMP-like innate immune response (see p. 135). For this reason, marginal zone lymphocytes have been termed *innate-like cells*. This functional aspect links in with the role of the spleen in responding to pathogens in the bloodstream, especially bacteria with a capsule such as *Streptococcus pneumoniae*.

Similar 'innate-like' lymphocytes are found in the subcapsular sinus of lymph nodes and amongst intraepithelial lymphocytes in the tonsils and Peyer's patches.

> **The splenic vasculature is arranged to filter blood through the red pulp.**

Central arteries run eccentrically in the white pulp of the spleen and lead to:

- Strands of arterioles and capillaries which supply the white pulp
- Arterioles and capillaries that run directly into a system of marginal zone fine vascular sinusoids (see Fig. 8.23)

The marginal zone sinusoids are arranged concentrically around the white pulp in the perilymphoid **marginal zone.** In human spleen, perfusion studies have defined three concentric systems:

- The marginal zone network
- The marginal sinuses
- The perimarginal cavernous sinus

The central arteries terminate in a series of straight arterial vessels, traditionally called **penicillar arteries.** These arteries are devoid of an investing layer of lymphoid cells and run in the red pulp. In turn, they give rise to arterioles and capillaries, which tend to leave the arterioles at right angles.

The postarteriolar splenic capillaries of the red pulp initially have a standard structure but then change into a specialized structure described as **ellipsoidal sheathed capillaries** (see Figs 8.21d and 8.21e). This part of the capillary has an inner endothelial layer which is surrounded by concentric layers of pericytes and specialized stromal cells called **sheath cells.** Intermixed in these concentric layers are macrophages and B lymphocytes. The function of the ellipsoidal sheathed capillaries is uncertain, but it has been proposed that they are involved in B-lymphocyte recirculation.

Most of the sheathed capillaries drain into the splenic parenchyma, which consists of a sponge-like network of spaces between stellate reticular cells (splenic cords). A small proportion of capillaries drain directly into the perimarginal cavernous sinuses.

◎ ADVANCED CONCEPT

Splenic Blood Circulation

Blood can be filtered by percolation through the parenchyma (splenic cords) and then into the sinusoids – **open** circulation – the main route of blood flow in the human spleen.

The **closed** circulation appears to be a minor component of human splenic blood flow. Blood from the perimarginal cavernous sinuses bypasses the slow route through the splenic parenchyma and enters the splenic venous sinus instead. This provides a system for blood to pass rapidly through the spleen without filtration. In humans, a small number of capillaries arising from the central arteries also open directly into the venous sinuses.

👥 CLINICAL EXAMPLE

Splenectomy

Removal of the spleen is necessary:
- When it is ruptured after abdominal trauma
- In some diseases; for example, lymphomas
- As part of major surgery; for example, removal of the stomach for cancer

Effects of Splenectomy
The effects of removing the spleen highlight its main functions.

Changes in the Blood
The blood film (Fig. 8.24) from a patient who has had a splenectomy shows increased numbers of platelets and abnormal red cells with deformed shapes (poikilocytosis) along with aged red cells contain blue-staining particulate inclusions of nuclear material (Howell–Jolly bodies).

These nuclear remnants would normally be removed by percolation through the splenic cords and into the splenic sinuses.

Infection
Patients who have had a splenectomy are at risk of developing life-threatening bacterial septicaemia. The most common organism involved is *S. pneumoniae*. The spleen filters the blood, and any blood-borne organisms are phagocytized by the macrophages in the splenic sinusoids. But in a person without a spleen, the organism can circulate in the blood and reproduce. It is therefore recommended that anyone undergoing a splenectomy should be immunized against *S. pneumoniae*.

Fig. 8.24 Postsplenectomy Blood Film. Micrograph of blood film from a patient after splenectomy. The red cells have bizarre shapes, and in this field some of the cells contain small particulate dark-staining inclusions [Howell–Jolly bodies (H)]. A nucleated red blood cell (RBC) is also present (N). (Courtesy Vishnu V.B. Reddy, MD, professor of pathology, University of Alabama at Birmingham, USA.)

MUCOSA-ASSOCIATED LYMPHOID TISSUE

> **Lymphoid cells may concentrate in mucosal surfaces and solid glands to provide defence.**

In addition to the mass of the peripheral lymphoid tissue encapsulated in the lymph nodes and spleen, the body contains an equally large amount of non-encapsulated lymphoid tissue, which is located in the walls of the gastrointestinal, respiratory and urogenital tracts; conjunctiva; and skin in addition to less defined populations within solid epithelial glands such as the thyroid and salivary glands.

This tissue is known as **mucosa-associated lymphoid tissue (MALT)** and takes the form of diffuse infiltrates or more discrete nodules; it provides immunological protection against invasion by pathogens via vulnerable exposed absorptive surfaces. In solid epithelial glands, MALT typically only forms visible structures in the presence of a disease stimulus, with normal tissues only showing inconspicuous scattered cells of the immune system.

The gut-associated lymphoid tissue (GALT) includes:
- The palatine, lingual and pharyngeal tonsils (adenoids)
- Mucosal nodules in the oesophagus
- **Peyer's patches** in the small intestine (see Chapter 11)
- Lymphoid aggregations in the large intestine and appendix
- A vast number of lymphocytes and plasma cells scattered throughout the lamina propria of the small and large intestines

The bronchus-associated lymphoid tissue (BALT) is located beneath the mucosa of the large respiratory passages (bronchi) in infancy and may be induced in disease states in adults. Nasal-associated lymphoid tissue (NALT) is present in the nasopharynx. An induced skin-associated lymphoid tissue (iSALT) comprising Langerhans' cells and scattered T and B cells in the epidermis and dermis can be associated with some disease states.

In these mucosa-associated sites, MALT comprises APCs (dendritic cells, macrophages), with the main population of lymphoid cells being $\gamma\delta$ T cells, NK cells and NKT cells (innate immune system). Other mature T cells and B lymphocytes are present, including a proportion of memory cells (adaptive immune system).

In large aggregations of MALTs, which are seen mainly in the tonsils and Peyer's patches, the lymphoid tissue is arranged into follicles, which often contain germinal centres and are similar to those of the lymph nodes. With immunohistochemical techniques, discrete B- and T-cell zones containing typical antigen-processing accessory cells can be identified and have functions analogous to those of the superficial cortex and paracortex of the lymph node, respectively.

Scattered lymphocytes in the lamina propria of the gut and respiratory tract include B cells, some of which mature into antibody-secreting plasma cells. All classes of antibody are produced, but IgA predominates.

IgA is secreted into the gut lumen in a form called *secretory IgA,* which is resistant to enzymatic digestion and provides protection against pathogens before they breach the tissues.

IgG and IgM are secreted into the lamina propria to deal with organisms eluding the surface protective mechanisms.

IgE mediates the release of histamine from mast cells, which are present in large numbers in the lamina propria.

The recirculation of lymphoid cells from MALTs is to local lymph nodes rather than to lymph nodes that drain non-mucosal tissues.

> **Intraepithelial lymphocytes are important components of MALT.**

It is increasingly recognized that there is a specialized population of lymphoid cells that inhabit the intercellular space within epithelial surfaces, termed **intraepithelial lymphocytes.** These cells are regarded as part of the MALT system.

Many of these cells are T-cell receptor $\gamma\delta^+$ T cells, which upon activation can secrete a range of cytokines with both inflammatory and protective functions and in this respect act as a component of the innate immune system. Other cells are components of the adaptive immune system, including memory cells.

> **Peyer's patches are large aggregations of lymphoid tissue found in the small intestine.**

Peyer's patches number about 200 in humans. They extend through the lamina propria and submucosa and often bulge into the gut lumen (Fig. 8.25). The overlying epithelium of a Peyer's patch (dome epithelium) is characterized by cuboidal rather than tall columnar cells (see Fig. 11.26) and contains large numbers of intraepithelial lymphocytes. Goblet cells are absent.

Some of the epithelial cells (microfold cells) exhibit numerous surface folds instead of the usual microvilli and have been designated *M cells.* These cells are derived from the mucosal crypts and function in the delivery of antigen from the gut lumen to lymphoid cells, which are wrapped in pockets at the basolateral cell membrane. M cells take in antigens at the folded apical membrane; they then internalize the antigen in vesicles from which they are transported to the basolateral membrane and delivered to the closely adjacent lymphoid cells.

Fig. 8.25 A Peyer's patch composed of lymphoid cells, including a germinal centre, associated with the bowel mucosa.

> **Tonsils are lymphoid tissues in the oropharynx.**

Waldeyer's ring of pharyngeal lymphoid tissue comprises four groups of tonsillar tissue. The largest is the palatine tonsils, which contain 12–15 deep tonsillar crypts lined by stratified squamous epithelium (Fig. 8.26). These crypts frequently contain plugs of lymphocytes, bacteria and epithelial debris, which may become calcified.

The tonsils contain numerous lymphoid follicles with germinal centres, and the lymphoid tissue appears to have a cellular make-up similar to that of Peyer's patches. The epithelium overlying the tonsillar tissue contains T cells and dendritic APCs. For other components of Waldeyer's ring, see page 201 and page 211.

 CLINICAL EXAMPLE

MALT may be the site of development of malignant tumours of lymphocytes termed *MALT lymphomas* (MALTomas). These tumours have distinct characteristics that distinguish them from other forms of malignant lymphoma derived from lymph node populations. MALT lymphoma belongs to a group called *marginal zone lymphoma* in which the malignant cells have characteristics similar to the B cells that are normally found in the marginal zone around germinal centres. In several settings, before the development of malignancy, there has been activation of MALT by a chronic inflammatory reaction; for example, lymphoma of the stomach may develop after inflammation of the gastric mucosa linked to infection by the bacterium *Helicobacter pylori*. In other settings the chronic inflammation is related to an organ-specific autoimmune disease such as Hashimoto's disease leading to a MALT lymphoma of the thyroid.

CLINICAL EXAMPLE

Tumours of the Lymphoid System

The main primary tumours of the lymphoid system are derived from lymphocytes and their precursors and are termed **lymphomas.** The diseases usually begin in lymph nodes, which become enlarged and firm; they may be localized or may involve several lymph node groups. In addition, lymphomas may also involve the spleen, bone marrow or liver. The first lymphoma was described by Thomas Hodgkin, and this specific type has subsequently been named *Hodgkin's lymphoma*. Thus the main categories of lymphoma are:

- Hodgkin's lymphoma (with the wit and intellectual rigour for which pathologists are renowned)
- Non-Hodgkin's lymphoma

Accurate identification of the specific type of lymphoma is very important in management and prognosis, and immunocytochemical methods are used to identify whether the tumour cells are B lymphocytes or T lymphocytes and further refined by use of a panel of markers for different cell subsets. Histological assessment of the cytological and nuclear characteristics of the tumour cells allows them to be identified as mature forms ('low grade') or immature precursor forms ('high grade'). High-grade lymphomas behave in a more malignant manner but are highly sensitive to cytotoxic chemotherapy. Increasingly, diagnosis is supplemented by analysis of gene expression profile of tumours that give additional prognostic and therapeutic information.

Fig. 8.26 Palatine Tonsil. (a) Low-power micrograph showing a typical tonsillar architecture with squamous epithelium folded into crypts (C) associated with dense lymphoid aggregates in which follicles are visible (F). **(b)** Medium-power micrograph of a tonsil showing a tonsillar crypt (C) lined by squamous epithelium and surrounded by tonsillar lymphoid tissue (L). The crypt contains colonies of oral commensal bacteria (B), which is a normal finding.

For online review questions, please visit https://studentconsult. inkling.com.

Blood and Lymphatic Circulatory Systems and Heart

INTRODUCTION

The main transport systems are the circulatory systems, in which substances are dissolved or suspended in liquid and carried from one part of the body to another in a series of tubes (vessels). There are two main circulatory systems: the blood circulatory system and the lymphatic system.

The **blood circulatory system** is the main method of transporting oxygen, carbon dioxide, nutrients and metabolic breakdown products, cells of the immune and other defence systems, chemical messengers (hormones) and many other important substances (e.g. clotting factors). Transfer of transported substances from blood to tissue and vice versa occurs in the systemic and pulmonary **capillary systems** (Fig. 9.1). These tiny thin-walled vessels permit the passage of fluid, small and large molecules, dissolved gases and even cells across their walls in both directions. The circulatory network that transports blood to the capillaries is called the **arterial system,** and the network that carries blood away from the capillaries is called the **venous system.**

The **lymphatic circulatory system** drains extracellular fluid from the tissues, returning it to the blood circulatory system after passage through lymph nodes. This system is also involved in absorption of nutrients from the gut.

BLOOD CIRCULATORY SYSTEM

> **The two main blood circulatory systems are the systemic and pulmonary systems.**

There are three types of blood circulatory systems, two of which (systemic and pulmonary circulations) depend on a central pump, the heart, to push the blood around (see Fig. 9.1). The third system is the portal system, discussed later.

The systemic circulation transfers oxygenated blood from a central pump (the heart) to all the body tissues (systemic arterial system) and returns deoxygenated blood with a high carbon dioxide content from the tissues to the central pump (systemic venous system).

The pulmonary circulation transfers deoxygenated blood with a high carbon dioxide content from a central pump (the heart) to the lungs (pulmonary arterial system) and transfers re-oxygenated blood from the lungs back to the central pump (pulmonary venous system).

The **portal systems** are specialized vascular channels that carry substances from one site to another, but do not depend on a central pump (see p. 166).

SYSTEMIC BLOOD VESSELS

There are two main types of large blood vessels:
- **Arteries,** which carry blood away from the heart toward the capillary systems at relatively high pressure
- **Veins,** which carry blood back to the heart from the capillary systems at relatively low pressure

The systemic arterial circulation is an extensive high-pressure system. The structure of its vessels reflects the high pressures to which they are subjected.

The output of the left ventricle is carried in large-diameter vessels with a high component of elastic tissue in their walls that smooths the systolic pressure wave. These are called the **large elastic arteries** (i.e. the aorta and its large branches, such as the carotid, subclavian and renal arteries).

Distal to these large elastic arteries are smaller vessels in which the artery walls become proportionately more muscular. These **muscular arteries** gradually decrease in size as they branch within tissues until they form **arterioles.** The arterioles then open into a system of very fine vessels termed **capillaries.**

From capillaries, blood moves into **venules** and then into **veins,** which become progressively larger as they approach the heart. The large veins carry blood at low pressure and hence have a small amount of muscle in their wall compared with arteries.

The pulmonary circulation transfers blood a short distance from the right ventricle of the heart to the capillary systems of the lung, and from there back to the left atrium of the heart. The pressures within the pulmonary circulation are lower and the walls of the main vessels are generally thinner than seen in the systemic circulation. The detailed histology of the pulmonary vasculature is discussed in Chapter 10.

> **The larger blood vessels are composed of three layers, which vary in prominence in the different vessel types.**

The walls of blood vessels are made up of three identifiable layers (tunica): **intima, media** and **adventitia.**

The tunica intima is composed of a lining layer of highly specialized, multifunctional, flattened epithelial cells termed

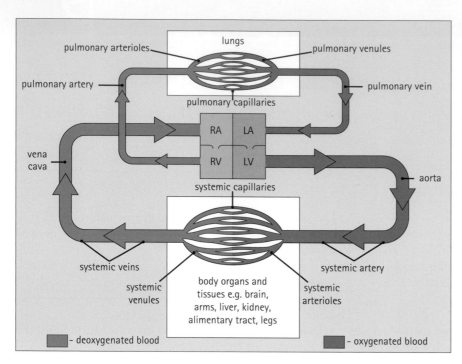

Fig. 9.1 Systemic and Pulmonary Blood Circulations. The main components and interrelationships of the systemic and pulmonary blood circulations. The heart is a four-chambered pump central to both systems. The direction of blood flow is indicated by *arrows*. Blood vessels that transport blood away from the heart are called *arteries* (arterial systems), and those that take blood to the heart are called *veins* (venous systems). The systemic venous and pulmonary arterial vessels carry deoxygenated blood; the pulmonary venous and systemic arterial vessels carry oxygenated blood. In organs and tissues other than the lung, the oxygenated blood gives up much of its oxygen and becomes deoxygenated; in the lungs deoxygenated blood is oxygenated. Gaseous exchange takes place in small, thin-walled vessels called *capillaries*. (*RA*, right atrium; *RV*, right ventricle; *LA*, left atrium; *LV*, left ventricle)

endothelium. This sits on a lamina (**the internal elastic lamina**); beneath this is a very thin subendothelial layer of fibrocollagenous support tissue containing occasional contractile cells with some of the properties of smooth muscle cells but which are also capable of synthesizing collagen and elastin (like fibroblasts) and which also can have phagocytic properties (like histiocytes/macrophages). These cells are called **myointimal cells** and become very important in the development of the most common arterial disease, atherosclerosis (see p. 162).

The media is the middle layer in a blood vessel wall and is composed predominantly of smooth muscle reinforced by organized layers of elastic tissue, which form elastic laminae. The media is particularly prominent in arteries, being relatively indistinct in veins and virtually non-existent in very small vessels. In vessels that are close to the heart, receiving the full thrust of the systolic pressure wave, elastic tissue is very well developed, hence the term **elastic arteries.** In muscular arteries and arterioles, the elastic lamina separating the tunica media and the tunica adventitia is the **external elastic lamina.**

The tunica adventitia is the outer layer of blood vessels. It is composed largely of fibroblasts and collagen, but smooth muscle cells may be present, particularly in veins. The adventitia is often the most prominent layer in the walls of veins. Within the adventitia of vessels with thick walls are small blood vessels, the **vasa vasorum,** which send penetrating branches into the media to supply it with blood. These are not seen in thinner vessels, which obtain their oxygen and nutrients by diffusion from the lumen. The adventitia also carries autonomic nerves, which innervate the smooth muscle of the media.

The differences between the layers in the wall of a small artery and a small vein are illustrated in Fig. 9.2. Although the

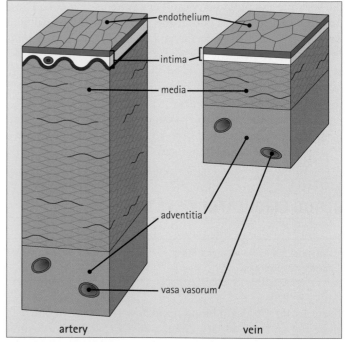

Fig. 9.2 General Structure of Blood Vessel Wall. The wall of a blood vessel is divided into intima, media and adventitia. In an artery, the intima contains elastic lamina and myointimal cells. In an artery, the media is much more developed than in a vein of the same diameter.

smaller vessels progressively lose the media and adventitia, all blood vessels have a tunica intima lined internally by the flat endothelial cells. The smallest vessels, the capillaries, have only a layer of endothelial cells sitting on a basal lamina. The endothelial cells lining the entire blood circulatory system are vitally important cells, with many functions.

> The endothelium is highly specialized, with endocrine, exocrine, cell adhesion, clotting and transport functions.

The endothelium is composed of flattened cells with diverse functional roles. In routine histological sections, the cytoplasm of most endothelial cells is barely visible and only the small flattened nuclei are seen. Ultrastructurally, each cell can be seen to be anchored to an underlying basal lamina; individual cells are anchored together by adhesion junctions, including prominent tight junctions, which prevent diffusion between cells. A prominent feature of endothelial cells is the presence of many pinocytotic vesicles, which are involved in the process of transport of substances from one side of the cell to the other. In small blood vessels of the nervous system, the endothelial cells express transport proteins, which are responsible for the active transport of all substances, for example, glucose, into the brain. Ultrastructurally, endothelial cells also contain smooth and rough endoplasmic reticulum and free ribosomes, with occasional mitochondria and variable numbers of microfilaments. The characteristic cytoplasmic organelle of the endothelial cell is an electron-dense ovoid structure called the **Weibel–Palade body,** which are storage granules containing von Willebrand factor, P-selectin and other vascular modulators (Fig. 9.3b).

Endothelial cells can sense changes in blood pressure, oxygen tension and blood flow. Each endothelial cell has chemoreceptors and mechanoreceptor elements linked to signalling structures of the primary cilium (see p. 37). In response to changes in local factors, endothelial cells respond by secreting substances which have effects on the tone of vascular smooth muscle. Vasodilators that cause relaxation of vascular smooth muscle and increase local blood flow include nitric oxide (NO), prostacyclin (PGI_2) and less well-defined factors that cause hyperpolarization of vascular smooth muscle (endothelium-derived hyperpolarizing factors [EDHFs]). Factors that cause vasoconstriction include thromboxane (TXA_2) and endothelin-1 (ET-1).

Endothelial cells are important for control of blood coagulation, and under normal circumstances the endothelial surface prevents blood clotting. This is done by high expression of factors that prevent blood clotting and low expression of factors that activate this process (see Fig. 9.3a).

▶ KEY FACTS

Endothelium

- Cells are bound together by junctional complexes and have many pinocytotic vesicles.
- Cells have many functional roles despite their apparent structural simplicity.
- Normally secretes factors which prevent blood clotting.
- Normally secretes factors which maintain the tone of vascular smooth muscle.
- Can be activated by cytokines to express cell adhesion molecules, which allow white blood cells to stick.

Factor secreted by endothelium	Activities
prostacyclin	vasodilation, inhibits platelet aggregation
nitric oxide	vasodilation, inhibits platelet adhesion and aggregation
tissue plasminogen activator (tPA)	regulates fibrinolysis
thrombomodulin	anticoagulant activity
thromboplastin	promotes coagulation
platelet activating factor (PAF)	activation of platelets and neutrophils
von Willebrand factor	promotes platelet adhesion and activation of blood coagulation

Fig. 9.3 Endothelial Cells. (a) Substances produced by endothelial cells that modulate blood coagulation and vasodilation. **(b)** High-power electron micrograph of part of an endothelial cell showing characteristic Weibel–Palade bodies (W) close to the surface contacting the vessel lumen (L). There are also pinocytotic vesicles (P) and smooth and rough endoplasmic reticulum.

Activated Endothelium

The endothelium can adapt rapidly to changes in its environment. Under certain circumstances, especially in response to inflammation, the endothelium may become activated and change its function.

The endothelium responds to blood flow and external stimuli to secrete factors which alter the state of contraction of vascular smooth muscle (vasoconstriction and vasodilatation).

Endothelium may become activated by cytokines and develop specialization for **emigration of lymphoid cells.** The endothelial cells become cuboidal in shape and express surface adhesion molecules, which facilitate lymphocyte adhesion and migration. This type of endothelium is normally seen in the specialized venules in the lymph node paracortex (high endothelial venules).

Endothelium may become activated by cytokines and express cell adhesion molecules for neutrophils. This normally occurs after any form of tissue damage and **allows neutrophils to migrate into local tissues** in the process of acute inflammation. The substance P-selectin, a cell adhesion molecule, is stored in special vesicles (Weibel–Palade bodies) inside the endothelium (see Fig. 9.3b). With appropriate stimulation, these vesicles dock with the endothelial cell membrane. P-selectin is then available on the cell surface for neutrophil adhesion.

Endothelium is normally locally impermeable to substances in the blood. Under the effects of certain factors – for example, histamine – endothelial cells lose attachment to each other and retract. This allows fluid and proteins to diffuse out into the local tissues, causing tissue swelling, termed **oedema.** This reorganization of cell–cell junctions is rapid and reversible and takes place in the space of a few minutes.

Elastic arteries are characterized by multiple elastic laminae in the media.

Elastic arteries are the largest arteries and receive the main output of the left ventricle; thus they are subjected to high systolic pressures of 120–160 mmHg. Furthermore, these large vessels are adapted to smooth out the surges in blood flow, as blood is impelled through them only during the systolic phase of the cardiac cycle. The elastic tissue in their walls provides the resilience to smooth out the pressure wave.

The intima of large elastic arteries is composed of endothelium with a thin layer of underlying fibrocollagenous tissue.

Elastic arteries have a thick, highly developed media of which elastic fibres are an important component. These are arranged in interrupted, lamellar circumferential sheets between layers of smooth muscle throughout the thickness of the media. In the largest artery, the aorta, there are often 50 or more layers (Fig. 9.4).

The elastic fibres are arranged in sheets so that they run circumferentially rather than longitudinally to counteract the tendency of the vessel to overdistend during systole. Return of the elastic fibres from the stretched to the unstretched state during diastole maintains a diastolic pressure within the aorta and large arteries of about 60–80 mmHg. Interposed between the elastic layers are smooth muscle cells and some collagen.

With age, and particularly in association with the common disease of the intima, atherosclerosis (see p. 162), the elastic fibres and smooth muscle fibres of the media of an elastic artery undergo degeneration and are replaced by non-elastic, non-contractile collagen. The most severe complication of the loss of elastic and smooth muscle is the permanent pathological dilatation of the elastic artery (usually the aorta). This is called **aneurysm** formation (see Clinical Example box, p. 162).

Fig. 9.4 Large Elastic Artery. (a) Low-power view of elastic van Gieson–stained large elastic artery (aorta). The predominant layer is the media (M), which is composed of elastic fibres *(black)* arranged as concentric sheets and separated by smooth muscle fibres and collagen. The red-stained tissues of the adventitia are included (A). **(b)** At a higher magnification this haematoxylin and eosin (H&E) image shows how layers of smooth muscle (M) are separated by the bright-pink elastic laminae (E), some of which show a characteristic wavy appearance, the tissue being in a non-distended state.

The adventitia of the large vessels carries vasa vasorum and nerves.

Muscular arteries have a media composed almost entirely of smooth muscle.

The large elastic arteries gradually merge into muscular arteries by losing most of their medial elastic sheets, usually leaving only two layers, an internal elastic lamina and an external elastic lamina, at the junction of the media with, respectively, the intima and the adventitia. The general structure of a muscular artery is shown in Figs 9.5a and 9.5b.

Fig. 9.5 Muscular Artery. (a) The most prominent layer of a muscular artery is the media. Composed of smooth muscle, it is bounded by an internal and an external elastic lamina. **(b)** Elastic van Gieson–stained transverse section through a muscular artery, which stains elastic black. The intima is visible inside the internal elastic lamina (I), which is crinkled because the vessel has contracted and is not perfused. The predominant layer is the muscular media (M) situated between an internal elastic lamina (I) and an external elastic lamina (E), which are composed of condensed sheets of elastic fibres. The outer adventitia (A) stains red, being composed largely of collagen. **(c)** A longitudinal section shows the muscular media (M) situated between the internal elastic lamina (IEL) and an external elastic lamina (EEL) *(black)*. **(d)** Medium-power view of the same artery showing the intima (I) and the fine black-staining elastic fibres running through the muscular media *(arrows)*. In this large muscular artery, the collagenous adventitia (A) is thick.

Atherosclerosis

Atherosclerosis is a disease of the arteries which starts in the intima. It is characterized by infiltration of the intima by oxidized lipids, which accumulate in macrophages and myointimal cells, accompanied by increased deposition of collagen. Such intimal thickening forms a so-called *atheromatous plaque.*

There are three common consequences of atheroma:

Impaired Blood Flow

Atheromatous change leads to a reduction in the size of the lumen of the vessel so that blood flow is decreased.

Thrombus Formation

Another complication of atherosclerosis is that it damages the smooth internal lining of endothelial cells, exposing circulating blood to the underlying intimal collagen. This can trigger coagulation to form a mass of blood clot, termed a *thrombus,* within the vessel. Thrombus further reduces the lumen of the vessel and may block it completely (Fig. 9.6), resulting in death of the tissue (infarction) supplied by the vessel. The myocardium is particularly vulnerable to infarction (see Fig. 9.22), as are the brain (stroke) and the feet and toes (gangrene).

Aneurysm Formation

As a plaque of atheroma enlarges, elastic fibres and smooth muscle are lost from the underlying media. In the large elastic arteries, such as the aorta, these specialized components become replaced by non-contractile, inelastic collagen, and the vessel dilates to form an abnormally wide sac termed an *aneurysm.* The danger of an aneurysm is that the vessel wall is greatly weakened and is prone to burst.

Fig. 9.6 Coronary Artery Atheroma and Thrombosis. Micrograph showing a transverse section from the coronary artery supplying the area of dead muscle shown in Fig. 9.22. The lumen has been greatly reduced by thickening of the intimal layer (I) by atheroma. The media (M) and adventitia (A) are normal. The intimal thickening and irregularity have led to the formation of a thrombus (T), which has blocked the vessel lumen.

In a muscular artery the media is composed almost entirely of smooth muscle. These arteries are therefore highly contractile, with their degree of contraction or relaxation being controlled by the autonomic nervous system and by endothelium-derived vasoactive substances. A few fine elastic fibres are scattered among the smooth muscle cells but are not organized into sheets. These are most numerous in the large muscular

arteries, which are a direct continuation of the distal end of the elastic arteries (see Figs 9.5c and 9.5d).

Muscular arteries vary in size from about 1 cm in diameter, close to their origin at the elastic arteries, to about 0.5 mm in diameter. In the larger arteries there may be 30 or more layers of smooth muscle cells, whereas in the smallest peripheral arteries there are only two or three layers. The smooth muscle cells are usually arranged circumferentially at right angles to the long axis of the vessel.

> **Arterioles are the smallest branches of the arterial tree.**

Arterioles vary in diameter, ranging from 30 μm to 400 μm (0.4 mm).

The intima of an arteriole is composed of endothelial cells lying on a basement membrane, with an underlying fine internal elastic lamina in the larger arterioles.

The arteriolar media is composed of one or two layers of smooth muscle cells (Fig. 9.7). As the arterioles become smaller,

Fig. 9.7 Arteriole. (a) Micrograph of a thin epoxy resin toluidine blue–stained section of three arterioles showing basement membrane (BM) as a pale-staining membrane surrounded by a layer of smooth muscle cells (SM). The inner endothelial cells (E) in the larger vessel appear rather cuboidal because it has contracted during the biopsy process. Note that the three arterioles differ not only in size but also with regard to the number of muscle cells. **(b)** The lower panel is made up of two images: on the left an arteriole immunostained to show smooth muscle (S) with endothelial cells (E) seen as blue counterstained nuclei and on the right an arteriole immunostained to show an endothelial marker (E) with non-stained smooth muscle (S) outside the endothelial layer. (Image used under Creative Commons License https://creativecommons.org/licenses/by-sa/3.0/ from the Human Protein Atlas Antibody to smooth muscle actin CAB013531 https://www.proteinatlas.org/ENSG00000107796-ACTA2/tissue/heart+muscle#img and Antibody to PECAM1 HPA004690 https://www.proteinatlas.org/ENSG00000261371-PECAM1/tissue/heart+muscle#img.)

the continuous layers of smooth muscle become progressively discontinuous. In the smallest arterioles, the endothelial cells have basal processes, which pierce the basement membrane and make junctional contacts with the smooth muscle cells. The adventitia of arterioles is insignificant.

Arterioles are highly responsive to vasoactive stimuli and make a major contribution to vascular resistance.

 KEY FACTS

Arterial System

- Large elastic arteries have a media composed of concentric layers of elastic and smooth muscle (e.g. aorta and subclavian arteries).
- Muscular arteries have a prominent media composed of smooth muscle, which is bounded by internal and external elastic laminae (e.g. coronary arteries).
- Arterioles are the smallest part of the arterial tree and have one to three complete layers of smooth muscle in their media.

The microvasculature starts at the level of the arterioles.

The microvasculature (Fig. 9.8) is composed of small-diameter blood vessels with partly permeable thin walls that permit the transfer of some blood components to the tissues and vice versa. Most of this exchange between blood and tissues occurs in the extensive capillary network, the smallest

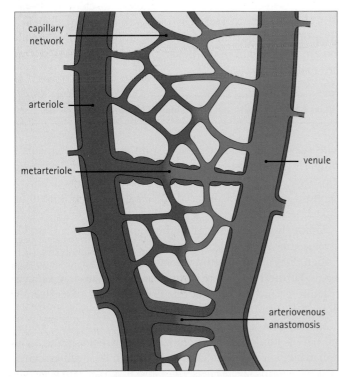

Fig. 9.8 Microvasculature. Blood flows from arteriolar to venular vessels through a complex network of capillaries, arising either directly from the arteriole or from the smaller metarteriole. Opening of the arteriovenous anastomosis directs blood flow out of the capillary network.

arterioles (metarterioles) emptying into the capillary system. The capillary networks drain into the first components of the venous system, the venules.

Capillaries are specialized for diffusion of substances across their wall.

Capillaries are the smallest vessels of the blood circulatory system (5–10 μm in diameter) and form a complex interlinking network.

Capillaries have the thinnest walls of all blood vessels and are the major site of gaseous exchange, permitting the transfer of oxygen from blood to tissues and carbon dioxide from tissues to blood. Fluids containing large molecules pass across the capillary wall in both directions.

The capillary wall (Fig. 9.9) is composed of endothelial cells, a basement membrane and occasional scattered contractile cells called *pericytes*.

Capillaries may be of two types: continuous or fenestrated.

Capillaries with **continuous** endothelium are the most common type, with the endothelial cells forming a complete internal lining to the capillary with no intercellular or intracytoplasmic defects (Fig. 9.10).

Capillaries with **fenestrated** endothelium are seen most commonly in the gastrointestinal mucosa, endocrine glands and renal glomeruli (see Figs 15.7 and 15.9). The endothelial cell cytoplasm is pierced by pores (fenestrations), which extend through its full thickness. In some fenestrations there is a thin diaphragm composed of fibrils which allows diffusion of small molecules.

Sinusoids are large-diameter channels with thin walls.

Highly specialized vascular channels, called *sinusoids,* are seen in some organs, for example, the liver (see Fig. 12.3) and spleen (see Fig. 8.21). They are endothelium-lined channels with a larger diameter than capillaries and scanty, discontinuous or absent basement membrane.

The endothelial cells in sinusoids are commonly highly fenestrated, often with large pores, and there may be substantial gaps between the cells.

 KEY FACTS

Capillaries

- Receive blood from arterioles and metarterioles (see Fig. 9.8)
- Are composed of a single layer of endothelium attached to a basal lamina
- Most have a continuous layer of endothelial cells which are tightly attached (continuous type)
- Some have pores which allow free diffusion from the lumen to tissues (fenestrated type)

Fig. 9.9 Capillary. (a) An epoxy resin section stained with toluidine blue of a capillary in longitudinal section. The wall is composed almost entirely of thin basement membrane (BM), the endothelial cytoplasm lining its internal surface not being visible at this magnification. An endothelial cell nucleus (EN) can be seen at one end. A similar but smaller capillary is seen in transverse section *(arrow)* between individual muscle fibres. **(b)** Electron micrograph of the capillary arrowed in **(a)**. At this low magnification, the endothelial cytoplasm (EC) is just visible, but the basement membrane is indistinct. **(c)** High-power electron micrograph of part of the capillary wall showing the basement membrane (BM), endothelial cytoplasm (C) and anchoring junction (J) between the cytoplasm of adjacent endothelial cells.

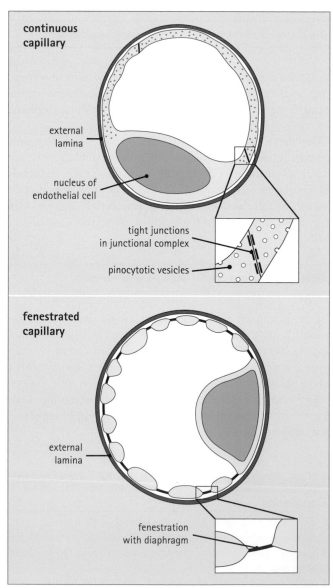

Fig. 9.10 Types of Capillaries. There are two types of capillaries: continuous and fenestrated. In continuous capillaries, substances are transported across the wall by pinocytosis.

| **Blood from capillaries enters a system of venules.** |

Capillaries drain into **postcapillary venules,** which are the smallest venules (10–25 μm in diameter). They resemble capillaries in structure but have more pericytes (Fig. 9.11).

Postcapillary venules drain into **large collecting venules,** 20–50 μm in diameter, in which the pericyte layer becomes continuous and surrounding collagen fibres appear.

As the collecting venules become larger bore, the pericytes are progressively replaced by smooth muscle cells, which form a layer one to two cells thick, and a fibrocollagenous adventitia becomes identifiable; these are **muscular venules** and are 50–100 μm in diameter. Muscular venules drain into the smallest veins.

| **Veins have thin walls and carry blood at low pressure.** |

Veins vary in size from less than 1 mm to 4 cm in diameter. In comparison with arteries of comparable external diameter, veins have a larger lumen and a relatively thinner wall and are therefore commonly collapsed in histological sections unless infusion-fixed.

Although intimal, medial and adventitial layers are present in veins, they are less clearly demarcated than in arteries, and it is often difficult to identify where one layer ends and another begins. Furthermore, there is considerable variation in vein wall structure according to location. The following description of veins of different sizes is therefore a generalization.

Small veins are a continuation of the muscular venules and have a similar wall structure but are larger – up to 1 mm in diameter – with more clearly defined muscle cell and outer fibrocollagenous layers (Figs 9.12a and 9.12b).

Medium-sized veins are 1–10 mm in diameter. They have an inner layer of endothelial cells on a basement membrane. This is separated by a narrow zone of collagen fibres from an indistinct condensation of elastic fibres producing a thin, discontinuous internal elastic lamina.

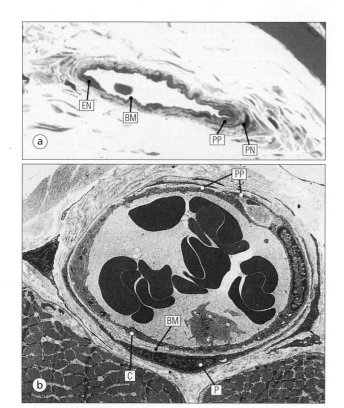

The inner layer is fairly consistent in structure, differing only in quantity of collagen and elastic fibres between the endothelium and the condensation of elastic fibres. However, the outer layers – still called *the media and adventitia*, but often arbitrarily and with little justification – vary considerably in thickness, proportions of collagen, elastic fibres and smooth muscle and in the orientation of the muscle fibres.

Large veins have an inner (intimal) layer similar to that of medium-sized veins, but there are usually more collagen and elastic fibres between the endothelial basement membrane and the elastic lamina, which is generally discontinuous. External to the elastic lamina there is a layer of smooth muscle embedded in collagen, and outside this is a thick layer of collagen in which there are bundles of longitudinally oriented smooth muscle fibres. Some elastic fibres intermingle with the collagen (see Fig. 9.12c).

Valves in large veins assist the flow of blood to the heart.

Venous circulation of blood is maintained by the contraction of venous smooth muscle, supplemented to varying degrees by external pressure from the contraction of the surrounding skeletal muscle responsible for arm and leg movement. Such assistance from skeletal muscle contraction is particularly important for maintaining the venous circulation of the arms and legs.

The veins in the arms and legs, which carry blood against gravity, are equipped with valves to prevent blood flowing back down the vein. These valves are thin flaps of intima that project into the lumen, with the free edges of the valve flaps pointing toward the heart; this allows blood to flow toward the heart but

Fig. 9.11 Postcapillary Venule. (a) Toluidine blue–stained epoxy resin section of a partly collapsed postcapillary venule. The endothelial cell nucleus (EN) and basement membrane (BM) can be identified. There are a few pericyte processes (PP) and a pericyte nucleus (PN) in the wall, but the details are not clearly visible. **(b)** Electron micrograph of a postcapillary venule showing the endothelial cell cytoplasm (C), basement membrane (BM) and pericytes (P) more clearly. Note that the finer pericyte processes (PP) apparently intervene between layers of the basement membrane.

Fig. 9.12 Veins. (a) H&E micrograph of a small vein. The media is composed of two to three layers of smooth muscle (thinner than in a small artery of this diameter). The endothelium is visible, but no distinct internal elastic lamina can be seen. Red cells and pink-stained plasma are in the lumen. **(b)** Micrograph showing an elastic van Gieson (EVG)–stained small vein. The rather variable and irregular arrangement of smooth muscle *(yellow)*, collagen *(red)* and elastic fibres *(black)* in its wall is evident. **(c)** Micrograph showing the wall of the largest vein in the body, the inferior vena cava. There is a distinct intima (I) and internal elastic lamina (EL), a layer of smooth muscle *(yellow, SM)* and an irregular layer of thick collagen *(red, C)*. This collagen indicates the approximate beginning of the adventitial layer, the thickest layer in large veins, being expanded by the presence of large bundles of longitudinally running smooth muscle (SML) (EVG stain).

prevents backflow. Incompetence of the valves in the veins of the legs causes varicose veins.

Valves are also present in other medium and large veins; their number varies depending on whether or not the vein is carrying blood against gravity.

> **Arteriovenous anastomoses allow blood to bypass capillary beds.**

In addition to the microvasculature (i.e. arterioles emptying into a capillary network, which drains into a venular system), there are additional vessels that bypass the capillary bed, allowing arterioles to communicate directly with venules; these are arteriovenous anastomoses (see Fig. 9.8).

At its arteriolar end, an arteriovenous anastomosis is thick-walled, mainly because of an abundant smooth muscle coat, which is richly innervated. Contraction of the thick smooth muscle layer closes off the lumen of the anastomosis at its origin and diverts blood into the capillary bed; relaxation opens the lumen, allowing blood to flow directly into a venule and thereby bypassing the capillary network.

Arteriovenous anastomoses are widespread but are most common in the skin in certain regions such as the fingertips, lips, nose, ears and toes. They are thought to play an important role in the skin's thermoregulatory function (see Chapter 18). Closure of the anastomosis diverts blood into the extensive dermal capillary system and permits heat loss, and opening of the vessel closes the capillary bed and conserves heat.

In the fingertips, there is a highly specialized type of arteriovenous anastomosis, the glomus body, which has a prominent arterial end (Sucquet–Hoyer canal) connecting directly to the venular end. The canal is surrounded by modified smooth muscle cells (glomus cells), which are richly innervated by the autonomic nervous system.

> **Blood vessels have both efferent and afferent innervation.**

Blood vessels that can significantly alter their lumen size by contraction and relaxation of their smooth muscle fibres have a major supply of adrenergic sympathetic fibres, stimulation of which causes muscle contraction and vasoconstriction.

Some blood vessels in skeletal muscles also have a cholinergic sympathetic innervation capable of producing vasodilation.

In certain areas, blood vessels have an afferent innervation, which provides information about the luminal pressure (baroreceptive information) and blood gas (i.e. carbon dioxide and oxygen) levels (chemoreceptive information). These are mainly located in the carotid sinuses and in the region of the aortic arch, pulmonary artery and large veins entering the heart.

Afferent fibres from the carotid sinus receptors travel in the glossopharyngeal nerve to the cardiorespiratory centres in the brain stem.

PORTAL BLOOD SYSTEMS

> **A portal system connects two capillary systems.**

Portal circulations are venous channels that connect one capillary system with another and do not depend on the central pumping action of the heart.

The nature of portal connecting vessels varies from site to site; for example, the vessels of the hepatic portal system (see Fig. 12.2), which connects capillaries in the intestine to the capillary-like sinusoids in the liver, are venous in nature, being small venules adjacent to the capillary beds and medium-sized and large veins in between. In the other main portal system, between the hypothalamus and the posterior pituitary (see Fig. 14.3), the connecting vessels are large capillaries and venules.

LYMPHATIC CIRCULATORY SYSTEM

> **The lymphatic system carries fluid that drains from the intercellular space of tissues.**

The intercellular spaces of almost all tissues contain small endothelial-lined tubes, which are blind-ending but otherwise identical in structure to blood capillaries. These are lymphatic capillaries and are permeable to fluids and dissolved molecules in the interstitial fluid.

In some areas, the lymphatic capillaries have a fenestrated endothelium and a discontinuous basement membrane, permitting the entry of larger molecules, such as large molecular weight proteins, triglycerides, and so on, and also some cells, particularly cells of the immune system.

The lymphatic capillary network acts as a drainage system, removing surplus fluid (lymph) from tissue spaces. Lymph is normally a clear colourless fluid, but lymph draining the intestine during absorption is often milky in appearance because of its high lipid content. This is called *chyle*.

The lymphatic capillaries merge to form thicker-walled vessels which resemble venules and medium-sized veins.

Lymph moves sluggishly from the capillary network into the larger lymphatic vessels; backflow is prevented by flap-like valves similar to those in veins (Fig. 9.13).

On its way to the larger vein-like lymphatics from the smaller lymphatics, lymph passes through one or more lymph nodes. It enters the lymph node at its convex periphery and leaves it through one or two lymphatic vessels at the concave hilum (see Fig. 8.11). During this passage, any antigens in the lymph can be processed by the immune system. Activated lymphocytes, which are important to immune defence, are added to the lymph.

The larger lymphatic vessels have muscular walls and pump the lymph into the following two main lymphatic vessels:

- The thoracic duct, which empties lymph into the venous system at the junction of the left internal jugular and left subclavian veins
- A more variable lymphatic vessel, the right main lymphatic duct, which empties into the junction between the right internal jugular and right subclavian veins

Fig. 9.13 Lymphatic Capillary. Micrograph showing a large lymphatic capillary (LC) running between pink-stained skeletal muscle fibres. The wall is very thin and lined by lymphatic endothelial cells. Note the delicate flap-like valves (V) controlling the direction of flow.

CLINICAL EXAMPLE

Spread of Cancer by Lymphatics

All lymphatic capillaries from an area drain into lymph nodes serving that particular area (regional lymph nodes). Such drainage is important in the spread of cancer, as cancer cells can enter the lymphatic capillaries and be carried to other sites. Cancer cells may also be trapped in the regional lymph node, where they can multiply and produce secondary tumours at some distance from the site of the primary cancer (see Fig. 8.19).

For example, cancers that originate in the breast may be carried in the lymph to the regional lymph nodes of the breast, most of which are in the axilla. Careful palpation of the axillary lymph nodes to detect possible tumour nodules is therefore a vital part of the physical examination of any patient with suspected breast cancer.

STEM CELLS AND THE VASCULATURE

Blood vessels are also known to be important components of the stem cell niche in various tissues and are seen as important in stem cell regulation.

Blood vessels themselves contain progenitor cells for endothelial cells and smooth muscle cells for renewal.

An interest in vascular stem cells and vascular growth is linked to understanding tissue development, tissue repair after injury and blood vessel formation in tumours. Inhibiting vascular growth is a target for cancer therapy.

However, the definitive identification of vascular stem cells, defined as self-renewing multipotent stem cells located in the wall of blood vessels that can form endothelial cells, pericytes, smooth muscle and adventitial cells to form a functional blood vessel, has been controversial. Adventitial progenitor cells have been identified with overlap with pericytes and mesenchymal stem cells. Cells that express stem cell antigen 1 (Sca-1) in adult blood vessels have stem or progenitor cell potential in model systems.

THE HEART

The heart is a muscular pump with four chambers. Two of these, the **atria,** receive blood from the systemic and pulmonary venous circulations, whereas the other two, the **ventricles,** pump blood into the systemic and pulmonary arterial circulations. In-between the cardiac chambers and at the two outflow portals of the heart are the **heart valves,** which prevent backflow of blood.

> **The wall of the heart is composed of the epicardium, the myocardium and the endocardium.**

The three layers of the heart wall are:
- A very thin outer **epicardium** (visceral pericardium) covered with flat mesothelial cells to produce a smooth outer surface
- A middle **myocardium** making up the vast bulk of the heart wall and composed of specialized muscle (cardiac muscle), which is responsible for the pumping action of the heart
- A very thin, inner smooth lining, the **endocardium,** covered by endothelial cells in direct contact with the circulating blood

The pericardium surrounds the heart and is lined by mesothelial cells.

The heart is enclosed within the pericardial sac, which is composed of compact fibrocollagenous and elastic tissue and lined internally by a layer of flat mesothelial cells, termed the **parietal pericardium.** This smooth mesothelial layer reflects over the outer surface of the heart to form the **visceral pericardium** (Fig. 9.14), also termed the **epicardium.**

The pericardial cavity is the space between the parietal and visceral pericardial layers. It contains a small amount of serous fluid to lubricate the surfaces and permit friction-free movement of the heart within the cavity during its muscular contractions.

When the visceral or parietal pericardium sustains structural damage as a result of disease, for example, inflammation, fibrin exudate covers the smooth lubricated surfaces and the friction-free movement is impaired. This can be detected clinically by listening over the heart area with a stethoscope, and a 'scratching' sound can be heard in time with each systolic contraction. This is called a **pericardial friction rub** and indicates inflammation of the pericardial surfaces, which can be further assessed by an ultrasound scan. This may occur when there has been a myocardial infarct (see Clinical Example box, p. 175) and is an indication that the full thickness of the myocardium of the left ventricular wall has been damaged from the inner endocardium to the outer pericardium.

Fig. 9.14 Visceral Pericardium (Epicardium). (a) Section of thin epicardium showing a narrow layer of fibrocollagenous tissue (F) containing elastic fibres *(black)*, covered by flat mesothelial cells (M) identical to those of the inner surface of the parietal pericardium (elastic van Gieson's stain). **(b)** H&E section of epicardium at higher magnification showing the detail of mesothelial cells (M). In many areas of the epicardium there is a layer of adipose tissue (A) (epicardial fat) beneath the fibrocollagenous tissue (F)

The epicardium forms the outer covering of the heart and has an external layer of flat mesothelial cells. These cells lie on a stroma of fibrocollagenous support tissue, which contains elastic fibres, as well as the large arteries supplying blood to the heart wall and the larger venous tributaries carrying blood from the heart wall. The large arteries (coronary arteries) and veins are surrounded by adipose tissue, which expands the epicardium.

The coronary arteries originate from the first part of the aorta just above the aortic valve ring and pass over the surface of the heart in the epicardium, sending branches deep into the myocardium. This superficial location of the arteries is of great practical importance, as it permits surgical bypass grafting to treat blocked arteries.

> **The myocardium is composed of specialized striated muscle termed cardiac muscle.**

The bulk of the heart is myocardium, which is the contractile element composed of specialized striated cardiac muscle (see Fig. 5.11).

The diameter of muscle fibres in the chambers of the heart varies according to the workload of the chamber (Fig. 9.15).

The left and right atria push blood into empty ventricles against minimal resistance during diastole and therefore have a thin wall composed of cells with a small diameter (see Fig. 9.15a).

The right ventricle pushes blood out through the pulmonary valve and through the pulmonary arteries to the lungs (see Fig. 9.1). It therefore has a moderately thick muscle layer composed of fibres intermediate in diameter between atrial and left ventricular muscle cells.

The left ventricle pumps blood through the high-pressure systemic arterial system and therefore has the thickest myocardium with the largest-diameter muscle fibres (see Fig. 9.15b).

Cardiac muscle fibres represent chains of individual cells linked together at intercalated discs, and cells may branch and connect adjacent fibres (see Figs 9.15c and 19.15d).

Because the myocardial muscle fibres of the left ventricle have the greatest workload (pumping blood throughout the body at a systolic pressure of 120 mmHg), they have a large energy requirement and therefore a high oxygen demand. If the blood supply to the myocardium is reduced, which is a common consequence of coronary artery disease, the muscle fibres become ischaemic and their function is impaired. This produces the symptoms of **angina** and, eventually, **myocardial infarction** (see p. 175).

The outer surface of the myocardium beneath the pericardium has a smooth contour, but the internal surface beneath the endocardium is raised into trabeculations, which are most marked in the ventricles. The trabeculations are covered by endothelial cells of the endocardium and do not interfere with the smooth flow of the blood.

In both ventricles, raised mounds of cardiac muscle (papillary muscles) protrude into the ventricular lumina and point toward the atrioventricular valves. Papillary muscles are the site of attachment of chordae tendineae, narrow tendinous cords that tether the atrioventricular valve leaflets to the wall of the ventricle beneath them.

> **Cardiac muscle cells secrete atrial natriuretic factor.**

Atrial myocardial fibres are smaller than those of the ventricles and contain small neuroendocrine granules, which are usually sparse and located close to the nucleus; they are most numerous in the right atrium. These granules secrete hormones in response to atrial muscle stretching called *cardiac natriuretic peptides* (cNPs), *atrial natriuretic peptide* (ANP) and *brain-type natriuretic peptide* (BNP).

Atrial natriuretic factor increases the excretion of water and sodium and potassium ions by the kidney. It also decreases blood pressure by inhibiting renin secretion by the kidneys and aldosterone secretion by the adrenals (see Chapter 14).

Serum levels of ANP and BNP are raised in some cardiac disorders – for example, in cardiac failure – and monitoring levels can be used in diagnosis.

Fig. 9.15 Myocardium. In transverse section, myocardial fibres from the atrium **(a)** can be compared to those from the left ventricle **(b)**. Although the fibres from both sites are lobulated with centrally placed nuclei, the ventricular fibres are larger. **(c)** Ventricular myocardium in longitudinal section. Myocardial cells form long fibres with centrally placed nuclei. There is a rich capillary network and minimal connective tissue in between cardiac muscle fibres. **(d)** Myocardial muscle may branch and bridge between adjacent fibres. At this magnification intercalated discs can be seen as eosinophilic structures separating individual cardiomyocytes *(arrows)*.

> **The endocardium lines the chambers of the heart and varies in thickness in different areas.**

The internal lining of all four heart chambers is the *endocardium,* which is composed of three layers (Fig. 9.16):
- The layer in direct contact with the myocardium
- The middle layer
- The innermost layer

The outermost layer is composed of irregularly arranged collagen fibres that merge with collagen surrounding adjacent cardiac muscle fibres. This layer may contain some Purkinje fibres, which are part of the impulse conducting system.

The middle layer is the thickest endocardial layer and is composed of more regularly arranged collagen fibres containing variable numbers of elastic fibres, which are compact and arranged in parallel in the deepest part of the layer. Occasional myofibroblasts are present.

The inner layer is composed of flat endothelial cells (see Fig. 9.16c), which are continuous with the endothelial cells lining the vessels entering and emerging from the heart.

The endocardium is variable in thickness, being thickest in the atria and thinnest in the ventricles, particularly the left ventricle. The increased thickness is almost entirely the result of a thicker fibroelastic middle layer (see Fig. 9.16). Localized areas of endocardial thickening (jet lesions) are common, particularly in the atria, and result from turbulent blood flow within the chamber.

> **The heart valves prevent blood flowing back into the heart chambers after emptying.**

During contraction of the ventricles (systole), blood is prevented from flowing back into the atria by two valves:
- The right atrioventricular (tricuspid) valve between the right atrium and right ventricle
- The left atrioventricular (bicuspid or mitral) valve between the left atrium and left ventricle

Similarly, to prevent blood flowing back into the two ventricles at the end of their contraction, there are valves between the ventricles and the large vessels into which they empty:
- The pulmonary valve between the right ventricle and its outflow vessel, the pulmonary artery
- The aortic valve between the left ventricle and its outflow vessel, the aorta

> **A central fibrocollagenous skeleton anchors the valves and chambers of the heart together.**

The heart has a fibrocollagenous skeleton, the main component being the **central fibrous body,** located at the level of the cardiac valves.

Extensions of the central fibrous body surround the heart valves to form the **valve rings,** which support the base of each valve. The valve rings on the left side of the heart surround the

Fig. 9.16 Endocardium. (a) Micrograph of elastic van Gieson (EVG)–stained right atrial endocardium (AE). The collagenous content stains red, elastic fibres stain black and myocardial muscle fibres (M) stain yellow. The nature of endocardial fibres is not apparent in a routine H&E-stained section. The atrial endocardium is much thicker than that which covers the ventricles. **(b)** Micrograph of EVG–stained left ventricular endocardium (VE) at the same magnification. It is a much thinner layer than in the atrium and contains much less elastic tissue; the muscle fibres (M) are large. The inner endothelial cell layer is usually poorly preserved in postmortem material, as here (E). **(c)** H&E micrograph of left ventricular endocardium (VE) with underlying cardiac muscle fibres (M). The elastic tissue seen in **(b)** is not visible without a special stain. The inner endothelial cell layer (E) is well preserved, as this sample is from a well-fixed diagnostic cardiac biopsy.

mitral and aortic valves and are thicker than those on the right side, which surround the tricuspid and pulmonary valves.

A short downward extension of the fibrocollagenous tissue of the aortic valve ring forms a fibrous septum between the right and left ventricles called the **membranous interventricular septum**. This is a minor component of the septum between the right and left ventricles, most of which is composed of cardiac muscle covered on both sides by endocardium. The membranous part is located high in the septal wall beneath the aortic valve.

> **The aortic and pulmonary valves have three cup-like cusps.**

The outflow valves of the right and left ventricles, the pulmonary and aortic valves, are composed of three cup-like cusps that fit closely together when closed. Because of their shape they are called *semilunar valves*.

The base of each valve is attached to a fibrocollagenous valve ring. The junctions between the cusps are called *commissures*.

> **The mitral and tricuspid valves are attached to heart muscle by tendinous cords.**

The atrioventricular valves are thin flaps attached to their respective valve ring at the base and tethered on their under-surface (ventricular surface) by the chordae tendineae. This prevents eversion of the valve leaflets into the atrium during ventricular contraction.

> **A heart valve is composed of fibroelastic tissue and is covered by endothelium.**

The heart valves all have the same general structure with a dense fibrocollagenous central plate (the fibrosa), which is an extension of the fibrocollagenous tissue of the central fibrous body and the fibrocollagenous valve ring. The fibrosa is covered on both surfaces by a layer of fibroelastic tissue and is covered by outer layers of flat endothelial cells. The thickness of the layers varies between valves, between sites within the same valve and with age (Fig. 9.17).

There are minor modifications to this general structure in the atrioventricular valves. Much of the lower ventricular surface of the atrioventricular valves is roughened, the roughening marking the points of insertion of the chordae tendineae. The chordae are not inserted solely at the free edge of the leaflet: some attach farther back, and a few small chordae insert near the base. The chordae fibres merge with the collagenous fibres of the central fibrosa of the valve leaflet. The atrioventricular valves may also have a thin layer of muscle fibres, continuous with those of the atrial wall, on their upper surface.

Fig. 9.17 Histology of Heart Valves. **(a)** High-magnification micrograph of H&E-stained aortic valve. The bulk of the valve leaflet is composed of loose fibrocollagenous tissue with non-staining glycosaminoglycans between the collagen fibres. There is a dense area of elastic tissue (El) on the superior surface. The flat endocardial cells (En) can be seen clearly on both surfaces of the valve. **(b)** High-magnification micrograph of elastic van Gieson (EVG)–stained aortic valve. The dense elastic tissue (El) stains black, and the collagen (C) stains red. **(c)** Micrograph of EVG-stained mitral valve close to its origin at the left atrioventricular valve ring. The leaflet is composed of red-staining collagen with some elastic fibres *(black)* running through it. The collagen is thickest, densest and most irregular on its inferior (ventricular) surface, where the chordae tendineae (CT) are attached. The chordae have a structure similar to that of tendon (see Fig. 13.9).

In addition to the general histological structure of heart valves, the aortic valve shows prominent fibroelastic thickening at the sites of cusp apposition during valve closure. This is sometimes visible as white lines (linea alba) just below the free edge of the cusps, with a central nodule at the midpoint of each cusp: the nodule of Arantius. These are also present but much less prominent on the pulmonary valve cusps.

Disorders of Heart Valves

There are several important abnormalities of the heart valves, all most commonly affecting the structure of the valves of the left side of the heart.

Rheumatic Valve Disease

Heart valves are damaged during the acute stage of a childhood illness called *rheumatic fever*. Healing of such damage results in progressive scarring of the valve leaflets, and their elastic content is replaced by irregular masses of collagen scar. The valves therefore become more rigid. The leaflets may also partially fuse, which limits their ability to open (stenosis) or close (incompetence).

Calcific Valve Disease

Calcific valve disease mainly affects the aortic valve, particularly if it is congenitally abnormal with only two cusps (i.e. bicuspid). Over time, the valves become thickened and distorted by fibrous scarring and deposition of calcium nodules (Fig. 9.18). This renders the valve leaflets immobile and impairs blood flow from the left ventricle during systole, leading to heart failure.

Infective Valvulitis

Heart valves may become colonized by bacteria or fungi, most commonly when the valve has been damaged previously, for example, by rheumatic disease. The damaged valve becomes covered in thrombus (blood clot), in which organisms proliferate. This causes signs of infection; the valve may become eroded and badly damaged; and fragments of thrombus may break off and enter the systemic circulation, where they can block smaller systemic arteries.

Fig. 9.18 Calcific Valve Disease. A bicuspid aortic valve that has become thickened and distorted by fibrous scarring and nodular calcium (CN) deposition.

The conducting system of the heart is composed of modified muscle fibres.

The heart contracts involuntarily, at a rate of around 70 beats per minute. The rhythmic contractions of atria and ventricles do not depend on nerve stimulation, but result from impulses generated within the heart itself. However, the autonomic

Fig. 9.19 Conducting System of the Heart. The opened right side of the heart trimmed to expose the septum between the two atria (AS) and the septum between the two ventricles (VS). The sinoatrial node (SA), internodal atrial muscle (IN), atrioventricular node (AV), bundle of His (BH) and right bundle branch (RBB) are indicated; the left bundle branch runs down on the left ventricular side of the interventricular septum.

nervous system can control the rate of heartbeat; stimulation of the parasympathetic (vagus) innervation slows the heart rate, and sympathetic stimulation increases it. The conducting system of the heart is composed of muscle fibres, which are modified to act as transducers rather than contractile cells. The impulse for contraction is initiated at a small group of specialized cells called the **sinoatrial (SA) node**, which acts as a pacemaker and stimulates atrial contraction. The impulse passes through the atrium and arrives at another node, the **atrioventricular (AV) node**. This node then initiates the later contraction of the ventricles, with the impulse passing down specialized bundles of cardiac muscle (the main bundle, the right and left bundle branches and the Purkinje fibres) to the farthest reaches of the ventricular muscle (Fig. 9.19).

Firing of the sinoatrial (SA) node regulates the cardiac rate as the primary cardiac pacemaker.

The SA node is located where the main vein from the upper part of the body (the superior vena cava) enters the right atrium (Fig. 9.20). Its position is constant, but the curved linear structure is so small that it is not visible to the naked eye, being only 1–1.5 cm long and only 0.1–0.15 cm wide on the

Fig. 9.20 Sinoatrial Node. (a) Micrograph showing the sinoatrial (SA) node situated in the atrial wall close to the entrance of the superior vena cava (SVC). The node is highlighted in this pentachrome stain by the pale blue-staining fibrocollagenous support tissue in which the cardiac pacemaker cells are embedded. Note the nodal artery (NA). **(b)** Medium-power H&E micrograph showing the irregular whorled network of small nodal fibres (F) embedded in the bulky fibrocollagenous stroma (S). A small nodal artery (NA) is present.

outer surface of the vena caval–atrial junction, just beneath the pericardium.

The SA node is composed of an irregular meshwork of specialized cardiac muscle fibres 3–4 μm in diameter. These are considerably smaller than normal atrial cardiac muscle fibres.

In contrast to other cardiac muscle cells, SA muscle cells do not have intercalated discs but connect with each other by gap junctions. They contain few myofibrils and lack an organized striation pattern.

The cells of the SA node are embedded in a bulky fibrocollagenous support tissue containing numerous blood vessels, including a prominent central artery, the nodal artery. Around the SA node is a paranodal area in which cells have characteristic in-between nodal cells and atrial muscle cells. Numerous nerve fibres can be seen peripherally.

The impulse generated by the SA node passes quickly to the AV node, stimulating atrial contraction in the process.

Impulses travel from the SA node to the AV node through the anterior, middle and posterior internodal tracts which are histologically indistinguishable from other atrial fibres.

> **The atrioventricular (AV) node is composed of specialized muscle fibres.**

The AV node is located beneath the endocardium of the medial wall of the right atrium, just in front of the opening of the coronary sinus and immediately above the tricuspid valve ring.

It is thus situated at the base of the interatrial septum, at the junction between atria and ventricles and between the central fibrous body and endocardium.

Histologically, the AV node is composed of a network of small muscle fibres identical to those of the SA node but less haphazardly arranged. As in the SA node, the fibres of the AV node are embedded in a fibrocollagenous stroma and have rich blood and nerve supplies.

> **The bundle of His, and the bundle branches arising from it, convey impulses to Purkinje fibres and the ventricles.**

The small fibres at the anterior end of the AV node are more regularly arranged and eventually become a distinct bundle of parallel fibres that forms the main bundle conducting the impulse from the AV node to the ventricles. This conducting bundle, the **bundle of His,** penetrates the collagen of the central fibrous body and then runs anteriorly for a short distance along the upper border of the muscle of the interventricular septum before dividing into right and left bundle branches.

The left bundle branch arises fan-like over a broad area as individual fibres, which leave the bundle of His; the remaining fibres form a distinct right bundle branch.

The left bundle branch fascicles run down beneath the endocardium of the left side of the interventricular septum in two main groups: a posterior group and a smaller anterior group.

Fig. 9.21 Purkinje Fibres. (a) Micrograph showing the large pale-staining Purkinje fibres (P) lying just under the endocardium (E) lining the interventricular septum and separated from the myocardium (M) by a zone of loose fibrocollagenous tissue. **(b)** The Purkinje fibres can be distinguished from normal cardiac muscle by a higher glycogen content as detected by a periodic acid–Schiff (PAS) stain and by high levels of the normal muscle protein αβ-crystallin, as shown in this immunohistochemical preparation.

The right bundle branch runs down beneath the endocardium of the right side of the interventricular septum as a single bundle.

The right and left bundle branches connect with a complex network of specialized conduction fibres, the **Purkinje fibres,** which are large muscle fibres with vacuolated cytoplasm owing to a high glycogen content, and scanty myofibrils. They lie in clusters of up to about six fibres (Fig. 9.21).

The Purkinje fibres, and other components of the conducting system, may be damaged during myocardial infarction (see Clinical Example box, p. 175, opposite). Like the normal myocardial fibres, they may degenerate and die as a result of a lack of oxygen when the arterial supply is cut off. This leads to abnormal heart rhythms (**dysrhythmias**), two of which (asystole and ventricular fibrillation) are almost instantaneously fatal unless rapidly corrected. These are important and common causes of fatality within the first few minutes and hours after a coronary artery occlusion.

The heart has a rich vascular supply.

Because of its constant contractile activity, the heart has enormous energy demands and therefore requires a substantial arterial supply. The left ventricle has the greatest oxygen demand and, consequently, the best arterial supply. Thus any interruption in the cardiac arterial supply mainly affects the structure and function of the left ventricle (see Fig. 9.22).

The heart is supplied by two coronary arteries that arise as direct side branches of the aorta, just above two of the cusps of the aortic valve. These are the left and right coronary arteries. Histologically, the main coronary arteries are medium-sized muscular arteries (see Fig. 9.5). They run in the epicardium and send branches into the myocardium, with a fine capillary bed running around the individual cardiac muscle cells. The least well-perfused part of the left ventricular muscle is the zone just below the endocardium: the subendocardium. This tenuous perfusion combined with the increased wall stress during systole makes the subendocardial region of the ventricular wall the most susceptible to ischaemic injury.

Venous tributaries run with the major coronary arteries before draining into a large venous channel, the coronary sinus, which runs in the atrioventricular groove on the posterior aspect of the heart, before opening into the right atrium at the coronary sinus opening.

⟫ KEY FACTS

The Heart

- Has a central fibrous core and is made up of epicardial, myocardial and endocardial layers.
- Epicardium (pericardium) covers the outer surface of the heart, contains the main coronary artery branches and is covered externally by smooth mesothelium.
- Myocardium is the contractile component of the heart and is composed of cardiac muscle cells, which are striated and linked by intercalated discs.
- The endocardium lines the internal surface of heart chambers and is covered by flat endothelial cells, which lie on a layer of fibroelastic tissue.
- The conduction system is composed of muscle fibres modified for impulse conduction rather than contraction.
- Valves have a central fibrous core covered by fibroelastic tissue with endothelium on their surfaces.
- Atrial muscle cells secrete the hormones ANP and BNP.
- The heart has a rich blood supply from two main coronary arteries (left and right), which arise as direct branches of the aorta just above the aortic valve ring.

CLINICAL EXAMPLE

Coronary Artery Disease

The most common and important disease of the heart is narrowing of the coronary arteries by atherosclerosis. This impairs the function of the left ventricle because it reduces the blood flow and hence the oxygen supply to cardiac muscle. The coronary arteries are particularly prone to this common disease, with two main consequences.

Angina

Slowly progressive reduction of the coronary artery lumen by atheroma reduces blood flow and impairs oxygenation of the left ventricular muscle, leading to a characteristic pattern of chest pain (angina), which is usually brought on by exertion (i.e. when the left ventricular muscle is working harder).

Myocardial Infarction

Complete obstruction of one of the coronary arteries or its branches (Fig. 9.23) results in one area of the heart muscle being deprived of blood and therefore oxygen. Such affected heart muscle fibres die via ischaemia and are not replaced. This process is called *myocardial infarction* (Fig. 9.22), colloquially known as a *heart attack*. Necrosis of cardiac myocytes causes breakdown of the cell contents and releases many proteins into the extracellular space. Cardiac troponins (T and I) are specific to cardiac myocytes and can be reliably measured in serum with very good sensitivity and specificity to diagnose myocardial infarction.

Fig. 9.22 Myocardial Infarction. A transverse slice across the left (L) and right (R) ventricles. The left ventricular myocardium is increased in thickness as a result of persistent high blood pressure (hypertension). The posterior part of the left ventricular wall and septum shows reddish-brown discoloration *(arrow)* caused by infarction (i.e. death of tissue after sudden deprivation of oxygenated blood supply) resulting from occlusion of the right coronary artery. Blood has seeped into the dead myocardium.

STEM CELLS AND THE HEART

Although there had been great interest in the possibility of finding stem cells in the adult heart which might be activated to promote repair after ischemic damage, as of yet this has not been found to be a clinically useful process. Cell lineage studies have, however, identified routes for the development of different cell types in the heart derived from human pluripotent stem cells (hPSCs), termed *hPSC-derived cardiac progenitor cells* (hPSC-CPCs) (see Fig. 9.23). These studies engender hope that stem cell methodologies can in the future be used to regenerate damaged heart tissues in clinical settings.

For online review questions, please visit https://studentconsult.inkling.com.

Fig. 9.23 Model of Cardiac Lineage Progression from Human Pluripotent Stem Cells. This diagram shows developmental stages and markers for cardiac cells derived from human pluripotent stem cells. Tripotent cardiac progenitors express signal regulatory protein A (SIRPA) and platelet-derived growth factor receptor α (PDGFRα) and differentiate towards SIRPA+/cluster of differentiation 34 (CD34)+/CD31+ endothelium, SIRPA+ smooth muscle or cardiomyocytes (CM) expressing SIRPA+/VCAM1+ (vascular cell adhesion molecule 1). Atrial and ventricular CMs can be identified by different expression of potassium voltage-gated channels Kv1.5 and Kir3.1, and pacemaker cells are found to express a special potassium channel (HCN4). Epicardial cells are self-renewing and differentiate towards smooth muscle and fibroblasts identified using a series of positive and negative selection markers. Whether some cells arise from multiple sources remains to be determined. (Reprinted and adapted from Skelton RJP, Kamp TJ, Elliott DA, Ardehali R. Biomarkers of human pluripotent stem cell-derived cardiac lineages. *Trends Mol Med.* 2017;23[7]:651–668. Copyright 2017, with permission from Elsevier.)

Respiratory System

INTRODUCTION

The respiratory system transfers oxygen from the air into the blood and carbon dioxide from the blood into the air.

Blood oxygen is used for cellular respiratory processes that generate carbon dioxide as a by-product. The gaseous exchange occurs in the distal part of the respiratory tract, where air-containing cavities (alveolar sacs) are in intimate contact with thin-walled blood vessels. The proximal part of the respiratory tract (upper respiratory tract) forms a series of transport passages by which air passes between the atmosphere and the gas exchange areas of the alveolar sacs (Fig. 10.1). On its way to the alveolar air sacs, the air is cleaned (by removal of particulate matter) and moistened, and its temperature is approximately equated to body temperature.

In addition, the proximal part of the respiratory tract has specialized structures involved in the perception of smell and flavour (olfactory mucosa) and the production of sound (larynx).

Upper Respiratory Tract

> **Ciliated, mucin-secreting epithelium lines the upper airways.**

The architecture of the nasal cavity and paranasal sinuses provides a large surface area for warming and moistening inspired air and for trapping particulate matter.

Air enters the respiratory system through the nostrils – the openings to the exterior at the front of the nasal cavity.

The external aspect of the nostrils is covered by skin, which extends for a short distance into the opening of the nostril (the vestibule) but then becomes a non-keratinizing squamous epithelium. Although occasional patches of stratified squamous epithelium persist, most of the nasal and paranasal sinus cavities are lined by a pseudostratified columnar epithelium, with many of the columnar cells bearing numerous cilia. Scattered among these columnar cells are mucus-secreting (goblet) cells with microvilli on their luminal surface. This pattern, with minor variations, is seen throughout most of the air-conducting part of the respiratory tract and is known as **respiratory-type epithelium** (Fig. 10.2).

> **The nasal and sinus submucosa is highly vascular and contains both mucous and serous glands.**

Beneath the nasal epithelium, the lamina propria contains many glands (Fig. 10.3) equipped with basal myoepithelial cells (see p. 93). Three main types of glands can be distinguished. Most are mucous glands, which secrete mucus to supplement that produced by the goblet cells in the lining epithelium. Some are serous cells containing basophilic granules (similar to those seen in the salivary glands, see p. 210), which produce small amounts of amylase. Finally, there are serous cells containing eosinophilic granules (similar to those seen in the lacrimal glands), which produce lysozyme.

Inspired air is moistened by the secretions of the serous glands, and a sheet of mucus secreted by the goblet cells lies on the mucosal surface and traps any inhaled particulate contaminants. The mucus is then wafted backwards (upwards) by cilia toward the pharynx, where it is swallowed or expectorated.

The lamina propria also contains variable numbers of immune cells (see Chapter 8), which are mainly lymphocytes, plasma cells and macrophages, together with a few neutrophils and eosinophils. Eosinophils are particularly numerous in people who have allergic rhinitis (hay fever).

A characteristic feature of the lamina propria is the presence of many blood vessels, which form an interconnecting network, the vessels being surrounded by a supporting stroma in which smooth muscle is prominent. This highly vascular submucosa makes a major contribution to the warming of inhaled air.

> **The paranasal sinuses are cavernous spaces in the maxillary, ethmoid, sphenoid and frontal bones of the face.**

Known, respectively, as the **maxillary, ethmoid, sphenoid** and **frontal** sinuses, each sinus communicates with the main nasal cavity through a series of orifices (Figs. 10.4a and 10.4b) and is lined by epithelium similar to that of the main nasal cavity. In addition to providing an increased surface area for the moistening and warming of inhaled air, the sinus cavities play a role in the nature of the sounds produced in speech and song.

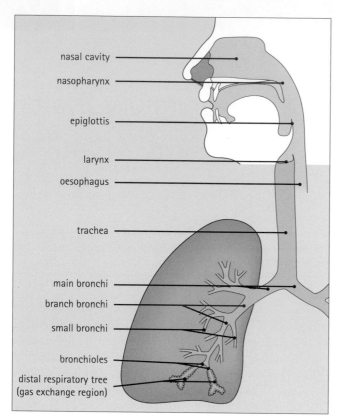

Fig. 10.1 Upper Respiratory Tract Transport Passages. The part of the respiratory tract that transports air from the atmosphere to the distal respiratory tract where gaseous exchange takes place.

Fig. 10.2 Nasal Epithelium. (a) H&E micrograph showing characteristic ciliated pseudostratified columnar epithelium (E) lining the nasal cavity. The surface cilia are seen as a fuzzy layer (C). The epithelial basement membrane (B) is seen above the subepithelial tissues in which scattered immune-related cells, including mast cells, plasma cells and lymphocytes, are present (S). **(b)** At higher magnification occasional goblet cells (G) can be seen, but these are not prominent unless a special stain is used. This type of epithelium lines the upper airways and is commonly referred to as *respiratory-type epithelium*.

> **The nasopharynx is a posterior continuation of the nasal cavities and becomes the oropharynx at the level of the soft palate.**

The nasopharynx, like most of the upper respiratory tract, is lined by columnar ciliated epithelium (Fig. 10.5a) containing occasional mucus-secreting goblet cells, but there are frequently patches of squamous epithelium, which arise by an adaptive process known as *metaplasia* (see Fig. 10.5b). The stratified squamous epithelium is normally non-keratinizing and increases in amount as the oropharynx is approached, and with increasing age. In this location, the presence of squamous epithelium is always indicative of disease, usually a persistent insult to the original columnar epithelium.

In the nasopharyngeal submucosa, there is abundant **mucosa-associated lymphoid tissue (MALT)**, forming part of the so-called *Waldeyer's ring* of pharyngeal lymphoid tissue. This MALT samples inhaled antigenic material and primes adaptive immune defences (see Chapter 8). Most of the nasopharyngeal lymphoid tissue is diffuse within the submucosa (see Fig. 10.5a), but larger nodular aggregates occur where the posterior wall of the nasopharynx meets its roof; these elevated areas of nasopharyngeal lymphoid tissue are called the **nasopharyngeal tonsils** or **adenoids** and are covered by ciliated columnar epithelium which clefts down into the lymphoid tissue mass, increasing the surface area of contact between lymphoid tissue and epithelium. Mucus-secreting goblet cells are more numerous within these clefts than on the surface.

Fig. 10.3 Nasal Lamina Propria. Micrograph showing subepithelial tissue of the nose. Numerous seromucous glands (G) discharge their secretions onto the epithelial surface through wide ducts (D).

Fig. 10.4 Nasal Cavity and Paranasal Sinuses. (a) Coronal section showing the relationship between the nasal cavity and ethmoid and maxillary sinuses. The frontal (anterior) and sphenoid (posterior) sinuses are not shown in this plane of section. The surface area of the respiratory mucosa is increased by long curved turbinate bones arising from the lateral walls of the nasal cavity and by the paranasal sinus system. Note the olfactory epithelium and its proximity to the olfactory nerves and bulbs. **(b)** Sagittal section showing the relationship between the nasal cavity, anterior nares (nostrils), vestibule, nasopharynx and frontal and sphenoid sinuses. The opening of the frontal sinus is not shown in this plane of section. Note the openings beneath the two upper turbinates of the ethmoid and maxillary sinuses and the opening in the nasopharyngeal fold of the eustachian tube from the middle ear.

Fig. 10.5 Nasopharynx. (a) Micrograph showing tall, ciliated columnar epithelium, with abundant lymphoid tissue in the submucosa. In this young non-smoking adult, there is no squamous metaplasia of the epithelium. **(b)** Micrograph from an adult smoker showing columnar ciliated nasopharyngeal epithelium (CC) undergoing metaplasia to transform into a non-keratinizing stratified squamous epithelium (S).

The **eustachian** or **auditory tubes** or **pharyngotympanic tubes** run from the middle ear cavities (see p. 397) down to the nasopharynx, opening into the lateral walls on either side; there is usually a small aggregation of lymphoid tissue in the nasopharyngeal submucosa where the eustachian tube opens into the nasopharynx, again part of the protective ring of MALT. The tube itself is lined by the same ciliated columnar epithelium, with mucous goblet cells, as the nasopharynx. The function of the tube is to ensure that the cavity of the middle ear (the tympanic cavity) is at atmospheric pressure: that is, the same pressure as the air in the nasopharynx.

As with all upper respiratory tract epithelium, the eustachian tube epithelium initially reacts to injury by excessive secretion of mucus from the goblet cells in the lining epithelium, with loss of cilia from the surface of the columnar epithelium cells. This excess of mucus, together with the reactive enlargement of the lymphoid tissue at the nasopharyngeal end of the eustachian tube, can lead to occlusion of the lumen of this narrow tube. This results in failure of the pressure equilibration function of the tube, with increased pressure and pain in the middle ear. Viruses and bacteria can also gain access to the middle ear from an infected nasopharynx, causing middle ear infection (otitis media).

The olfactory mucosa is located in the roof of the nasal cavity.

The olfactory mucosa, which senses smell and the more sophisticated aspects of taste, is located in the roof of the nasal cavity and extends a short way down the septum and lateral wall (see Fig. 10.4a).

The olfactory mucosa has a pseudostratified columnar epithelium composed of olfactory receptor cells, supporting (sustentacular) cells and basal cells. The disposition of these cells results in the pseudostratified appearance, as the nuclei of each type occupy different levels (Figs. 10.6a and 10.6b). Beneath the olfactory epithelium are small serous glands (of Bowman) with short ducts that penetrate the olfactory epithelium.

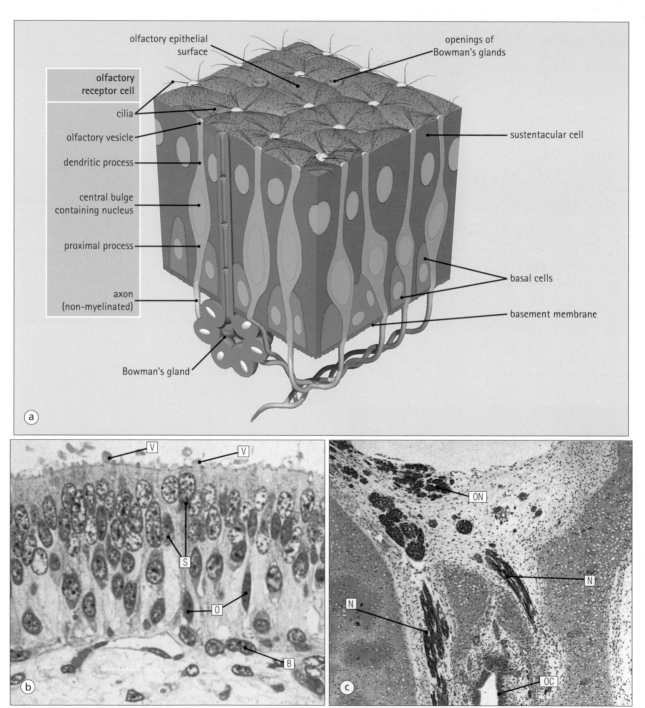

Fig. 10.6 Olfactory Mucosa. (a) This three-dimensional drawing shows the components of the olfactory mucosa, Bowman's glands and nerves leaving the base of the olfactory epithelial cells on their way to the main olfactory nerve. **(b)** Micrograph of a 0.5-μm acrylic resin section of human olfactory mucosa from an 18-week-old fetus before the associated bone plates have fully calcified. The nuclei of the basal (B), olfactory (O) and sustentacular (S) cells can be identified. The olfactory vesicles (V) on the luminal surface are just discernible. Compare with **(a)**. **(c)** Micrograph showing the nerve twigs (N) from the olfactory receptor cells (OC) fusing before passing upwards through the cribriform plate of the skull to join the olfactory nerve (ON), the first cranial nerve, demonstrated using the immunocytochemical method for neurofilament protein.

Their secretion may act as the solvent in which odorous substances dissolve.

> The olfactory epithelium is composed of basal, sustentacular and olfactory receptor cells.

Basal cells. The nuclei closest to the basement membrane of olfactory epithelium belong to the small basal cells. These cells are not in contact with the lumen and form the stem cells from which new olfactory cells can develop. Olfactory cells normally survive for about 1 month and regenerate after damage.

Sustentacular cells. The nuclei closest to the lumen in olfactory epithelium belong to tall sustentacular cells, which have a narrow base in contact with the basement membrane, expanding to more bulky cytoplasm near the lumen. The oval nuclei of sustentacular cells lie close to the lumen, and the perinuclear cytoplasm contains a moderate amount of rough endoplasmic reticulum and numerous mitochondria, implying a synthetic function. There are small cytoplasmic accumulations of yellow-brown pigment and numerous microvilli on the luminal surface.

Olfactory receptor cells. The olfactory receptor cells are bipolar neurons insinuated between the sustentacular and basal cells. They have a central bulge containing the nucleus; from this area extend two cytoplasmic processes: the dendritic and proximal processes. The **dendritic process** extends to the surface of the epithelium, where its tip is expanded into a club-shaped prominence, the **olfactory vesicle.** This bears cilia, some of which protrude into the nasal cavity, whereas other lateral cilia insinuate between the microvilli of the sustentacular cells. The cilia have the typical 9 + 2 arrangement (see Fig. 3.11) for some of their length, but there is a long distal portion, which contains only the two central fibres. The cilia are inserted into basal bodies in the olfactory vesicle. The **proximal process** is very narrow and passes down between the basal cells and basal portions of the sustentacular cells to penetrate the basement membrane. It then joins other non-myelinated processes to form the so-called **fila olfactoria,** which ultimately form synaptic connections in the **olfactory bulb** (the first cranial nerve; see Figs. 10.4 and 10.6c). The proximal processes are therefore regarded as axons.

> ### ▶ KEY FACTS
>
> #### *Nasal Cavity and Sinuses*
>
> * The nose and sinuses are lined by pseudostratified, ciliated columnar epithelium with goblet cells.
> * Main function is to filter, warm and moisten inhaled air.
> * Sinus cavities and turbinate bones provide a large surface area.
> * MALT is present in the nasopharyngeal tonsil (adenoid).
> * The nasopharynx communicates with the middle ear cavity through the auditory (eustachian) tube.
> * The roof of the nasal cavity is the site of olfactory mucosa, which includes bipolar olfactory neurons.

Larynx

On its way to the trachea, air from the nasopharynx passes through the laryngeal region.

The laryngeal region has an intricate architecture to:
* Prevent inspired air from entering the oesophagus
* Prevent ingested food and fluid from entering the trachea
* Permit the production of complex sounds

The laryngeal region therefore comprises:
* The **epiglottis,** which diverts inhaled air down through the larynx to the trachea and then to the lung, at the same time preventing ingested food and fluid from passing into the airways.
* The **true vocal cords,** which are responsible for the production of sound by vibrating in a stream of forcibly expressed air, with the nature of the sound being controlled by the vocalis muscle.
* The **false vocal cords (vestibular or ventricular ligament),** the **saccules** and **ventricles,** which modify the nature of the sounds produced by the vibrating true cords (Fig. 10.7).

The laryngeal architecture is maintained by a series of cartilaginous plates (mainly the thyroid, cricoid and arytenoid cartilages). These are joined together by densely collagenous ligaments and are mobilized by the action of small bands and sheets of striated muscle called the **intrinsic muscles of the larynx.**

The cartilages maintain the openness and shape of the airway and move to prevent food inhalation during swallowing, which is also partly the responsibility of the epiglottis.

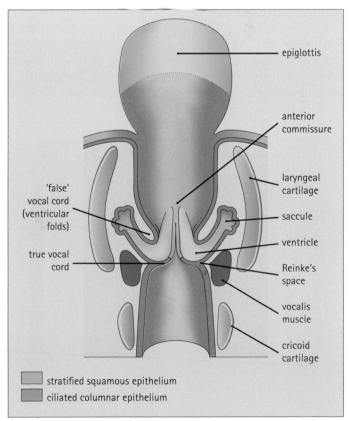

▨	stratified squamous epithelium
▨	ciliated columnar epithelium

Fig. 10.7 Structures of the Larynx.

> The epiglottis consists of a central sheet of elastic cartilage covered by mucosa on both sides.

Movement of the epiglottis prevents ingested food and liquids from passing into the trachea by covering the tracheal entrance during swallowing.

The anterior (lingual) surface is covered by stratified squamous epithelium continuous with that of the dorsal surface of the posterior part of the tongue.

The posterior surface, which faces the pharynx and larynx, is covered in its upper half by stratified squamous epithelium, and in its lower half by ciliated pseudostratified columnar epithelium. The lower half contains many seromucous glands, which penetrate deeply into the central elastic cartilage plate (Fig. 10.8).

> The false and true vocal cords are folds of mucosa.

Below the epiglottis, the laryngeal mucosa is everted into the laryngeal lumen to form two pairs of folds: an upper pair of false vocal cords and a lower pair of true vocal cords.

Between these cords, an outpouching of laryngeal mucosa forms the **ventricle** (Fig. 10.9) and its upward extension, the **saccule,** on each side.

The areas where the ends of the true cords are attached to the anterior and posterior walls of the larynx are called the **anterior** and **posterior commissures,** respectively.

The **false cords** are covered by ciliated columnar epithelium (see Fig. 10.9c), but islands of non-keratinizing stratified squamous epithelium are common in adults, becoming more extensive with increasing age.

Beneath the epithelium, a loose fibrocollagenous supporting stroma contains numerous blood and lymphatic vessels, in addition to seromucinous glands and fibres of skeletal muscle from the thyroarytenoid muscle. Small islands of elastic cartilage and adipose tissue may also be found in adults, adipose tissue being most commonly seen in the elderly.

Fig. 10.8 Epiglottis. Micrograph of epiglottis showing its central cartilaginous plate (CP) and seromucous glands (G), some of which split the cartilage, and the two types of epithelium (E) on its two faces.

The **true cords** are covered by stratified squamous epithelium, which shows a rete ridge formation (see Chapter 18) on its free edge and inferior surface, although its upper surface is flat. The epithelium contains occasional melanocytes, but no significant melanin is formed. The immediate subepithelial support tissue (**Reinke's space**) contains loose fibrocollagenous tissue, which is virtually devoid of lymphatic vessels. This is an important factor in limiting or delaying the spread of cancers arising in the true vocal cords.

Beneath Reinke's space are the fibroelastic fibres of the vocal ligament, to which the skeletal muscle fibres of the vocalis part of the thyroarytenoid muscle are attached (see Fig. 10.9c). There may be islands of elastic cartilage in the vocal ligament.

The **saccule and ventricle** are covered largely by respiratory-type ciliated columnar epithelium and contain seromucous glands in their subepithelial tissue (see Fig. 10.9d). In children, lymphoid aggregates are common, some with germinal centres.

The anterior and posterior commissures are covered with ciliated columnar epithelium, and their subepithelial zone consists of dense fibrocollagenous tissue containing seromucous glands. Lymphatics and blood vessels are common in both regions and are an important factor in the further spread of cancers of the vocal cords that invade locally to the commissures.

Phonation. The function of the larynx is to make noise for the purpose of communication. Air is forcibly expelled from the lungs and rushes upward past the laryngeal structures, particularly through the gaps between the true and false vocal cords. The distance between the right and left true vocal cords, and the tension within the cords, can be finely controlled at will using the vocalis muscle, which occupies much of the bulk of the true cords. Forced passage of air past the cords causes them to vibrate, generating noise, the nature and pitch of which depend on the rate of cord vibration, the degree of tension within them and the intercord space.

The sounds generated by the true cord are greatly modified by a combination of many factors, including resonance produced by the generated sound waves passing the false cords and entering the ventricle and saccule, reverberation of the sound around the nasal and oral cavities, and the control imposed on the sound emitted by movements of the tongue and lips.

> ▶▶ **KEY FACTS**
>
> *Larynx*
>
> - Comprises the epiglottis, false and true vocal cords, ventricles and sacculus.
> - The epiglottis prevents food and drink from entering the respiratory tract.
> - Vibration of the true cords generates sound, the character of which is modified by false cords, ventricles and sacculus and further by the mouth, tongue, nose, palate and lips.
> - Movement of true cords to create sound is under voluntary control, by the vocalis muscle.
> - Only the true cords and part of the epiglottis are covered by stratified squamous epithelium. All the other laryngeal structures are covered by ciliated columnar epithelium with mucus-secreting goblet cells.

Fig. 10.9 Laryngeal Region. (a) The laryngeal region opened in the midline posteriorly to show the epiglottis (E), the false cords (F), the true cords (T) and the openings of the ventricles (V) between them. This view also shows the anterior commissure (A). **(b)** The vocal cords as seen from above when examined clinically with a laryngoscope. Note the epiglottis (E), false cords (F), true cords (T), the opening of the ventricles (V) and the anterior commissure (A), where the true vocal cords meet in the midline anteriorly. **(c)** Low-magnification micrograph showing the histology of the false (F) and true (T) cords. The false cord (F) is covered by ciliated columnar epithelium and contains seromucous glands. The true (T) cord is covered by non-keratinizing stratified squamous epithelium and contains Reinke's space (R), fibres of the vocal ligament (VL) and the skeletal muscle fibres of the vocalis muscle (VM). Inset: Micrograph showing the epithelia of the true (T) and false (F) cords at a higher magnification. **(d)** Micrograph of the saccule, which is lined by ciliated columnar epithelium (CCE) and is rich in seromucous glands (G).

Lower Respiratory Tract

> **The trachea is lined with respiratory mucosa and is braced with cartilage.**

Below the larynx, the airway continues as the trachea, which runs down into the thoracic cavity where it divides into two main bronchi, one to each lung.

The trachea is a tubular structure about 10 cm long and 2–3 cm in diameter which is rendered rigid and non-collapsible by a number – usually 15–20 – of incomplete circular rings of cartilage that occupy 70%–80% of its circumference. Only a narrow strip of the posterior tracheal wall is deficient in cartilage; here the gap between the ends of each cartilage ring is bridged by a dense fibrocollagenous ligament rich in elastic fibres and bundles of smooth muscle (**trachealis muscle**), which permit some constriction of the tracheal lumen. The ligament linking the two cartilage ends prevents dilation (Fig. 10.10a).

The internal lining is a pseudostratified ciliated columnar epithelium containing scattered goblet cells. Subepithelial seromucous glands are particularly numerous in the posterior band devoid of cartilage (see Fig. 10.10b).

> **The trachea bifurcates into two main bronchi, which further subdivide.**

The **main bronchi** are extrapulmonary and enter each lung with the pulmonary arteries at the lung hilum. They then divide into **lobar bronchi,** one of which supplies each of the two lobes of the left lung (**left upper lobe bronchus and lower lobe bronchus**) and three lobes of the right lung (**right upper lobe bronchus, middle lobe bronchus and lower lobe bronchus**).

Each of the five lobar bronchi divides into a variable number of **segmental bronchi,** delivering air to one of the bronchopulmonary segments, where the bronchi divide for a further variable number of generations, eventually terminating in **bronchioles.** An overview of the architecture of the lung is shown in Fig. 10.1 and an orientation low-magnification micrograph in the Practical Histology section at the end of the chapter (see Fig. 10.25).

Fig. 10.10 Trachea. (a) Micrograph showing a child's trachea with an incomplete cartilage hoop (C), the free ends of the cartilage being joined by a band of muscle (M). The submucosa (S) contains numerous seromucous glands, particularly where the cartilage is deficient. **(b)** Micrograph showing tracheal mucosa with ciliated respiratory epithelium (E) on its surface and seromucous glands (G) in the submucosa (S). The inner part of the tracheal cartilage ring (C) can be seen at the base of the micrograph.

Fig. 10.11 Bronchial Wall. Medium-power micrograph showing a segment of the bronchial wall. Note the pseudostratified ciliated columnar epithelium (Ep), longitudinally running bands of elastin (El), bands of smooth muscle (SM), seromucous glands (G) and an isolated island of cartilage (C).

Throughout their course, the bronchi have a structure similar to that of the trachea (Fig. 10.11), but there are variations. The basic structure comprises:

- A pseudostratified columnar ciliated epithelium
- Subepithelial fibrocollagenous tissue containing variable quantities of seromucous glands
- Variable amounts of smooth muscle, with elastic fibres arranged in longitudinal bands
- Variable amounts of a partial cartilaginous ring

CLINICAL EXAMPLE

Acute bronchitis, caused by viral or bacterial infection of the lining of the tracheobronchial tree, damages the ciliated epithelium and permits the mucus to pass down (under the influence of gravity) into the distal portions of the respiratory tract. If the mucus contains inhaled pathogenic bacteria, this may lead to **bronchopneumonia** in which bacterial infection passes into the lungs through many small bronchioles. Because the direction of spread of infection is under the influence of gravity, the basal portions of the lower lobes of the lungs are most commonly affected.

> **Several cell types make up the epithelial lining of the bronchial tree.**

The bronchial tree is morphologically classified as being lined by a ciliated columnar epithelium (Fig.10.12a), which is pseudostratified in the larger bronchi and becomes less complex in smaller peripheral branches.

The understanding of cell types in the respiratory tract has been greatly advanced by recent studies applying the technique of single-cell RNA sequencing (scRNA-seq), which has both confirmed established morphological classifications and identified other cell types.

The respiratory epithelium contains ciliated columnar cells, basal cells, mucus-secreting goblet cells, protein-secreting club cells, neuroendocrine cells, ionocytes and tuft cells. The proportion of different cell types varies according to the level of the airway.

Basal cells lie on the basement membrane and are small cells that are not in contact with the lumen. They are important as stem cells to form different cells found in the bronchial epithelium and can proliferate and differentiate into various respiratory cells during healing after epithelial damage. This cell type can be identified by its expression of specific forms of keratin intermediate filaments (see Fig. 10.12b).

Ciliated cells are the most common cell type in respiratory epithelium (see Fig. 10.12a) and are columnar in most of the bronchial tree but are shorter and almost cuboidal in the most peripheral branches. They have a basal nucleus and lysosomes and numerous mitochondria in their supranuclear cytoplasm. The luminal surface of each cell bears about 200 cilia and some microvilli, each cilium being about 6 μm long. The ciliated cells play a key in protecting the airway from inhaled particulate material through mucociliary clearance. The importance of ciliated cell function is emphasized by the clinical syndromes associated with mutations in genes associated with cilial structure in the primary ciliary dyskinesias (see p. 56).

Goblet cells secrete mucin and are scattered between the ciliated cells (see Fig. 10.12a). They are most numerous in the main and lobar bronchi, becoming less common in the smaller branches. Their number increases in some chronic respiratory diseases.

Club cells (bronchial exocrine cells) are the main secretory cell within the airways. They vary in proportion to other cell types, increasing towards the smaller conducting airways where they are a major cell type in bronchioles. Their role is to secrete the protective protein uteroglobin into the airway and, importantly, they also act as a stem cell to form other cell types in the epithelium. Club cells are tall and have a dome-shaped apex with short microvilli. In routine histology they are not distinguished from other cell types in the respiratory epithelium. Electron microscopy shows organelles related to their exocrine function with prominent endoplasmic reticulum and secretory vesicles. Immunohistochemistry for their secreted product is recognized as the specific marker for club cells (see Fig. 10.12c).

Neuroendocrine cells are small round cells with dark-staining nuclei and clear cytoplasm, similar to those seen in the alimentary tract (see Fig. 11.32) and are located on the basement membrane. Pulmonary neuroendocrine cells (PNECs) are scattered throughout the tracheobronchial tree, but are most numerous in the smaller bronchi (see Fig. 10.12d). They are also seen in distal lung and can form clusters of cells termed *neuroepithelial bodies*. PNECs possess cytoplasmic processes and contain characteristic neuroendocrine granules. They receive sensory innervation and are understood to act as chemoreceptors. They secrete hormones and active peptides, including serotonin, calcitonin gene–related peptide and the mitogen bombesin, which are understood to have a paracrine effect on local cells, regulating local responses to environmental changes, including regulating pulmonary blood flow. PNECs are most numerous in the fetal lung; they may be scattered in the basal layer of the surface epithelium or congregate in small clumps.

Fig. 10.12 Bronchial Epithelium. (a) High-magnification H&E micrograph of the bronchial epithelium show-ing the various cell types present. Most of the cells are tall columnar ciliated cells (C) but scattered between them are occasional goblet cells (G). Basal cells (B) are located adjacent to the basement membrane. In routine sections it is not possible to distinguish the other cell types located in the epithelium. Longitudinal elastic fibres (E) of the bronchial wall can also be seen. **(b)** Basal cells can be identified by immunostaining for keratin 5, an intermediate filament present in this cell type. Basal cells can act as progenitor cells for other cell types in the epithelium. **(c)** Club cells are identified by immunostaining for the protein uteroglobin (CCSP) *(brown)* and shows them dispersed within the respiratory epithelium. **(d)** The population of neuroendocrine cells can be identified by immunostaining for chromogranin A *(brown)*, a protein present in neurosecretory vesicles. (Images (b), (c) and (d) used under Creative Commons License https://creativecommons.org/licenses/by-sa/3.0/ from the Human Protein Atlas: (b) Antibody to keratin 5 CAB080101 https://www.proteinatlas.org/ENSG00000186081-KRT5/tissue/bronchus#img; (c) Antibody to secretoglobin family 1A member 1 (SCGB1A1) CAB025686 https://www.proteinatlas.org/ENSG00000149021-SCGB1A1/tissue/lung#img; (d) Antibody to chromogranin A CAB040544 https://www.proteinatlas.org/ENSG00000100604-CHGA/tissue/bronchus#img.)

In the fetal lung they are responsible for the secretion of growth factors involved in pulmonary development.

Ionocytes are a recently described cell type identified by scRNA-seq. They are notable as the main cell type responsible for the expression of the cystic fibrosis transmembrane conduc-tance regulator gene (CFTR), which codes for a protein that transports chloride ions across cell membranes and where mutations are linked to the disease cystic fibrosis. This is a minority cell type, comprising 2%–3% of respiratory epithelial cells, and its involvement in normal function and disease is now being explored.

Tuft cells (brush cells), characterized by the presence of an apical tuft of cell projecting into the lumen, are also seen in the bronchial epithelium. This cell type is also present in a range of epithelial sites, including the alimentary tract, and has a chemosensing function.

Neuroendocrine cells of the bronchial mucosa are the cells of origin of one of the most important and highly malignant tumours of the bronchus, **small cell lung carcinoma** (also called *oat cell carcinoma*) (Fig. 10.13). Because they are neuroendocrine cells, some of these tumours secrete hormones or peptides, which can have significant metabolic effects, for example, adreno-corticotrophic hormone (ACTH)–like effects.

Fig 10.13 Small Cell Lung Cancer. This micrograph shows a small cell carcinoma. Cells have small nuclei, and hardly any cytoplasm is visible at this magnification. Immunohistochemistry can be used to confirm a neuroendocrine differentiation and assist in making a diagnosis.

Smooth muscle, lymphoid tissue and seromucous glands are present in the wall of bronchi.

The submucosa of the bronchial tree contains smooth muscle, seromucous glands and fibrocollagenous stroma with elastic fibres arranged in longitudinal bands.

In the main bronchi, the **smooth muscle** is largely confined posteriorly (as in the trachea), being attached to the ends of the incomplete cartilage rings, but in the intrapulmonary bronchi, the muscle is submucosal and arranged in an irregular spiral with two components: one spiralling to the left, the other to the right. It persists in the airway walls down to the smallest branches (bronchioles; see p. 188), long after the cartilage component has disappeared.

Hypertrophy of the smooth muscle is an important component of some lung diseases (see Clinical Example, p. 193).

The **submucosal bronchial glands** are seromucous glands which empty into the lumen through short ducts. Other deeper glands with longer ducts are located between and beneath the cartilaginous plates. The serous component is thought to secrete lysozyme and glycoprotein.

The submucosal mucous glands of the tracheobronchial tree produce thin mucus which passes on to the mucosal surface and traps inhaled particulate matter and micro-organisms. The cilia of the columnar epithelium constantly waft the thin sheet of mucus upward to the throat, so that none of it (and none of the entrapped material) normally passes down into the lower parts of the respiratory tract. This is referred to as the *mucociliary escalator*.

Myoepithelial cells (see p. 93) lie between the secretory and duct lining cells and their basement membrane, and some neuroendocrine cells are also present.

The bronchial wall contains MALT. Lymphocytes and IgA-secreting plasma cells are closely associated with the bronchial glands, and lymphoid aggregations are common, being most evident at bifurcations. The larger lymphoid aggregates occur in the proximal part of the bronchial tree and may have germinal centres.

Metaplasia in the Upper Respiratory Tract

The function of the epithelial lining of the upper respiratory tract (from nose to the end of the respiratory bronchioles) is to moisten the passing inhaled air and to remove any inhaled particulate matter by entrapment in the mucus secretions, which are then wafted proximally by the action of cilia. However, the ciliated and mucus-secreting epithelium that achieves this is, over a period of many years, subjected to a large number of insults, mainly chemical in the form of inhaled fumes from cigarettes, car exhausts, industrial pollution and so on. It is also repeatedly damaged by low-grade viral and bacterial infections. After many such destructive insults, the specialized epithelium may be replaced by stratified squamous epithelium, which is not specialized to remove particulate material but is much more resistant to damage. This is an example of **metaplasia** and is common in the epithelium of the upper respiratory tract. It has already been mentioned in the description of the nasopharynx (see p. 178), but also occurs in the trachea and proximal parts of the bronchial tree and is particularly common in cigarette smokers and people with recurrent bacterial bronchial infections.

Many examples of lung cancer originating in the bronchial tree are derived from areas of stratified squamous epithelium that have developed as a result of metaplasia. Hence, the tumours are squamous cell carcinoma.

Bronchi of all sizes contain some cartilage.

The main extrapulmonary bronchi have regular incomplete cartilage rings like the trachea, but the intrapulmonary bronchi have an irregular, roughly circumferential arrangement of cartilage plates connected by dense fibrocollagenous bands.

As the bronchi branch getting smaller and more peripheral, the cartilage plates decrease in size and number and are mainly concentrated at bifurcations.

The bronchioles are the smallest part of the conducting airways.

Bronchioles are distal airways located between the cartilage-walled bronchi and the site where the ciliated epithelium ceases (Fig. 10.14).

The bronchioles branch repeatedly, and as they do so, reduce their luminal size. With the absence of cartilage, smooth muscle becomes the major component of their wall (see Fig. 10.14b).

Fig 10.14 Bronchiole. (a) H&E micrograph showing part of a bronchiole (B) adjacent to a small branch of the pulmonary artery (P) with surrounding alveolar spaces. The bronchiole has a thin wall which does not contain cartilage. **(b)** A higher magnification of part of a bronchiolar wall. The bronchiole (B) is lined by a ciliated epithelium, which is a single layer and not pseudostratified as in the larger airways. A large proportion of cells are club cells but cannot be identified in such routine preparations – it is likely that the non-ciliated cells are club cells, but with section thickness, it is hard to tell which cells are non-ciliated. No goblet cells are present. The wall has a prominent layer of smooth muscle (S) responsible for bronchoconstriction. An adjacent small branch of the pulmonary artery is seen (P).

Bronchioles are lined by a respiratory epithelium containing all the different cell types as in the upper airways but in a different proportion. The morphological pattern is a ciliated columnar epithelium without pseudostratification, and the ciliated cells become lower and near cuboidal in the small peripheral branches.

In addition to ciliated cells, the other dominant cell type is club cells. This type of cell is not readily identified in haematoxylin and eosin (H&E) sections but can be identified by immunostaining for its secreted product (see Fig. 10.12c). Originally identified by electron microscopy, the club cell is not ciliated and is most numerous in the terminal bronchioles.

Occasional goblet cells can be seen in bronchioles, as are small numbers of neuroendocrine cells (sometimes clustered to form so-called *neuroepithelial bodies*) but there are no seromucous glands.

The final bifurcations of the bronchiolar tree produce terminal bronchioles, which are the smallest bronchioles, concerned solely with air conduction.

Distal Respiratory Tract

> **Gaseous exchange occurs in the distal respiratory tract.**

The terminal bronchiole leads into the distal respiratory tree, which is concerned with gaseous exchange. An overview of the histology is shown in the Practical Histology section at the end of the chapter (see Fig. 10.26).

The first elements of this system are the respiratory bronchioles, which are lined by cuboidal ciliated epithelium. This merges with the flattened epithelium lining ill-defined conduits outlined by a spiral of smooth muscle (alveolar ducts). The walls of these ducts are composed largely of the openings of laterally disposed air sacs (alveoli). Each alveolar duct terminates in two or three alveolar sacs formed from the confluence of the openings of several alveoli (Fig. 10.15a).

> **Alveoli are air sacs that are the main site of gaseous exchange.**

Alveoli number 150–400 million in each normal healthy lung and provide an enormous surface area (estimated at 70–80 m²) for gaseous exchange.

Each alveolus is a polygonal air space about 250 μm in diameter when normally inflated, with a thin wall which is covered with epithelial cells called **pneumocytes** and which contains pulmonary capillaries. The structures of the alveolar wall make up the diffusion barrier between the air and the blood (blood–air barrier).

Most alveoli open into an alveolar sac or an alveolar duct, but a few open directly into a respiratory bronchiole. Pores (of Kohn), which are 1–12 μm in diameter, permit communication between adjacent alveoli (see Fig. 10.15b).

The pores of Kohn provide direct communication from alveolus to alveolus, permitting rapid and even distribution of air throughout the lobe of the lung during inspiration. Unfortunately, some types of pathogenic bacteria can occasionally evade the protective mechanism of the mucociliary escalator in the trachea and bronchi and quickly gain access to the alveolar air spaces, where they may proliferate and pass rapidly from alveolus to alveolus through the pores of Kohn until an entire lung lobe is infected. This is **lobar pneumonia**.

The main cellular components of the alveoli include type 1 and type 2 pneumocytes, alveolar capillaries, and alveolar macrophages (Figs. 10.16 and 10.17).

Type 1 pneumocytes are very thin cells which allow gaseous diffusion.

Type 1 pneumocytes represent about 40% of the alveolar cell population but form 90% of the surface area lining the alveolar sacs and alveoli.

Type 1 pneumocytes are flat epithelial cells with greatly flattened nuclei (see Fig. 10.16) and are joined together by occluding or tight junctions (see p. 48). They contain scanty mitochondria and organelles, and their cytoplasm provides a very thin covering to the alveolar basement membrane, its thinness contributing to the efficiency of the blood-air barrier.

Type 2 pneumocytes secrete surfactant.

Type 2 pneumocytes represent 60% of the alveolar cell population numerically but occupy only 5–10% of the alveolar surface area.

Unlike the thin, flat type 1 cells, type 2 pneumocytes are rounded cells which are commonly located in obtuse angles in the polygonal alveolus (see Figs. 10.17a and 10.17b). Their nuclei are round and dark-staining, and their cytoplasm is rich in mitochondria and both rough and smooth endoplasmic reticulum. They also contain electron-dense vesicles and large spherical bodies of variably lamellated material, which is composed of phospholipid, protein and glycosaminoglycans and forms the basis of pulmonary surfactant. The granular surfactant material is extruded from the lamellar bodies through their microvillus luminal surfaces (see Figs. 10.17c and Figs. 10.17d).

◎ ADVANCED CONCEPT

Surfactant and the Type 2 Pneumocyte

The main function of type 2 pneumocytes is the production of pulmonary surfactant:

- Surfactant is a complex mixture of phospholipids (mainly dipalmitoyl phosphatidylcholine), carbohydrates (glycosaminoglycans) and proteins (including SP-A, SP-B, SP-C and SP-D).
- When released from the type 2 pneumocyte, surfactant produces a monolayer lining the internal alveolar surface, with a lower aqueous phase and a superficial lipid phase.
- Surfactant acts like a detergent by reducing alveolar surface tension, preventing collapse of alveoli during expiration and facilitating expansion during inspiration.
- Type 2 pneumocytes and surfactant are first detectable at about 28 weeks of gestation, after which time premature babies are theoretically capable of respiratory survival.
- Between 28 weeks and term, amounts of surfactant may be inadequate, and exogenous surfactant can be insufflated into the immature lungs of these premature infants.
- Surfactant deficiency leads to alveolar collapse, with type 1 pneumocyte damage leading to infantile respiratory distress syndrome, also referred to as *hyaline membrane disease*.

When the alveolar epithelium is exposed to certain toxic agents, particularly if there is extensive destruction of the sensitive type 1 pneumocytes, type 2 pneumocytes increase in size and number; it is believed that some type 2 cells can act as precursor cells for type 1 pneumocytes.

Fig. 10.15 Distal Respiratory Tree. (a) The relationships between the terminal bronchiole, respiratory bronchiole, alveolar ducts, alveolar sacs and alveoli. The *brown bands* are smooth muscle. **(b)** Low-power scanning electron micrograph of an alveolar sac looking into two of the alveoli (A) that open into it. The two alveoli are separated by a wall, which is covered by type 1 pneumocyte cytoplasm (T1). On the left is a pore of Kohn (PK), and a round type 2 pneumocyte (T2) can be seen in the right alveolus.

Fig. 10.16 Alveolar Wall Structure. **(a)** Micrograph showing alveolar walls immunostained to show podoplanin, a marker for pulmonary pneumocytes *(brown)*. The surfaces of each alveolar wall which face the air space are covered by a very thin sheet of pneumocytes. The pneumocyte is a type of specialized epithelium which covers the inside of the air exchange spaces. The thin, flattened cells are type 1 pneumocytes. **(b)** Micrograph of alveolar walls immunostained to show the endothelial marker PECAM1, marking small blood vessels *(brown)*, including alveolar capillaries. Each alveolar wall contains numerous capillaries, some cut in cross section while others in longitudinal section appearing as brown-stained linear streaks. The layer of pneumocytes shown in (a) covers the capillaries. **(c)** This micrograph has been stained to show the macrophage marker CD68. Brown-stained cells are alveolar macrophages. [Images used under Creative Commons License https://creativecommons.org/licenses/by-sa/3.0/ from the Human Protein Atlas Antibody: (a) Antibody to Podoplanin HPA007534 https://www.proteinatlas.org/ENSG00000162493-PDPN/tissue/lung#img; (b) Antibody to PECAM1 Antibody HPA004690 https://www.proteinatlas.org/ENSG00000261371-PECAM1/tissue/lung#img; (c) Antibody to CD68 CAB072862 https://www.proteinatlas.org/ENSG00000129226-CD68/tissue/lung#img.]

> **Alveolar macrophages phagocytose inhaled bacteria and particulate matter.**

Normally, alveolar macrophages lie on top of the alveolar lining cells and are also seen apparently free in the alveolar space, often containing phagocytosed material, particularly inhaled carbon particles.

Alveolar macrophages patrol the alveolar air spaces and the interalveolar septa (interstitium; see Figs. 10.16c and 10.18a), passing freely between the two. They phagocytose inhaled debris (e.g. fine dust, including carbon) and are an important defence mechanism against inhaled bacteria. They also remove excess surfactant and secrete a large number of agents, including enzymes such as lysozyme, collagenases, elastases and acid hydrolases.

After phagocytosis, macrophages may enter the respiratory and terminal bronchioles, where they either pass into lymphatic vessels and become transported to regional lymph nodes or they adhere to the ciliated mucus-coated epithelium, which is the first step on the mucociliary escalator. This eventually carries them up to the trachea and main bronchi, from which they are cleared in the mucus by coughing. Alternatively, the macrophages may remain in the interstitium.

Fig. 10.17 Type 2 Pneumocyte. (a) An H&E–stained thin acrylic resin section showing the confluence of the alveolar walls of three adjacent alveoli. In the angles are rounded cells with vacuolated cytoplasm; these are type 2 pneumocytes (T2). The nucleus of a thin type 1 pneumocyte (T1) is also seen. **(b)** Micrograph of alveolar wall immunostained to show keratin 18 *(brown)*, which is a marker of this type of epithelial cell. Type 2 pneumocytes are seen as plump cells adjacent to the junction of alveolar walls. The flat type 1 pneumocytes can also be seen covering both surfaces of the alveolar walls. Non-stained cells in the alveolar septa represent a mixture of capillaries and support cells. **(c)** Electron micrograph showing an active type 2 pneumocyte. The cell is round and has a convex luminal face, which is covered with microvilli. The most obvious intracytoplasmic organelles are large membrane-bound spherical bodies (B) containing lamellated lipoprotein material, which represents the surfactant substance. These can often be seen discharging their contents onto the luminal surface *(arrows)*. **(d)** Scanning electron micrograph of two type 2 pneumocytes. Note the microvilli (M) and small amounts of granular material *(arrow)*, which is recently disgorged surfactant. (Image (b) used under Creative Commons License https://creativecommons.org/licenses/by-sa/3.0/ from the Human Protein Atlas Antibody to cytosolic Keratin 18 CAB000008 https://www.proteinatlas.org/ENSG00000111057-KRT18/tissue/lung#img.)

Elastic tissue is an important functional component of the alveolar wall.	**Gaseous exchange occurs across the blood-air barrier in the alveoli.**

Elastin has remarkable properties of stretch and recoil (see p. 67) and has three important functions in the alveolar walls. First, it allows the lungs to stretch to accommodate the inhaled air. Then, having thus stored energy, it allows air to be expelled from the alveoli by recoiling. Finally, it acts as a spring, tethering the soft-walled bronchioles, which contain no cartilage, to the lung parenchyma and indirectly to the pleura, thus preventing bronchiolar and alveolar collapse during exhalation.

Oxygen diffuses from the alveolar cavity into the blood in the alveolar capillaries to become linked to red cell haemoglobin, and carbon dioxide diffuses from blood into the alveolar air. Each capillary is closely apposed to two alveolar cavities and is therefore located in the interalveolar septum or interstitium. Where the capillary contacts the alveolar wall, its basement membrane appears to fuse with that of the alveolar wall (Fig. 10.18). This is an example of a fusion basement membrane (see p. 72 in Chapter 4).

Fig. 10.18 Interalveolar Septum and Blood-Air Barrier. (a) The interalveolar septum showing the pulmonary capillaries coursing through the alveolar wall, sometimes in close contact with one wall, then the other. **(b)** A very high-magnification image of part of an alveolar septum immunostained for keratin 18, which is a marker of pneumocytes *(brown)*. The image is slightly fuzzy, as the optical resolution of the camera has been reached at this magnification. Capillaries (C) can be seen stained *blue* by the haematoxylin counterstain. The surface of the alveolar septum is covered by the thin layer of type 1 pneumocyte (T1) with some plump type 2 pneumocytes also seen. The blood–air barrier is made up of the type 1 pneumocyte, associated basement membrane and underlying capillary wall. **(c)** Transmission electron micrograph through the alveolar wall. It is largely occupied by a capillary (C) containing a red blood cell (RBC) and a monocyte (M). The monocyte will leave the capillary and ultimately enter the alveolar lumen to become an alveolar macrophage. Note the thin (Tn) and thick (Tk) parts of the alveolar wall. Both sides of the alveolar wall are covered by a thin layer of type 1 pneumocyte cytoplasm (T1). In the thick part, between type 1 pneumocyte cytoplasm and the capillary wall, there are collagen and elastic fibres (F). (Image (b) used under Creative Commons License https://creativecommons.org/licenses/by-sa/3.0/ from the Human Protein Atlas Antibody to Keratin 18 CAB000008 https://www.proteinatlas.org/ENSG00000111057-KRT18/tissue/lung#img.)

Parts of the interalveolar septum not occupied by the capillary contain fine collagen and elastic fibres together with some fibroblasts and macrophages.

Thus in some places the capillary is in direct contact with the alveolar wall (thin part) but in others is separated from it by cells and fibres (thick part). The thin part is the site of gas exchange, and the thick part is where liquids can move between the air spaces and the interstitium.

Macrophages move freely from alveolus to alveolus through the pores of Kohn. Both sides of the interalveolar septum are covered by a thin layer of type 1 pneumocyte cytoplasm (see Fig. 10.18).

CLINICAL EXAMPLE

Pulmonary Oedema

When the pressure in the pulmonary capillaries is increased, the fluid component of the blood, particularly water, can pass out of the capillary lumen first into the interstitium and then later into the alveolar spaces, so that the alveoli become filled with water (plus solutes and low molecular weight proteins). When this is extensive, there is no room for air to enter the alveoli, and the patient becomes extremely breathless and shows severe cyanosis because gaseous exchange is greatly reduced. This is the basis of **acute pulmonary oedema,** as may occur when the left side of the heart fails to empty and pressure builds up in the pulmonary veins draining into the left atrium; this increased pulmonary venous pressure is reflected back into the extensive pulmonary capillary system. This is the structural and physiological basis of **acute congestive left heart failure.**

CLINICAL EXAMPLE

Interstitial Fibrosis

In some lung diseases, the fibroblasts in the interalveolar septa increase in number and secrete excess collagen and elastin. This results in fibrocollagenous thickening of the septa (interstitial fibrosis).

Interstitial fibrosis increases the rigidity of the lung and limits expansion, but most importantly, impairs gaseous exchange because of the accumulation of collagen fibres between the capillary and alveolar walls, which impairs gas diffusion.

PULMONARY VASCULATURE

> **The lungs have a dual blood supply and venous drainage.**

Blood to the lungs is provided by the pulmonary and bronchial arteries and veins.

The more important of the two systems physiologically is the pulmonary vascular system, as this is the capillary component of the system and is the site of gaseous exchange. The bronchial system provides oxygenated blood to the larger components of the bronchial tree (see p. 196).

The pulmonary arteries supply the lung with relatively deoxygenated blood from the right side of the heart. This venous blood has supplied the body's tissues with oxygen and collected carbon dioxide (see Fig. 9.1).

The pulmonary arteries enter each of the lungs at the hilum and closely follow the course of the adjacent bronchus and its branches, dividing more or less with the bronchi. The vessels culminate in the extensive intimate **pulmonary capillary** network within the interalveolar septae (see Figs. 10.16b and 10.18).

The capillary network empties its re-oxygenated blood into **pulmonary venules and veins,** which eventually convey the blood to the left side of the heart for distribution to other organs.

Because the pulmonary arterial and venous system is a low-pressure system (i.e. pulmonary artery systolic pressure is 25 mmHg, whereas systemic arterial systolic pressure is 110–135 mmHg), the structure of its vessels differs considerably from those of the systemic circulation (see Chapter 9).

CLINICAL EXAMPLE

Chronic Obstructive Pulmonary Disease

The most common lung disease in the Western world is chronic obstructive pulmonary disease (COPD), which is characterized by difficulty in getting air into and out of the distal respiratory tree.

Two main disease processes cause COPD: chronic bronchitis and emphysema. These conditions may be present alone or in combination.

Chronic Bronchitis

In chronic bronchitis, the bronchial walls are thickened by a combination of muscle layer thickening and an increase in the number and size of the mucous glands. This correlates with excessive mucus, which is expectorated in this condition.

Emphysema

Emphysema is characterized by destruction of the walls of the alveolar ducts, sacs and alveoli, with permanent dilatation of air spaces (Fig. 10.19). This leads to loss of the elastic support for the bronchioles and results in their collapse, particularly during exhalation, and air trapping, as air is unable to pass the obstructed lumen.

Asthma

Asthma is an example of a reversible obstructive airways disease. It is caused by bronchoconstriction mediated by bronchiolar smooth muscle (see Fig. 10.14b) and excessive production of viscid mucus linked to immune-mediated factors, both of which obstruct the airways.

Fig. 10.19 Emphysema. Micrograph of lung from patient with severe emphysema, showing large air spaces (E) caused by extensive destruction of the alveolar walls. Only a few normal-sized alveolar spaces (A) remain for comparison. (Micrograph from digital pathology whole slide image provided by the University of Leeds Virtual Pathology Project https://www.virtualpathology.leeds.ac.uk. Reproduced with permission.)

The proximal pulmonary artery branches are elastic arteries.

From their origin at the pulmonary valve ring to the intrapulmonary branches at the level where the bronchi lose their cartilage plates to become bronchioles, the pulmonary arteries are elastic arteries.

These arteries have three main components (Fig. 10.20):
- A narrow intima composed of a single layer of endothelium lying on a narrow layer of scanty collagen fibres and myofibroblasts.
- A media composed of many layers of elastic fibres, which are irregular and fragmented in the pulmonary trunk and main pulmonary arteries but more regular and intact in the peripheral branches. Between the elastic fibres are smooth muscle cells and some collagen.
- Elastic laminae composed of longitudinally running fibres that form flat, interlinked strands of varying breadths. This particular orientation is probably an adaptation to counteract the stretching forces during lung expansion. In the aorta, which is exposed to circumferential stretch during systole, the elastic fibres are circumferential.

Fig. 10.20 Elastic Pulmonary Artery. Micrograph of an elastic pulmonary artery from a child. Note the endothelium (E), the scanty myofibroblasts (M) in the narrow intima (I), the thick media composed of fairly regularly organized alternating lamellae of elastic fibres (EI) and intervening smooth muscle (SM) cells and collagen (C). The elastic is easily seen in this H&E section because the lamellae are so thick.

The distal pulmonary arteries are muscular arteries.

At about the bronchial/bronchiolar junction, the medial elastic laminae largely disappear and the arteries become muscular.

These arteries continue to follow the bronchioles as far as the terminal and respiratory bronchioles, but also give off supernumerary arteries as side branches.

The media of the muscular pulmonary artery is composed largely of circularly orientated smooth muscle (Fig. 10.21a) and occasional collagen and elastic fibres. The organized laminated elastic tissue is confined to distinct internal elastic laminae (see Chapter 9).

Continuous branching of the muscular pulmonary arteries produces progressively smaller vessels with narrower bores and thinner walls because of diminishing smooth muscle in the media (see Fig. 10.21b). The muscle layer becomes discontinuous and finally disappears, the vessel then being called a *pulmonary arteriole* (see Fig. 10.21c).

Arterioles are difficult to distinguish from venules. The alveolar capillaries are discussed in Fig. 10.18.

Pulmonary veins drain into the left atrium.

Oxygenated blood from the alveolar capillaries enters small venules, then large venules, small veins, large veins and finally the main pulmonary veins, which empty into the left atrium.

The small venules are composed of a thin intima lying on a narrow zone of collagen and elastic fibres. These small tributaries fuse to form larger venules, which run in the fibrocollagenous septa and are associated with increasing numbers of myofibroblasts and smooth muscle cells in the media (Fig. 10.22).

Larger veins have a distinct media with a variably continuous internal elastic lamina and irregularly arranged smooth muscle fibres.

The largest pulmonary veins have a media in which elastic fibres are irregularly interspersed with collagen and smooth muscle fibres, rather than being confined to clearly defined elastic laminae.

Pulmonary vasculature varies considerably at the extremes of age.

Before birth, the pulmonary vasculature is barely perfused because of the bypass through the patent foramen ovale and ductus arteriosus. Thus the muscular pulmonary arteries have a small lumen, large endothelial cells and a thick media. In addition, there are small bundles of longitudinally running smooth muscle fibres in the intima.

These features change progressively to the adult pattern in the first few weeks of life, and new supernumerary arteries develop.

In old age, the veins and muscular pulmonary arteries thicken as a result of irregular fibrocollagenous thickening of the intima.

Fig. 10.21 Muscular Pulmonary Artery. (a) Micrograph of muscular pulmonary artery stained with H&E. Note the media (M) and adventitia (A). **(b)** Micrograph of a muscular pulmonary artery stained by the elastic van Gieson method to show the media (M) lying between two distinct dark-staining elastic laminae (EL). In addition to giving off a lateral supernumerary branch (S), this artery is bifurcating into two vessels with less well-formed arterial walls.

Fig. 10.22 Pulmonary Vein (a) in Transverse Section and **(b)** in Oblique Section. Pulmonary veins (V) are thin-walled vessels that run in fibrocollagenous septa (F) with paravascular pulmonary lymphatics (L). Small venules resemble pulmonary arterioles, but the small veins, as here, contain collagen and elastic fibres in the wall (W). Larger veins draining lobes develop smooth muscle cells and elastic fibres, and in large pulmonary veins these may form an interrupted or continuous elastic lamina. There are no valves in pulmonary veins of any size.

Fig. 10.23 Bronchial Artery. (a) Low-magnification micrograph of a bronchial artery from a 2-year-old child stained by the elastic van Gieson (EVG) method to show its muscular media (M) between the internal and external layers of elastic lamina (IEL) and (EEL). Elastic fibres appear *black* under the microscope. It is very similar to a normal systemic muscular artery and has a fibrocollagenous adventitial layer (A). **(b)** High-magnification micrograph of a bronchial artery from a healthy 50-year-old man stained by the EVG method. It shows marked thickening of the intima (I) by longitudinal smooth muscle cells *(yellow)*.

> **The bronchial arteries are direct lateral branches of the thoracic aorta.**

The bronchial arteries provide a secondary blood supply, which perfuses each lung at systemic arterial pressure to provide it with oxygenated blood.

The bronchial arteries follow the course of the bronchial tree and its branches to the level of the respiratory bronchioles, where they anastomose with the pulmonary artery branches. They also communicate with the pulmonary arterial system by capillary anastomoses in the bronchial submucosa.

In children, the bronchial arteries are histologically similar to other systemic muscular arteries (see Chapter 9). They have a muscular media and a distinct internal elastic lamina but no cohesive external elastic lamina (Fig. 10.23a).

In adults, the bronchial arteries develop smooth muscle, arranged longitudinally in small bundles within the intima. These are particularly prominent in some forms of chronic lung disease but are found from about 20 years of age in normal, healthy individuals (see Fig. 10.23b).

> **The bronchial veins drain into the azygos and hemiazygos veins.**

There are numerous anastomoses between the bronchial and pulmonary veins, with the bronchial veins running, with the bronchial arteries, in the adventitia of the airways.

> **There are no lymphatic vessels from the alveolar air sacs and interalveolar septa.**

Any fluid in the air spaces is absorbed into the thick part of the alveolar wall. This fluid diffuses proximally in the interstitium until it enters small lymphatics at about the level of the respiratory bronchioles. The small lymphatics (see Fig. 10. 22b) merge to form larger vessels that follow the bronchial tree proximally as far as the lung hilum, draining into a series of peribronchial lymph nodes on the way.

Another system of lymphatics runs in the visceral pleura and fibrocollagenous septa that divide the lung parenchyma into discrete lobules; these peripheral pleural lymphatics drain directly into the pleural space.

PLEURA

> **The pleurae are the linings of the thoracic cavity.**

The lungs are contained within the thoracic cavity, which is capable of increasing and decreasing in size by intercostal muscle relaxation and contraction. The internal lining of the thoracic cavity and the outer surface of the contained lungs are smooth, low-friction surfaces bathed with a small quantity of lubricating fluid. These surfaces are the pleurae. The outer surface of the lung is the visceral pleura, which is composed of five ill-defined layers:
- An outer layer of flat, mesothelial cells
- A narrow zone of loose, fibrocollagenous tissue, with no identifiable basement membrane between it and the mesothelium
- An irregular, external elastic layer
- An interstitial layer of loose, fibrocollagenous stroma containing lymphatics, blood vessels and nerves, together with some smooth muscle fibres
- An ill-defined internal elastic layer containing short lengths of elastic fibre, some of which merge with those of the interalveolar septa of the most peripheral alveolar groups

Fig. 10.24 Visceral Pleura. (a) Visceral pleura (stained H&E) showing some of the flat outer mesothelial cells (M) and the insertion of an interlobular septum (ILS) containing a lymphatic vessel (L) on its way to draining into the pleural cavity. Blood vessels and collagen fibres can be seen in the pleura. **(b)** The elastic van Gieson stain (elastic *black*, collagen *red*) reveals the ill-defined layered structure. The irregular external elastic layer (E) and ill-defined fragmented finer internal elastic layer (I) can be seen, as can the outer (OC) and interstitial (IC) collagenous layers, the latter containing blood vessels (BV).

These layers vary markedly from site to site (Fig. 10.24) but are particularly irregular in the region of a fibrocollagenous, interlobular septum, where the ill-defined elastic networks of the pleura often fuse into a single layer before extending partway into the septum.

Parietal pleura forms the internal lining of the thoracic cavity. Merging with the visceral pleura at the hilum of each lung, it has a similar structure but is usually simpler, with only one layer of elastic fibres.

Parietal pleura sits on a layer of adipose tissue, beneath which is a layer of dense fibrocollagenous tissue, which is, in turn, continuous with the periosteum of the ribs and the perimysium of the intercostal muscles.

CLINICAL EXAMPLE

Pleurisy

When the normally smooth and low-friction surfaces of the visceral and parietal pleura become abnormally roughened because of the presence of fibrin caused by local inflammation, they scrape against each other instead of sliding smoothly and effortlessly. This scraping can be heard through a stethoscope (pleural friction rub) as a scratching noise in time with inspiration and expiration. The pleura contains sensory nerves, so the condition is painful, the pain being most obvious when big inspiratory or expiratory movements are made, particularly from coughing. This condition is called *pleurisy* and occurs when the pleura is damaged by inflammation, particularly with bacterial infection of the lungs, where the infection spreads out to the pleural surface. Because of the pain on breathing, patients with pleurisy have shallow breathing and are reluctant to cough.

Fig. 10.25 Lung Architecture. Low-power micrograph showing the general architecture of the lung of a child. Bronchi (B), bronchioles (B1), the alveolar network (A) and the outer covering of pleura (P) are indicated.

Fig. 10.26 Distal Air Passages. Micrograph showing a terminal bronchiole (T) giving off a respiratory bronchiole (R), which has divided into three alveolar ducts (AD) with alveoli opening into them. They terminate in the alveolar sacs (AS), into which a number of alveoli open directly.

For online review questions, please visit https://studentconsult.inkling.com.

Alimentary Tract

INTRODUCTION

The alimentary tract is best considered as a muscular tube lined internally by an epithelium that varies in structure according to specialized functions required at particular sites along its length; with a few local variations, the structure of the musculature is similar throughout.

The function of the alimentary tract is to take in raw food material and to fragment it into small portions. These are then acted upon by a series of secretions, mainly enzymes, which convert the large molecules into smaller molecules, thus permitting their absorption into the blood and lymph circulation.

The small molecules are mainly amino acids, small peptides, carbohydrates, sugars and lipids, which are transported by the blood and lymph mainly to the liver, where they arc used as the building blocks in the synthesis of essential proteins, carbohydrates and lipids.

At the same time, the alimentary tract is designed to protect against pathogens gaining entry to the body.

> The alimentary tract can be divided into three functional components, with an additional auxiliary gland system.

The three functional components are the oral cavity, the simple transport passages and the digestive tract (Fig. 11.1).

The oral cavity is the area where food is ingested, broken up into smaller fragments by the action of the teeth and softened by secretions in the form of saliva from the salivary gland. The food material is moved around in the oral cavity by movement of the jaws and tongue to facilitate fragmentation. The moistened and fragmented bolus of food is then transferred by deglutition (swallowing) to the first of the simple passages, the oesophagus.

The simple transport passages have no function other than to act as a contractile conduit to pass semisolid material from one area to another. The first simple transport passage is the pharynx, through which food from the mouth passes into the oesophagus, which then transfers the moistened food bolus to the first part of the digestive tract, the stomach, before major digestion begins. The oesophagus is long, and the food bolus is forced along it by smooth muscle action in peristalsis under involuntary nervous control. The other simple transport passage is the anal canal at the end of the digestive tract. This transports semisolid undigested waste material (faeces) from the end of the digestive tract to the exterior. The initial stimulus to transport is involuntary as a result of increasing distension of the

rectum, but the timing of the evacuation of faeces can (usually) be controlled by voluntary (skeletal) muscle in an external sphincter. For semisolid material to pass easily through these simple transport passages, it is important that it is lubricated by mucus. For movement through the oesophagus, the mucus is incorporated into the food bolus in the mouth, having been secreted by mucous glands. In the anus, the faeces are lubricated by mucus secreted by the goblet cells in the colonic epithelium.

The digestive tract proper comprises the stomach, the small intestine and large intestine (colon and rectum). The stomach acts as a reservoir where the ingested fragmented food is held up by a sphincter until the acid and enzymatic secretions of the stomach mucosa have broken up the fragmented food into a semiliquid slurry (chyme), which then passes through the sphincter into the small intestine. Here, the process of digestion is continued by a combination of enzymes and other chemicals secreted by the small intestine itself and by the auxiliary glands, the liver and pancreas, the secretions of which enter the small intestine via ducts. In addition to this digestion function, the main function of the small intestine is absorption of the breakdown products of food digestion. The liquid food residue passes from the small intestine into the large intestine, where the majority of the fluid content is reabsorbed until the waste material is converted into semisolid waste material, lubricated for easy passage through the anal canal by mucus secreted by goblet cells in the colon and rectum.

All the components of the alimentary tract are structurally specialized to carry out their specific functions.

The auxiliary gland systems contributing to the function of the alimentary tract are the salivary glands, the liver and the pancreas, all of which pass their secretions into the main alimentary tract through ducts. The salivary glands are discussed on page 208; the pancreas on page 227; and the liver, which has many important functions other than those associated with digestion, merits a chapter of its own (see Chapter 12).

ORAL CAVITY AND ITS CONTENTS

> The oral cavity is lined throughout by stratified squamous epithelium but contains many highly specialized structures.

The mouth is lined by stratified squamous epithelium, the underlying submucosa containing varying numbers of salivary glands, which can secrete both a serous and a mucous fluid. Skeletal muscle fibres are common in the deeper layers and are responsible for altering the size and shape of the cavity and for moving food; skeletal muscle fibres form the bulk of the tongue and are also numerous and important in the cheeks.

In some areas, the deep tissues of the oral cavity consist of bone, either simple plates of bone (as in the hard palate) or modified bone (teeth). The immovable hard palate produces a rigid structure against which the tongue can move, and the teeth, which are embedded in bony supports (the mandibles and maxillae), are the main tools for fragmenting ingested food.

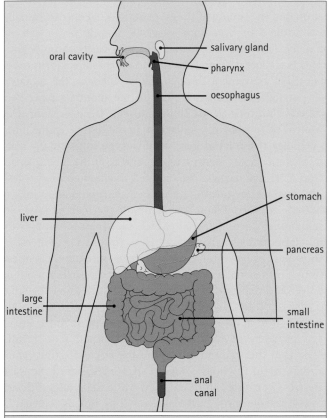

Three functional compartments		
	oral cavity	ingestion and fragmentation of food
	simple passages	transport of food or its residues without significant modification (oesophagus and anus)
	digestive tract	secretes enzymes induced in breakdown of food; absorbs molecules produced (stomach, small and large bowel)

Auxiliary gland system		
	secretory organs	located outside digestive tract and produce secretions which enter the gut via long ducts (salivary glands, pancreas, liver)

Fig. 11.1 The Alimentary Tract.

> **The lips are covered by squamous epithelium and contain glands and underlying muscle.**

The oral orifice is bounded by the lips, the external aspects of which are covered by hair-bearing skin with sebaceous glands and eccrine sweat ducts. Between the hair-bearing outer surface and the moist, fluid-bathed inner surface, there is a transitional zone known as the *vermilion* because of its pinkish-red appearance. Here, the epithelium is non-keratinizing stratified squamous with a prominent rete ridge system (see Chapter 18) and the papillae between the epithelial downgrowths contain prominent blood vessels, which are responsible for the pinkish-red colour.

The inner surface of the lips is lined by a non-keratinizing stratified squamous epithelium with a less well-developed rete ridge system, and small clumps of salivary tissue disgorge their secretions onto its surface through short ducts. In addition, occasional sebaceous glands (Fordyce's spots), which are particularly common near the angles of the mouth, open directly onto the mucosal surface, rather than into a hair follicle as in the skin.

In the deeper parts of the lips, bundles of striated muscle fibres (orbicularis oris muscle) are arranged mainly in a concentric manner around the oral orifice. This muscle is responsible for, among other things, opening and closing the oral orifice.

> **The cheeks are lined internally by squamous epithelium and contain glands and deep muscle.**

The cheeks are lined by thick, non-keratinizing squamous epithelium, the cells of which are often rich in glycogen. Areas of keratinization are common, usually as a result of chronic friction from ill-fitting dentures or from persistent cheek biting. The submucosa contains minor salivary glands (buccal glands), and the deep tissues contain the skeletal muscle fibres of the cheek muscles (buccinator).

> **The palate is rich in salivary gland tissue (palatine salivary glands).**

The epithelium of the palate is non-keratinizing, stratified squamous epithelium with, in the hard palate, a prominent rete ridge pattern, which reflects the frictional stresses this area is subjected to during mastication. Beneath the salivary gland tissue, the submucosa is firmly tethered to the periosteum of the palatal bone. The oral surface of the soft palate is covered with non-keratinizing stratified squamous epithelium extending to its posterior edge, where it meets ciliated columnar epithelium of the nasal surface.

> **The floor of the mouth contains salivary glands.**

The floor of the mouth is covered by thin, non-keratinized stratified squamous epithelium, which is continuous with that of the ventral surface of the tongue.

There are many minor salivary glands in the floor of the mouth (minor sublingual glands) and larger glands situated on either side of the midline frenulum of the ventral surface of the tongue (major sublingual glands, see p. 208).

The tongue is muscular and covered in squamous epithelium.

The tongue is a highly muscular organ that protrudes upwards and forwards into the oral cavity from its floor. The ventral surface of the tongue is covered by thin, non-keratinizing stratified squamous epithelium, continuous with that of the floor of the mouth. In contrast, the dorsal surface, which is commonly in contact with the hard palate during feeding, talking and at rest, is covered with a thick, keratinizing stratified squamous epithelium, which shows considerable specialization.

The upper surface of the tongue is divided into two main zones.

The dorsal surface of the tongue is divided into an anterior two-thirds and a posterior one-third. The two parts are separated by a V-shaped line of 6–10 dome-shaped protrusions, the *circumvallate papillae* (Fig. 11.2). Circumvallate papillae appear as flattened domes, the bases of which are depressed below the dorsal surface.

Each circumvallate papilla is surrounded by a narrow, moat-like channel, in the epithelium of which are numerous taste buds. These taste buds are thought to detect bitter taste. Small salivary glands discharge their secretions into the channels (Fig. 11.3).

The posterior third of the tongue is characterized by the presence of lymphoid tissue.

Low, smooth, dome-shaped elevations of the covering epithelium of the posterior third of the tongue are the result of lymphoid tissue (the lingual tonsillar tissue) in the submucosa (Fig. 11.4). This lymphoid tissue is part of the mucosa-associated lymphoid tissue (MALT, see p. 154) system protecting (with the palatine tonsils and the pharyngeal adenoids) the oral portal of entry.

Lymphocytes are numerous within the overlying, non-keratinizing stratified squamous epithelium, which extends down into the lymphoid tissue as narrow clefts. Small salivary glands open into the bottom of the narrow clefts, becoming more prominent and numerous near the line of circumvallate papillae.

Fig. 11.2 Dorsal Surface of the Tongue. The dorsal surface of the tongue can be divided into a posterior third (P) with smooth, dome-shaped elevations (E), and an anterior two-thirds (A) by a V-shaped line of circumvallate papillae (C). The surface of the anterior two-thirds is roughened by the presence of small filiform and fungiform papillae and by a surface keratin layer. In some places, the surface keratin may become thick and stained by food (coated tongue; *arrow*), particularly in the elderly (as here), and the coating may contain numerous bacterial colonies.

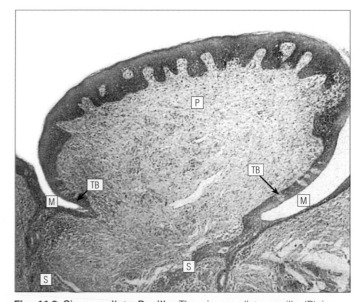

Fig. 11.3 Circumvallate Papilla. The circumvallate papilla (P) is surrounded by a moat (M) into the bottom of which empty prominent salivary glands (S). Taste buds (TB) are particularly numerous in the walls of the moat.

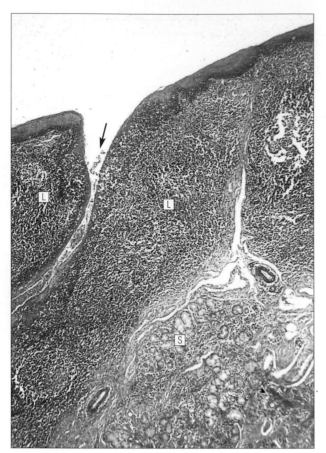

Fig. 11.4 Posterior Third of the Tongue. Posterior third of the tongue showing lymphoid tissue (L), cleft-like invaginations of the epithelium *(arrow)* and salivary glands (S) opening into the depths of the clefts.

The surface epithelium of the anterior two-thirds of the tongue is raised in a series of elevations called papillae.

The three types of papillae in man are circumvallate (described earlier), filiform and fungiform.

Filiform papillae are the most numerous papillae and are found all over the dorsum of the anterior two-thirds of the tongue. They are tall, narrow and pointed (Fig. 11.5) and are keratinized, particularly at their tips. Filiform papillae contain no identifiable taste buds.

Fungiform papillae (see Fig. 11.5) are scattered apparently randomly among the filiform papillae on the dorsal surface of the tongue and have a mushroom shape. Taste buds are present in their covering epithelium, with those at the anterior tip of the tongue detecting sweet taste and those just behind the tip and some way along the lateral borders detecting salty taste.

Taste buds are specialized sensory organs located in the epithelium of the tongue.

Each taste bud occupies the full thickness of the epithelium and comprises pale-staining, spindle-shaped cells in an oval cluster (Fig. 11.6). The luminal surfaces of the cells open into a small

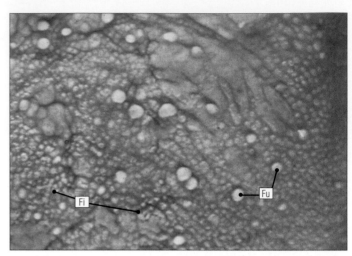

Fig. 11.5 Fungiform and Filiform Papillae. Part of the dorsal surface of the anterior two-thirds of the tongue showing the gross appearance of the mushroom-like fungiform papillae (Fu) and the smaller filiform papillae (Fi).

defect in the epithelium, the taste pore, and each cell bears a number of microvilli. Ultrastructurally, some of the spindle-shaped cells have synaptic vesicles and are associated with small afferent nerve fibres; these are the taste receptor cells. Other cells with more electron-dense cytoplasm and scanty secretory granules are supporting sustentacular cells. There are also cells resembling the taste receptor cells but lacking the synaptic vesicles and afferent nerve connections. The turnover of these cells is rapid (every 10–14 days), so there is a population of stem cells at the base of each taste bud.

The taste buds of the dorsal tongue detect acid, sweet, bitter and salty and provide early warning that food may be unpalatable.

▶ **KEY FACTS**

Anterior Two-Thirds of the Tongue

- Covered by stratified squamous epithelium, thin on ventral surface, thick and papilliform on dorsal surface
- Filiform, fungiform and circumvallate papillae on anterior two-thirds; the latter demarcate anterior and posterior parts of the tongue
- Taste buds are present on circumvallate and fungiform papillae
- Consists of striated muscle with a small amount of adipose tissue
- Salivary tissue in submucosa, mainly near circumvallate papillae

---

▶ **KEY FACTS**

Posterior Third of Tongue

- Covered by smooth, non-papillate stratified squamous epithelium
- Submucosa contains lymphoid aggregates (MALT), forming part of Waldeyer's ring
- Bulk is muscle and adipose tissue, with some salivary tissue in submucosa and muscle, mainly near circumvallate papillae

Fig. 11.6 Taste Buds in Circumvallate Papilla. (a) This thin acrylic resin section, stained with H&E, is from a circumvallate papilla of a surgically removed human tongue from an elderly man. It shows the oval taste buds (TB), which occupy the full thickness of the epithelium. The luminal aspect of the spindle-shaped cells opens on to the surface at the taste pore, the beginning of which is shown here (P). **(b)** An epoxy-resin section (0.5-μm thick) of a single taste bud, stained with toluidine blue to show the taste receptor cells with a mixture of spherical and spindle-shaped nuclei. A small bead of dark-staining glycosaminoglycan material is present in the taste pore.

Fig. 11.7 Musculature of the Tongue. (a) In the anterior two-thirds of the tongue, the striated muscle bundles (M) are tightly packed with relatively little intervening adipose tissue (A). Note that the muscle bundles run in many directions. In the bulkier, less mobile posterior third of the tongue, the adipose tissue is more abundant. **(b)** Collections of salivary glands (S) are numerous in the submucosa and muscular core of the posterior tongue, particularly close to the junction between the posterior one-third and anterior two-thirds.

Skeletal muscle in the tongue is arranged in many directions.

The musculature of the tongue comprises a complex pattern of skeletal muscle fibres. These fibres run in bands longitudinally, vertically, transversely and obliquely, with a variable amount of adipose tissue in between (Fig. 11.7). This arrangement gives the tongue great mobility to manipulate food in the mouth and for swallowing; it also provides the fine control of tongue movement for speech.

Islands of salivary tissue are present in the submucosa between the muscle and surface epithelium at the junction between the posterior one-third and the anterior two-thirds. Some of the deeper salivary gland extends down into the superficial muscular zone.

TEETH

Introduction

The main task of the oral cavity, the fragmentation of large food masses, is performed by the teeth, which are hard, heavily mineralized structures embedded in the raised alveolar ridges of the maxilla and mandible.

Teeth are arranged so that the free surface of those embedded in the mandible (lower teeth) oppose and contact those in the maxilla (upper teeth), allowing food material to be trapped between them.

The anterior teeth (incisor and canine teeth) have narrow, chisel-shaped or pointed free edges for chopping food into medium-sized pieces, whereas the posterior teeth (premolars and molars) have broader, flatter, free surfaces for grinding medium-sized food pieces into smaller fragments.

The mandible is joined to the body of the skull by the temporomandibular joint, which permits the mandible to slide backwards and forwards and from side to side, thus aiding the grinding of food between the broad surfaces of the opposing molar teeth.

> **Each tooth can be divided into two anatomical components: the crown and the root.**

The tooth is divided into two structural regions:
- The crown protrudes into the oral cavity.
- The root is embedded in the bone of the mandible or maxilla.

The junction between the crown and the root is called *the neck*. The mature tooth has five components: the central pulp cavity, dentine, enamel, cementum and periodontal ligament (Fig. 11.8).

> **The centre of each tooth comprises the pulp, which contains nutrient vessels and nerves.**

The pulp cavity is the soft central core of the tooth and contains collagen and fibroblasts embedded in an acellular matrix. The cavity approximates in shape that of the tooth as a whole, and its acellular matrix is composed of glycosaminoglycans.

Through the pulp cavity run the blood vessels that nourish the odontoblasts (see later) and the nerve twigs that provide dental sensation. These vessels and nerves enter and leave through a small **apical foramen** at the tip of the root.

The pulp cavity is narrow throughout most of the root (the **root canal**) but is expanded in the neck and crown (the **pulp chamber**). Its outer surface is lined by odontoblasts, which continually produce dentine. As dentine is progressively laid down, the pulp cavity diminishes in size.

Dentinogenesis and Odontoblasts

> **The specialized mineralized matrix of the tooth is called dentine and is secreted by odontoblasts.**

Dentine is composed of mineral salts and organic material. The mineral salts are calcium salts in the form of crystalline hydroxyapatite (about 70%–80%) arranged as long, hollow parallel tubules, the **dentinal tubules**. Within these run the organic

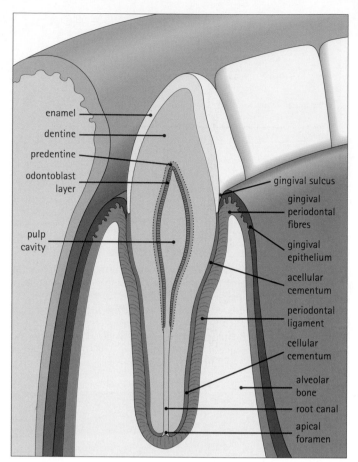

Fig. 11.8 Mature Incisor Tooth. The central pulp cavity, the outer layer of which contains cells (odontoblasts) that produce the specialized extracellular matrix components of the teeth, is surrounded by dentine, a relatively acellular mineralized material forming the bulk of each tooth. The dentine of the crown of the tooth is covered by enamel, a heavily mineralized material forming a resistant outer coat. At the neck of the tooth, enamel is continuous with cementum. This is a bone-like material forming an outer coat to the dentine in the root. Cementum is linked to the alveolar bone of the mandible or maxilla by the periodontal ligament, which is composed of tightly packed collagen fibres embedded at one end into the cementum of the tooth and at the other end into the bone forming the tooth socket.

material in the form of fine cytoplasmic processes of the odontoblasts and the type I collagen fibres and glycosaminoglycans that they produce (about 20%–30%).

Dentine is initially laid down by odontoblasts as a glycosaminoglycan matrix in which collagen fibres are linearly arranged. This non-mineralized predentine is synthesized by odontoblasts located at the outer limits of the pulp cavity (Fig. 11.9).

In humans, the odontoblast cytoplasmic processes extend only 25%–50% of the full length of the dentinal tubule; thus dentine close to the dentine–enamel border appears to contain empty tubules. In life, these empty tubules may contain fluid, which is lost during tissue processing.

As odontoblasts progressively synthesize new predentine at the inner surface of the pulp cavity (Figs. 11.9 and 11.10), the cavity slowly decreases in size throughout life.

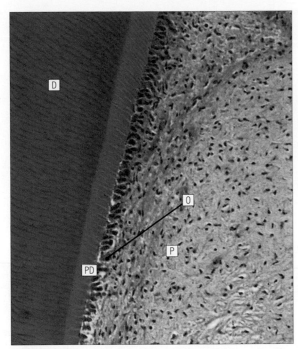

Fig. 11.9 Dentine, Predentine and Odontoblasts. Micrograph showing pulp cavity (P) lined externally by a layer of odontoblasts (O), external to which is a pale-staining band of predentine (PD). The outer layer is mineralized dentine (D), in which the pattern of dentinal tubules can be seen.

> **Dentinogenesis commences with the formation of predentine by odontoblasts.**

In predentine, randomly scattered collagen fibres (type I collagen) produced by the odontoblasts are embedded in an extracellular matrix of phosphoprotein and glycosamino-glycans (mainly chondroitin-6-sulfate).

Mineralization is initiated by the discharge of the matrix vacuoles from the odontoblast process and its branches running through the predentine layer.

Sometime after its formation, predentine becomes mineralized at its border with previously mineralized dentine; close to this predentine–dentine border the collagen fibres of predentine become more numerous and tightly packed. The dentine lining the dentinal tubules (peritubular dentine) is particularly compact and heavily mineralized (Fig. 11.11).

Ameloblasts and Enamel Formation

> **Enamel is the hardest material in the body.**

Enamel is composed almost entirely of the mineral hydroxy-apatite $[Ca_{10}(PO_4)_6(OH)_2]$, which is arranged in tightly packed hexagonal enamel rods or prisms (Fig. 11.12) about 4 μm in diameter, although some may measure up to 8 μm.

Each enamel rod extends through the full thickness of the enamel. The small interstices between adjacent rods

Fig. 11.10 Odontoblasts and Dentinogenesis. The functioning odontoblast is a tall, narrow cell, the base of which contacts cells and fibres of the pulp cavity (mainly fibroblasts and collagen). Its nucleus is basal and its cytoplasm is rich in mitochondria and rough endoplasmic reticulum. It has a large supranuclear Golgi complex. At the apex of the cell, the cytoplasm is drawn out into a long odontoblast process which runs through the predentine and dentine layers in the dentinal tubule, while small side branches penetrate the predentine. The cytoplasm of the odontoblast process and its branches contain numerous microtubules, along with small matrix vacuoles, which contain Ca^{2+} and PO_4^- ions. The matrix vacuoles play a key role in the mineralization of the dentinal matrix. The mechanism is almost identical to that whereby matrix vesicles from osteoblasts produce mineralization of osteoid matrix to produce bone mineralization (see Fig. 13.20).

are occupied by hydroxyapatite crystals. A small amount of organic matrix (protein and polysaccharide) represents the remnants of the matrix synthesized and excreted by the enamel-producing cells, the *ameloblasts*, before mineralization of the enamel.

Fig. 11.11 Dentinal Tubules. Scanning electron micrograph of dentine at a point well distant from the predentine layer. The mineral material contains regular empty dentinal tubules because the cytoplasmic processes of the odontoblasts extend only a short way into the tubules. Note the more compact dentine lining the tubules.

Enamel is formed during tooth development by the ameloblasts.

Ameloblasts degenerate when the tooth erupts, after which time the enamel cannot be replaced by new synthesis. In the developing tooth (see Fig. 11.17), the functioning ameloblast is a tall, narrow cell, with its base attached to the cells of the stratum intermedium (Fig. 11.13). The nucleus is located basally, and basal cytoplasm contains abundant mitochondria. The supranuclear cytoplasm contains a large, active Golgi complex and abundant rough endoplasmic reticulum, together with microtubules, which are predominantly longitudinally arranged, and secretory vacuoles which become larger and more numerous near the upper pole.

At the upper pole, the cell elongates into a single large Tomes's process and forms a fringe of smaller processes around its neck. The Tomes' process contains numerous microtubules and large numbers of secretory vacuoles.

The rough endoplasmic reticulum synthesizes various proteins and glycoproteins (including amelogenin and enamelin), which form the organic matrix of enamel (pre-enamel) and are packaged by the Golgi complex into secretory vacuoles. These then move into the Tomes' process and the small neck processes, discharging their contents onto the surface.

Mineralization of the matrix proteins by hydroxyapatite occurs almost instantaneously, producing small enamel crystallites and, with progressive mineralization, the enamel rods or prisms.

Fig. 11.12 Enamel. (a) H&E-stained section of early forming enamel (E) being produced by a layer of ameloblasts (A). The enamel shows a distinctive pattern owing to the arrangement of enamel prisms and abuts the dentine (D). **(b)** Scanning electron micrograph showing the characteristic arrangement of tightly packed enamel prisms or rods.

The compact structured enamel prisms are probably derived from the surface of the main Tomes' process, whereas the small amount of less compact interprism enamel, which has a larger organic matrix component, is probably derived from the small neck processes.

Enamel covers the dentine only in the region of the exposed crown (Fig. 11.14); in the root, the dentine is covered by cementum (see Figs. 11.8 and 11.15).

Fig. 11.13 Ameloblasts and Enamel Formation. The functioning ameloblast is a tall, narrow cell, with its base attached to the cells of the stratum intermedium. The Tomes's process at the upper pole is rich in secretory vacuoles containing organic matrix proteins and numerous microtubules. Each Tomes's process has small associated cytoplasmic processes around it; these also produce some enamel, but the main enamel prisms are produced by the Tomes's process.

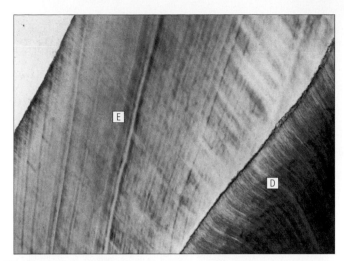

Fig. 11.14 Formed Enamel. Unstained ground section of a mature human tooth showing the characteristic patterns of enamel (E) and dentine (D); the tightly packed dentinal tubules are clearly seen. The linearity of the compact parallel enamel prisms runs from the dentinal–enamel interface in straight lines to the surface. The coarse, slightly curved, oblique lines seen in this photomicrograph are an artifact produced by the grinding process used to make this section.

Fig. 11.15 Cementum. Micrograph showing the dentine (D), cementum and fibrous periodontal ligament (P) of the root of a tooth at the junction between the narrow compact acellular cementum (AC) and the broader cellular cementum (CC), in which osteocyte-like nuclei can be seen (O).

Cementum and Periodontal Ligament

> **Cementum is a bone-like tissue; it is calcified and contains collagen.**

A thin layer of cementum covers the root of the tooth, being thin, compact and acellular (acellular cementum) over the upper region, but thicker and containing lacunae and cementocytes (cellular cementum) lower down (see Fig. 11.15).

Cementocytes resemble osteocytes (see Chapter 13) and remain viable throughout life, being nourished through canaliculi which link the lacunae. They can become activated to produce new cementum when required.

In addition to the cementocytes, which are scattered throughout the cellular cementum, there is a layer of cells called *cementoblasts*, which are similar to the actively synthetic osteoblasts of bone (see Fig. 13.17).

Fig. 11.16 Periodontal Ligament. H&E-stained section showing the relationship between the tooth (T), bony socket (B) and fibrous periodontal ligament (PL) at the neck of the tooth.

Cementoblasts lie against the surface of the periodontal ligament and probably produce most new cementum by appositional deposition.

> **The periodontal ligament is a suspensory ligament tethering the tooth in the bony alveolar socket of the mandible or maxilla.**

The periodontal ligament is composed of dense collagen and fibrocytes, with the fibres running across the gap between the cementum of the tooth and the bone of the alveolar socket (Fig. 11.16). As the collagen fibres are embedded in a ground substance, this ligament also acts as a shock absorber, in addition to permitting limited movement of the tooth within the bony socket.

At its cemental and alveolar limits, some of the collagen fibres are inserted into the cementum and bone. The alveolar bone at the inner margin of the socket is composed of woven bone rather than compact lamellar bone. Above the upper limit of the alveolar bone, the fibres of the periodontal ligament become the gingival periodontal fibres and blend with the submucosa of the gingivae.

Tooth Development

> **Teeth develop from both ectoderm and mesoderm.**

Teeth develop from both ectoderm and mesenchyme of mesodermal origin, the ectodermal component being the enamel derived from the enamel organ, and the mesenchyme producing the rest of the tooth.

The enamel organ originates as a cellular downgrowth of the oral epithelium, initially in the form of a cap-shaped epithelial tooth bud connected to the overlying oral epithelium by the dental lamina. Beneath the epithelial tooth bud, a condensation of mesenchyme contributes to the rest of the tooth.

The stages in tooth formation are summarized in Fig. 11.17.

THE GUMS

> **The gingiva (gum) is the portion of oral mucosa covering the alveolar bone ridge surrounding the tooth.**

The gingival mucosa is continuous with the alveolar mucosa covering the rest of the bone. A small sulcus lies between the tooth and the bulk of the gingiva.

The sulcal epithelium is thin stratified squamous, whereas that on the outer surface of the gingiva is thick and keratinized, with a prominent rete ridge pattern.

The submucosa in the region of the gingival sulcus is commonly infiltrated by chronic inflammatory cells and also contains gingival periodontal fibres, which are an extension of the upper limit of the periodontal ligament.

SALIVARY GLANDS

> **There are three main salivary glands and many minor glands.**

The mouth receives secretions from salivary gland tissue located both inside and outside the mouth. These glands may contain mucus-secreting cells, serous cells or a mixture of both. The serous glands secrete a watery solution containing enzymes (e.g. amylase, lysozyme), an IgA secretory piece and lactoferrin, an iron-binding compound.

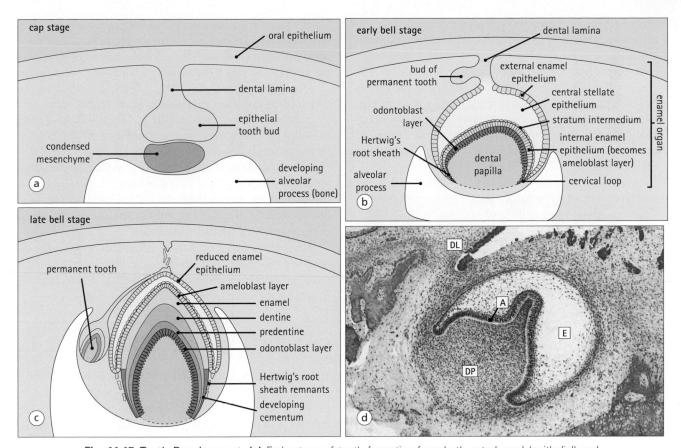

Fig. 11.17 Tooth Development. (a) Early stage of tooth formation from both ectodermal (epithelial) and mesenchymal components. **(b)** The cells of the epithelial tooth bud develop into the enamel organ, differentiating into a bell-shaped structure with a central core of loosely arranged stellate cells (stellate epithelium) and a peripheral layer of cuboidal or low columnar epithelium. The outer cell layer of the convex surface is the external enamel epithelium and that of the concave surface the internal enamel epithelium. The internal enamel epithelium differentiates into an outer layer of tall, columnar ameloblasts (see Fig. 11.13) and a two- to three-cell-thick inner layer called the *stratum intermedium*. Where the external and internal enamel epithelium meet is called the *cervical loop*. An extension downward of cells of the external enamel epithelium forms the so-called *Hertwig's root sheath*, which defines the final size of the tooth root, being later replaced by the cementum. In the concavity of the enamel organ, the mesenchyme continues to condense to form the dental papilla, and a row of odontoblasts develops at its junction with the enamel organ, in contact with the ameloblast layer. In deciduous teeth, like the incisor shown here, the permanent tooth arises from a side-growth from the dental lamina. **(c)** Odontoblasts begin to produce predentine, and this stimulates the production of enamel by the ameloblasts. Calcification of the predentine and pre-enamel begins almost immediately, and dentine and enamel continue to be laid down until the form of the tooth is complete. The dental papilla becomes enclosed by dentine to form the dental pulp. The non-ameloblast components of the enamel organ become much reduced and eventually atrophy. When enamel formation is complete, the ameloblasts degenerate to form a thin layer of irregular cells, which ultimately disappear when the tooth erupts. The cells of Hertwig's root sheath begin to degenerate as the cementum is deposited by cementoblasts on the surface of the dentine of the tooth root. Partial development of the permanent tooth continues alongside the deciduous tooth in the same manner. **(d)** Micrograph of a resin section of a developing tooth at the early bell stage, showing the enamel organ (E), including the ameloblast layer (A), the dental papilla (DP) and the degenerating dental lamina (DL).

The largest salivary glands are located outside the mouth and transfer their secretions into the oral cavity by long ducts; smaller glands, sited mainly in the submucosa of the oral lining, are less well-defined and empty their secretions into the mouth by short ducts.

The main salivary glands are the submandibular, the parotid and the large sublingual glands.

> **The submandibular salivary gland secretes a mixed serous/mucous product.**

The submandibular glands are roughly ovoid in shape and are situated on either side of the neck just below the mandible. Their ducts open into the floor of the mouth, one on each side of the frenulum of the tongue.

The submandibular glands are typical mixed glands containing both serous and mucous elements, with serous elements predominating.

The secretory acini are composed mainly of epithelial cells, which are responsible for the serous secretion, and are plump cells filled with prominent, purplish-staining zymogen granules.

The mucus-secreting cells are pale-staining with abundant clear cytoplasm and often form blind-ending tubules, the blind end bearing a demilune or crescent of zymogen-rich serous cells (Fig. 11.18).

Fig. 11.18 Submandibular Salivary Gland. (a) This low-magnification image shows the gland composed of lobules of cellular acini, each of which has fibrous septa (F) containing ducts. **(b)** The submandibular salivary gland has both a mucous and a serous component. The serous component (S) contains numerous large zymogen granules, whereas the mucous component (M) is often arranged in duct-like structures, the ends of which are capped by the so-called *serous demilunes* (D). A striated duct (SD) shows the characteristic features of an ion exchange epithelium. (Micrograph from digital pathology whole slide image provided by the University of Leeds Virtual Pathology Project https://www.virtualpathology.leeds.ac.uk. Reproduced with permission.)

The secretory acini empty into intercalated ducts, which are lined by cuboidal or low columnar epithelium and merge to form intralobular ducts. These are characterized by tall columnar epithelium, which stains pale pink and shows a characteristic striated pattern (see Fig. 3.14) of basal cytoplasm. Hence, intralobular ducts are commonly called *striated ducts*.

Intralobular duct epithelium is biochemically active and modifies the concentration and content of the fluids produced by the secretory acini.

The intralobular striated ducts fuse to form larger interlobular ducts, which are lined by a non-striated, often pseudostratified epithelium. Interlobular ducts then join to form the major ducts, some of which (particularly the main submandibular duct) may have a ciliated epithelium.

There is a network of myoepithelial cells between the epithelium and the basement membrane of the acini and much of the ductular system, with contraction of the myoepithelial cells squeezing the secretion toward the major ducts.

> **The parotid salivary glands secrete a serous product.**

The parotid glands are situated below and in front of the pinna on each side of the face. They are flat and well encapsulated, and the facial nerve runs through them, dividing them into superficial and deep portions. Their long ducts open into the oral cavity opposite the second upper molar tooth on each side.

The parotids are composed entirely of serous glands rich in zymogen granules, with a variable amount of adipose tissue in the interstitium between parotid lobules (Fig. 11.19).

> **The sublingual glands secrete a mainly mucous product.**

The large sublingual glands are located in the floor of the mouth, one on either side of the frenulum of the tongue. Their short ducts open into the mouth near to, or with, the submandibular ducts. These glands are composed predominantly of mucous cells.

> **There are numerous smaller groups of salivary gland tissue.**

The oral cavity contains a large amount of salivary gland tissue scattered diffusely in the submucosa.

The most important are:
- Lingual glands in the submucosa and muscle layers of the dorsal surface of the tongue (see Fig. 11.7b)
- Minor sublingual glands close to the larger major sublingual glands (other tongue glands are found on the inferior surface of the tip of the tongue and on its lateral borders)
- Labial glands on the inner surface of the lips
- Palatine glands in the submucosa of the soft and hard palates
- Tonsillar glands in the mucosa associated with the palatine and pharyngeal tonsils
- Buccal glands in the submucosa lining the cheeks

Fig. 11.19 Parotid Salivary Gland. (a) Low-magnification image showing the gland comprises lobules separated by fibrous septa (S) containing large ducts. (b) The parotid salivary gland is composed entirely of basophilic granular serous cells (S), with variable amounts of intervening adipose tissue (A). Note the small ducts (SD) and part of a major duct (MD). (Micrograph from digital pathology whole slide image provided by the University of Leeds Virtual Pathology Project https://www.virtualpathology.leeds.ac.uk. Reproduced with permission.)

The labial, sublingual, minor lingual and buccal glands are composed predominantly of mucous cells, but some serous cells may be present. The palatine and lateral lingual glands are entirely mucus secreting.

TRANSPORT PASSAGES

The pharynx, oesophagus and anal canal are comparatively simple transport tubes through which ingested food is transmitted by peristalsis without undergoing significant metabolic change. They are muscular tubes lined internally by stratified squamous epithelium and some mucous glands which provide lubricating mucus.

The pharynx is divided into oropharynx and nasopharynx.

The pharynx is located at the back of the mouth and transfers partly fragmented food from the oral cavity into the upper end of the oesophagus. It also connects the nasal system of air chambers and the upper end of the trachea. The opening of the mouth into the pharynx is the **oropharynx**, and the nasal opening is the **nasopharynx**. The eustachian tube from the middle ear (see Chapter 10) opens into the pharynx on each side.

The oropharynx and pharynx proper are lined by largely non-keratinizing stratified squamous epithelium. The nasopharynx is lined mainly by ciliated columnar epithelium, but stratified squamous epithelium occurs at its lower end where it joins the oropharynx.

The submucosa of the pharynx is well endowed with lymphoid tissue.

There is a particularly prominent aggregation of lymphoid tissue in the nasopharynx forming the pharyngeal tonsil (adenoids). At the junction between the mouth and pharynx, in the oropharynx, are large lymphoid tonsillar masses in the gap between the glossopalatine and pharyngopalatine arches on each side. These are the palatine tonsils. The tonsils are discussed on page 156.

OESOPHAGUS

Introduction

The oesophagus lies between the pharynx and the stomach. It transports food in an undigested but fragmented form to the stomach, where digestion begins. It is about 25-cm long, originating from the pharynx at the level of the cricoid cartilage and extending down the posterior mediastinum in the midline to the level of the diaphragm; it penetrates the left crus of the diaphragm before opening into the stomach at the oesophago-gastric junction.

The oesophagus is lined by squamous epithelium, which lies over a lamina propria and a muscularis mucosae.

The oesophageal mucosa is composed of non-keratinizing stratified squamous epithelium, lamina propria and muscularis mucosae (Fig. 11.20). The basal zone of the epithelium may be several cell layers thick and consists of cuboidal or rectangular cells with dark nuclei and purple-staining cytoplasm, in which there is no glycogen. Scattered in this layer are occasional melanocytes and neuroendocrine cells.

Above the basal zone, the epithelial cells are larger and may be rich in glycogen, gradually becoming more flattened as the lumen is approached (Fig. 11.21).

Fig. 11.20 Oesophageal Mucosa and Submucosa. The oesophagus is lined by non-keratinizing stratified squamous epithelium (E), beneath which is a thick lamina propria (LP) and muscularis mucosae (MM). The submucosa contains abundant vessels and nerves, together with oesophageal mucous glands (EMG), which are characteristically surrounded by lymphocytic infiltrate.

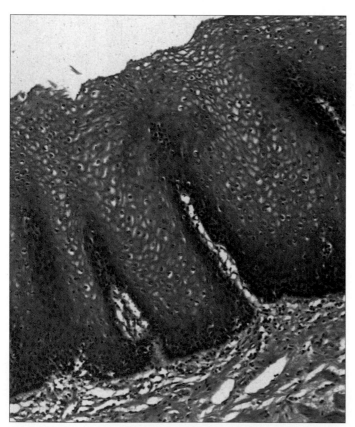

Fig. 11.21 Oesophageal Epithelium. At high magnification, the oesophageal squamous epithelium contains some pale-staining cells distended with glycogen; its lower border is irregular.

The average epithelial thickness is 500–800 μm, but this is difficult to measure accurately because the lower border is irregular and tongues of lamina propria extend up toward the luminal surface, giving an appearance similar to the rete ridge arrangement in the epidermis of the skin (see Chapter 18).

The oesophageal lamina propria consists of loosely arranged collagen fibres and fibroblasts embedded in an acellular glycosaminoglycan matrix, with a normal scattering of lymphocytes and eosinophils, in addition to occasional mast cells and plasma cells.

The muscularis mucosae is of variable thickness, being particularly thick at the lower end where it approaches the oesophagogastric junction. In the upper oesophagus, the fibres appear to be arranged haphazardly, but in the lower third, there are continuous sheets of longitudinal and circular smooth muscle.

> **The submucosa of the oesophagus contains mucous glands, lymphoid tissue, nerves and blood vessels.**

The submucosa of the oesophagus is broad and contains mucous glands (see Fig. 11.20) that secrete acid mucins. Each gland has two to five lobes, which drain into a short duct lined by stratified columnar epithelium, with the duct penetrating the muscularis mucosae, lamina propria and epithelial layer to open into the lumen. Lymphocytes, plasma cells and eosinophils are particularly common around the glands and their ducts (see Fig. 11.20). Aggregations of lymphoid cells forming small follicles are common in the oesophageal submucosa near the squamous/columnar epithelial junction.

Oesophageal submucosa is also particularly rich in blood vessels, lymphatics, nerves and ganglion cells.

> **The muscle of the oesophagus contains both striated and smooth types.**

The muscularis propria (externa) of the oesophagus varies along its length, although it is generally arranged in discrete circular and longitudinal layers. In the upper third of the oesophagus, the layers are composed almost entirely of striated muscle, but a gradual transition to smooth muscle occurs in the middle third, where both striated and smooth muscle fibres are found together. The muscle layers in the lower third are composed entirely of smooth muscle and are continuous with the smooth muscle layers of the stomach.

> **The oesophagogastric junction is an important site of pathological abnormality.**

Unlike the rest of the oesophagus, which is lined by stratified squamous epithelium, the short length (1–1.5-cm long) of oesophagus below the diaphragm is lined by columnar epithelium similar to that of the cardiac region of the stomach; this is the oesophagogastric (squamous/columnar) junction (Fig. 11.22). Disease results from exposure of the squamous epithelium of the lower oesophagus to acid and digestive enzymes from the stomach (Fig. 11.23).

Fig. 11.22 Oesophagogastric Junction. (a) Macroscopic appearance of the junction between the oesophagus and stomach. Most of the oesophagus is lined by a stratified squamous epithelium (pale), whereas the stomach epithelium appears brown. **(b)** H&E section of the squamous/columnar junction in the region of the oesophagogastric junction showing the abrupt transition between oesophageal squamous epithelium (EE) and columnar gastric epithelium (GE). In the region of the junction, lymphoid aggregates (L) and oesophageal mucous glands (EMG) are particularly prominent.

KEY FACTS

Oesophagus

- Lined by non-keratinizing stratified squamous epithelium
- Submucosa contains mucous glands, lymphoid aggregates and prominent blood vessels, particularly at the lower end
- Muscle is striated type in upper third, smooth muscle in lower third and both in middle third
- Lower oesophagus is an important site of common diseases, particularly ulceration, stricture and cancer

CLINICAL EXAMPLE

Oesophageal Ulceration and Barrett's Oesophagus

The squamous epithelium of the oesophagus is protected from exposure to gastric acid by:
- The anatomical arrangement of the oesophagogastric junction.
- The small oesophagogastric muscular sphincter, which in most cases prevents reflux of gastric contents into the lower oesophagus.

However, the system is not foolproof, and reflux of acid gastric secretions may occur into the lower oesophagus causing inflammation and pain. Under the constant irritating effect of reflux of acidic gastric secretions, the epithelium in the lower oesophagus changes its form from stratified squamous epithelium to a gastric type of glandular epithelium. This condition is called *Barrett's oesophagus* and is an example of epithelial metaplasia (see p. 178).

The islands of columnar epithelium in Barrett's oesophagus are particularly prone to ulceration and inflammation (see Fig. 11.23) and are also predisposed to the development of one type of oesophageal cancer.

Fig. 11.23 Barrett's Oesophagus. The lower half of the oesophagus (E) and the upper part of the stomach (S). Compare with Fig. 11.22a. At the oesophagogastric junction (OGJ) are four ulcers (U), which lie in inflamed metaplastic glandular (columnar) mucosa that extends up as far as the *arrow*. Above the *arrow*, there is normal oesophageal stratified squamous epithelium, which shows yellowish discolouration as a result of repeated vomiting. Healing of such ulcers can lead to scarring of the lower end of the oesophagus, and thereby narrowing of its lumen (i.e. an oesophageal stricture), so that swallowing becomes almost impossible.

ANAL CANAL

> **The anal canal is a muscular conduit transporting faeces for elimination.**

The anal canal transports the residue of ingested food after it has been digested and most of its water content has been extracted (i.e. faeces) from the rectum to the exterior in the process known as *defecation*.

Anatomically, the anal canal is a tube 3–4-cm long (Fig. 11.24), the diameter of which is controlled by two sphincter systems.

The internal anal sphincter is composed of smooth muscle and is a localized thickening of the circular muscle of the lower rectum. It is under autonomic control and responds to distension of the rectal reservoir.

The external anal sphincter is composed of skeletal striated muscle and is continuous with the fascia and muscles of the pelvic floor. It is under voluntary control.

> **The anal canal is mainly lined by stratified squamous epithelium.**

At its upper end, the anal canal is lined by columnar epithelium identical to that of the rectum. This changes to a non-keratinizing stratified squamous type at the level of the pectinate (or dentate) line, which marks the site of the anal membrane of the fetus (i.e. the junction of gut endoderm and the ectodermal invagination of the proctodeal pit).

The pectinate line is a line of small, crescentic, valve-like mucosal extrusions, with small vertical folds – the anal columns – arising from their junctions.

Small branched tubular glands, the anal glands, open into the anal canal just above the pectinate line, and another set of glands, the prominent apocrine glands of the perianal skin, lie at the lower end of the anal canal (circumanal glands).

> **Two prominent venous plexuses are associated with the anal canal.**

The internal haemorrhoidal plexus lies in the submucosa of the upper end of the canal above the level of the pectinate line.

The external haemorrhoidal plexus lies in the submucosa at the lower end in the region of the junction between the anal canal and perianal skin.

CLINICAL EXAMPLE

The internal haemorrhoidal plexus is particularly prone to become greatly enlarged as a result of chronic congestion secondary to raised intrapelvic pressure, such as may occur during pregnancy and repeated excessive straining to defecate as a result of constipation. This enlargement causes the veins to bulge into the anal canal and even to become so large that they protrude outside the anal orifice. Here, they are subject to trauma and inflammation and may become extremely painful. These protrusions are called **haemorrhoids** or *piles,* and when they protrude from the anal orifice, *prolapsed piles.*

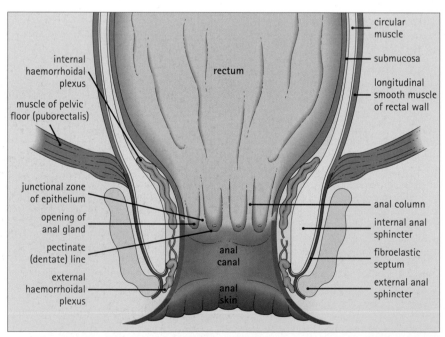

Fig. 11.24 Anal Canal. The anal canal showing the epithelial linings of the rectum (columnar), anal canal (non-keratinizing stratified squamous) and anal skin (keratinizing epidermis rich in hair follicles, eccrine and apocrine glands). There is a variable junctional zone of epithelium at the pectinate line. The internal sphincter is a continuation of the circular smooth muscle layer of the rectum, and the external sphincter is composed of skeletal muscle under voluntary control. The rectal longitudinal muscle loses its fibres at the level of the puborectalis muscle of the pelvic floor and continues as a fibroelastic septum between the internal and external sphincters. Note the positions of the internal and external haemorrhoidal plexuses; haemorrhoids (piles) result from enlargement of the internal haemorrhoidal plexus.

DIGESTIVE TRACT

The digestive tract is the site of several processes:

- Major digestion of food material (some digestion begins in the mouth as a result of salivary secretion of diastase)
- Absorption of the end products of digestion
- Absorption of ingested fluids and reabsorption of secreted fluids

The digestive tract comprises the stomach, small intestine (i.e. duodenum, jejunum and ileum) and large intestine (i.e. caecum, appendix, colon and rectum). Its basic structure is shown in Fig. 11.25.

The digestive mucosa, composed of lining epithelium, lamina propria and muscularis mucosae, is the most variable component of the digestive tract and usually contains a mixture of epithelial cell types, both absorptive and secretory. The epithelium is supported by a variable layer, the lamina propria, which is composed of supporting cells and their products (including collagen). Within the lamina propria are small blood vessels, lymphatics, nerve fibres and cells belonging to the immune and defence systems (see Chapter 8), particularly eosinophils, macrophages and lymphocytes. The deep aspect of the lamina propria rests on a usually thin muscle layer, the muscularis mucosae.

> **The surface area of the digestive passages is increased by the formation of folds and glands.**

The efficiency of absorptive and secretory processes is improved by increasing the surface area of contact between the epithelial cells and the lumen. This is achieved by:

- Intrusions or folding of the lining epithelium into the lumen (i.e. villi or plicae)
- Inversions of the epithelium to form tubular structures, the lumina of which communicate with the main lumen
- Formation of complex glands within or exterior to the tract wall

Examples of these structural modifications will be discussed in relation to specific areas of the digestive tract.

> **The submucosal layer contains vessels, nerves and a specialized nerve plexus.**

The submucosa lies between the mucosa and the main muscle layer of the digestive tract wall. It is composed of fibroblasts, collagen and acellular matrix and contains blood vessels, lymphatics and nerves, which supply or drain their smaller equivalents in the lamina propria of the mucosa.

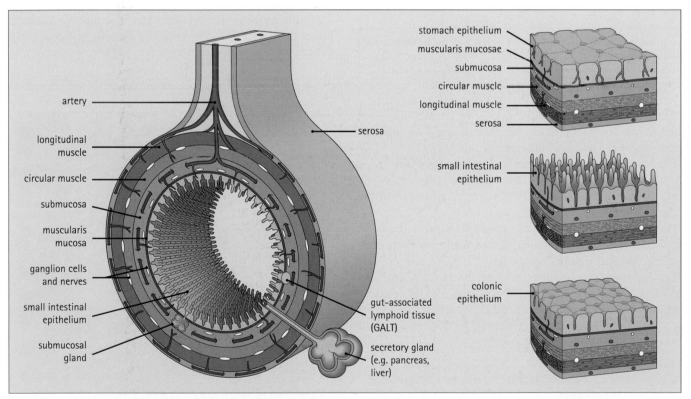

Fig. 11.25 Basic Structure of the Digestive Tract. The digestive tract is a muscular tube lined internally by specialized epithelium which, for most of its length, has a combined secretory and absorptive function. Three patterns of epithelial structure (stomach, small intestine and colon) are shown in this diagram. Externally, the tract has an outer layer of flat mesothelium, where it runs through the peritoneal cavity. Various secretory organs, which are derived embryologically as outgrowths of the putative alimentary tract, lie partly or completely outside it. These organs (e.g. pancreas and liver) produce secretions which are vital for the tract to function normally; they are transferred to the digestive tract lumen by one or more ducts.

In addition, the submucosa contains clumps of ganglion cells associated with the autonomic nerve supply of the tract, and in some areas contains lymphoid aggregates and follicles, which are part of the gut-associated lymphoid tissue (GALT) (see later).

> **The smooth muscle in the bowel wall is arranged in distinct layers, each of which is oriented in different directions.**

The musculature of the alimentary tract is responsible for moving the luminal contents gradually along the tract from mouth to anus. It therefore extends beyond the digestive part of the tract into the transport passages (i.e. the oropharynx, oesophagus and the anal canal). Movement is achieved by peristalsis.

There are two layers of smooth muscle throughout most of the digestive tract and a third layer in the stomach (see later). Traditionally identified as an outer longitudinal layer and an inner circular layer, they are in fact arranged spirally, with the inner circular layer being a compact spiral and the outer longitudinal layer being a more elongated helix (i.e. an arrangement similar to that of the smooth muscle of the ureter; see Fig. 15.37).

Between the two main smooth muscle layers of the digestive tract are small blood and lymphatic vessels, together with the nerves and ganglion cells of the autonomic nervous system.

The basic pattern of two muscle layers that extend into the transport passages of the alimentary tract, proximally into the oesophagus and distally into the anal canal, is modified by the presence of some skeletal muscle.

> **Localized thickenings of muscle in the bowel wall act as valves and are called sphincters.**

In some areas, the basic muscle pattern is also modified by a localized increase in the circular muscle to act as a sphincter. Sphincter contraction occludes the lumen and thus prevents the passage of the luminal contents.

The pyloric sphincter is the most important sphincter and is located at the junction between the stomach and duodenum. By contracting, it delays stomach emptying, thereby permitting continued food breakdown in the stomach.

The oesophagogastric sphincter is located between the lower oesophagus and proximal stomach; it normally prevents reflux of gastric contents into the oesophagus.

The ileocaecal valve is situated between the terminal ileum and caecum; it delays the discharge of ileal contents into the caecum.

The internal anal sphincter, sited at the upper end of the anal canal, retains faecal waste material in the rectum until controlled defecation is possible.

> **The outer coat of the bowel wall is called the adventitia, being covered in some parts by peritoneum.**

The adventitia is the outer coat of the digestive tract and surrounds the external layer of muscle. It is composed of loosely arranged fibroblasts and collagen embedded in matrix, with variable numbers of adipocytes.

The adventitia contains large blood and lymphatic vessels and nerves, with the major arterial supply and venous drainage of the tract wall passing through it.

Some of the digestive tract is retroperitoneal, but most is within the peritoneal cavity, and here the outer surface of the adventitia over much of its circumference is covered by a layer of flattened epithelium: the mesothelium (visceral peritoneum). This is identical to and continuous with the mesothelium lining the peritoneal cavity internally and covering the mesenteric attachment of the alimentary tract to the posterior abdominal wall (parietal peritoneum).

Adventitia covered by mesothelium (i.e. adventitia of the stomach, most of the small intestine and the large intestine) is commonly called the *serosa*. Where adventitia is not covered by a mesothelium (i.e. adventitia of part of the duodenum and some of the colon), it merges with adjacent tissues.

> **Immunological defence against antigens ingested in the digestive tract is provided by the GALT.**

Throughout the digestive tract, the lamina propria contains cells of the immune system (see Chapter 8), including lymphocytes, plasma cells and macrophages. In addition to these cells, there are individual intraepithelial lymphocytes (Fig. 11.26).

The lymphoid cells are commonly arranged as large follicles, often with germinal centres, and are partly located in the mucosa and partly in submucosa, thus splitting the muscularis mucosae. In the ileum, the follicles aggregate to form substantial nodules called *Peyer's patches* (see p. 155).

Fig. 11.26 Gut-Associated Lymphoid Tissue (GALT). Micrograph showing the typical arrangement of a nodule of GALT in the lamina propria. The epithelial cells (M cells), closely associated with the lymphoid aggregate, are cuboidal and show no cytoplasmic specialization such as mucin droplet formation. Note the intraepithelial lymphocytes (IEL).

Although lymphoid follicles and Peyer's patches contain both B and T lymphocytes, the diffuse, nonfollicular infiltrate in the lamina propria is composed largely of T lymphocytes.

The mucosal epithelial cells that overlie the lymphoid follicles and Peyer's patches differ from the usual epithelial cells in both structure and function and are called *M cells* (see Fig. 11.26). They are cuboidal or flat rather than tall and columnar and have luminal microfolds rather than tall microvilli.

M cells are believed to take up antigenic macromolecules from the intestinal lumen, incorporating them into endocytotic vesicles and then transporting them to the lateral intercellular space in the region of an intraepithelial lymphocyte.

> **The gut has both intrinsic and extrinsic innervation.**

The intrinsic innervation of the gut is located in two zones of the bowel wall (Fig. 11.27a) Collections of nerves and ganglion cells in the submucosa form an interconnected network called the *submucosal (Meissner's) plexus* (see Fig. 11.27b), whereas collections of nerves and ganglion cells between the inner circular and outer longitudinal components of the muscularis proper form a network called the *myenteric (Auerbach's) plexus* (see Fig. 11.27c).

The extrinsic system comprises an autonomic input from parasympathetic (stimulatory) and sympathetic (inhibitory) abdominal plexuses that modulates the activity of the intrinsic innervation of the gut. In addition, sensory nerves terminate in the bowel as tendril-like sensory endings.

The afferent autonomic impulses mediate visceral reflexes and sensations such as rectal fullness.

> **Interstitial cells of Cajal act as pacemaker cells for bowel contraction.**

A network of indistinct spindle cells is present in the wall of the gut called *interstitial cells of Cajal* (ICCs).

These cells act as the source of excitation for rhythmic smooth muscle contraction that forms peristalsis, being the origin of slow waves in gut motility. These cells act as transducers of neuronal activity coming from nerve plexus layers, and excitation originating in ICCs is passed to smooth muscle cells. There is also evidence that these cells respond to stretching of the bowel wall and, in response, increase peristalsis.

ICCs appear as spindle cells with cell processes (bipolar or stellate) indistinguishable in routine histological sections from the background of smooth muscle spindle cells and other types of spindle cell such as fibroblasts. Immunohistochemistry for the receptor tyrosine kinase, Kit (CD117) acts as a marker that shows the extent of this important cell network and identifies submuscular, intramuscular, myenteric and subserosal groups. On electron microscopy, ICCs have a discontinuous basement membrane and caveolae and have communicating gap junctions with neuronal processes and smooth muscle cells.

STOMACH

From the oesophagus, food enters the stomach, a dilated portion of the digestive tract where fragmented food is retained while it is macerated and partially digested. At the lower end of the stomach, the pyloric sphincter (see Fig. 11.33) prevents the passage of food until it is converted into a thick, semiliquid paste or pulp (chyme).

Fig. 11.27 Intrinsic Innervation. (a) Orientation image showing the location of the nerve plexus in the bowel wall. The myenteric plexus, highlighted here as a yellow band (MP), is located between the two muscle layers (M). The submucosal plexus (SP), highlighted here in *green*, is distributed in the submucosa (S). **(b)** High-power micrograph showing a cluster of ganglion cells (G) in the small bowel submucosa (S) of the small intestine forming part of the submucosal plexus (Meissner's plexus). Note the muscularis mucosae (mm) and the small intestinal mucosa (Mu). **(c)** High-power micrograph showing myenteric plexus (Auerbach's plexus) (P) composed of nerves and Schwann cells surrounding ganglion cells (G) and its location in between the two layers of the muscularis propria (M).

> **There are three layers of muscle in the stomach wall.**

The muscular wall of the stomach differs from the standard digestive tract pattern by the presence of a third layer of oblique muscle fibres. These lie internal to the circular layer and assist in the complex churning action necessary to mix food thoroughly with the secretions of the gastric mucosa.

The stomach muscle layers are thick. When contracted, they decrease the stomach capacity and the mucosa is thrown up into longitudinal folds called *rugae,* which are most prominent on the convexity of the stomach (the greater curvature). This is the state of the stomach when it is empty; when it is full, the musculature relaxes and thins and the rugae stretch flat as the stomach distends.

The stomach is ideally equipped for its role as a reservoir by its distensibility, the presence of the pyloric sphincter and the mechanisms preventing reflux at its upper end.

> **The gastric epithelium secretes hydrochloric acid, digestive enzymes and mucus. It also contains a population of hormone-secreting cells.**

Food is converted into chyme by the secretions of the gastric mucosa into the lumen.

These are:
- A dilute solution of hydrochloric acid (approximately 0.16 N)
- Solutions of proteolytic enzymes, mainly pepsin
- Small amounts of other enzymes (e.g. rennin and gastric lipase)
- Mucins, mainly in the form of neutral mucins

The major functions of the gastric epithelium are the secretion of acid and digestive enzymes. It also secretes mucus to lubricate ingested food and to protect itself from the corrosive effects of the acid and enzymes. The surface area of the stomach epithelium is increased by downgrowths that form glands.

The secretions are produced by three main cell types. In addition, there is a population of endocrine cells and a population of stem cells from which the other cell types are derived. The cell types are:
- Mucous cells
- Acid-producing cells (oxyntic or parietal cells)
- Enzyme-producing cells (chief cells or peptic cells)
- Stem cells
- Enteroendocrine cells

> **Gastric mucous cells are of two types: surface mucous cells and neck mucous cells.**

Surface mucous cells (Fig. 11.28a) are tall and columnar with basal nuclei and clear-staining luminal cytoplasm distended by numerous small mucin vacuoles, which are discharged into the stomach lumen by exocytosis. The cells also have prominent endoplasmic reticulum, and the Golgi complex is located above the nucleus.

The luminal surface of surface mucous cells shows scanty short microvilli with a surface glycocalyx, and junctional complexes join adjacent cells near the luminal surface.

Fig. 11.28 Gastric Mucous Cells. (a) In this high-power micrograph, the gastric surface mucous cells have basal nuclei and bulky luminal cytoplasm filled with pale-staining mucus. **(b)** In contrast to the very tall surface gastric mucin cells, the neck region of the gastric pits contains smaller mucin-secreting cells, which appear crowded together. On the left of this micrograph are specialized cells of the gastric glands (chief cells and parietal cells).

The lateral borders of the cells are often separated by a considerable intercellular gap, which is traversed by cytoplasmic protrusions of the lateral walls; this separation disappears as the apical surface is neared, where the binding of adjacent cells is very tight. Surface mucous cells are also thought to produce blood group substances.

Neck mucous cells (see Fig. 11.28b) are smaller and less regular in shape than surface mucous cells, mainly because they are compressed and distorted by adjacent cells. They have a basal nucleus and finely granular cytoplasm, owing to the presence of small mucin vacuoles, which are smaller than those in the surface mucous cells.

The vacuoles can be distributed throughout the cytoplasm and are not aggregated near the luminal surface as they are in the surface mucous cells. By light microscopy it is not always apparent that neck mucous cells contain mucin, and a periodic–acid Schiff (PAS) stain is often necessary to highlight it.

> **The acid-producing cells of the stomach are called parietal cells.**

The acid-producing cells are large pyramidal cells with central nuclei and pale eosinophilic cytoplasm (Fig. 11.29a). The cytoplasm often appears vacuolated, particularly around the nucleus. The cell attachment to the basement membrane is broad, but their luminal aspect is narrow, being compressed between adjacent cells. Despite this, these cells have a vast luminal surface area as a result of deep microvilli-lined invaginations producing so-called *canaliculi* (see Fig. 11.29b).

In the cytoplasm close to the canaliculi are clusters of round or oval vesicles that have clear centres and distinct membrane borders and which are thought to be involved in the transfer of substances from the cytoplasm to the lumen of the canalicular system. The rest of the cytoplasm is packed with round or oval mitochondria with closely packed cristae (see Fig. 11.29c). This high concentration of mitochondria is responsible for the eosinophilia of the cell cytoplasm, particularly at the periphery.

A small Golgi and some rough endoplasmic reticulum are also present.

Parietal cells also produce intrinsic factor, the glycoprotein that avidly binds to vitamin B_{12} to render it absorbable by the digestive tract.

> **Chief cells secrete the enzyme pepsin.**

The enzyme-producing cells of the stomach are also known as *chief* or *peptic cells*. They have characteristics of a protein-secreting cell with large basal nuclei, basophilic basal cytoplasm resulting from a rich, protein-producing, rough endoplasmic reticulum, and at their apex near the gland, lumen contain refractile pink-stained cytoplasmic granules (Figs. 11.30 and 11.31); they therefore resemble the exocrine cells of the pancreas (see p. 228). The granules contain the inactive enzyme precursor pepsinogen, which is disgorged into the gastric lumen, where it is converted by gastric acid into the active proteolytic enzyme pepsin.

Pepsin is a potent enzyme, breaking down large protein molecules into small peptides and converting almost all of the structural proteins into soluble small molecular weight substances; it is largely responsible for the conversion of solid food particles to fluid chyme.

Fig. 11.29 Acid-Producing Cells. (a) The acid-secreting cells (parietal cells) (P) have pale-stained eosinophilic cytoplasm with some cells showing faint vacuolation running in a crescent close to the nucleus. Basophilic chief cells make up the rest of this gastric gland. **(b)** The acid-producing cell has an intricate system of invaginations (canaliculi) lined by microvilli, which produce the perinuclear vacuolated appearance seen on light microscopy. The rest of the cytoplasm is packed with mitochondria, particularly at the cell periphery. A small Golgi and some rough endoplasmic reticulum are also present, with vesicles close to the canaliculi. **(c)** Electron micrograph showing the intricate canalicular system (C) of an acid-producing cell; the cytoplasm is largely occupied by tightly packed mitochondria (M).

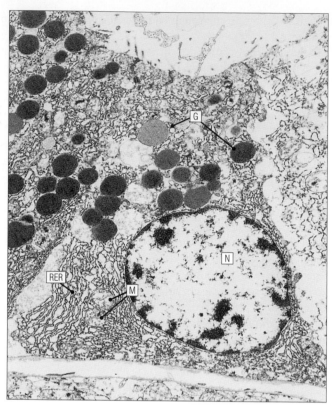

Fig. 11.30 Enzyme-Producing Cells. Electron micrograph of an enzyme-producing cell showing its large basal nucleus (N), abundant mitochondria (M), abundant rough endoplasmic reticulum (RER) and the grey-staining spherical granules (G), which contain pepsinogen and are responsible for the granular appearance of these cells in H&E-stained sections (see also Fig. 11.31).

◎ **ADVANCED CONCEPT**

Acid-Producing Cells

The acid-producing cells have abundant carbonic anhydrase, which is thought to play a vital role in generating H^+ ions for the production of hydrochloric acid (HCl).

Carbon dioxide (CO_2) diffuses across the basement membrane from blood capillaries into the cell, where it links with water molecules (a reaction catalysed by carbonic anhydrase) to produce carbonic acid (H_2CO_3); this instantly dissociates into an H^+ ion and an HCO_3^- ion. The latter passes back into the blood, whereas the H^+ is pumped into the lumen of a canaliculus. Chloride ions (Cl^-) are actively transported across the cell into the canaliculus from the capillaries in the lamina propria.

◎ **ADVANCED CONCEPT**

Stem Cells

The epithelial cells of the gastric mucosa are formed from stem cells. Stem cells are the precursor cells of all epithelial cells of the gastric mucosa. They are small cells with oval basal nuclei and show no cytoplasmic specialization when completely undifferentiated, but are capable of differentiating into mucous, acid-producing, enzyme-producing or endocrine cells.

Normally present in very small numbers in humans, they increase in number and activity when the gastric epithelium is continually damaged, for example, in chronic irritation of the gastric mucosa (i.e. chronic gastritis). A surge of stem cell activity enables an ulcerated area of the stomach to be rapidly re-epithelialized. Such regeneration is an important final step in the healing of a stomach ulcer.

Fig. 11.31 Gastric Gland. H&E appearance of a gastric gland from the body of the stomach. In the upper part of the micrograph, most of the cells are acid-producing parietal cells (P) with pale eosinophilic cytoplasm. In the lower part most of the cells are enzyme-producing chief cells (C), which have basophilic basal cytoplasm. The apical portion of cells close to the gland lumen contain numerous eosinophilic granules of a secretory product.

Endocrine cells in the gastric mucosa secrete a variety of hormones.

Enteroendocrine cells (see Chapter 14) of the stomach are small and round and are situated on the epithelial basement membrane. In haematoxylin and eosin (H&E) paraffin sections, they have a round, central dark-staining nucleus and a rim of clear cytoplasm (Fig. 11.32a).

Ultrastructurally, the cytoplasm contains membrane-bound neurosecretory granules, with the shape, size, number and electron density varying according to the substance secreted.

- Cells secreting gastrin (G cells) are concentrated in the pyloric mucosa in the base of glands.
- Endocrine cells in the stomach also secrete somatostatin (see Fig. 11.32b), cholecystokinin, vasoactive intestinal peptide, endorphins and substance P.

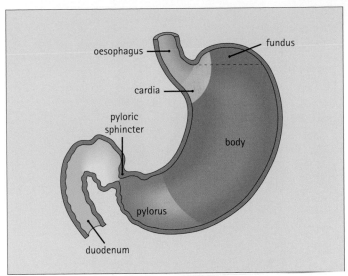

Fig. 11.33 **Areas of the Stomach.** The stomach, showing the three histologically distinguishable areas. The cardia extends from the squamous/columnar junction at the lower end of the oesophagus for a variable distance into the upper stomach, usually 2–3 cm down the lesser curve; cardiac mucosa may also extend partway into the fundus, which is an anatomical rather than a histological feature. Pyloric mucosa lines a roughly conical area in the lower third of the stomach, starting about halfway down the lesser curve. The area is variable and tends to begin higher on the lesser curve in women. Body mucosa occupies the rest of the stomach, including most of the anatomical fundus. The transition between the various mucosal patterns is commonly gradual, with a narrow junctional zone showing features of both.

Fig. 11.32 **Gastric Endocrine Cells. (a)** Micrograph of the base of glands in the body of the stomach showing the H&E appearance of gastric enteroendocrine cells (END). They are small with a pale cytoplasm and a small, dark-staining central nucleus. Acid-producing (A) and enzyme-producing (E) cells are also evident. **(b)** Micrograph of a section stained by immunohistochemistry to show the distribution of somatostatin-secreting endocrine cells in the pyloric gastric mucosa. Endocrine cells are numerous in the neck region, with a few scattered cells in the deep glands.

The neck zone between the superficial and deep zones is narrow and composed largely of immature stem cells mixed with some neck mucous cells. The immature stem cells proliferate and migrate upward to replenish the predominantly mucous cells of the superficial zone and downward to replenish the cell types in the glands of the deep zone.

The deep zone is composed of glands, the bases of which lie close to or in the muscularis mucosae, whereas the upper ends open into the bases of the superficial zone pits.

The structure of the deep zone varies, there being three main histological patterns that delineate three main areas of the stomach: the cardia, the body and the pylorus (Figs. 11.33 and 11.34).

> **The gastric mucosa can be divided into three histological zones: a superficial zone, a neck zone and a deep zone.**

There are three zonal divisions of the gastric mucosa. The superficial zone is composed of a layer of surface mucous cells with downgrowths which are variously called *foveolae, pits* or *crypts*.

The mucous cells lining the pits are not as tall and columnar as those on the surface; they also contain less mucin.

The superficial zone is roughly constant in its content and structure throughout the stomach.

▶▶ KEY FACTS

Stomach

- There are three layers of smooth muscle in the wall.
- Mucosa is divided into cardia, body and pyloric regions.
- Parietal cells are specialized to produce acid and also secrete intrinsic factor.
- Chief cells secrete the enzyme pepsin as an inactive precursor: pepsinogen.
- Endocrine cells in the mucosa secrete gastrin, somatostatin and vasoactive intestinal peptide (VIP).

Fig. 11.34 Gastric Mucosa. (a) Cardiac mucosa. The superficial and deep zones of the cardiac mucosa are about equal in thickness. The surface and crypt epithelium is composed of mucous cells, and the deep zone is composed of tubular and branched glands lined by mucous cells, with scattered endocrine and acid-producing cells becoming more numerous near the junction with the body mucosa. Some of the more complex glands are coiled. The muscularis mucosae is thick and irregular and often sends bundles of fibres toward the surface, interdigitating with the glands. The histological appearance of cardiac mucosa surface is shown in Fig. 11.28. **(b)** Body mucosa. The superficial zone of the body mucosa accounts for only 25% or less of the mucosal thickness. Most pits open directly and singly onto the surface, but some fuse before opening to form a wider crevice. The deep zone is composed of tightly packed, long, straight tubular glands that end blindly at the muscularis mucosae. At their upper ends the glands open into the bases of the crypts through a variably constricted neck region. The glands may open into single or larger fused crypts. The superficial zone is covered by surface mucous cells, with neck mucous cells covering the deeper parts of the pits. At the neck region, neck mucosa cells are mixed with stem cells. The glands are composed of acid-producing cells, enzyme-producing cells, neck mucous cells and scattered endocrine cells. **(c)** Body mucosa. H&E section of body mucosa showing the superficial zone (S) composed of mucus-secreting cells, a narrow neck zone (N) containing mainly stem cells and neck mucous cells and the deep zone (D), largely composed of acid-producing and enzyme-producing cells. **(d)** Pyloric mucosa. The superficial zone of the pyloric region occupies slightly more than 50% of the mucosal thickness, and the crypts are often branched. The deep zone is composed of tortuous single or branched glands extending down to the muscularis mucosae. The cell content of the superficial and neck zones is the same as in the cardiac and body mucosa. The glands are lined by mucous cells, but scattered acid-producing cells and numerous endocrine cells are also present. Acid-producing cells become more numerous close to the pyloric sphincter. **(e)** Pyloric mucosa. H&E section of pyloric mucosa showing the superficial zone (S) occupying about 50% of the mucosal thickness. The narrow neck (N) and substantial deep (D) zones are composed of mucous cells, which form branching glands in the deep zone.

CLINICAL EXAMPLE

Gastric Ulcer

The stomach normally contains an acid solution but is protected from the damaging effects of the acid by various mechanisms, including the presence of a thin layer of mucus over the surface of the epithelial cells.

In some circumstances, particularly in association with *Helicobacter pylori* infection, these protective mechanisms break down and the acidic gastric contents damage the mucosa. The resulting death of epithelial cells and lamina propria leads to the formation of a shallow ulcer. Continued exposure of such an unprotected area leads to the formation of a deep ulcer (chronic gastric ulcer), which can extend through the submucosa and the muscle layers (Fig. 11.35) and takes a long time to heal.

Because gastric acid also enters the first part of the duodenum, this area may also be subject to ulceration (duodenal ulcer), as may the lower oesophagus if reflux of gastric acid occurs (see Fig. 11.23).

Fig. 11.35 Chronic Gastric Ulcer. Micrograph of an H&E section through a chronic gastric ulcer, which has extended through the mucosa (M), submucosa (SM) and muscularis propria (MP).

SMALL INTESTINE

Introduction

When the pyloric sphincter opens, partially digested food (chyme) empties from the stomach into the small intestine, which is the main site for the absorption of amino acids, sugars, fats and some larger molecules produced by digestion. The small intestine also secretes enzymes to complete the digestive processes begun in the stomach. It begins at the pylorus, the distal limit of the stomach, and ends at the ileocaecal valve, the proximal limit of the large intestine. At autopsy, when the longitudinal muscle is relaxed, the small intestine usually measures about 6 m, but in life it measures only about 3-m long. It is divided into three sections (duodenum, jejunum and ileum), although the transitions from one to the other are not precise.

The duodenum is the proximal 20–25 cm of small intestine and is entirely retroperitoneal. It has the shape of a letter C, with the head of the pancreas fitting into its concave edge. The bile and pancreatic ducts open into the duodenum in this concavity.

The jejunum begins where the duodenum emerges from behind the peritoneum and extends to an ill-defined junction with the ileum.

The ileum extends from the jejunum to the ileocaecal valve.

> **The small bowel has several modifications to increase its surface area.**

As the major absorptive site, the small intestine shows architectural modifications to optimize its surface area.

The mucosa and submucosa are thrown up into a large number of folds, or plicae, arranged circularly around the lumen. These are most prominent in the jejunum (Fig. 11.36a).

Fig. 11.36 Small Intestine – General architecture. (a) Macroscopic view of the small intestine mucosal surface showing tightly packed circumferential mucosal folds (plicae) (F). The white box shows the plane of section of the next image. **(b)** Low-power micrograph of the mucosal folds (F), which are filled with tissue from the submucosa (S), beyond which are the two muscular layers (M). Supported by the collagenous submucosal tissues, the plical folds remain even when the bowel is in a relaxed state. The black box shows an area of mucosa and submucosa similar to the next micrograph for orientation. **(c)** The small intestinal mucosa is thrown into projections called *villi* (V), below which are the glandular crypts (C) of the small intestine. The core of villi is formed from the mucosal lamina propria, which also surrounds the crypts. The muscularis mucosae (MM) separates the mucosa from the submucosa (S).

Fig. 11.37 In two dimensions, the villi appear to have the same structure, but in three dimensions their structure can be seen to correspond to one of three main patterns: they are either finger-like (F), leaf-like (L) or ridge-like (R), as shown in this scanning electron micrograph. There are also occasional intermediate forms. The proportions of these patterns vary from site to site and also with age. In babies and young children, the villi of the duodenum and proximal jejunum are almost entirely leaf- or ridge-like, with finger-like villi appearing with age. The adult pattern is present by 10–15 years.

The surface of the plicae is further arranged into villi, which protrude into the intestinal lumen (see Figs. 11.36b and 11.36c and Fig. 11.37). The small intestine has the standard arrangement of musculature (i.e. an external layer of longitudinal muscle and an inner circular layer) and a substantial submucosa in which GALT (see p. 155) is prominent.

CLINICAL EXAMPLE

Gluten Enteropathy (Coeliac Disease)

The absorptive function of the jejunum depends on the integrity of the villi. If enough villi are damaged, food material cannot be absorbed, leading to weight loss, abdominal bloating and diarrhoea.

One important cause of extensive loss of villi is coeliac disease, caused by an allergy to the wheat protein, gluten. The resulting immune-mediated inflammation leads to flattening of the jejunal surface with extensive loss of villi (Fig. 11.38).

Gluten enteropathy commonly presents in babies and young children with failure to thrive and to gain normal height and weight for their age. It also commonly presents in adults with malabsorption, including weight loss, diarrhoea and anaemia. Systemic features can also lead to neurological abnormalities and joint disease.

The villi usually assume their normal structure when gluten-containing food is excluded from the diet, and the malabsorptive state subsequently improves.

Fig. 11.38 Gluten Enteropathy (Coeliac Disease). Micrograph of villous damage resulting from gluten sensitivity. The jejunal mucosal surface is flattened owing to extensive loss of villi. Compare with Fig. 11.36c. (Micrograph from digital pathology whole slide image provided by the University of Leeds Virtual Pathology Project https://www.virtualpathology.leeds.ac.uk. Reproduced with permission.)

There are three functional zones of small intestinal epithelium.

The small intestinal epithelium can be divided into three functional zones. These are the villi, the crypts and the neck zone, where villi and crypts merge. (The features of the villi are discussed with Fig. 11.39, and the crypt structure is illustrated in Figs. 11.40 and 11.41.)

The cells of the epithelium are enterocytes, mucous cells, Paneth cells, endocrine cells and stem cells, and their numbers and distribution vary in the different zones of the epithelium.

Enterocytes are the main cell in the villi and are absorptive in function.

Enterocytes are tall, columnar cells with round or oval nuclei in the lower third of the cell.

The luminal surface of enterocytes is highly specialized; each cell bears 2000–3000 tightly packed, tall microvilli, which are coated by a glycoprotein: the glycocalyx (see Fig. 11.39c). This is composed of fine filamentous extensions of the microvillus cell membrane.

The glycocalyx contains a number of enzymes (brush border enzymes, e.g. lactase, sucrase, peptidases, lipases and alkaline phosphatase), which are important in digestion and transport (see Fig. 11.39e).

Beneath the microvillus surface, the enterocyte cytoplasm contains lysosomes and smooth endoplasmic reticulum and paired centrioles in the terminal bar region (see p. 49). Nearer the nucleus, the cell is rich in rough endoplasmic reticulum and mitochondria and there is a prominent Golgi. Between the nucleus and the basement membrane are mitochondria and many ribosomes and polyribosomes. The lateral walls of enterocytes show complex interdigitations and are the sites of Na^+ and K^+ ATPase activity. The lateral walls are separated from the microvillus surface by desmosomes and tight junctions (see Fig. 3.6).

The ultrastructural features of the enterocyte are linked to its absorptive function, and therefore many of the features and mechanisms are common to other active absorptive cells, such as those of the proximal convoluted tubule cell of the kidney. These absorptive mechanisms are illustrated and discussed in Chapter 15.

Mucous (goblet) cells are found mainly in the upper two-thirds of the crypts.

Occasional mucous cells are scattered among the enterocytes of the villi (see Figs. 11.39a and 11.39b).

Mucous cells contain globules of mucin in their luminal cytoplasm, the mucin being discharged onto the surface when the cytoplasm is fully expanded by mucin granules. The scanty basal cytoplasm is rich in rough endoplasmic reticulum.

Mucous cells are least frequent in the duodenum and increase in number in the jejunum and ileum, being most numerous in the terminal ileum close to the caecum.

Fig. 11.39 Small Intestine Villus. (a) Thin acrylic resin stained with H&E, showing a single villus, which is covered by tall enterocytes (E) bearing a prominent microvillus brush border (MV). Scattered among the enterocytes are occasional goblet mucous cells (M) and intraepithelial lymphocytes (L). The stromal core contains small capillaries and lymphatics (not shown) and a number of lymphocytes, plasma cells and macrophages. **(b)** Electron micrograph of a row of enterocytes. Note the microvillus border (MV), part of a mucous cell (M) and the endocrine cell with basal granules (E). **(c)** Electron micrograph of microvillus brush border (MV) at high magnification. The glycocalyx (G) can be seen as a faint greyish haze on the surface of the microvilli. **(d)** Scanning electron micrograph of part of the villus surface. Note the tightly packed enterocytes, the microvilli of which are partly obscured by the layer of glycocalyx. Mucous cells discharging their mucus (M) are clearly seen. **(e)** Enzyme histochemical preparation of small intestine showing the distribution of the enzyme lactase (*blue* staining), which is localized to the luminal surface of the enterocytes. Like many other cell-surface enzymes responsible for food breakdown in the small intestine, the enzyme sits in the glycocalyx.

Paneth cells are found in the lower third of the crypts.

Paneth cells have basal nuclei and prominent large eosinophilic granules in their luminal cytoplasm (see Fig. 11.40). Ultrastructurally, these granules are spherical and electron dense, with the remaining cytoplasm being rich in rough endoplasmic reticulum; these are features of a protein-secreting cell (see Fig. 3.14).

Paneth cells contain substances called *defensins*, which are secreted and protect against infection. The secreted factors also modulate stem cell activity in epithelial growth.

Endocrine cells are located mainly in the lower third of the crypts but are also seen higher up in the villi.

Endocrine cells in the small bowel resemble those seen in the stomach (see Fig. 11.32), being roughly triangular in shape, with the broad base being in contact with the basement membrane and the narrow apex reaching the lumen. Their nuclei are spherical and their cytoplasm pale staining (see Fig. 11.41).

Fig. 11.40 Paneth Cells. H&E micrograph of the base of a small intestinal crypt showing numerous Paneth cells (P) containing large numbers of brightly eosinophilic, red-staining granules. A small endocrine cell (E) with ill defined fine basal eosinophilic granules can also be seen. Three mitotic figures are present in the image, seen as basophilic structures in the epithelial cells

Ultrastructurally, the cytoplasm contains neuroendocrine granules, and the luminal surface bears microvilli.

Small intestinal endocrine cells secrete a number of hormones and peptides, including serotonin (5HT), motilin, cholecystokinin, neurotensin, secretin and vasoactive intestinal peptide (VIP).

> **Stem cells are found in the lower third of the crypts.**

The replication of stem cells replenishes the stock of the other cells, including the Paneth and endocrine cells. Most replication is to replace the mucous cells and enterocytes of the villi, as these cells have a rapid turnover, being shed from the tips of the villi about 5 days after production.

Before developing into the mature form of the two cell types, the stem cells differentiate into intermediate cells, which show some features of both mucous cells and enterocytes. This process involves the Wnt signalling pathway. These cells occupy much of the upper two-thirds of the crypts.

Stem cells and intermediate cells are particularly numerous when there is increased cell loss from the villi, which is a common feature of many diseases affecting the small intestine; the crypts increase in length and show increased numbers of cells in mitosis (i.e. crypt or gland hyperplasia).

> **The lamina propria of the small intestine is most clearly seen in the core of the villi, but also surrounds and supports the gland crypts.**

The lamina propria of the small bowel is composed of collagen, reticulin fibres, fibroblasts and glycosaminoglycan matrix, through which run blood capillaries, lymphatics and nerves. It contains some smooth muscle fibres.

The blood vessels and lymphatics are particularly prominent in the villi, with a central lymphatic (lacteal) running vertically down the centre of the core of each villus.

The lamina propria also contains lymphocytes, plasma cells, eosinophils, macrophages and mast cells.

The lymphocytes are largely T lymphocytes with a proportion of gamma delta cells (see Chapter 8); most of the plasma cells produce IgA. Lymphocytes are also present in the villous epithelium, usually in a basal position between the lateral intercellular spaces, and, like those in the lamina propria, they are also T lymphocytes.

Eosinophils are common in the lamina propria throughout the digestive tract.

Macrophages are found mainly beneath the basement membrane in the upper reaches of the villi. In addition to roles in innate immunity, they are thought to engulf particulate antigens and to ingest soluble antigens before presenting them to T lymphocytes.

Mast cells are seen mainly in the crypt region.

Fig. 11.41 Endocrine Cell. (a) H&E micrograph of the base of a small intestinal crypt showing a typical pale-staining enteroendocrine cell (E). In this thin acrylic resin section, the Paneth cell (P) granules are difficult to see. **(b)** Small bowel mucosa immunostained to show endocrine cells secreting motilin *(brown)*, a gut hormone that stimulates peristalsis after a meal. These motilin-producing gut endocrine cells have been termed *Mo-cells*. (Image used under Creative Commons License https://creativecommons.org/licenses/by-sa/3.0/ from the Human Protein Atlas. Antibody to motilin HPA069392 https://www.proteinatlas.org/ENSG00000096395-MLN/tissue/duodenum#img.)

> **The submucosa of the small bowel contains vessels, lymphoid tissue and nerves.**

The small intestinal submucosa contains lymphatics, blood vessels and the submucosal plexus of nerves and ganglion cells. In addition, it contains part of the larger lymphoid aggregates of the GALT, which cross the muscularis mucosae.

In the first part of the duodenum, the submucosa contains mucus-secreting Brunner's glands.

⟫ KEY FACTS

Small Bowel

- Characterized by a mucosa raised into finger-like villi which contain abundant blood vessels and lymphatics
- Lined by columnar epithelium with goblet cells
- Glycocalyx of surface epithelium has enzymes, for example, lactase and alkaline phosphatase
- Duodenum is associated with submucosal mucous glands (Brunner's glands)
- Contains mucosal endocrine cells which secrete gut hormones
- Has two layers of muscularis propria separated by a myenteric nerve plexus

> **The small intestine has regional specializations in the duodenum, jejunum and ileum.**

The duodenum differs from the rest of the small intestine as follows:

- It is entirely retroperitoneal.
- Its villous pattern contains a high proportion of leaf and ridge forms (see Fig. 11.37).
- It contains prominent mucus-secreting submucosal glands (Brunner's glands; Fig. 11.42), which penetrate and split the muscularis mucosae so that some acini are located within the lamina propria of the mucosa.
- It receives secretions of glands located outside the digestive tract through long ducts; these glands are the liver (see Chapter 12) and the exocrine component of the pancreas.

Brunner's glands are similar to the submucosal glands of the pyloric region of the stomach, being composed of mucous cells lining short ducts that open into the bases or sides of the crypts of the mucosa. Brunner's glands secrete an alkaline mucoid material (pH 8.0–9.5), which may protect the duodenal mucosa from the acid chyme, bringing its pH toward the level at which the pancreatic enzymes are most effective.

Brunner's glands are also thought to secrete urogastrone, a peptide that inhibits acid secretion by the stomach. Endocrine cells can be demonstrated in these glands immunocytochemically.

The **jejunum** is the main absorptive site of the digestive tract and shows not only the greatest development of plical folds (see Fig. 11.36a) but also the most complex villous system, with finger-like villi being predominant.

The **ileum** is characterized by the greatest development of GALT. The lymphoid cells aggregate into large nodules (Peyer's patches), which expand the lamina propria of the mucosa, split the muscularis mucosae and extend into the submucosa.

EXOCRINE PANCREAS

> **The exocrine pancreas is a glandular organ that secretes into the gut via a main duct system.**

The pancreas is a long, thin, tapering structure extending from its head, which occupies the space formed by the concavity of the duodenum, to its tail, which is situated in the left hypochondrium near the hilum of the spleen.

Fig. 11.42 Brunner's Glands. The first part of the duodenum is characterized by the presence of large, fluid-secreting mucous glands. **(a)** This low-power view shows duodenal mucosa with Brunner's glands (B) both below and above the layer of the muscularis mucosae (MM). **(b)** The glands open into the duodenal crypts (C). (Micrograph from digital pathology whole slide image provided by the University of Leeds Virtual Pathology Project https://www.virtualpathology.leeds.ac.uk. Reproduced with permission.)

The main pancreatic duct joins the distal end of the bile duct to open into the lumen of the duodenum at a small, raised mound, the **ampulla of Vater**.

The pancreas has a thin, ill-defined fibrocollagenous capsule, from which narrow irregular septae penetrate it, dividing it into lobules (Fig. 11.43a). Each lobule is composed of roughly spherical clusters (acini) of secretory exocrine cells (see Fig. 11.43b). Each acinus has an individual intra-acinar duct, which drains into progressively larger ducts (see Figs. 11.43c and 11.43d).

Fig. 11.43 Exocrine Pancreas. (a) This low-magnification micrograph shows the pancreas is composed of lobules of cells separated by septa containing adipose tissue (A). Towards the centre of each lobule is a large duct (D), which converge to form a main pancreatic duct. Just visible at this low power are pale-staining islets of Langerhans (I). The majority of the pancreas is composed of basophilic exocrine acini. **(b)** Acini are composed of pancreatic acinar cells (PA). These contain abundant rough endoplasmic reticulum reflected in basophilia in the basal cytoplasm adjacent to the nucleus. The pink-stained apical cytoplasm contains eosinophilic zymogen granules (Z) **(c)** Part of the ductular system with centroacinar cells (C) arising from the acini (A) as the intra-acinar component of the intercalated duct (ID). **(d)** Intercalated ducts lead into larger intralobular ducts (TD), which run in fine collagenous trabeculae within the lobules. These small ducts are lined by a cuboidal epithelium. Eventually, ducts converge to drain from each pancreatic lobule to form larger interlobular ducts, eventually forming the main pancreatic duct. (Micrograph from digital pathology whole slide image provided by the University of Leeds Virtual Pathology Project https://www.virtualpathology.leeds.ac.uk. Reproduced with permission.)

Pancreatic exocrine cells are protein-secreting cells.

The acini are composed of protein-secreting cells (pancreatic acinar cells), which have a broad base and narrow apical surface, covered by a few short microvilli.

The cells are rich in rough endoplasmic reticulum, which is concentrated mainly in the lower half of the cell and is responsible for their cytoplasmic basophilia. The upper half of the cell, close to the lumen, contains variable numbers of eosinophilic zymogen granules, which contain the pre-enzymes synthesized by the cell (see Fig. 11.43b). Some cells contain large numbers of these granules, whereas others, which contain few or none, are thought to have recently disgorged their granules by exocytosis into the acinar lumen. It is thought that the pre-enzymes are synthesized by the rough endoplasmic reticulum and then transferred to the Golgi, which packages them into granules.

The pancreatic acinar cells produce and secrete the precursors of a wide range of enzymes.

The secretions of pancreatic exocrine cells are involved in the breakdown of food in the lumen of the duodenum and include proteolytic enzymes (particularly trypsinogen, chymotrypsinogen, procarboxypeptidases A and B and proelastase) and lipolytic enzymes (pro-phospholipase and pro-lipase). The pancreas also secretes amylase, cholesterol esterase and ribonucleases.

Activation of the proenzymes occurs only in the duodenal cavity, with the conversion of trypsinogen to active trypsin by an enterokinase located in the duodenal brush border triggering a cascade of reactions in which the inactive precursors are converted to active enzymes.

Pancreatic secretion is alkaline owing to the selective secretion of bicarbonate ions, which is thought to be performed by the ductular system rather than by the acinar cells.

The control of pancreatic exocrine secretion is regulated by both hormonal and neural mechanisms. Interaction of receptors on acinar cells with hormones (termed *secretagogues*) activates secondary messenger systems and stimulates secretion. Secretagogues include secretin and VIP. Serotonin and cholecystokinin (CCK) stimulate vagal cholinergic pathways and stimulate pancreatic secretion.

> **Pancreatic secretions run in a ramified ductal system which merges into a main pancreatic duct.**

The pancreatic ductal system begins in the acinus. Pale-staining centroacinar cells represent the intra-acinar component of the intercalated duct, are lined by a simple monolayer of cuboidal epithelium and form a complex network which links to intercalated ducts (see Fig. 11.43c).

The intercalated ducts from individual acini fuse to form larger intralobular ducts that in turn drain into interlobular ducts which run in the fibrocollagenous septa between the pancreatic lobules and are lined by columnar epithelium.

Interlobular ducts join the main pancreatic ducts, which run longitudinally from the tail of the pancreas to its head and empty into the duodenal lumen at the ampulla of Vater. The main pancreatic ducts are lined by tall columnar epithelium containing a number of mucin-secreting goblet cells.

LARGE INTESTINE

> **The large intestine modifies the fluid content of faeces as it passes for elimination.**

The large intestine comprises the:
- Caecum
- Ascending, transverse and descending colons
- Sigmoid colon
- Rectum

The structure of the large intestine is fairly constant throughout, although there are regional variations, particularly between the caecum and the rectum.

The main function of the large intestine is to convert the liquid small intestinal contents to solid indigestible waste material: faeces. This is achieved by extensive reabsorption of water and soluble salts from the bowel content until it is semisolid. With increasing solidity, mucin is required to lubricate its passage along the bowel. The **appendix** is a small appendage arising from the caecum.

> **The large intestinal epithelium is specialized for mucus secretion and salt and water absorption.**

The epithelial component of the mucosa of the large bowel is a mixture of absorptive cells and mucous cells. These are arranged as simple, straight, nonbranching tubular downgrowths extending from the surface to the muscularis mucosae. The cell types present are columnar cells, mucous cells, stem cells and endocrine cells (Fig. 11.44). Around the epithelial crypts is a layer of myofibroblasts forming the pericryptal sheath (see Fig. 5.15), which has roles in homeostasis of the mucosa.

Other epithelial cells are found adjacent to the lymphoid aggregates in the lamina propria and are tightly packed cuboidal or columnar epithelial cells, which have a relatively high nucleus-to-cytoplasm ratio and do not contain mucin. These cells are similar to the M cells associated with the lymphoid tissue in the small intestine.

Columnar cells are the most numerous type of epithelial cell in the large intestine. They are narrow, slender cells and appear to be in a minority because they are compressed between the much larger mucous (goblet) cells. Their luminal surfaces have a microvillus brush border, and there is evidence that they can produce and secrete a neutral polysaccharide, possibly glycocalyx material.

Columnar cells carry out the salt and water absorptive function of the colon. They lack brush border enzymes and so play no part in digestive breakdown, but have prominent lateral intercellular spaces, which suggests active fluid transport. Furthermore, they are well equipped with Na^+ and K^+ ATPases in the lateral cell membranes.

Mucous cells possess large numbers of mucin granules, which produce the bulging, rounded, cytoplasm responsible for their synonym: **goblet cells**. The mucin vacuoles are larger in the sigmoid colon and rectum than in the caecum and ascending colon, and there appears to be a difference in the type of mucin secreted. Mucin from the colon and rectum is highly sulphated; that from the caecum and ascending colon is less sulphated and contains sialic acid radicals.

As the goblet cells approach the surface of the large intestine, they begin to discharge their mucus and continue to migrate upwards to form part of the surface epithelium, which is mainly composed of columnar cells.

> **Stem cells are the precursors of other cell types.**

Stem cells form all of the specialized cells of the large bowel mucosa. They are located at the bases of the tubular glands and can develop into either mucous or columnar cells or into large intestinal endocrine cells.

Although the main function of the stem cells is to maintain the cell populations of the colonic tubular glands during normal wear and tear and cell turnover, they are also vital in the rapid replacement of cells damaged by disease.

Fig. 11.44 Large Intestine. (a) Micrograph showing large intestine mucosa. The surface is flat and simple, straight tubular glands (TG) extend down to the muscularis mucosae (MM). **(b)** The glands are lined by two populations of cells, the most numerous but less obvious being compressed tall columnar cells (C). The more easily seen cells are the mucous cells (mucus-secreting goblet cells, G), here stained *blue* by Alcian blue. **(c)** High-power micrograph showing both columnar cells (C) and goblet cells (G) in the upper part of the tubular gland, whereas the surface cells (S) are mainly columnar and contain little mucin. **(d)** At the bases of the glands, the cell population is a combination of uncommitted stem cells (S), goblet cells (G), columnar cells (C) and occasional small pale-staining endocrine cells (E).

CLINICAL EXAMPLE

When only the epithelial cells of the colonic tubular glands are destroyed in disease, the stem cells restock them, and the appearance of the glands is restored as straight tubular glands. When the damage is more severe and persistent, with destruction of the support cell and stromal architecture of the lamina propria supporting the glands, the stem cells produce new epithelial cells, but the glands so formed are architecturally distorted, often being short and branched instead of a long, straight tube. In addition, the proportions of the various cell types in the regenerated glands may be abnormal, a reduction in the number of mucin-secreting goblet cells being the most common. Histological identification of these changes in a colonic biopsy is an indication of an episode of severe mucosal damage in the past, for example, in chronic ulcerative colitis (see p. 232).

Endocrine cells are comparatively few in number in the large bowel and are scattered among the other cells.

In the large bowel, endocrine cells are mainly in the lower half of each tubular downgrowth and have a broad base, narrowing to a small luminal surface covered with microvilli. Their neuroendocrine granules are situated basal to the nucleus and can sometimes be seen as small eosinophilic dots in H&E paraffin sections.

Immunocytochemical methods have shown that these cells contain a number of substances related to their endocrine function, including chromogranin, substance P, somatostatin and glucagon.

The large intestinal lamina propria consists of collagen, reticulin and fibroblasts embedded in a glycosaminoglycan matrix.

There is a very thin layer of compact collagen immediately beneath the basement membrane of the surface epithelium.

The cell content of the lamina propria includes lymphocytes and scattered eosinophils, the lymphocytes being mainly T cells. Also present are small lymphoid follicles (part of the GALT, see p. 155), the larger of which breach the muscularis mucosae and extend into the submucosa. Cells containing PAS-positive granules, known as *muciphages,* are a common finding, particularly in the rectum.

The muscularis mucosae consists of a two-layered smooth muscle arrangement.

The muscularis mucosae of the large bowel has an inner circular and an outer longitudinal layer, but this distinction is usually only clear in abnormally thickened muscle layers. Elastic fibres are also present.

The muscularis mucosae is penetrated by fine nerve twigs from the submucosal plexus, with these nerves continuing vertically into the lamina propria. The innervation of the colon is particularly important in the diagnosis of Hirschsprung's disease (see Fig. 11.47).

The muscularis propria is responsible for the main propulsive forces in the bowel wall.

The muscularis propria of the large intestine consists of an inner circular muscle layer and an outer longitudinal layer, which is not continuous, being concentrated into three bands: the taeniae coli. These muscle layers are responsible for propulsion of the gut contents by peristalsis.

▶▶ KEY FACTS

Large Bowel

- Mucosa specialized for water and salt absorption and mucus secretion.
- Mucosa characterized by long straight tubular glands of columnar epithelium containing goblet cells and absorptive cells.
- Two layers to muscularis propria with intervening myenteric nerve plexus. Outer longitudinal muscle arranged as narrow bands (taeniae coli).

APPENDIX

The appendix has the same basic structure as the large bowel.

The appendix is a small, blind-ending tubular diverticulum arising from the caecum. It is normally 5–10 cm-long and about 0.8 cm in diameter. Both measurements vary from person to person, but its diameter decreases with increasing age, being at its greatest at 7–20 years of age.

The wall of the appendix is composed of a muscularis propria, which has an outer longitudinal and an inner circular component

like the rest of the digestive tract. The submucosa contains blood vessels, nerves and variable amounts of lymphoid tissue.

In children, the lamina propria and the submucosa contain abundant lymphoid tissue with prominent follicle formation (Fig. 11.45a). This is not present at birth, but progressively populates the appendix over the first 10 years of life, thereafter progressively disappearing, so that the normal adult appendix shows only traces of this tissue (Fig. 11.45b).

As the lymphoid tissue atrophies in the adult, the submucosa becomes progressively more collagenous, and in the elderly, the mucosa itself may become more fibrotic, particularly near the tip.

(a)

(b)

Fig. 11.45 Appendix. (a) Transverse section of the appendix from a 10-year-old child. It is lined by large-bowel-type mucosa (M), in which there are large lymphoid follicles (F) extending into the submucosa (SM). (b) Transverse section of the appendix from a 36-year-old man at the same magnification as in (a). Note the relative reduction in size and the virtual disappearance of the lymphoid follicles (F). Mucosa (M); submucosa (SM).

CLINICAL EXAMPLE

In children, the abundant lymphoid tissue in the appendix can increase in bulk in response to a transient generalized viral infection or infection localized to the bowel and cause obstruction of the appendix. The lumen may also become blocked off by inspissated faecal material, which can solidify to become hard (a faecolith). Obstruction of the drainage of the distal part of the appendix causes stasis of the secretions in the blocked-off distal end and predisposes to bacterial infection. This is the basis of the common surgical emergency in children of acute appendicitis.

The mucosal epithelium of the appendix is colonic in nature.

The mucosa of the appendix is composed of straight tubular glands containing tall, columnar absorptive cells, mucin-secreting goblet cells and some enteroendocrine cells, which are mainly found in the bases of the glands. Enteroendocrine cells are also found in the submucosa, closely related to nerves and ganglion cells, particularly near the closed tip of the appendix.

CLINICAL EXAMPLE

Disorders of the Large Bowel

The colon and rectum are subject to a number of disorders, many of which are transient and the result of dietary indiscretion, for example, after the ingestion of large quantities of beer! The three most important diseases of long duration in adults are:
- **Cancer** of the large bowel epithelium (adenocarcinoma)
- **Benign polyps** of the bowel epithelium (adenomas)
- **Diverticular disease,** in which increased pressure in the bowel lumen forces mucosa through the muscle layers
- **Ulcerative colitis**, which is a severe ulcerating disease of the colonic mucosa

Ulcerative Colitis

The cause of ulcerative colitis is not known, but large bowel mucosa is lost over an extensive area, with ulceration and destruction of the absorptive epithelium (Fig. 11.46).

This mucosal damage impairs water resorption from the colonic contents, and thus the normal solid faeces are replaced by large quantities of watery diarrhoea, which is similar in content and texture to the contents of the ileum. Destruction of the mucosa also leads to bleeding, so the watery diarrhoea is often mixed with blood.

Hirschsprung's Disease

In infants and children, the most important disease of the large bowel is **Hirschsprung's disease,** in which defecation is not possible because a segment of the lower rectum is completely devoid of ganglion cells in the submucosa and muscularis layers. Normal innervation is described on page 217 and illustrated in Fig. 11.27.

The affected segment of bowel is narrowed, and the child's abdomen distends with unpassed faeces, with fatal perforation occurring if it is not treated.

Although the abnormality primarily affects the lower rectum, the aganglionic segment may be extensive, involving much of the distal colon.

Diagnosis is confirmed by rectal biopsy, establishing that submucosal ganglion cells are absent. A characteristic feature is hypertrophy of preganglionic nerve twigs in the muscularis mucosae, submucosa and lamina propria (Fig. 11.47).

Fig. 11.46 Ulcerative Colitis. Micrograph of wall of sigmoid colon from a patient with ulcerative colitis. Note the complete destruction of the mucosa and some submucosa (SM) with infiltration of inflammatory cells (small blue cells). Only a few scattered remnants of absorptive and mucus-secreting epithelium remain *(arrow)*.

Fig. 11.47 Hirschsprung's Disease. Micrograph showing prominent nerve twigs in the lamina propria (LP), muscularis mucosae (MM) and submucosa (SM). This rectal biopsy from a child with Hirschsprung's disease has been stained by the cholinesterase enzyme histochemical technique.

For online review questions, please visit https://studentconsult.inkling.com.

Liver

INTRODUCTION

The liver acts as a vast biosynthetic chemical factory, synthesizing large complex molecules from substances brought to it in the blood, particularly substances recently absorbed by the intestine and transported by a portal blood system.

> The liver has a wide range of functions, which accounts for its complex structure.

All of the biochemical functions of the liver are carried out by the epithelial parenchymal cells of the liver, the hepatocytes, and are dependent on close interrelationships between:
- The vasculature (hepatic artery and portal vein branches, sinusoids and central veins)
- The hepatocytes
- The bile drainage systems (the canaliculi and intrahepatic bile ducts; Fig. 12.1).

Bile synthesis and secretion. The liver produces bile, an alkaline secretion containing water, ions, phospholipids, bile pigments (mainly bilirubin glucuronide) and bile acids (glycocholic and taurocholic).

Excretion of bilirubin. Bilirubin is produced in the spleen from the breakdown of the haem component of haemoglobin. In the liver the bilirubin is conjugated with glucuronic acid, and the conjugate (bilirubin glucuronide) is excreted in the bile and thence the faeces.

Protein metabolism. The liver is centrally involved in protein metabolism. It brings about deamination of amino acids; it produces urea from circulating ammonia; it also interconverts amino acids and produces the so-called *nonessential amino acids*. The liver synthesizes many proteins, including most of the plasma proteins such as albumin, and blood clotting factors, such as fibrinogen and prothrombin.

The profile of proteins secreted by the liver can be influenced by cytokines circulating in the blood. In patients with inflammatory disorders, circulating cytokines can increase the concentration of several liver-produced proteins in the blood, such as fibrinogen, transferrin and serum-amyloid A protein. The production of some other proteins is downregulated, for example, albumin. This is called an *acute-phase response*.

Carbohydrate metabolism. Lipids and amino acids are converted into glucose in the liver by gluconeogenesis. The liver makes and stores glycogen and forms intermediary compounds in carbohydrate metabolism.

Lipid metabolism. The liver is involved in the synthesis of cholesterol, lipoproteins and phospholipids. It synthesizes fat from other precursors. It also oxidizes fatty acids to provide energy.

Storage. The liver acts as a store for vitamins A, D and B_{12}. It stores iron as ferritin.

Conjugation and elimination of metabolites and toxins. The smooth endoplasmic reticulum of the liver possesses large numbers of enzymes that break down or conjugate metabolites or toxic substances (e.g. alcohol and barbiturates). Certain hormones are eliminated by the liver.

LIVER VASCULATURE

> The liver receives blood from two vessels: the hepatic artery and the hepatic portal vein.

The liver receives blood from two sources:
- The hepatic artery perfuses the liver with oxygenated blood from the coeliac axis branches of the aorta.
- The hepatic portal vein carries blood from the digestive tract and spleen to the liver, the blood from the digestive tract being rich in amino acids, lipids and carbohydrates absorbed from the bowel and that from the spleen being rich in haemoglobin breakdown products.

In the liver, the two input circulations (hepatic artery and hepatic portal vein) discharge their blood into a common network of anastomosing small vascular channels, the sinusoids (Fig. 12.2). The terminal parts of the hepatic portal and arterial systems run together in a connective tissue framework called **portal tracts,** which also contain bile ductules.

After entering the liver at the porta hepatis, the portal vein divides within the liver into progressively smaller branches (interlobar, segmental and interlobular branches), which then branch further, eventually forming an extensive anastomosing network of terminal portal venules. Lateral side branches (inlet venules) of the terminal portal venules empty blood into the sinusoids, where it blends with blood from the terminal hepatic artery branches.

The hepatic artery divides into successively smaller branches, with the terminal elements running with the terminal branches of the hepatic portal vein before emptying into the hepatic sinusoids by short side branches (the arteriosinusoidal branches). A peribiliary plexus of small arterial branches supplies oxygenated blood into the large intrahepatic bile ducts before draining into the sinusoids, where it blends with blood from the portal venous system.

Fig. 12.1 Architecture of the Liver. (a) Hepatocytes (liver cells) are arranged as interconnecting sheets of cells that surround sinusoids containing blood supplied by small side branches of the hepatic artery and portal vein. Sinusoidal blood drains into a central terminal hepatic venule, each of which empties into an intercalated (sublobular) vein. Bile produced by hepatocytes enters narrow canaliculi, which drain into small bile ducts running with the hepatic artery and portal vein branches. Larger bile ducts and branches of the hepatic artery and portal vein are surrounded by collagenous tissue to form portal tracts. **(b)** Portal tracts contain a small bile duct (BD), a terminal branch of the hepatic artery (HA) and a component of the distal part of the hepatic portal venous system (PV). All are contained within a fibrocollagenous supporting stroma. Surrounding the portal tract are hepatocytes arranged in sheets.

Fig. 12.2 Hepatic Microcirculation. Blood from the terminal branches of the hepatic artery and the portal vein enters the sinusoidal system via small side branches, the arteriosinusoidal branch and inlet venule, respectively. It then passes along the sinusoid lumina toward the terminal hepatic venule (central vein). Although highly simplified here, in reality, the sinusoidal system is an interconnecting system of capillary-like channels in close contact with the functioning liver cells (hepatocytes).

The sinusoids are surrounded on all sides by hepatocytes. In this way, blood flowing through the liver is exposed to a massive surface area of liver cells.

> **Hepatic sinusoids are the highly specialized liver capillary equivalents.**

The hepatic sinusoids permeate the whole of the liver. They are lined by a thin, discontinuous, highly fenestrated endothelium, which is closely related externally to plates and cords of hepatocytes (Fig. 12.3), albeit separated from them by a space. This perisinusoidal space of Disse is the main site where material is transferred between the blood-filled sinusoids and hepatocytes. This transfer is in both directions, with some material being taken up by hepatocytes in addition to being secreted.

The hepatic sinusoids are partly lined by phagocytic cells (**Küpffer cells**), which are a form of macrophage and are derived from circulating blood monocytes.

> **Stellate cells are mesenchymal cells with functional roles in vitamin A storage, liver cell regeneration and collagen production in disease states.**

Within the perisinusoidal space is a population of small cells with scant cytoplasm called *hepatic stellate cells* (formerly called *perisinusoidal cells* and *Ito cells*). These represent around 5% of the total liver cell population. In conventional histological

Fig. 12.3 Hepatic Sinusoids. (a) High-power H&E micrograph showing the relationship between the sinusoidal channels (S) and the plates of cuboidal hepatocytes (H). Note the terminal hepatic venule (V). **(b)** Micrograph of liver stained to demonstrate reticulin fibres *(black)*, which run in the space of Disse between the hepatocyte surface and the endothelial cells lining the sinusoid (see also Figs. 12.6c and 12.6d). This method delineates the outline of the sinusoid (S) and the hepatocyte columns (H) and is used in the histological diagnosis of liver disease on small cores of liver tissue obtained by needle biopsy (see Fig. 1.1). **(c)** Immunohistochemical staining of liver for VAP-1 *(brown)*, which is a marker for hepatic endothelial cells and shows them lining the sinusoids in-between the blue-stained plates of liver cells. **(d)** Immunostaining of liver for CD68 *(brown)*, a macrophage marker showing the distribution of Küpffer cells in relation to hepatic sinusoids (Images (c) and (d) used under Creative Commons License. https://creativecommons.org/licenses/by-sa/3.0/. From the Human Protein Atlas (c) Antibody to amine oxidase copper containing 3 HPA000980. https://www.proteinatlas.org/ENSG00000131471-AOC3/tissue/liver#img. (d) Antibody to CD68 HPA054158. https://www.proteinatlas.org/ENSG00000129226-CD68/tissue/liver#img.)

Fig. 12.4 Hepatic Stellate Cells. Hepatic stellate cells can be stained using immunohistochemical techniques and are not easily seen on routine histology. This image shows smooth muscle actin (alpha-SMA) immunostaining of liver in which stellate cells are seen as linear, brown-stained structures adjacent to sinusoids and hepatocytes. (Image used under Creative Commons License. https://creativecommons.org/licenses/by-sa/3.0/. From the Human Protein Atlas. Antibody to smooth muscle actin HPA041264. https://www.proteinatlas.org/ENSG00000107796-ACTA2/tissue/liver#img.)

preparations they are hard to see and are best identified using special staining with immunohistochemical methods (Fig. 12.4).

Stellate cells are located between the lateral surface of hepatocytes and the sinusoidal endothelial cells with an elongated spindle and multiprocessed ramified shape. Cell processes bear protrusions termed *spines,* which have a functional role as chemosensing structures. A characteristic feature of stellate cells is the presence of cytoplasmic lipid vacuoles at the site of intracellular storage of vitamin A.

Stellate cells have several roles, including acting as support cells in the developing liver, acting as support cells for hepatocytes, in liver cell regeneration and as an immunomodulator regulating local inflammatory responses.

In response to liver damage stellate cells can transform to a myofibroblast-like cell with contractile and collagen-secreting properties. In these circumstances stellate cells become activated by cytokines and change their morphology to develop more cytoplasm along with expression of alpha smooth muscle actin. Stellate cells are understood to be responsible for the production of collagen in the process of fibrous scarring in the liver (see Fig. 12.9).

> **Blood leaving the sinusoids enters the central venules of the liver lobules.**

Blood which has passed through the functioning liver parenchyma enters terminal hepatic venules (central veins of the lobules; discussed later on p. 240), which in turn unite to form intercalated veins; these then fuse to form larger hepatic vein branches. Hepatic veins are devoid of valves and open separately into the inferior vena cava.

> **Lymphatic fluid drains from the liver to the thoracic duct.**

The liver produces a large volume of lymph. Fluid drains from the space of Disse into the portal tracts, in which it travels in fine channels. These lymphatic channels increase in size as portal tracts merge toward the hepatic hilum. Finally, lymph drains into the thoracic duct. Such is the extent of lymph production by the liver that it comprises about half of the total lymph flow in the body under resting conditions.

HEPATOCYTES

> **The main functional cell of the liver is the hepatocyte.**

Hepatocytes (liver cells), which are intimately associated with the network of blood vessels (sinusoids), are polarized polyhedral cells with three identifiable types of surfaces (see later). As would be expected in cells that are so metabolically active, their cytoplasm is packed with a wide range of organelles.

The nuclei are large, spherical and central and contain scattered clumps of chromatin and prominent nucleoli. Many cells are binucleate, and nuclei are frequently polyploid; progressively more tetraploid nuclei develop with age.

The Golgi is either large and active or small and multiple and is mainly seen near the nucleus, with an extension lying close to the canalicular surface.

There are numerous free ribosomes in the cytosol, along with large glycogen deposits and some lipid droplets, the glycogen being closely related to the smooth endoplasmic reticulum.

Lysosomes (see p. 31) of various sizes are numerous, some containing lipofuscin and lamellated lipoprotein. They are particularly large and numerous near the canalicular surface.

Peroxisomes (see p. 33) usually number 200–300 per cell.

Mitochondria are abundant, numbering more than 1000 per cell, and scattered randomly. This vast mitochondrial component gives the hepatocyte cytoplasm its eosinophilic granular appearance in haematoxylin and eosin (H&E)–stained sections.

> **Hepatocytes have three important surfaces.**

The hepatocyte surfaces are important because they are involved in the transfer of substances between hepatocyte, blood vessels and bile canaliculi.

The three types of surfaces are sinusoidal, canalicular and intercellular (Figs. 12.5 and 12.6).

> **Sinusoidal surfaces are separated from the sinusoidal vessel by the space of Disse.**

Sinusoidal surfaces account for approximately 70% of the total hepatocyte surface. They are covered by short microvilli, which protrude into the space of Disse. Between the bases of the microvilli are coated pits (see Fig. 2.5), which are involved in endocytosis.

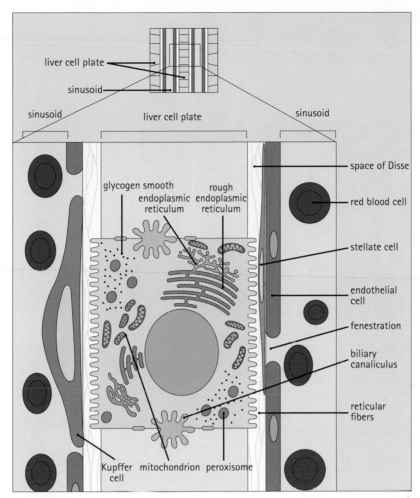

Fig. 12.5 Hepatocyte. Hepatocytes are epithelial cells linked together by epithelial junctions. They have three types of cell surfaces, but in this two-dimensional diagram, only two of the three hepatocyte surfaces are shown: one that faces the sinusoid with a microvillar surface and one that forms a biliary canaliculus. Each hepatocyte contains abundant rough endoplasmic reticulum and smooth endoplasmic reticulum, reflecting biosynthetic roles. Mitochondria and peroxisomes are numerous. Glycogen is stored within the cytosol. The space of Disse separates the hepatocytes from a discontinuous layer of endothelial cells lining the sinusoids. Phagocytic Küpffer cells also line the sinusoids. Stellate cells are also located adjacent to the space of Disse.

The sinusoidal surface is the site where material is transferred between the sinusoids and the hepatocyte.

> **Canalicular surfaces are the surfaces across which bile drains from the hepatocytes into the canaliculi.**

These account for approximately 15% of the hepatocyte surface and are closely apposed, except at the site of a canaliculus, which is a tube formed by the exact opposition of two shallow gutters on the surface of adjacent hepatocytes.

Canaliculi are about 0.5–2.5 μm in diameter, being smaller close to the terminal hepatic venule, and are lined by irregular microvilli arising from the canalicular surfaces of the hepatocytes.

Hepatocyte cytoplasm close to the canaliculi is rich in actin filaments, which are possibly capable of influencing the diameter of the canaliculus and thus the rate of flow.

The cell membrane around the canalicular lumen is rich in alkaline phosphatase and adenosine triphosphatase, and the canalicular lumen is isolated from the rest of the canalicular surface by junctional complexes (Fig. 12.7b).

> **The intercellular surfaces are the surfaces between adjacent hepatocytes that are not in contact with sinusoids or canaliculi.**

Intercellular surfaces account for about 15% of the hepatocyte surface. They are comparatively simple but specialized for cell attachment and cell-to-cell communication via communicating junctions (see Fig. 3.7).

Fig. 12.6 Hepatocyte. (a) Micrograph of a thin H&E section of liver showing hepatocytes which are roughly cuboidal and stacked into regular plates of cells. The have a pale granular eosinophilic cytoplasm corresponding to prominent cell organelles with much of the pallor being caused by the presence of glycogen. The nuclei are central with a distinct nuclear membrane and prominent nucleoli. One binucleate hepatocyte can be seen *(bottom left)*. Some of the hepatocyte surface lines the sinusoidal channel (i.e. sinusoidal surface, SS), whereas other surfaces are in contact with adjacent hepatocyte (i.e. intercellular surfaces, ICS), and some of the adjacent hepatocyte surfaces have bile canaliculi running between them. Details of the canaliculi cannot be distinguished on routine staining (see Fig. 12.7). **(b)** Low-power electron micrograph showing some of the cytoplasm of two adjacent hepatocytes (H), joined by their canalicular surfaces (CS) in which a bile canaliculus (BC) can be seen. The other surfaces of the hepatocyte are the sinusoidal surfaces (SS) bordering the sinusoid lumen (S). The space between the hepatocyte surface and the sinusoid is the space of Disse (SD). **(c)** Medium-power electron micrograph showing the space of Disse (SD) between the sinusoidal surface of the hepatocyte (H) and the endothelial cell (E) lining the sinusoid. A number of irregular microvilli (MV) protrude into the space of Disse from the hepatocyte surface. The microvilli are much less regular in humans than in rodents. Some of the support fibres of the reticulin network (R) can be seen. **(d)** The space of Disse lying between the hepatocyte and the discontinuous endothelium lining the sinusoid. The space contains microvillus processes from the hepatocyte surface and collagenous reticulin fibres, which form a supportive mesh.

Fig. 12.7 Bile Canaliculi. (a) Micrograph showing bile canaliculi highlighted by immunostaining for CEA, which shows the canaliculi as brown lines or dots, depending on whether they have been sectioned longitudinally or transversely. The nuclei and outlines of hepatocytes (H) can be seen, as can an occasional sinusoid (S). **(b)** Electron micrograph of the canalicular surface of two apposed hepatocytes. Note the canaliculus (C) filled with microvilli and the junctional complexes (JC) separating the canalicular lumen from the rest of the apposed hepatocyte.

⯈ **KEY FACTS**

Hepatocytes

- Metabolically highly active and rich in cytoplasmic organelles
- High energy requirement with numerous mitochondria
- Much of the cell surface is related to sinusoids, where exchange of materials with blood takes place
- Part of the surface is in contact with bile canaliculi, where bile excreted from hepatocytes enters the biliary drainage system

Hepatocyte Stem Cells and Liver Regeneration

The ability of the liver to regenerate itself has made it the prototype for mammalian organ regeneration. There are two main forms of regeneration in response to different types of liver injury. The main cells involved are mature, normally non-dividing adult hepatocytes that can proliferate and regenerate the liver, as seen after the majority of liver injuries caused by drugs, toxins, surgical resection or acute viral diseases. The second tier of reserve lies in a progenitor cell population, activated when injury is severe or when the mature hepatocytes can no longer regenerate the liver because of senescence. Studies of liver resections in humans have demonstrated restoration of the residual liver size in 3–6 months.

FUNCTIONAL ORGANIZATION OF HEPATOCYTES

Hepatocytes have different metabolic profiles depending on how close they are to portal tracts.

All hepatocytes are not equal, having different metabolic profiles depending on their distance from portal tracts.

Hepatocytes close to the portal tracts are exposed to blood that contains the highest oxygen concentration and contain enzymes involved in oxidative reactions. These cells make and store glycogen and produce and secrete proteins.

Hepatocytes farthest from the portal tracts – those adjacent to the central venules – are most distant from the oxygenated arterial blood supply. These hepatocytes have little capacity for oxidative activities and contain many esterases, being involved in conjugating and detoxifying reactions.

Hepatocytes in-between these extremes have intermediate metabolic properties.

These different metabolic profiles partly explain why different sets of hepatocytes are susceptible to different disease processes, especially responses to certain toxins.

The microanatomy of the liver has been described in two ways, termed the *lobular* and *acinar* concepts, respectively.

The liver can be functionally divided into structures termed *lobules*.

The components of the liver (i.e. the hepatocytes, terminal hepatic venules, portal triads and sinusoids) are arranged in a fairly constant pattern, which has been described as lobular (Fig. 12.8). The classic lobule is a roughly hexagonal structure in cross-section, being composed of:

- A central terminal hepatic venule, into which drains a converging series of sinusoidal channels like the spokes of a bicycle wheel
- Interconnecting plates of hepatocytes which surround sinusoidal channels and run between the central terminal hepatic venule and the periphery of the lobule
- Peripherally arranged portal tracts, each containing terminal branches of the hepatic artery and portal vein and a small tributary of the bile duct

Thus a ring of portal tracts forms the outer limit of each classic lobule.

The channels within each portal tract are surrounded by a small amount of fibrocollagenous tissue, and in some animals, particularly the pig, fibrocollagenous septa extend from one portal triad to another, clearly outlining the limits of each lobule. In humans, however, these fibrous septa are absent and so the lobule is less clearly defined.

In the lobule, three main zones of hepatocytes are identified, termed *centrilobular*, *periportal* and *mid-zones*. Most of the nomenclature used in the descriptions of disease processes (e.g. centrilobular necrosis) is based on the lobular concept.

Fig. 12.8 Hepatic Architecture: Lobule and acinus. (a) The architecture of the liver and the relationship between the vessels and ducts in the portal tract, the sinusoids and the central veins. The lobular *(orange)* and acinar *(green)* concepts are overdrawn. **(b)** Low-power micrograph showing the general liver architecture. Note the central terminal hepatic venules (CV), portal tracts (PT) and interconnecting cords of hepatocytes. The concepts of the hepatic lobule (L) and hepatic acinus (A), discussed below, are overdrawn.

The outer layer of periportal hepatocytes adjacent to the portal tract is called the *limiting plate;* it is the first group of hepatocytes to be damaged in inflammatory liver disorders that primarily involve the portal tracts.

> **The liver can also be functionally divided into structures called *acini*.**

The lobule concept has stood the test of time; however, it has also been proposed that the structure of the liver is best considered in terms of another structural unit, the acinus (see Fig. 12.8). The proposal is based on observations made on injection studies of the microcirculation of the liver; the acinus concept is based on the volume of liver receiving its blood supply from a single

terminal branch of the hepatic artery contained within a portal tract. In this structural unit, the periphery of the acinus is the central vein, whereas the centre is the portal tract. In the acinar model, hepatocytes are divided into three zones:

Zone I: Those hepatocytes closest to the portal tract, which synthesize glycogen and proteins

Zone II: Hepatocytes between zones I and III

Zone III: Those hepatocytes adjacent to the central venule, which contain esterases and conjugating enzymes

The lobular and acinar concepts are simply two different ways of looking at the structure of the liver. In humans, neither lobules nor acini have a clearly visible outline in histological sections.

Cirrhosis

Many slowly progressive diseases destroy hepatocytes and lead to distortion of liver architecture, particularly the relationships between the sinusoids, the portal venous system and the bile ducts.

Death of hepatocytes is followed by scarring, and although hepatocytes can regenerate and produce a new population of cells, their connections with the portal system and the biliary drainage are destroyed. This pattern of liver disorder, known as *cirrhosis* (Fig. 12.9), is a common cause of chronic liver failure.

Cirrhosis is characterized by:
• Continuing death of hepatocytes.
• Collapse of normal architecture.
• Increased production of fibrocollagenous tissue, leading to irregular scarring.

Fig. 12.9 Cirrhosis (Masson Trichrome Stain). Micrograph of cirrhotic liver. Note the fibrous scarring *(blue)*, which has distorted the normal architecture. There are nodules of regenerating liver cells, but their connections with the vascular supply and bile drainage system are cut off by the coarse bands of blue-stained scar.

• Attempted regeneration of surviving hepatocytes, which form irregular nodules and have abnormal relationships with the microvasculature and bile drainage system. Regenerating hepatocytes can continue some synthetic functions but eventually fail to keep pace with normal demands, and the symptoms of liver failure begin to develop.

Cirrhosis produces chronic liver failure and symptoms appear progressively over a period of some years, usually culminating fatally in coma or as a result of the complications of portal hypertension.

Portal Hypertension

In cirrhosis, the sinusoidal connections between the portal venous system and the draining central terminal hepatic venules and hepatic veins are blocked or destroyed.

Portal venous blood cannot therefore flow through its normal channels (i.e. through sinusoids into central terminal hepatic venules). Thus the blood pressure in the portal venous system increases considerably and causes portal hypertension.

One escape route for portal venous blood is via anastomoses with the systemic venous system; these are normally closed when portal pressure is low, but open when portal pressure rises.

When these anastomotic channels are distended with blood, they are called *varices*.

One of the sites of such an anastomosis is at the lower end of the oesophagus, which is unfortunate, as the distended submucosal blood vessels (oesophageal varices) bulge into the lumen of the oesophagus and are easily eroded by gastric acid, resulting in torrential haemorrhage.

Bleeding from oesophageal varices is a severe complication of portal hypertension and cirrhosis and may be fatal.

Cirrhosis and portal hypertension most commonly follow persisting hepatocyte destruction caused by alcohol toxicity, some forms of viral hepatitis and autoimmune liver disease.

INTRAHEPATIC BILIARY TREE

Bile produced by hepatocytes passes into bile canaliculi.

The bile canaliculi carry the bile back to the portal tracts (i.e. in the opposite direction to the blood).

As the canaliculi approach the bile ductules (Fig. 12.10a) in the portal tracts, they open into short passages lined by small cuboidal cells (the canals of Hering). From here, bile flows into the bile ductules in the portal tract.

Bile ductules anastomose freely and converge to form the bile ducts in the larger portal tracts (see Fig. 12.10b); these ducts in turn converge and link with others to form larger ducts, the *trabecular ducts* (see Fig. 12.10c).

Many of these ducts fuse to form large intrahepatic bile ducts, which converge near the liver hilum into the main hepatic ducts.

Bile formed in the liver is passed into the gut through the extrahepatic bile ducts.

The small tributaries of the intrahepatic biliary tree fuse to become increasingly larger channels, eventually fusing to become two large ducts: the right and left lobar bile ducts. These join at the hilum of the liver to form the common hepatic duct, which is the first part of the extrahepatic bile duct system.

About 3–4 cm after leaving the liver, the common hepatic duct receives the cystic duct (a small duct from the gallbladder) and becomes the common bile duct.

The common bile duct is about 6–7-cm long and opens into the duodenum at the ampulla of Vater, having passed through the head of the pancreas and combined with the pancreatic duct.

Fig. 12.10 Intrahepatic Bile Ducts. (a) Micrograph showing a small bile ductule in a small portal tract sectioned both along its length (L) and transversely (T). The ductule has a simple structure with low cuboidal epithelium and a narrow surrounding zone of collagen (C) and some smooth muscle fibres. **(b)** In larger portal tracts, small bile ducts (D) are larger than the ductules in the smaller portal tracts. It is common to see even smaller ducts (SD) in the same larger portal tract. A larger branch of the hepatic artery (A) and hepatic portal vein (V) run in the collagenous tissue of the portal tract. **(c)** Bile ducts converge to form larger duct structures progressing towards the hilum of the liver. This micrograph shows a trabecular duct (TD), which is significantly larger than a small bile duct, with a larger lumen and a lining of columnar epithelium. It is surrounded by dense fibrocollagenous tissue of the trabecular septum (TS) in which it runs.

> ⟫ **KEY FACTS**
>
> ### Biliary System
>
> - Bile is produced by hepatocytes from breakdown products of haemoglobin.
> - Bile passes from the canalicular surface of hepatocytes → bile canaliculi → bile ductules in portal tracts → trabecular ducts → intrahepatic bile ducts → lobar ducts → common hepatic duct.
> - Bile is concentrated in the gallbladder by extraction of water by absorptive epithelium, then stored, having passed through the head of the pancreas.

GALLBLADDER

Introduction

The gallbladder is an ovoid sac with a muscular wall and is capable of moderate distension. It concentrates and stores bile, receiving dilute watery bile from the common hepatic duct and emptying thick, concentrated, variably mucoid bile into the common bile duct.

Bile is transported into and out of the gallbladder through a short duct: the cystic duct. This duct contains a spirally arranged outgrowth of mucosa, which forms the spiral valve of Heister.

> **The gallbladder has a muscular wall.**

The gallbladder wall has a mucosa which comprises an absorptive epithelium resting on a highly vascular lamina propria. There is no muscularis mucosa. The muscle layer is normally thin and apparently haphazardly arranged but with a tendency to be circumferential. There is an outer dense fibrous layer, which is partly covered by peritoneal serosa, but partly loosely binds one aspect of the gallbladder to the underside of the liver (Fig. 12.11).

Fig. 12.11 Gallbladder Wall. The gallbladder receives bile from the liver through the common hepatic duct via the cystic duct. The bile is concentrated (by absorption of water) and stored in the gallbladder until required, when it is squirted out into the common bile duct by contraction of the gallbladder wall to eventually pass into the duodenum. The gallbladder has an internal lining of absorptive epithelial cells (E) (see Fig. 12.12), thrown into folds to increase the surface area for absorption. The lamina propria (LP) contains prominent blood vessels and a scattering of lymphocytes and plasma cells. The smooth muscle layers (M) are thin in a healthy gallbladder but become thickened if there is any obstruction to bile outflow (see Fig. 12.13b). There is an outer layer of compact fibrous tissue (F), which has a serosal (S) surface over part of the gallbladder surface. Where the gallbladder wall lies against the underside of the liver, this fibrous layer loosely merges with the fibrous tissue of the liver capsule, though they can be easily separated by blunt dissection during surgical removal of the gallbladder (cholecystectomy).

Fig. 12.12 Gallbladder. (a) Low-power micrograph of the gallbladder showing the mucosa (M) with its ridged mucosal folds, the submucosa (SM) and the muscular wall (MW). **(b)** High-power micrograph of gallbladder epithelium. The cells are tall and columnar with basal nuclei and a luminal surface bearing microvilli. The microvilli are discernible as a faint brush border (BB).

> **The gallbladder mucosa is covered by tall, columnar epithelial cells specialized for absorption.**

The lining cells have numerous microvilli on their luminal surfaces and complex interdigitations of their lateral walls (Fig. 12.12). These differently specialized surfaces are separated by junctional complexes (see Fig. 3.6).

Gallbladder epithelial cells are adapted for salt and water absorption and have abundant basal and apical mitochondria; Na^+ and K^+ transport ATPases in their lateral walls.

Na^+ and Cl^- ions are actively pumped from the cell cytoplasm into the lateral intercellular space to produce an osmotic gradient between it and the gallbladder lumen. Water is therefore drawn into the space from the lumen and then enters the abundant capillary network in the lamina propria.

This mechanism is similar to that employed by the proximal convoluted tubule epithelial cell in the kidney to absorb water and ions (see Chapter 15).

Gallbladder epithelium is thrown up into folds, or plicae, which flatten when the gallbladder is distended.

CLINICAL EXAMPLE

Gallstones

Gallstones (i.e. stones or calculi in the gallbladder or biliary tree) form when solid concretions of bile act as a nidus for calcium salt deposition. Small gallstones are often asymptomatic; larger gallstones can cause obstructive jaundice or inflammation of the gallbladder termed *cholecystitis*.

Obstructive Jaundice

Obstructive jaundice results from the blockage of a bile duct, for example, by a gallstone that has passed from the gallbladder and become impacted in the common bile duct on its way to the duodenum.

Blockage of the bile duct impedes the flow of bile into the duodenum. This results in:

- Damming of bile in the proximal biliary tree, intrahepatic bile ducts and eventually bile canaliculi
- Passage of retained canalicular bile into the hepatic sinusoids and thence into the bloodstream, producing jaundice

- Impaired intestinal breakdown of fat owing to lack of the emulsifying bile acids normally present in bile
- Pale faeces, the normal faecal colour being caused by the presence of bile and its breakdown products

Cholecystitis

Gallstones may become impacted in the cystic duct (Fig. 12.13a) and obstruct the flow of bile at this point. This has the following consequences, which are the basic features of so-called *chronic cholecystitis* (see Fig. 12.13b):

- The gallbladder contracts more strongly to try to overcome the obstruction, and consequently its musculature thickens.
- Resulting high pressure within the gallbladder lumen pushes pouches of mucosa into the muscle layers (Rokitansky–Aschoff sinuses).
- Stasis of bile within the gallbladder predisposes to infection, and episodes of pain and fever are common.

Fig. 12.13 Obstructive Biliary Disease. (a) A greatly enlarged gallbladder with a gallstone (GS) impacted in its neck, close to the cystic duct. Obstruction of bile drainage has led to bile stasis and consequent infection, producing red inflamed mucosa *(arrow).* **(b)** Micrograph of a chronically obstructed gallbladder. The muscle layer (M) is thickened by hypertrophy and a pouch of epithelium-lined mucosa (Rokitansky–Aschoff sinus, ARS) has bulged through it. Compare with Fig. 12.11.

CLINICAL EXAMPLE

Liver Failure

Liver disease can affect any of the liver's functions, although when large numbers of hepatocytes are damaged, all of the functions tend to be disturbed.

Failure of Synthetic Functions

The liver fails to produce important proteins, such as albumin and the various protein clotting factors.

The reduced synthesis of albumin leads to a reduced oncotic pressure of the blood, which results in oedema and accumulation of watery fluid in the peritoneal cavity (ascites).

Failure of clotting factor synthesis leads to spontaneous bleeding.

Failure of Detoxification Functions

The liver fails to convert metabolic waste products into innocuous substances. Toxic substances therefore circulate in the blood and cause a number of symptoms, including confusion, altered consciousness and eventually hepatic coma, which is rapidly fatal.

Failure of Bile Secretion

Failure of adequate bile secretion into the alimentary tract leads to retention of bile in the liver, with some of the components of the retained bile entering the blood and producing yellowing discolouration of the blood plasma and tissues (jaundice).

Chronic Hepatic Failure

If hepatocyte damage is slowly progressive, the abnormalities outlined earlier develop insidiously over a period of years. This is called *chronic hepatic failure* and is most commonly associated with cirrhosis (see Fig. 12.9).

Acute Hepatic Failure

If the liver disease is severe and of sudden onset, the metabolic abnormalities appear suddenly. This is acute hepatic failure and is most commonly associated with some acute virus infections (e.g. hepatitis B virus infection) or exposure to liver toxins (e.g. paracetamol/acetaminophen). In either case, acute hepatic failure results from the widespread death of liver cells.

CLINICAL EXAMPLE

Tumours of the Liver and Biliary Tree

The most common tumour to involve the liver is metastatic disease as a result of spread of tumour from another primary site. Tumours of the gastrointestinal system commonly spread by the portal venous system to the liver, for example, carcinoma of the colon or carcinoma of the stomach. Metastasis to the liver by bloodstream spread is also common from carcinoma of the lung and carcinoma of the breast.

Primary malignant tumours of the liver can be derived from hepatocytes (hepatocellular carcinomas). This type of tumour is predisposed by the presence of cirrhosis and by infection by hepatitis B or C virus.

Tumours derived from the biliary tree are uncommon. When they do occur, they are generally adenocarcinomas, as they are derived from the glandular epithelium that normally lines the biliary tract.

For online review questions, please visit https://studentconsult.inkling.com.

Musculoskeletal System

INTRODUCTION

The musculoskeletal system, which provides mechanical support and permits movement, is composed of skeletal muscle, tendons, bones, joints and ligaments.

Skeletal muscles act as contractile levers and are connected to bone by **tendons. Bones** act as rigid levers, articulating with other bones through **joints,** which are kept in relationship by **ligaments.**

A special characteristic of muscle, tendons and joints is the possession of a rich sensory nerve supply, which detects the position of the body and the velocity of movement. The integration of this sensory information by the central nervous system is vital for the musculoskeletal system to function normally.

The main functional attribute of bone is its specialized extracellular matrix, which is hardened by the deposition of calcium, enabling it to function as a rigid lever.

The rigid, hard character of bone belies its importance as a metabolic reservoir of mineral salts and the fact that it is in a constant state of dynamic remodelling.

SKELETAL MUSCLE

> **Skeletal muscle is responsible for voluntary movement.**

The histological characteristics of skeletal muscle cells and the structural basis of muscle contraction are described on pages 82-86.

Individual muscle cells are arranged into large groups to form anatomically distinct muscles. These are characterized by:

- An orderly alignment of the constituent cells to generate a directional force after contraction
- Anchorage to other structures by highly organized fibrocollagenous support tissues
- A rich blood supply reflecting high metabolic demands
- Innervation and control by specialized neurons (motor neurons) that terminate on muscle cells at specialized nerve endings (motor endplates)
- Incorporation of specially adapted skeletal muscle cells into structures called *spindles* to act as sensors of muscle stretch

> **Embryologically, muscle fibres develop from mesenchymal tissues.**

In embryogenesis, skeletal muscle develops from primitive mesenchymal tissues of the mesoderm. Small spindle-shaped or strap-shaped cells with a single nucleus and abundant pink-staining cytoplasm develop from primitive mesenchymal cells. These are skeletal muscle cell precursors, the rhabdomyoblasts (Fig. 13.1). Numerous individual rhabdomyoblasts then fuse to form multinucleate muscle fibres, with the cells enlarging in size when they become connected to the nervous system and receive motor stimulation. Cells that are differentiating into muscle express a transcription factor in the nuclei called *MyoD*, and immunostaining for this protein can be used in diagnosis to determine a muscle origin for a tissue sample.

Residual cells with the function of rhabdomyoblasts (i.e. capable of differentiating further into functional striated muscle cells) persist in adult skeletal muscle as **satellite cells** (see Fig. 13.6). After muscle damage and loss of fibres, these cells proliferate and may produce new muscle cells.

Fig. 13.1 Development of Skeletal Muscle. This photomicrograph shows elongated rhabdomyoblasts, with abundant pink-staining cytoplasm, developing in primitive mesenchyme in human embryonic tissue.

A muscle is composed of many muscle fibres.

A mature muscle fibre is composed of large numbers of myofibrils bounded by a cell membrane termed *the sarcolemma* (see p. 82 and Fig. 13.2).

Each skeletal muscle cell is typically extremely long (up to 10 cm in length), and it is therefore more usual to use the term *skeletal muscle fibre* rather than cell.

Many muscle fibres are arranged together to form a muscle (Fig. 13.3). Despite being elongated, individual muscle cells do not extend the full length of a muscle, but are arranged in overlapping bundles, with the force of contraction being transmitted through the arrangement of the support tissues.

Different muscles are characterized by different physiological and metabolic properties.

The physiological and metabolic properties of individual skeletal muscles are determined by differences in the structure of their constituent muscle fibres.

Fig. 13.2 Skeletal Muscle Fibres. (a) Micrograph of skeletal muscle fibres in a longitudinal section showing prominent cross-striations. The dark bands are termed *A bands* (anisotropic, i.e. birefringent in polarized light), and the light bands are termed *I bands* (isotropic, i.e. no interference with polarized light). These bands correspond to the arrangement of thick and thin filaments in myofibrils (see Fig. 5.2). Nuclei (N) appear as elongated structures just beneath the cell membrane, and each fibre contains many nuclei. **(b)** Micrograph of skeletal muscle fibres in a transverse frozen section showing roughly hexagonal profiles with flattened sides where they are compressed by adjacent fibres. Nuclei (N) appear as small circular profiles at the periphery of each fibre. Individual myofibrils are generally not identifiable by light microscopy.

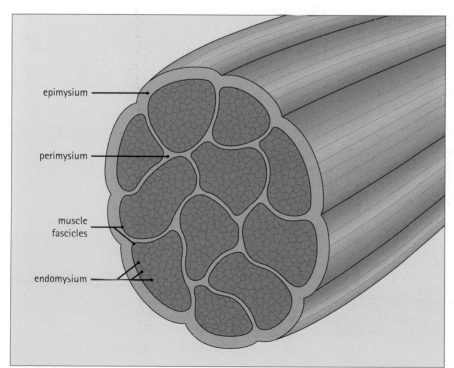

Fig. 13.3 Organization of Muscle Fibres Into Muscle. Individual muscle fibres are surrounded by endomysium, which is composed of sheets of external lamina identical to basement membrane (see p. 69). Endomysium secures the muscle fibres to each other and contains both capillary blood vessels and individual nerve axons (see Chapter 6). Clusters of muscle fibres are held together by fine sheets of fibrocollagenous support tissue (perimysium) to form fascicles. Blood vessels, lymphatic vessels and nerves run in the endomysial support tissues. An anatomically defined muscle is composed of many fascicles, which are surrounded externally by a thick layer of fibrocollagenous support tissue, the epimysium.

In both animals and humans, it has been possible to define several subtypes of muscle fibres by macroscopic, physiological, biochemical and histochemical criteria, but there are marked interspecies variations.

Histochemical staining for specific enzymes delineates several types of fibres and is a useful method for analysing muscle. Two main types of fibres are identified (types 1 and 2), and type 2 fibres can be subdivided into types 2A, 2B and 2C (Fig. 13.4). Type 2C fibres are thought to be a primitive form of type 2 fibre and, with appropriate innervation, are probably capable of developing into 2A or 2B fibres. Such histochemical staining is used routinely in the study of muscle pathology and allows the histological diagnosis of certain muscle diseases.

Histochemical staining can also be correlated with other functional and biochemical attributes of muscle (see Fig. 13.4c).

Not all muscles have the same proportions of type 1 and type 2 fibres. In general, muscles with a role in maintaining posture (e.g. calf muscles) have a high proportion of type 1 fibres, whereas muscles used for short bursts of power have abundant type 2 fibres.

Different individuals are genetically endowed with variable proportions of muscle fibre types in defined muscles, and this may limit athletic prowess at a particular sport; training does not affect the proportion of fibres in any given muscle but does influence their size.

> **Muscle has a rich blood supply because of the high energy demands of contraction.**

Large arteries penetrate the epimysium and divide into small branches that run in the perimysial support tissues, forming perimysial arteries and veins. These branches terminate in a vast capillary network, which runs in the endomysium. Each muscle fibre is served by several capillary vessels.

> **Normal adult skeletal muscle cells do not undergo cell division.**

Any increased demands placed on a muscle, for example, by weight training, result in increased muscle size because the cells themselves increase in size (i.e. hypertrophy).

It is possible, however, for skeletal muscle cells to regrow because the pool of inactive stem cells in adult muscle, called *satellite cells*, can be stimulated to divide after damage. These cells are not discernible by light microscopy but may be seen ultrastructurally (Fig. 13.5). They are infrequent and appear as small spindle-shaped cells lying just beneath the external lamina of a muscle fibre.

Fibre type	Metabolism	Contractile behaviour
1	oxidative	slow twitch
2A	oxidative and glycolytic	fast twitch, fatigue resistant
2B	glycolytic	fast twitch, fatigue sensitive

Fig. 13.4 Fibre Types. (a) Micrograph of a transverse frozen section of muscle stained by an enzyme histochemical method to demonstrate NADH transferase, which indicates oxidative capacity. Two different subtypes of fibres are evident. Type 1 fibres (1) show a high level of activity and stain darkly, whereas type 2 fibres (2) are paler because of their lower level of activity. **(b)** Micrograph of muscle stained for one form of myofibrillar ATPase at pH 4.2. This technique also delineates two fibre types. Type 1 fibres stain darkly, having a high level of activity, whereas type 2 fibres have a low level of activity and stain lightly. Note that the type 1 and 2 fibres are arranged in a haphazard or check pattern. **(c)** Table detailing the physiological features of different fibre types.

Fig. 13.5 Satellite Cells. Electron micrograph showing a satellite cell. These cells, small and spindle-shaped, are found immediately beneath the external lamina of a muscle fibre and act as stem cells in adult muscle.

Fibres that have regenerated in adult life after damage to a muscle can be detected histologically because they commonly contain centrally placed nuclei, rather than the peripheral nuclei typical of normal fibres.

Muscle contains stretch receptors.

Although there are no pain receptors in skeletal muscle, there are receptors sensitive to stretch, which function as part of a feedback system to maintain normal muscle tone (i.e. the spinal stretch reflex arc).

Sensory fibres that provide information on the tension of skeletal muscle arise from two sources:

- Encapsulated nerve endings responding to stretch in the tendon associated with a muscle
- Spiral nerve endings (sensory afferent fibres) sensing stretch and tension of specialized muscle fibres contained in a special sense organ in muscle called the *muscle spindle* (Fig. 13.7)

The muscle spindle sensory mechanism maintains normal tone and muscle coordination.

Motor nerves to muscle terminate in motor endplates.

Large nerves, containing both motor and sensory axons, enter muscles by penetrating the epimysium and branch to form small nerves, which run in the perimysium.

Perimysial nerves contain axons to fulfil both motor and sensory functions. The motor axons destined to innervate skeletal muscle (α efferent fibres) enter the endomysium as nerve twigs and branch to innervate several fibres.

At the end of each twig, the axon becomes modified to form a *motor endplate*, and it is this that activates skeletal muscle contraction (Fig. 13.8).

Activation of the motor axon causes the release of acetylcholine from its storage granules by exocytosis. Acetylcholine then diffuses across the gap between the axon and muscle fibre and interacts with specific membrane receptors to cause depolarization of the muscle fibre, which initiates contraction (see p. 84).

(see p. 84)

CLINICAL EXAMPLE

Diseases of Muscle

Several diseases of muscle have been attributed to specific metabolic or structural abnormalities. In many instances disease is linked to a mutation in a gene coding for one of the proteins involved in anchoring the muscle contractile proteins to the cell membrane (Fig. 13.6a).

Duchenne's muscular dystrophy is the most common inherited muscle disease and characteristically affects male children. Such individuals become unable to stand unaided in early childhood and develop progressive muscle weakness, becoming wheelchair-bound by their mid-teens and typically dying in early adult life.

The abnormality in Duchenne's muscular dystrophy is caused by a defect in the gene coding for a protein called *dystrophin* (see Fig. 13.6b). This protein links the actin cytoskeleton of muscle to the external lamina; its absence leads to abnormal muscle fibre fragility.

Fig. 13.6 Diseases of Muscle. (a) Micrograph of frozen section of skeletal muscle from a child showing the typical appearance of dystrophy, which is an inherited primary disorder of muscle. There is marked variation in fibre size, with some large fibres (L) and some abnormally small fibres (S). Some fibres are dead (D) and are being removed by phagocytic cells. **(b)** Micrograph of normal skeletal muscle stained by an immunocytochemical method for dystrophin (which stains *brown*), showing its localization in the sarcolemma. In Duchenne's muscular dystrophy, this protein is absent.

The activity of secreted acetylcholine is rapidly curtailed by the activity of an enzyme called *acetylcholinesterase*, which is bound to the basement membrane investing the junctional folds.

In addition to nerve fibres controlling voluntary movement, specialized motor axons (γ efferent fibres) innervate fibres in the muscle spindle.

Fig. 13.7 Sensory Innervation of Skeletal Muscle. (a) The sensory innervation of muscle, which arises from two sources: encapsulated nerve endings in the tendons respond to stretch, and spiral nerve endings in muscle spindles sense stretch and tension. The muscle spindle is composed of a fusiform capsule of fibrocollagenous tissue (continuous with the perimysium) surrounding a group of 8–15 thin muscle fibres. These fibres are termed *intrafusal fibres* to distinguish them from normal skeletal muscle fibres (extrafusal fibres). Two types of intrafusal fibres can be distinguished: those with a fusiform shape and a central aggregate of nuclei (nuclear bag fibres) and those of uniform width with dispersed nuclei (nuclear chain fibres). Specialized motor nerve fibres (gamma [γ] efferent fibres) innervate the intrafusal fibres and adjust their length according to the state of stretch of the muscle, which is detected by spiral nerve endings. The spiral nerve endings are wrapped around the intrafusal fibres and form special sensory afferent fibres running back to the spinal cord. **(b)** Micrograph of frozen section from a child's muscle showing a muscle spindle, identified by its circular fibrocollagenous capsule (C) and its content of intrafusal muscle fibres (M).

🏃 CLINICAL EXAMPLE

Myasthenia Gravis

Myasthenia gravis is a disease caused by the formation of antibodies to the acetylcholine receptor on the sarcolemma in the junctional folds of the motor endplates. The antibodies bind to the acetylcholine receptors and thereby prevent released acetylcholine from interacting with the receptors and causing depolarization.

Affected individuals develop tremendous muscle weakness manifested by fatiguability, inability to lift the arms, failure to maintain an upright posture of the head and drooping of the eyelids.

Treatment is by the administration of drugs (anticholinesterases) that inhibit the action of the enzyme acetylcholinesterase. This potentiates the action of released acetylcholine and allows it to bind to receptors not blocked by antibody.

Myasthenia gravis is an autoimmune disease.

MUSCLE ATTACHMENTS

To transmit the force of contraction, the cell surface at the end of the muscle fibres is adapted for attachment to highly organized fibrocollagenous support tissues, which anchor the muscle to other structures.

Such anchorage may be provided by:

- Anatomically distinct tendons
- Broad areas of anchorage to a bony surface
- Broad areas of anchorage to sheets of fibrocollagenous support tissue (fascia) which run between muscles

> **Tendons attach some muscles to bone.**

Muscles are connected to bone by dense compact collagenous tissue called *tendinous tissue,* which may be in the form of short sheets attaching to bone over a large area, often linear, or long cylindrical structures which connect some muscles to the bones of the hands and fingers and feet and toes. The largest and most distinct of the cylindrical type of tendons is the Achilles tendon, which connects the substantial muscle masses of the back of the calf with the bones at the back of the foot, involved in flexion and extension of the foot. A series of long cylindrical tendons run through the hands to the fingers.

Tendinous tissue is composed of tightly packed, longitudinally running collagen fibres, with the elongated flattened nuclei of inactive fibroblast-like cells scattered between them (Fig. 13.9) called **tenocytes.**

Tendinous tissue is relatively acellular and has both low oxygen/nutrient requirements and a very limited blood supply. Because of this poor vascularity, tendons that have been damaged by trauma (usually because of acute overstretching, particularly in sporting injuries) are extremely slow to heal, for example, Achilles tendon rupture and extensor tendonitis in the elbow ('tennis elbow').

> **Tendons attach to skeletal muscles at specialized structures called myotendinous junctions.**

The collagen fibres of tendons are firmly tethered to the muscle fibres of skeletal muscles at specialized areas called **myotendinous insertions** or **junctions** (Fig. 13.10). At these sites, individual muscle fibres develop a complex interdigitating surface, which is tightly anchored to the collagen fibres of the intramuscular portion of the end of the tendon.

> **Many tendons lie within fibrocollagenous tendon sheaths.**

Where the long cylindrical type of tendon has to run over the bone surface, it must be protected from damage resulting from repeated friction. An example is the long flexor tendons of the hand running to the fingers. This protection from friction damage is achieved by the tendon having a thin outer fibrous capsule sometimes called the **epitendineum,** coated on its outer surface by flat mesothelial cells, which are synovial in type and

Fig. 13.8 Motor Innervation of Skeletal Muscle. (a) A thin resin section of skeletal muscle stained with toluidine blue showing a small perimysial nerve, which contains both motor (efferent) and sensory (afferent) fibres. **(b)** A methylene blue-stained teased preparation of muscle showing several nerve twigs (T) branching from a single axon to innervate muscle fibres. There is a bulbous swelling (the motor endplate, MEP) at the end of each twig at the site of connection with the muscle. The group of fibres innervated by a single axon is a motor unit. **(c)** Micrograph of a thin resin section of skeletal muscle stained with toluidine blue to show the motor endplate (MEP). The axon terminates in a dome-shaped swelling of the nerve terminal in direct apposition to the cell membrane of the muscle fibre to form the MEP. This is invested by a layer of Schwann cell cytoplasm (S). **(d)** Electron micrograph of a motor endplate showing the cell membrane of the muscle fibre thrown into a series of deep folds (junctional folds, JF) beneath which the sarcoplasm (Sa) contains numerous mitochondria (M). In the terminal swelling of the motor axon, neurosecretory granules (G) containing the transmitter substance acetylcholine and mitochondria are abundant. The terminal swelling of the axon is separated from the muscle cell membrane by a gap of 30–50 nm (the synaptic cleft, C), which includes the external lamina of the muscle. **(e)** The motor endplate. The sarcoplasmic membrane in the region of the motor endplate contains specialized receptors which, when activated by acetylcholine, permit muscle cell membrane depolarization.

secrete small amounts of lubricating fluid similar to that which lubricates synovial joints (see p. 267). Such tendons are surrounded by a thin collagenous sheath which is lined internally by similar synovial-type mesothelial cells, also secreting lubricating fluid. This structure is called the **tendon sheath**, and the synovium related to the epitendineum and the tendon sheath is called **tenosynovium**. Thus the tendon can slide effortlessly and without friction within a lubricated sheath (Fig. 13.11).

Despite these preventive measures, repeated overuse of some tendons (particularly in the hands) can lead to structural

Fig. 13.9 Tendon. Micrograph of tendon showing highly organized regular bundles of collagen (C) with a few interspersed tenocytes.

Fig. 13.10 Myotendinous Junction. This micrograph of a myotendinous junction (MTJ) shows apparent splitting of the rounded contour of a muscle fibre to form several small, rounded structures separated by fibrocollagenous tissue. Such splitting of the terminal portion of the fibre increases the surface area available for anchorage to support tissues and thus contributes to the mechanical strength of insertion.

damage to both epitendineum and tendon sheath, which manifests as a painful condition localized to the affected tendon (*tendonitis*). Various forms of tendonitis, particularly those affecting the hands and arms, are often regarded as components of so-called *repetitive strain injury*.

Fig. 13.11 Tendon Sheath. This long flexor tendon (T) from the finger has an epitendineum (E) coated by flat lining cells on its outer surface. A thin fibrous tendon sheath (S) has a similar layer of flat lining cells on its inner surface. The tendon sheath space (TSS) contains thin lubricating fluid secreted by the lining cells. The lining cells are like those forming the intima of synovium (p. 267).

> **Tendon is attached to bone by fibres which pass through the periosteum and penetrate into the bone.**

At the attachment to bone, the type I collagen fibres of a tendon merge with the type I collagen of the periosteum and send fibres that penetrate into the bone (Fig. 13.12). These are called *Sharpey's fibres*.

The original tendon collagen is probably incorporated into bone when the periosteum makes new bone, initially in bone development in intrauterine life, and is continually reinforced in periods of high periosteal activity during bone growth in childhood.

Maintenance of the tendon at the site of the bone attachment is the responsibility of the collagen-synthesizing fibroblasts of the periosteum. These cells have the capacity to convert into chondroprogenitor cells (chondroblast precursors) or osteoprogenitor cells (osteoblast precursors, see Fig. 13.16). For this reason, the tendon close to its attachment to the bone may contain small islands of cartilage or bone.

> **Other important structures in the musculoskeletal system have a structure similar to that of tendons.**

Ligaments join one bone to another (see Fig. 13.29). Like tendons, they are composed of tightly packed collagen fibres running predominantly in the same direction but less regularly than in long cylindrical tendons, with inactive elongated fibrocytes

Fig. 13.12 **Tendon Insertion Into Bone.** Collagen fibres *(arrows)* from a tendon (T) insert obliquely into bone (B). These are called *Sharpey's fibres.* Other tendon collagen fibres merge with collagen fibres of the periosteum.

lying between the collagen bundles. In some areas there is a need for the ligaments to have elasticity, for example, in the prominent and extensive ligaments that help to bind the bones of the vertebral column together (e.g. ligamentum flavum). In such areas the ligament contains abundant elastic fibres which also run regularly spaced and parallel with the collagen fibres; these are sometimes called **elastic ligaments.**

Aponeuroses are flat sheets, often extensive, of tendon-like compact fibrocollagenous tissue, which may connect muscle to muscle (e.g. in the anterior abdominal wall), muscle to bone at an insertion or muscle to long cylindrical types of tendon. Thus many aponeuroses can be considered to be part of the tendinous system. Because the muscle fibres are attached to an aponeurosis in different directions, the component collagen of the aponeurosis is arranged in layers that run in different directions. Large aponeuroses are found in the palms and soles.

BONE

Introduction

Bone is a highly specialized support tissue which is characterized by its rigidity and hardness. Its four main functions are to provide **mechanical support** (e.g. ribs), to permit **locomotion** (e.g. long bones), to provide **protection** (e.g. skull) and to act as a **metabolic reservoir** of mineral salts.

Bone is composed of:
- Support cells (osteoblasts and osteocytes)
- A non-mineral matrix of collagen and glycosaminoglycans (osteoid)
- Inorganic mineral salts deposited within the matrix
- Remodelling cells (osteoclasts)

> **Bone contains a specialized extracellular matrix material called osteoid.**

Osteoid is a collagenous support tissue of type I collagen embedded in a glycosaminoglycan gel containing specific glycoproteins (e.g. osteocalcin) that strongly bind calcium. Deposition of mineral salts in the osteoid gives bone its characteristic rigidity and functional strength.

Osteoid is synthesized by specialized support cells called *osteoblasts,* which have the same collagen synthesis capacity as fibroblasts (see p. 73). Formed calcified bone can be eroded by osteoclasts – modified multinucleate phagocytic cells belonging to the monocyte/macrophage family (see p. 123).

Coordinated activity of osteoclasts (eroding formed bone) and osteoblasts (synthesized new osteoid) is important in maintaining bone structure and any structural modifications necessary to meet increased or altered demands. This is called *bone remodelling.*

> **Bone is constantly being remodelled.**

Bone is a dynamic tissue, being continually formed and destroyed under the control of hormonal and physical factors. This constant activity permits the process of modelling (i.e. modification of the bone architecture to meet physical stresses).

Bone turnover is normally low in adults, but in babies and children it is high to allow the growth and active remodelling required to cope with new demands, for example, with the onset of walking.

In the adult, bone turnover can increase from its normal basal level to meet any increased demand, for example, to increase bone bulk necessary for coping with increased physical activity, like running, jumping and climbing in sporting activities, and in the repair of bone fracture. In addition, increased bone turnover and remodelling can be the result of pathological processes, for example, after the excessive secretion of parathyroid hormone by overactive parathyroid glands or a parathyroid tumour (see p. 282). Another example is Paget's disease (see later and p. 263 in the Clinical Example box). In these cases, the bone remodelling is chaotic and random and not related to the need to counter physical stress; thus the bone architecture is seriously damaged, and symptoms such as pain and predisposition to fracture ensue.

Bone modelling is discussed in greater detail later.

> **The two main patterns of bone are called *woven* and *lamellar*.**

Two types of bone can be identified according to the pattern of collagen forming the osteoid:
- **Woven** bone is characterized by haphazard organization of collagen fibres and is mechanically weak.
- **Lamellar** bone is characterized by a regular parallel alignment of collagen into sheets (lamellae) and is mechanically strong (Fig. 13.13).

Fig. 13.13 Woven and Lamellar Bone. Polarizing micrograph of repairing bone showing both recently formed woven bone (W) at the centre and original lamellar bone (L) on either side. Note the haphazard arrangement of the collagen fibres in the woven bone and the regular parallel arrangement in the lamellar bone.

Woven bone is produced when osteoblasts produce osteoid rapidly; the collagen fibres are deposited in an irregular, loosely intertwined pattern. This occurs initially in all fetal bones (see Fig. 13.25), but in this case, the resulting woven bone is gradually replaced by remodelling and the deposition of more resilient lamellar bone.

In adults, woven bone is created when there is rapid new bone formation, as occurs in the repair of a fracture or in Paget's disease (see Fig. 13.24). After a fracture, woven bone is remodelled and lamellar bone is deposited, but in Paget's disease the woven bone persists and leads to mechanical weakness and bone deformity. Virtually all bone in the healthy adult is lamellar.

Bones have a dense outer cortex and an inner trabecular region.

Most bones have a basic architecture composed of:
- An outer cortical or compact zone
- An inner trabecular or spongy zone

Cortical bone forms a rigid outer shell that resists deformation, whereas the inner trabecular meshwork provides strength by acting as a complex system of internal struts. The spaces between the trabecular meshwork are occupied by bone marrow (see Chapter 7).

In bones with a substantial weight-bearing function, the trabecular pattern is arranged to provide maximum resistance to the physical stresses to which that bone is normally subjected.

The specialized support cells of the bone reside either on its surfaces or within small spaces in formed bone termed *lacunae*.

The details of normal bone architecture are shown in Figs. 13.14 and 13.15.

Fig. 13.14 Bone Architecture: Cortical and Trabecular Bone. **(a)** Low-power scanning electron micrograph showing the architecture of bone (cortical and trabecular) and its relationship to bone marrow (see Chapter 7). The cortical bone (C) is dense and forms a compact outer shell, which is bridged by narrow, delicate plates of trabecular bone (T). The spaces between the trabecular bone are occupied by yellow marrow (adipose tissue) or haemopoietic red marrow. Here the marrow (M) has retracted from the bone during tissue preparation. **(b)** Medium-power scanning electron micrograph showing more detail of cortical (C) and trabecular bone (T). The outlines of a number of Haversian systems (H) of various sizes, each with a central canal, can be seen. **(c)** Polarizing micrograph of a single osteon (Haversian system). A central Haversian canal (H) is surrounded by concentric layers of lamellar bone, which contains a number of *dark black* spaces marking the sites of osteocytes (O). Outside the Haversian system are less regularly arranged interstitial bone lamellae (I), which act as packing between adjacent Haversian systems.

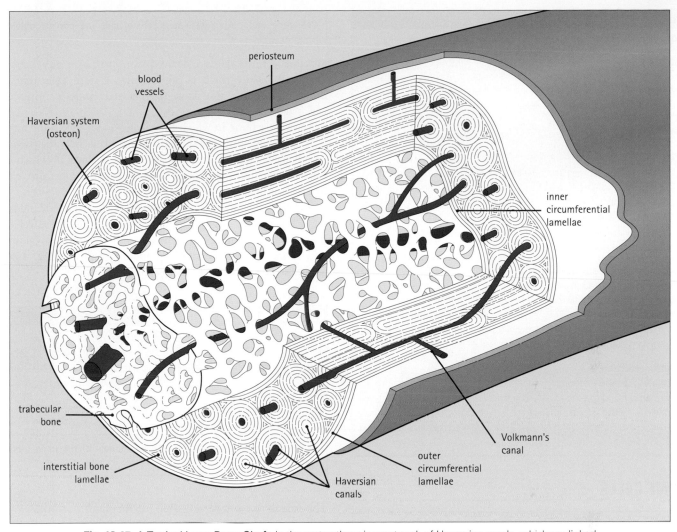

Fig. 13.15 A Typical Long Bone Shaft. In the cortex there is a network of Haversian canals, which are linked by transverse Volkmann's canals. The canals contain blood vessels and some nerves. Each Haversian canal is surrounded by concentric layers of lamellar bone. These layers contain concentrically arranged rings of osteocytes, each lying in its small lacuna and communicating with osteocytes in its own and adjacent layers through cytoplasmic processes lying in narrow canaliculi. The Haversian canal and its concentric bone and osteocyte system are called a *Haversian system* or *osteon*. The interior of each Haversian canal is lined by flat osteoprogenitor cells or bone-lining cells, as are the inner surface of the cortical bone plate and the outer surfaces of the bone trabeculae. This layer, called the *endosteum*, provides a source of new osteoblasts necessary for new bone formation if remodelling is needed. Cortical remodelling in the Haversian canals is common. The Haversian canal systems, interspersed with irregularly arranged interstitial bone lamellae which act as packing, occupy the bulk of the cortex; inner and outer circumferential bone lamellae separate the Haversian systems from the endosteum and the outer surface of the bone, the fibrocollagenous periosteum. The strong, dense cortical bone encloses the medullary cavity comprising bone marrow and an interconnecting network of trabecular bone, providing strength with lightness.

▶▶ KEY FACTS

Osteoid

- Is a specialized form of type I collagen embedded in a glycosaminoglycan gel.
- The supporting gel contains specific proteins (e.g. osteocalcin), which have an affinity for calcium.
- Is synthesized and secreted by osteoblasts, which also orchestrate deposition of mineral salts.

- May be deposited by osteoblasts in regular parallel sheets (lamellar) or haphazardly (woven).
- Healthy bone formed from lamellar osteoid is strong and efficient.
- Bone formed from woven osteoid is comparatively weak, bulky and inefficient and is usually pathological, resulting from fracture or Paget's disease.

Abnormalities of Bone Architecture

Abnormal bone architecture may result from:
- Damage both to cortical and trabecular bone because of fracture
- Decreased cortical and trabecular bone because of osteoporosis
- Destruction of trabecular bone because of cancer
- Maldevelopment of bone
- Metabolic bone disease (see Clinical Example boxes, p. 262).

Osteoporosis

In old age, both cortical and trabecular bone become thinned (osteoporosis, see Fig. 13.23) and are therefore more fragile and more prone to fracture. Fracture of the neck of the femur is common in the elderly. Osteoporosis may also develop after disuse, for example, in the leg bones of a wheelchair-bound person.

There is evidence that hormonal disturbances may induce osteoporosis in postmenopausal women.

Bone Involvement in Cancer

The bone marrow is a common site of spread of some forms of cancer, particularly cancers that originate in the breast (see Fig. 18.27), bronchus, prostate, thyroid and kidney. Proliferation of tumour cells frequently destroys the trabecular bone and thus leads to an increased tendency to bone fracture (pathological fracture), an important complication of widespread cancer.

Maldevelopment

There are a number of diseases arising from impaired bone formation during embryological development. Many of these are incompatible with survival, and such children commonly die in utero or shortly after birth. The most common maldevelopment of bone that is compatible with life is achondroplasia, resulting in a form of dwarfism characterized by a normal-sized trunk but short limb bones.

BONE CELLS

Four main types of cells maintain bone.

Cells concerned with the production, maintenance and modelling of the osteoid are:
- Osteoprogenitor cells
- Osteoblasts
- Osteocytes
- Osteoclasts

Osteoprogenitor cells are the stem cells of bone and form osteoblasts.

Osteoprogenitor cells are derived from primitive mesenchymal stem cells. They form a population of stem cells that can differentiate into the more specialized bone-forming cells (i.e. osteoblasts and osteocytes).

In mature bone in which there is no active new bone formation or remodelling, the osteoprogenitor cells become flattened spindle cells closely applied to the bone surface, in which case they are termed *bone-lining cells* and sometimes also called *inactive osteoblasts*.

In actively growing bone, however, for example, in fetal bone or in a period of high turnover in adult bone, these cells are much larger and more numerous, containing plump oval nuclei and more abundant spindle-shaped cytoplasm (Fig. 13.16), converting to cuboidal active osteoblasts.

Mesenchymal stem cells must first turn on a set of genes to develop into an osteoprogenitor cell type. This transformation involves synthesis of several specific transcription factors essential for osteoblast differentiation, including Runx2 as a key gene in osteoblast differentiation and the production of bone morphogenetic proteins (BMPs).

Osteoblasts synthesize the organic component of the bone matrix (osteoid).

The osteoblasts are responsible for formation of bone. When fully active, osteoblasts are cuboidal or polygonal cells. They have basophilic cytoplasm, which reflects the abundance of rough endoplasmic reticulum in their cytoplasm, resulting from their role as active protein-synthesizing and secreting cells. For details of osteoblast structure and function, see Fig. 13.17 and also see Fig. 13.20.

Osteoblasts adhere to the bone matrix through surface expression of integrins, which bind to proteins in osteoid.

Fig. 13.16 Osteoprogenitor Cells. Micrograph of toluidine blue–stained epoxy resin section showing numerous plump spindle-shaped osteoprogenitor (Op) cells in the developing skull bone of a 15-week human fetus. Derived from primitive mesenchymal cells, they are transformed into osteoblasts (Ob), which are larger and more cuboidal. The osteoblasts have begun to deposit osteoid collagen (C).

Fig. 13.17 Osteoblasts. (a) Micrograph of an acrylic resin section of actively growing fetal bone stained by Goldner's method, which distinguishes mineralized bone *(turquoise)* from unmineralized osteoid. Note the zone of unmineralized newly formed osteoid (OS) adjacent to the row of actively synthesizing osteoblasts (Ob) on one side of the trabeculum. On the other side, a layer of now-flattened osteoblasts has entered an inactive resting phase (ROb), and its recently formed osteoid is now almost fully mineralized *(arrow)*. **(b)** Micrograph of a toluidine blue–stained thin epoxy resin section of actively growing bone, with a row of cuboidal osteoblasts (Ob) actively synthesizing and secreting organic matrix (osteoid, OS); the cells have bulky basophilic cytoplasm owing to their protein-synthesizing rough endoplasmic reticulum. Some of the osteoid is lightly mineralized (mOS). **(c)** Low-power electron micrograph showing an osteoblast (Ob) at the face of newly forming bone. Note the zone of unmineralized osteoid (OS), which has recently formed between the active osteoblast and the older mineralized bone (mB). **(d)** High-power electron micrograph showing the characteristic cytoplasmic features of an active osteoblast. The cytoplasm is rich in rough endoplasmic reticulum (RER) and there are prominent mitochondria (M); the collagenic protein precursors and glycosaminoglycans are synthesized in the RER and then packaged in the Golgi before transfer to the cell surface in secretory vesicles. The cell surface shows numerous cytoplasmic processes (CP), particularly on the face in contact with existing osteoid (OS). The secretory vesicles discharge their contents from this surface to form identifiable osteoid collagen fibres (OC) embedded in an electron-lucent matrix (Mx) of glycosaminoglycans and proteoglycans. The formation and secretion of collagen is described on page 64.

In order to respond to local and systemic signals, osteoblasts have receptors for parathyroid hormone (PTH), 1,25-vitamin D$_3$, corticoids, prostaglandins and oestrogen.

The main product of osteoblasts is osteoid, which consists of type I collagen; non-collagen proteins such as osteocalcin, osteonectin, bone sialoprotein and osteopontin; and proteoglycans including decorin and biglycan.

CLINICAL EXAMPLE

A radioisotope bone scan involves administration of technetium 99 followed by imaging its location after uptake into bone. Technetium 99 is taken up by osteoblasts and incorporated into newly formed mineralized bone. 'Hot spots' on a bone scan can therefore be interpreted as areas with high activity of osteoblasts and may be the site of disease activity in bone involving abnormal bone turnover.

Osteocytes are inactive osteoblasts trapped in mineralized bone.

When osteoblasts have completed a burst of osteoid-producing activity, most return to a relatively inactive state, becoming flattened and spindle-shaped and closely applied to the now-inactive bone surface, termed *bone-lining cells.* Some osteoblasts, however, become surrounded by mineralizing bone matrix and lie within small cavities (lacunae) in the bone. When this happens, the cell is called an *osteocyte* and comprises around 90% of the total cellular component of bone (Fig. 13.18). Usually, osteocytes are

arranged haphazardly, but in cortical bone they assume a regular pattern (see p. 254). Osteocytes had been considered inactive cells, but there is considerable evidence that they are metabolically highly active and act as essential sensors for mechanical stress in bone, being central for signalling to other cells involved in maintaining bone structure.

Adjacent osteocytes can communicate with each other via long cytoplasmic processes that lie in narrow channels called *canaliculi.* This communication is via gap junctions between adjacent osteocytes involving the protein connexin 43. It is understood that systems for sensing mechanical stress in bone are located on osteocyte processes, possibly mediated by an ability to detect shear stress in pericellular fluid in canaliculi. The importance of this is that it allows for cell signalling to modulate local bone remodelling depending on mechanical stresses encountered.

Osteocytes under certain conditions, including during lactation, can modify their local environment to cause bone resorption and thereby increase serum calcium levels for use in milk production. This process is termed *osteocytic osteolysis.*

Fig. 13.18 Osteocytes. (a) Micrograph of a toluidine blue–stained acrylic resin section of bone showing osteocytes trapped within mineralized bone matrix. Note their fine cytoplasmic processes, which lie in narrow canalicular channels in the mineralized bone and link one osteocyte with another. **(b)** Electron micrograph of a recently entrapped osteocyte. It shows some of the cytoplasmic rough endoplasmic reticulum (RER) and mitochondria (M) of the osteoblast from which it is derived. Note the origin of one of its cytoplasmic processes (CP), with the rest being out of the plane of section.

CLINICAL EXAMPLE
Tumours of Osteoblasts

Osteosarcoma

The most important tumour derived from bone cells is osteosarcoma, which is a malignant tumour of osteoblasts. It is most common in children and adolescents and usually involves the bones around the knee joint, either the lower end of the femur or the upper end of the tibia.

The tumour cells resemble osteoblasts in both structure and function, in that they synthesize osteoid; however, the production of osteoid is scanty, haphazard and irregular, and it does not mineralize normally.

The malignant osteoblasts are largely primitive and more closely resemble immature osteoprogenitor cells than mature osteoblasts.

Osteosarcoma spreads extensively via the bloodstream, often producing secondary (metastatic) tumours in the lungs.

Benign tumours of osteoblasts (osteoid osteomas) occur as localized swellings in bones, which are often painful. They may enlarge slowly, but do not spread to distant sites.

Osteoclasts erode mineralized bone.

Osteoclasts are large cells with multiple nuclei and abundant cytoplasm derived from precursors in the myeloid/monocyte lineage that circulate in the blood after their formation in the bone marrow. Osteoclast precursors develop at sites on bone surfaces destined for resorption and fuse with one another to form multinucleated cells.

Mature osteoclasts are found attached to the bone surface at sites of active bone resorption, often in cavities where they have eroded into the bone. These cavities are called *resorption bays* or *Howship's lacunae* (Fig. 13.19).

Fig. 13.19 Osteoclast. (a) Micrograph of a toluidine blue–stained epoxy resin thin section showing a single osteoclast (Oc), which has alighted on an irregular spur of bone before reabsorption. At a later stage, the spur of bone will have been eroded and levelled as a result of osteoclast activity. **(b)** Micrograph of Goldner-stained acrylic resin section of bone showing active resorption of bone on one face, with a multinucleate osteoclast (Oc) lying in a Howship's lacuna. There is active osteoblast deposition of new osteoid on the other face *(arrow)* in a bone that is undergoing active modelling (see Fig. 13.21). **(c)** Electron micrograph of an osteoclast demonstrating its richness in Golgi, lysosomes, secretory vesicles and mitochondria. At its interface with the bone, highly complex cytoplasmic protrusions from the osteoclast's surface appear as a ruffled border (R). **(d)** High-power electron micrograph of the ruffled border region where numerous fine cytoplasmic processes (CP) extend from the surface of the osteoclast, some interdigitating with the collagenic fibres (C) of the osteoid. Fragments of mineralized osteoid (mOS) can be seen between the cytoplasmic processes. **(e)** Micrograph of a frozen section of bone demonstrating abundant acid phosphatase activity *(red)* in an osteoclast (Oc), which is actively eroding the bone surface.

MINERALIZATION OF OSTEOID

> The rigidity of bone is determined by deposition of minerals.

The hardness and rigidity of bone are the result of the presence of mineral salt in the osteoid matrix. This salt is a crystalline complex of calcium and phosphate hydroxides called *hydroxyapatite* $[Ca_{10}(PO_4)_6(OH)_2]$.

For mineralization to occur, the combined local concentrations of Ca^{2+} ions and PO_4^- ions must be above a threshold value in the form of a supersaturated concentration. There are two phases in mineralization called *vesicular* and *fibrillar* phases:

- Vesicles called *matrix vesicles* between 30 and 200 nm in diameter bud from the apical membrane of osteoblasts. These vesicles bind to proteoglycans in osteoid and are rich in the enzymes alkaline phosphatase and pyrophosphatase, both of which can cleave PO_4^- ions from phosphate-containing substrates.

- A high local concentration of calcium ions is present in osteoid mediated by a glycoprotein (osteocalcin), which binds extracellular Ca^{2+} ions. In the process of mineralization, osteoblasts are the source of enzymes that degrade the calcium-binding proteoglycans, causing free calcium ions to be mobilized. This free extracellular Ca^{2+} then actively enters the matrix vesicles through calcium channels composed of proteins called *annexins*.

- The enzyme alkaline phosphatase, which is produced by osteoblasts, increases the PO_4^- ion concentration within matrix vesicles.

- Through these processes, the matrix vesicles accumulate Ca^{2+} and PO_4^- ions, which achieve supersaturation concentrations and then nucleate to form hydroxyapatite crystals.

- In the fibrillar phase of mineralization, crystals cause rupture of matrix vesicles with spread of hydroxyapatite into the surrounding matrix. The fibrillar phase continues with accretion of further crystals through foci growing from other matrix vesicles. In this way, a wave of mineralization sweeps through new osteoid (Fig. 13.20).

Fig. 13.20 Mineralization of Bone. (a) The events believed to occur in a newly formed osteoid. Immediately adjacent to the irregular osteoblast surface is a zone A of freshly deposited osteoid collagen and glycosaminoglycan containing newly formed matrix vesicles. Next is a zone B in which early crystals of hydroxyapatite are being deposited in slightly older matrix vesicles, and beyond it a zone C in which the foci of mineralization rapidly enlarge by accretion of mineral salts. In zone D, the individual foci of mineralization, each centred on a matrix vesicle remnant, have become almost completely confluent. In zone E, mineralization is complete, and the underlying osteoid collagen is obscured. The junction between zones C and D is the so-called *calcification front,* but as this term is used inaccurately in an entirely different context in pathological studies of bone disease, it is best avoided unless carefully defined. **(b)** High-power electron micrograph showing early mineral deposition in a zone of recently formed osteoid from fetal bone. Note the early crystalline pattern of mineralization of a matrix vesicle *(arrows)* in zone B and enlargement of foci of mineralization in zone C, becoming confluent in zone D. Zones A and E are not shown.

Other cells that produce matrix vesicles are the ameloblasts and odontoblasts of the developing tooth (see p. 205) and chondrocytes; hence the frequent mineralization of cartilage.

In states of high turnover of bone, osteoblasts produce large amounts of osteoid in a short time and mineralization lags behind, catching up only when the rate of new osteoid production falls. In this situation, distinct layers of unmineralized osteoid can be seen between the layer of active osteoblasts and the previously mineralized bone. This is evident in the phases of rapid bone growth in fetal life and also in adult life during periods of active remodelling of bone, such as after fracture or as part of some disease processes.

> **Selective resorption of formed bone occurs where the osteoclast is in contact with the bone surface.**

Mature osteoclasts are highly specialized cells that become polarized to form functionally distinct cell surfaces.

The sealing zone is an area in the periphery of the osteoclast responsible for adhesion of the cell to the bone surface. It is formed by a local organization of actin fibrils and actin-binding proteins and is the site of membrane expression of specialized adhesion molecules (the $\alpha_v\beta_3$-integrin and CD44) which bind to proteins in the bone matrix, including sialoprotein and osteopontin.

The ruffled border is the site of active membrane fusion events mediating resorption of bone and is formed by microvilli in contact with the bone matrix. Vesicles from the endosome/lysosome system fuse with the cell membrane at the ruffled border and secrete lytic enzymes such as tartrate-resistant acid phosphatase (TRAP) and matrix metalloproteinase-9 (MMP-9) onto the bone surface. The membrane in this zone is also the site for a H^+-ATPase, which produces hydrogen ions that reduce the pH at the bone surface beneath the osteoclast to dissolve mineral hydroxyapatite crystals.

Resorption of bone is believed to proceed as follows:

- Osteoclasts are recruited to sites of bone resorption by local signalling from osteocytes and other cell types.
- Lytic enzymes are released from the osteoclast cytoplasm by exocytosis from the ruffled border where it is in contact with the bone.
- The released enzymes hydrolyse the collagenous protein and glycosaminoglycans of the adjacent bone matrix.
- The disrupted bone matrix yields up its attached mineral salts.
- Local acidic conditions, created by the osteoclast H^+ membrane pump, break up the hydroxyapatite, thereby releasing soluble Ca^{2+} and PO_4^- ions.
- Some of the soluble breakdown products of demineralization and protein hydrolysis are resorbed by the osteoclast by endocytosis.

Osteoclasts are highly mobile and resorb bone as they move along the bone surface. In some bone diseases, the osteoclasts are stimulated into inappropriate resorptive activity and at the same time appear to lose their mobility so that they remain localized to one area of the bone surface. In this situation, they bore deeply into the bone at one site (tunnelling resorption) instead of sweeping bone away from a wide area.

◎ ADVANCED CONCEPT

The differentiation of monocytes into osteoclasts is stimulated by signals that promote the activation of specific transcription factors. These signals come from osteoprogenitor cells and osteoblasts in the bone that produce **macrophage colony-stimulating factor (M-CSF)** and from osteoblasts, osteocytes and stromal cells, which produce **RANK ligand (RANKL)** which, if it binds to its receptor called **receptor activator of nuclear factor κB (RANK)** expressed on osteoclast cell membrane, results in activation to bone-resorbing osteoclasts. The production of RANKL by osteoblasts can be stimulated by parathormone-related peptide (PTHrP), vitamin D, prostaglandin E_2 (PGE2) and interleukins 1 and 2. Osteoblasts and stromal cells produce another factor called **osteoprotegerin (OPG)** that binds to RANKL and in turn prevents it from binding to RANK, thus inhibiting formation of osteoclasts. The balance in activity within the RANKL/RANK/OPG system therefore regulates the activity of osteoclastogenesis.

▶ KEY FACTS

Bone Cells

Osteoprogenitor Cells
- Are precursors of osteoblasts

Osteoblasts
- Synthesize osteoid collagen, then mineralize it by depositing calcium and phosphate hydroxides (hydroxyapatite)
- Produce matrix vesicles rich in Ca^{2+} and PO_4^- ions and the enzymes alkaline phosphatase and pyrophosphatase, essential for mineralization
- Are only large, metabolically active cells when there is a requirement for new osteoid deposition; when inactive, they are insignificant spindle cells lying on the bone surface (bone surface cells)
- Act as a component of the stem cell niche for haemopoietic cells of the bone marrow

Osteocytes
- Are derived from osteoblasts trapped within the bone they have made
- Regulate bone remodelling by secretion of several factors that act on other cell types such as RANKL, OPG and sclerostin

Osteoclasts
- Are multinucleate cells derived from blood monocytes
- Are highly mobile cells capable of eroding mineralized bone by enzymic hydrolysis of osteoid collagen, with release of bone minerals
- Express RANK receptor which, when bound to its ligand, activates osteoclast formation
- Osteoclastic resorption of bone can be stimulated by PTH in response to a low serum calcium level

BONE REMODELLING

> After initial deposition, the bone matrix and the struts forming trabecular bone are remodelled.

In rapid bone growth during fetal development and childhood, large quantities of bone are produced by osteoblastic synthesis of bone matrix, which is subsequently mineralized. The subsequent pattern of remodelling is determined by local mechanical stresses, so that the bone matrix is aligned to resist local shearing and compressive stresses.

Modelling (Fig. 13.21) is achieved by a carefully balanced combination of:
- New bone deposition and mineralization by active osteoblasts (see Fig. 13.17)
- Selective resorption of formed bone by osteoclasts (see Fig. 13.19)

◎ ADVANCED CONCEPT

- Bone remodelling involves coordinated activity of all the main cell types in bone, the activity of which is controlled by both local and systemic factors.
- There is constant turnover and remodelling of bone in response to mechanical stresses and metabolic factors.
- Local factors include effects of growth factors, cytokines and prostaglandins produced by the bone cells.
- Systemic factors include PTH, calcitonin, 1,25-dihydroxyvitamin D_3 (calcitriol) and steroids (corticoids, androgens and oestrogens).

A bone remodelling cycle has been characterized as mediated by transient microscopic structures called **basic multicellular units (BMUs)** as part of a **bone remodelling compartment (BRC)**. This consists of a leading edge of destructive osteoclasts, a following group of restorative osteoblasts and a covering sheath of bone-lining cells together with blood vessels. The BRC receives cell signals from osteocytes and bone-lining cells believed to coordinate and regulate the activity of remodelling.

> Osteoclast resorption of bone can be stimulated by PTH (parathormone).

Parathormone is secreted by the parathyroid glands, which maintain a constant level of Ca^{2+} ions in the blood by increasing their output of parathormone in response to low serum Ca^{2+} ion concentration (see p. 280).

Parathormone increases the serum Ca^{2+} ion level by stimulating osteoclastic activity. In addition, parathormone can increase blood Ca^{2+} by reducing Ca^{2+} ion loss by the kidney and by increasing Ca^{2+} absorption by the small intestine.

The effect of parathormone activity in the bone is not usually detectable histologically unless there is prolonged and excessive parathormone secretion.

The elevation of blood Ca^{2+} produced by osteoclast-driven bone resorption is not matched by a rise in serum PO_4^- because parathormone also stimulates PO_4^- excretion by the kidney.

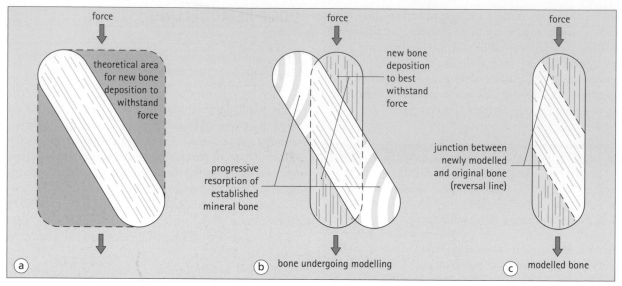

Fig. 13.21 Bone Modelling. (a) A piece of bone inappropriately orientated to best withstand the direction of the force to which it is exposed. The force could be resisted by deposition of new bone on the old in the area indicated, but this would produce a large heavy block of bone which, if repeated throughout the body as a whole, would result in such a bulky mass that movement would be impossible. A more efficient strength-to-weight ratio is achieved by remodelling. **(b)** How the bone can be modelled to become more efficient. The junctions between original bone and newly modelled bone are not easily seen in histological sections of mineralized bone, but are evident when decalcified sections are examined, particularly if the section is examined in polarized light, which accentuates the different directions of the osteoid collagen fibres. The junctions between different phases of bone deposition in different directions are called *reversal lines* and are particularly numerous and haphazard when bone modelling has been random and uncontrolled, as in Paget's disease. **(c)** Final remodelled bone with reversal lines.

> **Osteoclast activity and bone resorption are inhibited by calcitonin.**

Calcitonin is a hormone produced by thyroid C cells (see Fig. 14.18). It antagonizes parathormone and is secreted in response to a high serum Ca^{2+} level. It has a direct effect on osteoclasts by inhibiting their activity in resorbing bone, but also has an effect on the kidney, where it increases the rate of excretion of both calcium and phosphate. The sum effect of calcitonin is to lower the levels of both calcium and phosphate ions in the blood. The ability of calcitonin to suppress the activity of osteoclasts in resorbing bone has been used in the treatment of Paget's disease; treatment with salmon calcitonin sometimes reduces the level of activity of the disease.

CLINICAL EXAMPLE

Osteomalacia (Failure of Mineralization)

Mineralization of osteoid can take place only if there are sufficient Ca^{2+} and PO_4^- ions.

If the blood level of Ca^{2+} ions is low because of disorders causing hypocalcaemia or if PO_4^- ion levels are low (which is uncommon and usually the result of excessive PO_4^- ion loss in the urine), then mineralization is impaired. This leads to the condition known as *osteomalacia* (Fig. 13.22).

Patients with osteomalacia develop softening of the bone, which comes to contain a larger proportion of unmineralized osteoid, and patients can experience bone pain and bone fractures.

Osteomalacia in the growing bones of children leads to the disease called *rickets* and produces permanent deformity of the soft, poorly mineralized bones.

Fig. 13.22 Osteomalacia. Micrograph of iliac crest bone embedded in acrylic resin without prior decalcification from a patient with osteomalacia. Note the broad zone of unmineralized osteoid *(purple)* and the central zone of mineralized bone *(black)* in this section stained by von Kossa's silver technique. The reduced mineralized content of the bone leads to it being abnormally weak.

CLINICAL EXAMPLE

Osteoporosis and Paget's Disease

Osteoporosis (Fig. 13.23) can occur because of disuse (e.g. prolonged bed rest, limb paralysis) but also in people who are otherwise healthy, particularly post-menopausal women. In this condition there is loss of the mass of bone, and this leads to bone fragility with an increased tendency to bone fracture, particularly compression fractures of vertebrae.

Paget's disease is characterized by an increase in bone remodelling affecting one or more bones. There is a phase of excess osteoclast activity, leading to resorption of bone and a later phase of osteoblastic attempts to fill in the remaining erosions (Fig. 13.24). The condition is increasingly linked to genetic predispositions with mutations in the genes *SQSTM1* and *RANK* and linkage to regions of chromosome 5 and 6 identified. It is felt that causation is linked to factors that interfere with normal cell signalling between osteoclasts and osteoblasts.

When the wave of osteoclastic resorption dies down or moves elsewhere, the osteoblasts continue to produce new bone to repair the damage. Thus, paradoxically, the affected piece of bone usually ends up larger than it was originally.

The repaired bone is, however, less able to resist physical stress because the new bone deposition is haphazard and reparative, rather than organized and constructive; it is therefore more prone to fracture.

Fig. 13.23 Osteoporosis. (a) Micrograph of a resin section of a bone biopsy from the iliac crest showing normal cortical and trabecular bone stained with a silver method, which makes calcified bone show up as *black*. **(b)** Micrograph of bone from a patient with osteoporosis. When compared with **(a),** which shows bone mass of a healthy patient of the same age, it is clear that the cortical zone is narrower and that the trabeculae are thinner and less numerous.

Fig. 13.24 Paget's Disease. Micrograph of a resin-embedded Goldner-stained section from a patient with active Paget's disease. There is uncontrolled osteoclast (Oc) resorption of a bone, and osteoblasts (Ob) are attempting to fill in sites of recent osteoclast erosion in an adjacent site.

In the fetus, new bone formation may be intramembranous or endochondral.

Bone develops in the fetus by two mechanisms:
- Condensation from sheets of mesenchymal cells, which act as bone-forming membranes (intramembranous ossification)
- Transformation of previously deposited cartilage (endochondral ossification)

In intramembranous ossification, bone is formed within pre-existing membranes.

Intramembranous ossification results in the formation of flat bones, such as those of the skull, and also contributes to some of the cortical bone shafts of long bones. In intramembranous ossification (Fig. 13.25), some of the primitive mesenchymal spindle cells of the mesenchymal membrane enlarge and

Fig. 13.25 Intramembranous Ossification. (a) Micrograph of an acrylic resin, Goldner-stained section from the skull of a developing fetus. Within the fibrocollagenous membrane, islands of primitive mesenchymal cells develop into clusters of osteoprogenitor cells (Op, see also Fig. 13.16), which mature into osteoblasts. The osteoblasts then lay down osteoid (OS), which becomes mineralized *(blue)*. Although the initial bone islands are irregular in shape, remodelling by synchronized osteoblast and osteoclast activity produces flattened sheets of bone. **(b)** Micrograph of fetal skull showing a slightly later stage in the same process. The bone is now roughly fashioned in the shape of a plate, with almost continuous outer and inner layers bridged by trabeculae (T). The spaces between the bone are occupied by primitive mesenchymal tissue, developing fibrocollagenous tissue and a system of interconnecting vascular channels (V). Later still, the bone plates thicken and haemopoietic marrow fills the spaces.

develop abundant rough endoplasmic reticulum to become active osteoprogenitor cells and eventually osteoblasts.

The resulting osteoblasts begin to deposit bone in isolated islands, and remodelling begins instantly by combined osteoblast and osteoclast activity to form a network of trabecular bone.

Intervening residual mesenchymal tissue develops prominent blood vessels, and some mesenchymal cells eventually develop into haematopoietic bone marrow (see Chapter 7).

Further development is associated with increased bone formation on the outer and inner surfaces to form complete plates of bone (the outer and inner tables).

The external surfaces of cortical bone are continuously maintained in adult life by intramembranous ossification from the periosteum, particularly in response to changing stresses or injury.

> **Endochondral ossification is the method whereby the fetus forms long and short bones using preformed cartilage models.**

In this process, hyaline cartilage (see Fig. 4.20) is deposited in the shape of the required bone and is subsequently transformed into bone by osteoid deposition and mineralization.

Endochondral ossification permits elongation and thickening of the bone during fetal development and throughout childhood until bone growth ceases.

Hyaline cartilage develops from a mass of immature mesenchymal tissue and assumes the approximate shape of the bone. In the case of a long bone, this will include a shaft (diaphysis) with club-shaped expansions (the epiphyses) at either end (Fig. 13.26).

A layer of spindle-shaped mesenchymal cells, chondroblasts and some osteoprogenitor cells surrounds the hyaline cartilage model and forms a perichondrium. Later, as osteoprogenitor cells outnumber chondroblast precursors, this layer is termed the *periosteum*.

At the midshaft of the diaphysis osteoprogenitor, cells transform into osteoblasts and lay down osteoid, which becomes mineralized to form a collar of bone around the diaphysis. Concurrently, the chondrocytes in the cartilage model multiply, so that it increases in length and breadth; chondroblasts in the perichondrium/periosteum produce new cartilage. Calcium salts are then deposited in the cartilage matrix.

Once the bony collar has been formed, the diaphysis increases in diameter by bone deposition on the outer surface of the collar and resorption of bone on the inner surface.

Capillaries grow into the diaphysis of the model by penetrating the periosteum; they carry osteoprogenitor cells, which then establish a primary ossification centre in the centre of the diaphysis.

The osteoprogenitor cells in the primary diaphyseal ossification centre transform into osteoblasts and begin to deposit osteoid, which progressively replaces the calcified cartilage of the original model.

Mineralization of the osteoid, followed by some remodelling, produces a network of trabecular bone, which progressively occupies the core of the diaphysis and merges with the denser compact bone of the peripheral bone collar.

At about the time of birth, blood vessels and osteoprogenitor cells grow into the cartilaginous club-shaped ends of the developing bone (epiphyses) at either end of the diaphyseal shaft and form secondary (or epiphyseal) ossification centres.

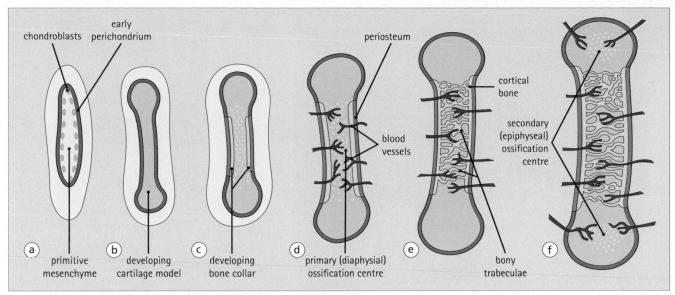

Fig. 13.26 Prenatal Long Bone Development (Endochondral Ossification). (a) Chondroblasts develop in primitive mesenchyme and form an early perichondrium and cartilage model. **(b)** The developing cartilage model assumes the shape of the bone to be formed, and a surrounding perichondrium becomes identifiable. **(c)** At the midshaft of the diaphysis, the perichondrium becomes a periosteum through the development of osteoprogenitor cells and osteoblasts, with the osteoblasts producing a collar of bone by intramembranous ossification. Calcium salts are deposited in the enlarging cartilage model. **(d)** Blood vessels grow through the periosteum and bone collar, carrying osteoprogenitor cells within them. These establish a primary (or diaphyseal) ossification centre in the centre of the diaphysis. **(e)** Bony trabeculae spread out from the primary ossification centre to occupy the entire diaphysis, linking up with the previously formed bone collar, which now forms the cortical bone of the diaphysis. At this stage, the terminal club-shaped epiphyses are still composed of cartilage. **(f)** At about term (the precise time varies between long bones), secondary or epiphyseal ossification centres are established in the centre of each epiphysis by the ingrowth, along with blood vessels of mesenchymal cells, which become osteoprogenitor cells and osteoblasts.

Long bones continue to grow throughout childhood and adolescence.

Increase in length is the result of continued endochondral bone formation at each end of the long bones.

An actively proliferating plate of cartilage (the epiphyseal plate) remains across the junction between the epiphysis and diaphysis. This gives rise to the apposition of new cartilage to the ends of the diaphysis, which is converted to trabecular bone, leading to a progressive increase in length (Fig. 13.27). Activity of the epiphyseal plate normally ceases after puberty.

New bone forms on the diaphyseal side of the epiphyseal plate as follows:
- Cartilage on the epiphyseal face of the epiphyseal plate proliferates to produce columns of chondrocytes embedded in matrix.
- Chondrocytes approaching the diaphyseal face of the epiphyseal plate become greatly enlarged and pale staining and begin to produce alkaline phosphatase, which facilitates calcification of the matrix.
- Osteoblasts lay down osteoid on the calcified cartilaginous matrix as the first stage in the ossification of the calcified cartilaginous trabeculae.
- The deposited bone is remodelled as it is incorporated into the diaphysis.

The epiphyseal plate and the zone of ossifying cartilaginous matrix trabeculae form the metaphysis.

Increase in circumference of the diaphysis is achieved by formation of new bone on the outer surface of the cortical bone, which is subjected to slightly less active resorption on its inner aspect. This increases not only the diameter of the diaphysis but also the thickness of the cortical bone.

JOINTS

Introduction

Bones are connected to each other by joints, which permit varying degrees of movement between the joined bones.

Joints can be divided into two main groups:
- Those that permit limited movement
- Those that permit free movement (diarthrodial joints)

Some joints between bones are formed by fibrocollagenous or cartilaginous tissue.

In joints that permit only limited movement, the bones are connected by flexible fibrocollagenous or cartilaginous tissue. Such joints generally occur between bones subserving a primary supportive or protective role, for example, between:
- The flat bones of the skull, which are joined by fibrous or ligamentous tissues (syndesmoses)
- The ribs and the sternum, which are joined by cartilage (synchondroses)

Fig. 13.27 Postnatal Development of Long Bones (Endochondral Ossification). (a) The initial enlargement of the secondary (epiphyseal) ossification centre within the epiphyseal cartilage, leaving an epiphyseal plate of cartilage and a surrounding of cartilage which will ultimately become the articular cartilage. **(b)** The fine detail of the epiphyseal plate between the secondary epiphyseal ossification centre on one side and the developing diaphyseal trabecular bone on the other. Chondrocytes in the epiphyseal plate proliferate in columns towards the diaphysis, becoming hypertrophied as they deposit cartilage matrix. The matrix becomes progressively mineralized before osteoblasts deposit osteoid on the calcified matrix model. **(c)** Low-power micrograph of decalcified H&E-stained epiphyseal region from a long bone of a fetus, for comparison with **(b)**. Epiphyseal plate cartilage (E), the proliferative zone (PZ), the hypertrophic zone (HZ), the calcified cartilage zone (CCZ) and the beginning of the ossification zone (OZ) can be seen. At this stage, there is haemopoietic marrow in the spaces between the ossifying plates of cartilage (OC). Secondary ossification centres develop in the epiphyseal cartilage at a later stage of development.

In old age, the support tissue forming both syndesmoses and synchondroses tends to be replaced by bone to form a rigid immobile joint (synostosis).

> **A clinically important group of joints with limited movement are those between vertebrae.**

The bodies of the vertebrae are joined to each other by the intervertebral discs to form a long uninterrupted column (vertebral column). The discs are thick rubbery pads which not only act as shock absorbers but also permit some movement, so that the column is flexible within limits.

Intervertebral discs are composed of fibrocollagenous tissue containing some chondrocytes and cartilage matrix (fibrocartilage, see p. 79). The two surfaces in contact with the vertebral bodies each consist of a thin layer of hyaline cartilage covering a concentrically lamellated rubbery structure of fibrocartilage

(the annulus fibrosus). At the centre of the disc is a soft, semifluid core of gelatinous matrix (the nucleus pulposus, Fig. 13.28).

CLINICAL EXAMPLE

Sciatica

Wear and tear on the intervertebral discs may lead to degeneration of the annulus fibrosus, with outward protrusion of the nucleus pulposus. This results in:

- Impaired efficiency of the disc as a shock absorber
- Expansion of the annulus fibrosus, causing it to bulge

If the annulus fibrosus bulges in the region of the spinal nerves as they emerge from the spinal cord, the nerves may be stretched and damaged, producing peripheral nerve symptoms.

Intervertebral disc degeneration is most common in the lumbar region of the vertebral column and causes pressure on the nerves, producing sciatica – pain travelling down the back and outer side of the leg.

Fig. 13.28 Intervertebral Disc. (a) Micrograph of an acrylic resin section of an intervertebral disc (I) between two vertebrae (V) stained with H&E. **(b)** Micrograph of part of the same intervertebral disc at higher magnification, showing the annulus fibrosus (AF) forming a compact outer region adjacent to vertebral bone and the soft, semifluid at the centre, the nucleus pulposus (NP).

Joints that allow free movement between adjacent bones are termed synovial joints.

The bone ends are held together by bands of collagenous tissue (ligaments), which may be external or internal to the joint cavity; external ligaments surround a fibrous capsule enclosing the heads of the bones, which are separated from each other by a lubricant fluid, synovial fluid.

Because the bone ends move against each other (diarthrodial joints), they are coated with a smooth, friction-free layer of hyaline cartilage (articular cartilage), and the synovial fluid provides a thin lubricant film between the opposing articular cartilages.

The internal lining of the joint capsule is a specialized secretory epithelium, the synovium, which produces synovial fluid.

Synovium lines the spaces of diarthrodial joints but also lines tendon sheaths and bursae. A surface intimal layer overlies an underlying subintima and provides a lubricated surface allowing movement between adjacent tissues.

The synovial intima is composed of one to four layers of cells which vary from flat, mesothelial-like cells to spindle-shaped, polyhedral or cuboidal cells. Two cell types have been defined in synovial intima: type A cells are phagocytic and contain numerous lysosomes with cell markers showing a macrophagic origin, whereas type B cells contain abundant rough endoplasmic reticulum, are derived from fibroblasts and are adapted for production of hyaluronan.

The subintimal layer consists of a zone of loosely arranged fibrocollagenous tissue containing fibroblasts, mast cells and macrophages. There are blood and lymphatic vessels together with a nerve supply. A small number of lymphoid cells are usually present in the subintima, mainly T lymphocytes.

In some areas, the subintima is composed largely of adipocytes, for example, in association with fat, when the structure may be termed *adipose synovium.*

The term *fibrous synovium* is used to describe synovium covering tendons and structures such as the annular pads seen in finger joints and the meniscus structures in the knee joint. In these sites, the intimal layer lies directly on the underlying specialized structure separated by an ill-defined, thin collagenous layer.

Ligaments, composed of dense collagenous tissue, stabilize joints.

Structures around the joint that prevent excess movement include collagenous external ligaments and tendinous muscle attachments (Fig. 13.29). External ligaments surround articular (synovial) joints, attaching one bone to the other over the outer surface of the joint capsule.

Ligaments are composed of tightly packed collagen fibres all running in the same direction, with compressed fibrocytes in-between; thus they resemble tendon, but differ from tendon in that they contain elastic fibres. Ligaments strengthen the joint; they permit normal movement but prevent overflexing or overextension. The attachment of ligament to bone is like that of tendons.

In some complex joints, there are internal ligaments (e.g. cruciate ligaments in the knee joints) to prevent overstretching or twisting and fibrocartilaginous menisci (also in the knee) to stabilize and guide gliding movements.

Fig. 13.29 Synovial Joint. (a) A simple synovial joint showing the two articulating bone ends separated from each other by synovial fluid and enclosed within a fibrocollagenous capsule. Surrounding ligaments and tendinous muscle attachments prevent excess movement. **(b)** Low-power micrograph of an interphalangeal joint of the finger. Note the ends of the articulating bone (B), the articular cartilages (AC) and the joint capsule enclosing the synovial cavity (SC), which contains synovial fluid. The synovial cavity is lined internally by synovium.

CLINICAL EXAMPLE

Arthritis

Osteoarthritis

Some synovial joints, particularly the hip and finger joints, are exposed to persistent wear and tear over many years. This sometimes leads to degeneration of the articular cartilage, which loses its normal complement of hydrated glycosaminoglycans and so is unable to resist compressive forces. This leads to erosion of the cartilage and rubbing together of adjacent bone surfaces.

Eventually the surface bone becomes highly compacted and ivory-like; this is called *eburnation*.

The constant bone-to-bone trauma and excessive movement at the joint lead to a painful swollen joint with:

- Thickening of the joint capsule
- Irregular protuberances of abnormal new bone at the edges of the articular surfaces (osteophytes)
- Reduction in the synovial space

These are the typical changes of osteoarthritis.

Rheumatoid Arthritis

The synovium is the seat of another common form of arthritis called *rheumatoid arthritis*, an autoimmune disease causing immune-mediated damage to the synovial membrane, which then causes inflammatory destruction of adjacent articular cartilage.

The synovial membrane becomes thick and extensively infiltrated by cells of the immune system (mainly lymphocytes and plasma cells), and the damaged articular cartilage is replaced by vascular fibrocollagenous tissue (pannus). The condition leads to loss of the radiological joint space because of the loss of articular cartilage and deformity of affected joints.

CLINICAL EXAMPLE

Bursitis

Joint bursae can become inflamed (bursitis) and lead to pain on movement around a joint, tenderness and swelling as a result of accumulation of synovial fluid in the lumen. In many cases, bursitis is attributed to repetitive trauma (Fig. 13.30). Less commonly a bursa may become inflamed because of an infection or an autoimmune condition such as rheumatoid disease. In bursitis, the synovial lining of the bursa shows thickening caused by increased numbers of both type A (macrophages) and type B (fibroblast-like) synoviocytes. There is also proliferation of small blood vessels in the outer fibrous layer together with infiltration by inflammatory cells such as lymphocytes and macrophages. With chronicity, there is thickening of the outer fibrous layer caused by collagen deposition.

Fig. 13.30 Bursitis of Prepatellar Bursa. Bursitis can affect the prepatellar bursa, which lies over the knee between the patella and the overlying skin. The most common cause is chronic trauma, often the result of frequent kneeling, and is commonly referred to as *housemaid's knee*. On magnetic resonance imaging prepatellar bursitis appears as a fluid collection. **(a)** The drawing shows a fluid collection within the prepatellar bursa *(blue)*, located anteriorly to the patella (P) and the proximal part of the patellar tendon *(arrowheads)*. **(b)** Sagittal MRI showing a fluid signal collection anterior to the patella (P) indicating prepatellar bursitis *(arrowheads)*. (From Marra MD, Crema MD, Chung M, et al. MRI features of cystic lesions around the knee. *Knee.* 2008;15:423–438. Copyright 2008, with permission from Elsevier.)

For online review questions, please visit https://studentconsult.inkling.com.

Endocrine System

INTRODUCTION

Cell communication is vital for any multicellular organism to function efficiently.

At a local level, cells communicate via cell surface molecules and gap junctions, whereas remote communication is mediated by the secretion of chemical messengers, which activate cells by interacting with specific receptors. Such secretion may be one of four main types: autocrine, paracrine, endocrine or synaptic (Fig. 14.1).

Autocrine secretion occurs when a cell secretes a chemical messenger to act on its own receptors. This is particularly evident in the local control of cell growth by substances such as epidermal growth factor.

Paracrine secretion describes the secretion of chemical messengers to act on adjacent cells. This is also concerned mainly with the local control of cell growth and is a mode of action of many of the cells of the diffuse neuroendocrine system (see p. 288).

Endocrine secretion is the secretion of chemical messengers (hormones) into the bloodstream to act on distant tissues.

Synaptic secretion refers to communication by direct structural targeting from one cell to another via synapses, and this is confined to the nervous system.

The chemical messengers belong to four main molecular classes:
- Amino acid derivatives (e.g. epinephrine [adrenaline], norepinephrine [noradrenaline], thyroxine)
- Small peptides (e.g. encephalin, vasopressin, thyroid-releasing hormone)
- Proteins (e.g. nerve growth factor, epidermal growth factor, insulin, growth hormone, parathormone, thyroid-stimulating hormone)
- Steroids (e.g. cortisol, progesterone, oestradiol, testosterone)

Most chemical messengers are water-soluble hydrophilic molecules that diffuse freely and usually interact with a cell surface receptor protein. However, steroids and thyroxine are hydrophobic: after carriage to a cell by special proteins in the blood, they pass through its membrane to interact with receptor proteins inside.

Fig. 14.1 Secretion of Chemical Messengers. The four mechanisms of chemical messenger secretion.

ENDOCRINE CELL AND TISSUE SPECIALIZATION

> **Cells whose main role is to secrete messenger substances are termed *endocrine cells*.**

Endocrine cells are found in three distinct anatomic distributions:

- Gathered together in one specialized organ to form an endocrine gland (e.g. adrenal, pituitary, and pineal glands)
- Forming discrete clusters in another specialized organ (e.g. ovary, testis, pancreas)
- Dispersed singly among other cells in epithelial tissues, particularly in the gut and respiratory tract, in which case they form part of what is referred to as the *diffuse neuroendocrine system*

> **Endocrine cells and tissues have special characteristics related to their secretory function.**

Certain cells termed *neuroendocrine cells* have membrane-bound vesicles, which are granules containing the chemical messenger. Secretion is achieved by exocytosis, in which the membrane of the vesicle fuses with the cell membrane, thereby discharging its contents outside the cell. Neuroendocrine cells transiently store the messenger as specific neuroendocrine granules, which can be identified in cells using immunohistochemical staining techniques.

Endocrine tissues are usually highly vascular to facilitate rapid dissemination of secreted products into the bloodstream. In contrast to other types of secretory cells, the secretory pole of endocrine cells is adjacent to the capillary vessel wall and the nucleus is found at the opposite pole.

Autocrine and paracrine messengers act relatively quickly because they interact with local cell receptors and then are rapidly destroyed once secreted, thereby limiting their activity.

Endocrine messengers act relatively slowly, having to diffuse into the bloodstream, circulate to a target organ, and then enter a target cell. Many neuroendocrine cells secrete amines or peptides and have common metabolic features involving the uptake of amines, which then undergo decarboxylation in the process of hormone synthesis. This has led to the term *APUD cells* (amine precursor uptake and decarboxylation cells).

Cells containing neuroendocrine granules and of neuroendocrine lineage have a restricted set of specific metabolic isoenzymes and structural proteins, which can be detected histochemically. γ-Enolase is an isoenzyme in the glycolytic pathway that is present in high concentrations in neuroendocrine cells together with PGP 9.5 (ubiquitin-C-terminal hydrolase). In the neuroendocrine granules, chromogranin is a component of the core protein, and synaptophysin is a glycoprotein in their membrane. Histochemical detection of these substances enables their use as markers of neuroendocrine differentiation.

PITUITARY

> **The pituitary is a multifunctional endocrine gland.**

The pituitary gland secretes a large number of hormones to activate many peripheral endocrine cells: for example, those in the adrenal glands, thyroid, testes and ovaries.

The pituitary is a bean-shaped gland approximately $12 \times 10 \times 9$ mm in size and weighing 0.4–0.9 g in the adult. It is situated beneath the brain, to which it is linked by the pituitary stalk, and is surrounded by the bone of the base of the skull in a depression of the sphenoid bone termed the *sella turcica* (Fig. 14.2a).

Fig. 14.2 Pituitary Gland. (a) The pituitary gland and its relationship to surrounding structures. **(b)** Low-magnification H&E image showing the junction between the anterior pituitary (A) and the posterior pituitary (P). The adenohypophysis is composed of islands of pink-staining neuroendocrine cells, and the neurohypophysis is composed of pale-staining neuropil. Small cysts are seen (I) and represent part of the intermediate lobe. Some groups of neuroepithelial cells (T) are seen on the *left* of the image and represent part of the tuberal lobe.

The anterior pituitary (adenohypophysis) is an epithelial-derived tissue with three distinct components: the distal lobe (pars distalis) forms the major portion of the gland; the intermediate lobe (pars intermedia), which is a rudimentary zone in man but prominent in other mammals; and the tuberal lobe (pars tuberalis), which is a layer of cells running up the pituitary stalk (see Fig. 14.2a).

The posterior pituitary (neurohypophysis) is composed of neuronal processes and glia and has three components: the neural lobe (pars nervosa, infundibular process), lying behind the anterior pituitary in the sella turcica; the pituitary stalk (infundibular stem), in which axons run from the brain above; and the median eminence (infundibulum), a funnel-shaped extension of the hypothalamus (see Figs. 14.2a-14.2b).

The anterior pituitary is composed of islands of neuroepithelial cells, and the posterior pituitary is composed of axons and associated glial cells (see Fig. 14.2b).

Embryologically, the anterior pituitary is thought to be derived from an outgrowth of the foregut ectoderm called *Rathke's pouch*. This connects with a downgrowth of the developing hypothalamus, which forms the posterior pituitary and comes to lie in the base of the skull.

The vascular supply of the pituitary integrates the functions of the endocrine and nervous systems.

A special network of blood vessels (pituitary portal system, Fig. 14.3) carries hormones from the hypothalamus of the brain to stimulate or inhibit the hormone secretion of the anterior pituitary.

The major blood supply to the anterior pituitary is derived from vessels that run down the pituitary stalk. These are easily damaged in severe head injury, resulting in death of the anterior pituitary and consequent ablation of its endocrine function.

ANTERIOR PITUITARY

The anterior pituitary secretes several hormones into the bloodstream.

The anterior pituitary is served by a fine capillary network (see Fig. 14.3) which, bringing blood from the hypothalamus, contains both stimulatory and inhibitory hormones. These hormones control the neuroendocrine cells of the anterior pituitary. In turn, their secretions diffuse back into the capillary network, which subsequently drains into the pituitary veins and thence into the carotid venous sinus and systemic circulation.

The anterior pituitary is composed of islands of endocrine cells associated with a capillary vascular system (Fig. 14.4). The gland contains five distinct types of endocrine cells, which are not uniformly distributed within the gland (Fig. 14.5). Cells were originally named by their staining characteristics

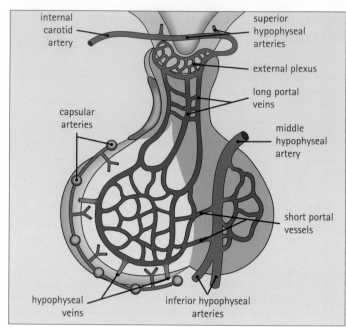

Fig. 14.3 Vascular Supply of the Pituitary. The blood supply of the pituitary arises from three paired arteries originating from the internal carotid arteries. The superior hypophyseal arteries enter the median eminence and form the external plexus close to nerve endings from neuroendocrine cells in the hypothalamus. This gives way to a parallel capillary network which surrounds larger central muscular vessels and runs down the pituitary stalk to form the long portal vessels. Arising from the portal vessels, capillary vessels run forward into the anterior pituitary, providing a direct vascular link between the hypothalamus and the neuroendocrine cells of the anterior pituitary. Additional blood supply to the posterior pituitary is derived from the small middle and inferior hypophyseal arteries. A minor blood supply to the periphery of the anterior pituitary is derived from small blood vessels in the capsule of the gland.

(Fig. 14.6), but it is now usual to name pituitary endocrine cells according to their specific hormone product. Pituitary endocrine cells have the same basic ultrastructure (Fig. 14.7). These cells are:

- Somatotrophs (Fig. 14.8), which secrete growth hormone (GH)
- Lactotrophs (Fig. 14.9), which secrete prolactin (PRL)
- Corticotrophs (Fig. 14.10), which secrete adrenocorticotropic hormone (ACTH), β-lipotropin (β-LPH), α-melanocyte stimulating hormone (α-MSH) and β-endorphin
- Thyrotrophs, which secrete thyroid-stimulating hormone (TSH)
- Gonadotrophs (Fig. 14.11), which secrete the gonadotropic hormones, follicle-stimulating hormone (FSH) and luteinizing hormone (LH)

The intermediate lobe of the anterior pituitary is relatively small in humans.

The intermediate lobe of the anterior pituitary is located between the posterior pituitary and the distal lobe (see Fig. 14.2). It is poorly developed in humans compared with other mammals, consisting of a series of gland-like acini lined by a cuboidal epithelium. These cells are usually immunoreactive for

Fig. 14.4 Anterior Pituitary Cells and Vessels. (a) H&E section showing a thin, indistinct capsule (C) beneath which there are endocrine cells arranged in islands. The endocrine cells vary in size, with both small (S), large (L) and intermediate-sized cells (M) in different islands. Cells also vary in their staining characteristics, with large cells typically being eosinophilic and granular, whereas smaller cells are amphophilic. These differences correspond to cells with different types of hormone secretions. (b) More detail can be seen in this toluidine blue resin section showing pituitary endocrine cells (E) arranged in groups and surrounded by capillaries (C). A dense capillary network facilitates hormone secretion.

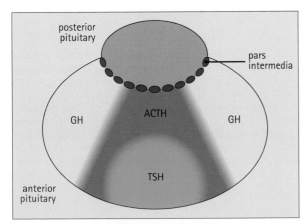

Fig. 14.5 Regional Distribution of Anterior Pituitary Cells. A horizontal cross-section of the distal lobe of the pituitary. The lateral wings contain mainly somatotrophs, which secrete GH, whereas corticotrophs, which secrete ACTH, β-lipotropin, α-MSH and β-endorphin, are concentrated in the median portion of the gland just in front of the posterior pituitary. Thyrotrophs, which secrete TSH, are concentrated anteriorly. Lactotrophs secreting PRL and gonadotrophs secreting FSH and LH are uniformly scattered throughout the gland.

Fig. 14.6 Traditional Methods for Demonstrating Cells of the Anterior Pituitary. Traditionally, cells of the anterior pituitary were classified into three types: acidophils (cytoplasm staining with acidic dyes), basophils (cytoplasm staining with basic dyes and the periodic acid–Schiff [PAS] method) and chromophobes (cells with no cytoplasmic staining). In the PAS orange-G haematoxylin stain shown here, acidophils (A) stain bright yellow, basophils (B) stain darkly and chromophobes (C) do not stain. Nuclei are stained black using haematoxylin. The acidophils correspond to production of GH or PRL (i.e. somatotrophs and lactotrophs), basophils correspond to thyrotrophs, corticotrophs and gonadotrophs. Basophils stain well with haematoxylin and PAS, which detect glycosyl groups, because TSH, LH and FSH are glycoproteins and the ACTH precursor protein is glycosylated. Chromophobes fail to stain because they contain very few granules and may be lactotroph, somatotroph, thyrotroph, gonadotroph or corticotroph in nature. Some cells, which contain sparse dense-core granules with no recognizable immunostaining, have been termed *null cells*.

Fig. 14.7 Ultrastructure of Anterior Pituitary Cells. Electron micrograph of anterior pituitary cells showing their numerous hormone-containing dense-core granules (G). It is possible to identify different types of endocrine cells by fine ultrastructural details of secretory vesicles and the pattern of distribution.

corticotropic hormones, and it has been suggested that they may be producing one of the minor subunits of the pre-pro-opiomelanocortic peptides, such as β-LPH, α-MSH or β-endorphin, rather than ACTH.

> **The tuberal lobe is an upward extension of the anterior pituitary around the pituitary stalk.**

The tuberal lobe consists of a thin layer of cuboidal epithelial cells. Immunohistochemically, most of the cells are gonadotrophs.

Occasionally, nests of squamous cells can be seen, from which cysts and even tumours may develop. It has been assumed that these are embryological remnants of the ectodermal Rathke's pouch.

Fig. 14.8 Somatotrophs. Somatotrophs make up about 50% of the anterior pituitary and are generally large, ovoid or polygonal in shape, as shown in this section stained to show GH by an immunoperoxidase method. Ultrastructurally, somatotrophs contain abundant, randomly distributed electron-dense granules, which measure from 300 to 600 nm in diameter, but the majority are between 350 and 450 nm. The rough endoplasmic reticulum is arranged in parallel stacks, many positioned parallel to the cell membranes. Tumours which are derived from somatotroph cells contain spherical bundles of intermediate filaments called *fibrous bodies*.

Fig. 14.10 Corticotrophs. Accounting for 15%–20% of the entire anterior pituitary cell population but tending to cluster, corticotrophs are large and polygonal in shape, as shown in this micrograph stained to show ACTH by an immunoperoxidase technique. Many corticotrophs possess an unstained perinuclear vacuole called the *enigmatic body,* which is derived from secondary lysosomes. Granules in corticotrophs are large and typically measure 250–700 nm in diameter. Large perinuclear bundles of intermediate cytokeratin filaments are prominent ultrastructurally, and these become even more prominent in glucocorticoid excess, when they are visible under the light microscope as pink-staining inclusions (Crooke's hyaline).

Fig. 14.9 Lactotrophs. Lactotrophs make up about 25% of the anterior pituitary. Although some are rounded and polygonal, most are compressed by adjacent cells into narrow angular profiles, as shown in this section of gland stained by an immunoperoxidase method to show prolactin. They increase in size and number during pregnancy and lactation. Ultrastructurally, lactotrophs have a prominent Golgi compared with all other anterior pituitary cells, and their granules measure 200–350 nm in diameter. Of interest, exocytosis may be seen at their lateral borders (misplaced exocytosis) and in the usual site adjacent to capillary basement membrane. This feature can be used in diagnostic assessment, as it is limited to lactotroph-derived tumours.

Fig. 14.11 Gonadotrophs. Constituting around 10% of anterior pituitary cells, gonadotrophs are scattered as single cells or small groups throughout the gland, as seen in this section which has been stained to show the β subunit of FSH by an immunoperoxidase technique. Both FSH and LH may be evident within the same cell. Ultrastructurally, the granules are 150–400 nm in diameter. After ablation of the ovaries or testes, gonadotrophs develop extensive cytoplasmic vacuolation. This is the result of dilation of the endoplasmic reticulum by stored product and caused by the loss of feedback inhibition by gonadal steroids. Such cells – large, rounded and vacuolated on light microscopy – are called *castration cells.*

CLINICAL EXAMPLE

Tumours of the Anterior Pituitary

The most important tumour of the anterior part of the pituitary gland is the benign **pituitary adenoma**. Although benign, this tumour causes severe symptoms for two reasons. First, it may grow large enough to push out of the small pituitary fossa and compress the optic chiasma and nerves that run over the top of the pituitary fossa; this causes severe visual disturbances and eventual blindness. The second reason is that some pituitary adenomas secrete excessive amounts of hormone, causing various endocrine syndromes. For example, the tumour illustrated in Fig. 14.12 was composed mainly of somatotrophs, which secreted large amounts of GH. In children this would produce gigantism; in adults the syndrome is called *acromegaly*.

Fig. 14.12 Pituitary Adenoma. An adenoma is a benign tumour of epithelial-type cells, including neuroepithelial cells. This H&E photomicrograph shows endocrine cells in a pituitary adenoma which was surgically removed from a patient by entering the pituitary fossa through the sphenoid sinus, via the nose. In contrast to normal pituitary, cells are of one morphological type and are not arranged in small islands. In areas, cells are arranged along capillaries, with the granule-filled secretory pole facing the vessel, which is characteristic of neurosecretory cells. Immunostaining showed growth hormone production.

POSTERIOR PITUITARY

> The posterior pituitary is a continuation of the hypothalamic region of the brain.

The posterior pituitary extends down into the pituitary stalk and sella turcica (see Fig. 14.2) and secretes oxytocin and antidiuretic hormone (vasopressin).

It is pale-staining in haematoxylin and eosin (H&E) sections, being composed of the axons of neuronal cells lying in the supraoptic and paraventricular nuclei of the hypothalamus, together with supporting glial cells termed *pituicytes* (Fig. 14.13).

Fig. 14.13 Posterior Pituitary. The posterior pituitary is composed of axons which originate from cells in the hypothalamus and possess numerous neurosecretory granules containing either oxytocin or vasopressin, together with a carrier protein termed *neurophysin*. Where axons are adjacent to capillaries, they form fusiform swellings filled with neurosecretory granules (Herring bodies) (H). The posterior pituitary also contains specialized stellate glial cells, similar to astrocytes, called *pituicytes* (P). In the micrograph, axons are seen as a pale fibrillary background neuropil (N) in which the pituicytes (P) and capillary vessels filled with red blood cells are present.

The axons terminate in the posterior pituitary as varicosities called **Herring bodies** located adjacent to a rich network of capillary vessels.

HYPOTHALAMUS

> The actions of the endocrine and nervous systems are coordinated by the hypothalamus.

The hypothalamus is a region of the brain composed of several clusters of neurons that secrete hormones. These hormones act as either releasing or inhibiting factors for the hormones secreted by the anterior pituitary and are transported to the pituitary gland by two routes as follows:

- A specialized system of blood vessels transports hypothalamic hormones to act locally on neuroendocrine cells in the anterior pituitary (Fig. 14.14).
- Axons project down from the hypothalamus to form the pituitary stalk, which terminates as the posterior pituitary.

⟫ KEY FACTS

Pituitary Gland and Hypothalamus

- Anterior pituitary secretes PRL, GH, ACTH, TSH, FSH, and LH
- Posterior pituitary stores and secretes oxytocin and ADH, which are made in hypothalamic nuclei
- Hypothalamus is in direct communication with the posterior pituitary via the pituitary stalk and the anterior pituitary via the pituitary portal vessels
- Hypothalamus produces hormones that stimulate or inhibit the release of anterior pituitary hormones

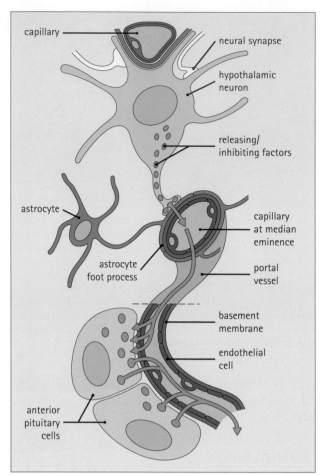

Fig. 14.14 Hypothalamic Control of Anterior Pituitary Hormone Production. Hypothalamic neurons secrete releasing/inhibiting factors in response to chemoreceptive and neural inputs. These hormones diffuse into capillaries at the median eminence and are carried to the anterior pituitary in the portal vessels. Astrocyte foot processes surrounding the capillary vessels form part of their diffusion barrier.

◎ ADVANCED CONCEPT

Hypothalamic Hormones

At least eight hormones are known to be secreted by hypothalamic neurons. Two of these are the peptides **oxytocin** and **arginine vasopressin**, synthesized in the cell bodies of neurons in the supraoptic and paraventricular nuclei of the hypothalamus. They pass down axons into the posterior pituitary via the pituitary stalk and are released into the capillaries of the posterior pituitary.

The other hypothalamic hormones are inhibiting or releasing hormones controlling the secretion of anterior pituitary hormones. They are transported via the pituitary portal vessels (see Fig. 14.14). These are:

- Thyrotropin-releasing hormone (TRH) – mainly from paraventricular nucleus
- Gonadotropin-releasing hormone (GnRH) – mainly from arcuate nucleus and preoptic area
- Growth hormone–releasing hormone (GHRH) – mainly from arcuate nucleus
- Corticotropin-releasing hormone (CRH) – from anterior part of paraventricular nucleus
- Growth hormone–inhibiting hormone (GIH) – also known as **somatostatin** (SS) – from paraventricular nuclei
- Prolactin release–inhibiting hormone (PIH) – also known as **dopamine** (DA) – from arcuate nuclei.

No single prolactin-releasing hormone has been found, but other hormones have this action (e.g. oxytocin, vasoactive intestinal polypeptide [VIP] and TRH).

PINEAL GLAND

> **The pineal gland secretes melatonin.**

The pineal gland is located just below the posterior end of the corpus callosum of the brain. It is a flattened conical structure 6–10-mm long and 5–6-mm wide; it is covered by leptomeninges and composed of lobules of specialized cells, which are separated by septa containing unmyelinated nerves and blood vessels (Fig. 14.15). The gland consists of two major cell types: pinealocytes and glial cells.

Pinealocytes are neuron-like cells that produce melatonin, which induces rhythmic changes in the secretions of the hypothalamus, pituitary and gonads, and is said to act as an endocrine transducer. They have pink-staining cytoplasm and dark-staining rounded nuclei and are often arranged in rosettes, where several cells surround a central fibrillary area composed of cell processes directed toward a small capillary vessel.

Glial cells tend to be bipolar elongated cells that run between nests of pinealocytes. They are indistinct unless specially stained.

A common age-related change in the pineal is the accumulation of calcium particles, which are visible on a skull radiograph; thus the gland can be used as a radiological midline landmark.

The pineal gland is innervated by sympathetic and parasympathetic nervous systems. In addition, signals from the retina arrive indirectly, as shown in Fig. 14.15a.

THYROID GLAND

Introduction

The thyroid gland secretes two hormones, thyroid hormones (triiodothyronine [T_3] and thyroxine [T_4]) and calcitonin. Thyroid hormones have a major role in the regulation of the basal metabolic rate, whereas calcitonin is involved in calcium homeostasis.

> **The thyroid gland consists of two lateral lobes and an isthmus.**

The lateral lobes of the thyroid are arranged on either side of the thyroid cartilage and upper trachea in the anterior portion of the neck. These lobes are joined near their lower poles by the isthmus crossing in front of the lower larynx; occasionally, a small triangular pyramidal lobe projects upward from the midpoint of the isthmus.

Each lateral lobe is about 5-cm long, 3–4-cm wide and 2–3-cm deep. In the healthy adult, the thyroid weighs 15–20 g and is slightly heavier in males, although many factors influence its weight at any one time, for example, pathological abnormalities.

The thyroid is enclosed by a thin collagenous capsule from which internal septa penetrate the parenchyma, dividing it into irregular lobules.

Fig. 14.16 Thyroid. (a) Micrograph showing normal human thyroid composed of variable-sized follicles (F) filled with pink-staining thyroid colloid. In this illustration the thyroid follicles are in a storage phase, so the lining epithelium (E) is cuboidal or flat and the stored colloid fills the follicle. There is a complex intimate capillary network between adjacent follicles. The details of the thyroid epithelial cell in an active phase are illustrated in Fig. 14.17 and the calcitonin-secreting component of the thyroid in Fig. 14.18. **(b)** Micrograph showing thyroid acinus composed of specialized thyroid epithelium (TE) resting on a basement membrane (BM). These epithelial cells enclose a lumen filled with thyroid colloid (TC) and are surrounded by a fine network of capillaries (C) associated with thin fibrous septa.

Embryologically, the thyroid develops from a downgrowth of endoderm arising near the root of the tongue and called the *thyroglossal duct,* which atrophies and leaves a nodule of thyroid tissue at its correct anatomic site.

Occasionally, the thyroglossal duct fails to atrophy completely, and thyroglossal duct tissue persists in the midline of the neck, usually as a cyst or a sinus tract (thyroglossal duct cyst).

> **The thyroid gland contains colloid, which is rich in thyroglobulin.**

The glandular component of the thyroid is composed of epithelium arranged as tightly packed spherical units called *acini* (Fig. 14.16).

Each acinus is lined by a single layer of specialized thyroid epithelium, which rests on a basement membrane and encloses a lumen filled with thyroid colloid, a pink-staining (eosinophilic) homogeneous proteinaceous material rich in thyroglobulin.

Fig. 14.15 Pineal Gland. (a) The location of the pineal gland. Output of pineal melatonin is modulated by light through nervous pathways which input as sympathetic innervation to the gland. **(b)** Low-power micrograph of a reticulin-stained section of pineal showing the septa (S) that divide it into discrete lobules (L) of pinealocytes. **(c)** High-power micrograph of an H&E-stained section of pineal showing a single pineal lobule surrounded by septa composed of glial processes and small vessels. In the centre of the lobule, pinealocyte cell bodies are found in a background of pink-staining cell processes, some of which form a rosette structure.

Thyroglobulin is the storage form of thyroxine and is an iodinated glycoprotein (Fig. 14.17). The size of an acinus depends on whether it is in a secretory or a storage phase.

During an active secretory phase, the thyroid follicular cells show the following changes:

- The endoplasmic reticulum becomes more prominent.
- Free ribosomes become more prominent.
- The Golgi enlarges.
- The surface microvilli increase in number and length.
- Intracytoplasmic droplets appear (representing colloid in endocytotic vesicles generated by pseudopodial extensions of cytoplasm at the luminal surface).

> **The synthesis and breakdown of thyroglobulin are controlled by the hypothalamus and pituitary gland.**

Low blood thyroxine levels stimulate the hypothalamus to produce Thyrotropin-releasing hormone (TRH) which then stimulates the anterior pituitary to produce Thyroid-stimulating hormone (TSH). In turn, TSH stimulates both thyroglobulin synthesis and breakdown, with a consequent increase in thyroxine release into the capillary circulation. When thyroxine levels rise, TRH and TSH production decreases.

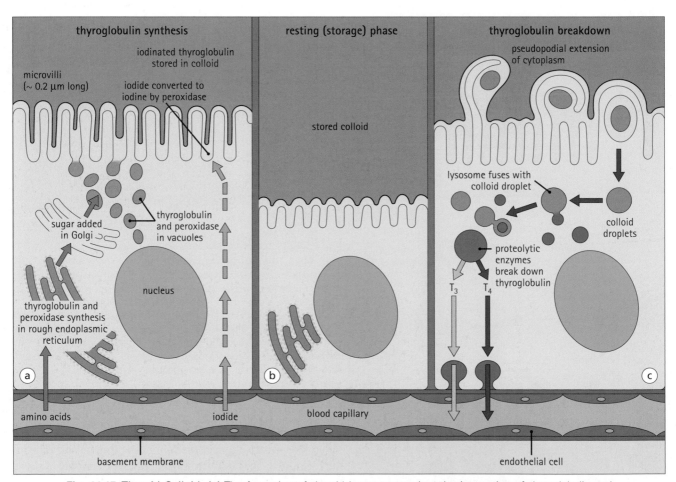

Fig. 14.17 Thyroid Colloid. (a) The formation of thyroid hormone requires the interaction of thyroglobulin and iodine. Thyroglobulin is produced by the thyroid epithelial cells, with its protein component being synthesized in the rough endoplasmic reticulum and transported by the Golgi, where most of its sugar component is added by glycosylation. The thyroid epithelial cell is able to transport iodide against a concentration gradient from the capillary blood to where it is concentrated in the lumen of the follicle. However, iodide requires conversion to iodine, which is performed by the enzyme thyroid peroxidase. This enzyme is also synthesized in the epithelial cell and enters the same secretory vesicles as contain thyroglobulin. Thyroglobulin and thyroid peroxidase leave the exit face of the Golgi from small vacuoles, which are transported to the luminal surface. They are released into the lumen by exocytosis. Once secreted at the cell membrane, thyroid peroxidase becomes active and converts iodide into iodine. Iodine is then added to the tyrosine component of thyroglobulin. **(b)** Thyroglobulin acts as a reservoir from which thyroxine can be produced and secreted into the capillary circulation when required. **(c)** To release thyroxine from the stored colloid, the thyroid epithelial cell extrudes pseudopodial extensions of cytoplasm from its luminal surface; these enclose small droplets of colloid, which are then incorporated into its cytoplasm. Lysosomes fuse with the small vacuoles, and hydrolysis and proteolysis of the thyroglobulin occur, breaking it into smaller units, the most important of which is tetraiodothyronine (T_4) or thyroxine. Another product is triiodothyronine (T_3). Both are iodinated amino acids.

◎ ADVANCED CONCEPT

Thyroid Hormones

The two hormones are triiodothyronine (T_3) and thyroxine, which is tetraiodothyronine (T_4), both of which are iodinated derivatives of tyrosine. The thyroid follicular cells produce and secrete mainly T_4 (only 5%–10% of the thyroid's output is T_3), but T_3 is functionally much more potent than T_4. Most of the active T_3 is produced in other tissues by the removal of one iodine molecule from T_4; the kidney and liver are particularly important deiodinators of T_4. In the plasma, both T_3 and T_4 are largely bound to a protein, thyroxine-binding globulin (TBG); probably only the free non-bound hormones are physiologically active.

The thyroid also produces the hormone calcitonin.

Calcitonin inhibits calcium resorption from bones by osteoclasts, thus antagonizing the action of parathormone (see p. 280) and lowering blood calcium levels. It may increase the rate of osteoid mineralization.

Calcitonin-producing cells (C cells) are scattered between the thyroid acinus (follicle) lining cells and are occasionally seen in small clusters in the interstitial spaces between adjacent acini. The latter location, most common in animals, such as the dog, explains the archaic name *parafollicular cells*.

C cells are small pale-staining cells, which are difficult to see by routine light microscopy but can be identified either by electron microscopy or by immunohistochemical techniques (Fig. 14.18). Ultrastructurally, they contain the dense-core neurosecretory granules that are characteristic of neuroendocrine cells.

Calcitonin secretion seems to be controlled directly by blood calcium levels.

Fig. 14.18 Thyroid C Cells. Micrograph showing the distribution of thyroid C cells *(brown)* stained using an immunohistochemical method for calcitonin in the adult thyroid; they are present amongst the thyroid acinus lining cells and in some interstitial clusters. (Image used under Creative Commons License. https://creativecommons.org/licenses/by-sa/3.0/. From the Human Protein Atlas. Antibody to calcitonin HPA064453. https://www.proteinatlas.org/ENSG00000110680-CALCA/tissue/thyroid+gland.)

◫ CLINICAL EXAMPLE

Thyroid Cancer

Most malignant thyroid tumours are derived from the glandular epithelial cells lining the thyroid follicles and are therefore thyroid adenocarcinomas. A rare tumour, called *medullary carcinoma*, is derived from the thyroid C cells and secretes excessive amounts of calcitonin. Both tumours can spread by lymphatics and present clinically as enlarged lymph nodes in the neck. Certain types of thyroid cancer spread by the bloodstream to lung and bone.

◫ CLINICAL EXAMPLE

The Most Common Cause of Thyrotoxicosis Is an Autoimmune Disease

In thyrotoxicosis there is overproduction of thyroid hormones. The most common cause is Graves' disease, in which autoantibodies develop and target the TSH receptors found on thyroid epithelial cells. The cells are stimulated and increase in size and number, producing excess thyroid hormones (Fig. 14.19).

Hyperthyroidism linked to Graves' disease manifests clinically by weight loss and heat intolerance (caused by an increased basal metabolic rate), tremor and rapid pulse. There is bulging of the eyes (exophthalmos) owing to an increase in the orbital support tissues, linked to the autoimmune process.

Fig. 14.19 Thyrotoxic Hyperplasia. Micrograph showing the characteristic features of hyperplastic thyroid in Graves' disease. The epithelial cells lining thyroid acini have been stimulated to proliferate (hyperplasia) and, instead of being cuboidal (see Fig. 14.16), are tall and columnar. There is less colloid seen in acini (A) than in normal thyroid. In some acini the increased number of thyroid epithelial cells causes development of papillary folds of acinar epithelium. The increased stimulation of the thyroid leads to excess secretion of thyroid hormones and thyrotoxicosis. (Micrograph from digital pathology whole slide image provided by the University of Leeds Virtual Pathology Project https://www.virtualpathology.leeds.ac.uk. Reproduced with permission.)

PARATHYROID

> **The parathyroid glands secrete parathormone, which is involved in calcium homeostasis.**

The parathyroid glands, of which there are at least four and, in some people, up to eight, are small, pale, tan endocrine glands. They are usually ovoid in shape but are occasionally flattened by moulding from adjacent organs or tissues.

Each gland is approximately 5-mm long, 3-mm wide and 1–2-mm thick, although size varies considerably with age and calcium metabolic status. In adults, each gland weighs approximately 130 mg, with those in women being slightly heavier than in men.

The parathyroid glands are sited in the neck in the region of the thyroid gland, but their precise location is variable. They are derived from the third and fourth branchial pouches, with the glands from the third pouch being located near the lower pole of the thyroid, whereas those from the fourth pouch lie close to the upper pole, either behind it or at the cricothyroid junction; those behind the upper pole are often sited inside the thyroid capsule and are therefore apparently intrathyroidal.

The parathyroids at the lower pole have a much more variable location. Approximately half are sited on the anterior or posterior surface of the lower pole of the lateral lobes, with the other half being located in the thymic tongue just beneath the lower pole. Occasionally, parathyroid glands may be found in the mediastinum, within thymic remnants.

The parathyroid glands secrete the hormone parathormone, which is important in maintaining calcium homeostasis. It increases calcium ion concentration in the blood by mobilizing the calcium stored in mineralized bone. Parathormone achieves this by stimulating osteoclasts to erode bone from the surfaces of bone trabeculae (see p. 258). When the serum calcium level falls, an increase in parathormone secretion equalizes it by mobilizing the stored calcium in bone. Excessive secretion of parathormone leads to structural damage to bone and excess calcium in the blood (hypercalcaemia, see Clinical Example box, p. 282).

> **Three main histological cell types are seen in the parathyroid.**

The normal adult human parathyroid is surrounded by a thin fibrous capsule and is composed of three cell types:

- Adipocytes
- Chief cells, which produce parathormone
- Oxyphil cells

Adipocytes appear in the parathyroid at puberty and gradually increase in number until about the age of 40, from then on remaining a fairly constant proportion of the entire gland, although their number may decrease in old age. They form a background stroma in which the chief and oxyphil cells are arranged in cords and nests close to a fine network of capillary vessels (Fig. 14.20b).

When there is a continuous increased requirement for parathormone, for example, when the serum calcium level is persistently low in renal failure, the chief cells increase in number (hyperplasia) at the expense of the adipocytes.

> **Parathyroid chief cells are the active endocrine component of the gland.**

Chief cells are about 8–10 μm in diameter and are roughly spherical in shape. Their nuclei are small, round, dark staining and central, and their cytoplasm is usually pale pinkish-purple (see Fig. 14.20c), although at certain stages, they become vacuolated with glycogen and lipid, when they are sometimes referred to as *clear cells*.

Their ultrastructural appearance depends largely on whether they are in a resting, synthesizing or secreting stage of hormone response. They contain membrane-bound neuroendocrine granules of parathormone, commonly arranged toward the periphery of the cell. In the synthesizing phase, there are stacks of rough endoplasmic reticulum and an active Golgi. In the resting phase, the neuroendocrine granules are still present, but the Golgi is small and the rough endoplasmic reticulum less prominent; glycogen granules and small lipid droplets are also seen. The glycogen and lipid become less apparent during hormone synthesis but reappear when the cells are secreting the packaged hormone.

In the healthy adult with a normal calcium balance, approximately 80% of the chief cells are in the resting phase. If hypercalcaemia develops, this proportion increases to 100% (and the cells contain numerous fine lipid droplets), but it decreases with transient or permanent hypocalcaemia. On light microscopy a synthesizing or secreting chief cell can be identified by its purplish cytoplasm and the absence of fine lipid droplets (see Fig. 14.20c).

> **Parathyroid oxyphil cells are larger than chief cells and have abundant eosinophilic cytoplasm.**

Parathyroid oxyphil cells are greater than 10 μm in diameter, and the cytoplasm is markedly eosinophilic and granular owing to the presence of many mitochondria. Their nuclei are small, spherical and dark staining (see Fig. 14.20c).

Ultrastructurally, oxyphil cell cytoplasm is packed with large active mitochondria, with intervening cytoplasm containing only scanty free ribosomes and glycogen granules; endoplasmic reticulum and neurosecretory vacuoles are uncommon, suggesting that the cells are not endocrinologically active (see Fig. 14.20d). Transitional cell forms with features of both oxyphil and active chief cells are occasionally seen.

Fig. 14.20 Parathyroid. (a) Micrograph showing a child's parathyroid gland (P) closely associated with lymphoid tissue (L). The gland is almost entirely composed of endocrine cells separated by fibrocollagenous septa (S) rich in blood vessels. With increasing age, progressively more adipose tissue develops in the parathyroid gland. **(b)** Low-power micrograph of an H&E-stained section of parathyroid. Note the adipocytes (A), which are seen as non-staining areas. **(c)** High-power micrograph of an H&E-stained section of parathyroid showing chief cells (C) and oxyphil cells (O). **(d)** Electron micrograph of parathyroid showing the edge of an oxyphil cell and its nucleus (N). Note the scanty peripheral neurosecretory granules (G) and numerous mitochondria (M) in this resting phase cell. (Micrograph (b) and (c) from digital pathology whole slide image provided by the University of Leeds Virtual Pathology Project https://www.virtualpathology.leeds.ac.uk. Reproduced with permission.)

Oxyphil cells are rare before puberty but appear in increasing numbers in early adult life, either singly or in clumps. In the elderly, they are often numerous and sometimes form variably sized oval or rounded tumour-like nodules within a normal-sized parathyroid. They also increase in number in people who have chronic kidney disease.

CLINICAL EXAMPLE

Disorders of Parathormone Secretion: Hypocalcaemia

Secretion of parathormone by the parathyroid glands is finely controlled by a feedback loop based on the level of calcium ions in the blood. When Ca^{2+} in the blood falls below an acceptable level, a burst of parathormone secretion stimulates osteoclasts to erode just enough bone to release the appropriate amount of calcium to bring the blood level back to normal, when a feedback mechanism stops further parathormone secretion. When calcium loss is excessive and persistent (e.g. in some examples of kidney disease, when calcium ions are constantly lost in large amounts in the urine), the persistently low serum calcium levels (hypocalcaemia) act as a constant stimulus to parathormone production in an attempt to compensate. All parathyroid glands become filled with actively hormone-secreting chief cells and enlarge. This increase in cell number is called **parathyroid hyperplasia**. This massive consistent outpouring of parathormone stimulates extensive erosion of bone by osteoclasts, and the architecture of the bone is destroyed, leading to severe bone disease. Parathyroid hyperplasia in response to hypocalcaemia is called **secondary hyperparathyroidism**; despite the enormous release of calcium in this way, it usually does not compensate for the vast amounts being lost in the urine by the diseased kidneys, and the serum calcium level rarely rises back to normal limits.

Hypocalcaemia can also occur when all the parathyroid glands are inadvertently removed surgically during total removal of the thyroid, usually for cancer. It may also be the result of inadequate absorption of dietary calcium.

Tumours of the Parathyroid

The main tumour that occurs in the parathyroid glands is the benign **parathyroid adenoma** (Fig. 14.21). These tumours are almost always solitary and cause enlargement of the affected parathyroid gland. This tumour constantly secretes excess parathormone, irrespective of the serum calcium level, and constant osteoclastic erosion of the bone leads to extensive bone destruction and very high levels of calcium ions in the blood (**hypercalcaemia**). This is called **primary hyperparathyroidism**.

Fig. 14.21 Parathyroid Adenoma. (a) This very low-magnification image shows a parathyroid gland removed surgically. It was the only enlarged gland found using imaging. It is replaced by a solid mass of endocrine cells, which is a benign tumour, termed an *adenoma*. **(b)** Micrograph showing the cells of the parathyroid adenoma. Note that the tumour is composed of sheets of chief cells and that the usual adipose tissue component has been replaced by tumour cells. (Micrograph from digital pathology whole slide image provided by the University of Leeds Virtual Pathology Project https://www.virtualpathology.leeds.ac.uk. Reproduced with permission.)

ADRENALS

Introduction

The adrenal glands are located on the upper poles of the kidneys and combine two distinct endocrine systems within one organ. The adrenal cortex synthesizes and secretes steroid hormones produced from cholesterol. The adrenal medulla is a neuroendocrine component, synthesizing and secreting the vasoactive amines epinephrine (adrenaline) and norepinephrine (noradrenaline).

Adrenal Cortex

> The adrenal cortex secretes steroid hormones.

The adrenal cortex – the outer layer of the adrenal gland in the adult – is composed of three distinct zones. These zones, the zona glomerulosa, zona fasciculata and zona reticularis, are bound externally by a thin fibrous capsule and internally by the adrenal medulla (Fig. 14.22).

Fig. 14.22 Adrenal Cortex. (a) Low-power micrograph showing adrenal cortex (C) and medulla (M). Three distinct zones can be seen in the cortex, the zona glomerulosa (ZG), zona fasciculata (ZF) and zona reticularis (ZR). **(b)** Micrograph showing the adrenal cortex at higher magnification. Note the zona glomerulosa (ZG), zona fasciculata (ZF) and zona reticularis (ZR). The zona fasciculata is the middle zone and is composed of pale-staining cells rich in lipid droplets. The histological details of the cells in these zones are shown in greater detail in Figs. 14.23, 14.24 and 14.25.

Fig. 14.23 Zona Glomerulosa. (a) The zona glomerulosa is composed of small compact cells (C) arranged in clumps and separated by stroma composed largely of thin-walled capillaries. The cells contain scanty lipid droplets associated with well-developed smooth endoplasmic reticulum and comparatively little rough endoplasmic reticulum. **(b)** Immunostaining for CD56 highlights the zona glomerulosa as a zone of intensely stained cells, contrasting with less intense staining of the membrane of the zona fasciculata below (Image used under Creative Commons License. https://creativecommons.org/licenses/by-sa/3.0/. From the Human Protein Atlas. Antibody to CD56 CAB000142. https://www.proteinatlas.org/ENSG00000149294-NCAM1/tissue/adrenal+gland#img.)

Fig. 14.24 Zona Fasciculata. (a) These cells are arranged in vertical columns, which are usually two to three cells wide, the columns being separated by capillaries (Cap). **(b)** Ultrastructurally, the cells have prominent rough endoplasmic reticulum, characteristic small round or ovoid mitochondria with tubular cristae and extensive lipid vacuoles. The surfaces of cells adjacent to capillaries may show small microvilli extending to the capillary wall.

The outer zona glomerulosa (Fig. 14.23) synthesizes and secretes mineralocorticoids, mainly aldosterone and deoxycorticosterone. The zona glomerulosa is the thin subcapsular zone of adrenal cortex that merges imperceptibly on its inner surface with the middle zona fasciculata. It is not always a complete layer and has a patchy distribution.

The middle zona fasciculata (Fig. 14.24) secretes glucocorticoids, mainly cortisol and corticosterone, and also small amounts of the androgenic steroid dehydroepiandrosterone (DHA). The zona fasciculata occupies most of the adrenal cortex and is composed of large rectangular cells with light-staining clear or finely vacuolated cytoplasm caused by intracytoplasmic accumulation of lipid droplets containing cholesterol and intermediate lipids, in addition to formed glucocorticoids.

The inner zona reticularis (Fig. 14.25) produces androgenic steroids and some glucocorticoids, but normally only in small amounts. This inner zone of adrenal cortex is thinner than the zona fasciculata but thicker than the zona glomerulosa. It is composed of cells with eosinophilic cytoplasm arranged in an anastomosing network of clumps and columns with a capillary network closely apposed to the cell membranes. A characteristic feature of this layer when stained with H&E is the presence of brown pigment (lipofuscin). To the naked eye, the layer appears pale brown, whereas the zona fasciculata is bright yellow.

Ultrastructurally, the cells possess prominent smooth endoplasmic reticulum and electron-dense irregular aggregations of lipofuscin, along with lysosomes and oval or long mitochondria, with tubular cristae similar to those seen in the cells of the zona fasciculata.

Fig. 14.25 Zona Reticularis.

> **The adrenal in the fetus has an extra outer cell layer.**

In the fetus and neonate, the adrenal cortex is proportionately much larger than in the adult and has an additional external cortical zone. This additional outer layer involutes after birth, with the three layers of the adult cortex developing from the remaining cells. The cells that involute have the appearance of steroid-secreting cells, possessing a large Golgi and many lipid droplets; furthermore, they have round mitochondria with tubular cristae similar to those of the adult zona fasciculata.

Activity of the fetal adrenal cortex is controlled partly by the fetal pituitary through the feedback of cortisol on pituitary ACTH secretion and partly by the placenta.

Adrenal Medulla

> **The adrenal medulla secretes catecholamines.**

The adrenal medulla, the centre of the adrenal gland, is surrounded by adrenal cortex. The adrenal medulla is derived from the neural crest and is part of the neuroendocrine system, secreting epinephrine (adrenaline), norepinephrine (noradrenaline) and associated peptides, including enkephalins. Epinephrine and norepinephrine synthesis is controlled by sympathetic and parasympathetic nerve twigs present in the gland.

Adrenal medullary cells have large, commonly pale-staining nuclei, and their cytoplasm is usually finely granular, with a purplish-staining reaction. They are usually polyhedral in shape, arranged in clumps, cords or columns and surrounded by a rich network of capillaries (Fig. 14.26a).

> **Cells of the adrenal medulla contain neurosecretory granules.**

Ultrastructurally, cells of the adrenal medulla contain neuroendocrine granules. These vary in size and appearance, ranging from 150 to 350 nm in diameter.

Cells secreting epinephrine (adrenaline) have small, spherical neuroendocrine granules almost entirely occupied by electron-dense material with a narrow, clear halo between the central material and the thin surrounding membrane.

Cells secreting norepinephrine (noradrenaline) have larger neuroendocrine granules with a more obvious electron-lucent layer inside the membrane, with the granules containing irregular and often angulated electron-dense material (see Fig. 14.26b).

Adrenal medullary cells synthesize and store their respective peptide hormones, normally releasing only small amounts at a time, although during periods of acute stress or excitement, larger quantities are secreted under the influence of the autonomic nervous system.

Because of their high catecholamine content, adrenal medullary cells develop an intense brown colour when exposed to air or to a strong oxidizing agent, such as potassium dichromate, owing to the formation of brown pigment when the amines are oxidized. This is the basis of their antiquated name *chromaffin cells.*

Fig. 14.26 Adrenal Medulla. **(a)** Micrograph of adrenal medullary cells showing their large nuclei and finely granular cytoplasm. **(b)** Electron micrograph showing large dense-core granules corresponding to norepinephrine (noradrenaline) (N) and epinephrine (adrenaline) (E).

 CLINICAL EXAMPLE

There are two tumours of the adrenal medulla; they are uncommon but very important.

Phaeochromocytoma is usually benign, in that it enlarges but does not spread to distant sites. Although benign, it produces severe symptoms and may be fatal. This is because it is derived from cells that produce epinephrine (adrenaline) and norepinephrine (noradrenaline), and the tumours produce these active chemicals in excessive amounts, leading to uncontrollable high blood pressure, which may be fatally complicated by a stroke or severe heart failure.

Neuroblastoma is a highly malignant tumour of the adrenal medulla usually seen in childhood and that is derived from primitive neural crest embryonic stem cells (neuroblasts), from which the adrenal medulla develops in embryonic life. Occasionally, some of these cells persist after birth and may develop into this tumour. This is an example of a so-called *embryonal* tumour; another type is seen in the kidney in children (nephroblastoma, see p. 323).

There is a rich vascular supply to both the cortex and medulla.

The adrenal glands receive a rich arterial supply, which forms an arterial plexus of capsular arteries over their surface. Two types of vessels are derived from these arteries: cortical arterioles and medullary arterioles; they supply blood to the cortex and medulla, respectively, although there is communication between the two systems at the interface between the cortex and medulla. The vascular supply is shown in Fig. 14.27.

▶ **KEY FACTS**

Adrenal

- Zona glomerulosa (narrow, subcapsular zone of cortex) secretes mineralocorticoids, mainly aldosterone.
- Zona fasciculata (broad, yellow mid-zone of cortex) secretes glucocorticoids, mainly cortisol and corticosterone.
- Zona reticularis (narrow inner zone of cortex) secretes mainly androgenic steroids.
- Adrenal medulla (central, enclosed by cortex, brown) is neuroendocrine and secretes epinephrine (adrenaline) and norepinephrine (noradrenaline).

PANCREAS

Introduction

The neuroendocrine component of the human pancreas exists in three forms:

- Islets of Langerhans are distinct structures accounting for most of the hormone-producing cells.
- Isolated nests or clumps of neuroendocrine cells form a minority population of cells gathered into small groups, which are distinct from islets.
- Single cells are scattered within the exocrine (see p. 227) and ductular components of the pancreas and are demonstrable by immunocytochemical methods.

Pancreatic endocrine cells are grouped into clusters called *islets of Langerhans.*

Islets of Langerhans are discrete, rounded clusters of cells scattered throughout the pancreatic tissue (Fig. 14.28a). They are embedded in its exocrine component and are most numerous in the tail region. They vary considerably in size and in the number of cells they contain. Individual cells within the islets are smaller and paler than the exocrine cells and assume spherical or polygonal shapes owing to moulding by adjacent cells. Each islet has a capillary network which is in contact with each cell (see Fig. 14.28b).

Pancreatic islets develop as cellular buds from the same small ducts that ultimately supply the exocrine pancreatic components. Occasionally in humans, variably sized islets can be seen in association with a pancreatic duct in the supporting fibrous tissue.

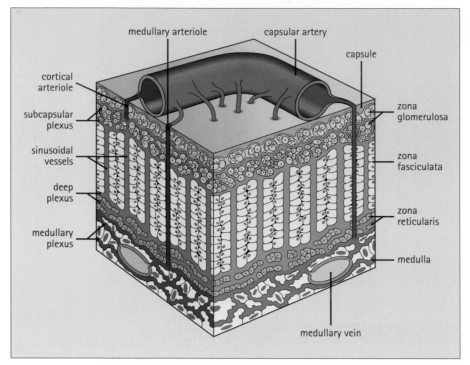

Fig. 14.27 Vascular Anatomy of the Adrenal Gland. Cortical arterioles form a subcapsular plexus. This gives rise to sinusoidal vessels running down between the columns of the zona fasciculata of the adrenal cortex before forming a further deep plexus in the zona reticularis. This deeper plexus communicates with the plexus of vessels supplying the medulla. Medullary arterioles arise directly from the capsular arteries and run straight down through the cortex into the medulla, where they form a medullary plexus. The deep medullary plexus drains by small venous vessels into the large medullary vein.

🧍 CLINICAL EXAMPLE

Diabetes Mellitus

Diabetes mellitus is a disease in which there is inadequate action of the hormone insulin. It is a multisystem disease that affects carbohydrate, fat and protein metabolism.

Two main types of diabetes mellitus are identified on clinical grounds:
- **Type 1** diabetes (insulin-dependent diabetes mellitus [IDDM]). This usually develops in childhood or adolescence but is increasingly recognized in older patients. It is an autoimmune disorder in which the insulin-secreting pancreatic islet cells are destroyed. The pancreas shows loss of β cells with infiltrating lymphocytes responsible for their destruction. This is a β-cell–specific autoimmune process that may be caused by an abnormal immune response to certain viral infections. The destruction of insulin-secreting cells leads to insulin deficiency, which in turn leads to hyperglycaemia and other secondary metabolic complications.
- **Type 2** diabetes (non–insulin-dependent diabetes mellitus [NIDDM] or maturity-onset diabetes). This type of disease is more common than type 1 diabetes. Unlike type 1 diabetes, where there is a loss of insulin-secreting cells from the pancreatic islets, in type 2 diabetes, disease is the result of the phenomenon of peripheral insulin resistance.

In diseases that destroy the pancreas, islet cells are lost in addition to the exocrine part of the pancreas. Patients with chronic pancreatitis or patients with cystic fibrosis may develop diabetes mellitus as a result of such pancreatic pathology.

Each pancreatic islet contains a number of different neuroendocrine cells.

Each different cell type is mainly concerned with the secretion of a single hormone. The nomenclature of these individual cell types is confusing, and so next, each type is identified by its main hormone (with other terms given in parentheses).

There are four main cell types and at least two minor ones. Of the total number of pancreatic endocrine cells, the proportions of the main cell types are as follows:
- Approximately 70% are insulin- and amylin-secreting cells (B or β cells) (Fig. 14.29)
- Approximately 20% are glucagon-secreting cells (A or α cells) (Fig. 14.30)
- Approximately 5%–10% are somatostatin-secreting cells (D, δ or type III cells) (Fig. 14.31)
- Approximately 1%–2% are pancreatic polypeptide–secreting cells (PP or F cells)

The PP cells, which are comparatively scanty when a random block of the pancreas is examined, are found in greater numbers in the posterior lobe of the pancreas, in the head and neck region. They are also found as scattered cells in duct walls.

Fig. 14.28 Islets of Langerhans. (a) Medium-power photomicrograph of an islet of Langerhans (I) embedded in the exocrine component (E) of the pancreas. The islets, roughly spherical, are composed of much smaller cells than the exocrine pancreas, from which they are separated by a fine fibrocollagenous capsule (C). **(b)** High-power micrograph showing islet cells. Note that each cell is in contact with the capillary network (C).

Fig. 14.29 Insulin-Secreting Cells. (a) Immunocytochemical method for insulin. **(b)** Immunocytochemical method for amylin (same islet). Insulin/amylin-secreting cells occupy the central area of the pancreatic islets and are the most common cell type. These cells have well-developed rough endoplasmic reticulum, a prominent Golgi, and numerous neurosecretory vesicles about 300 nm in diameter. The vesicles have a central electron-dense core in the form of a rhomboidal or polyhedral crystalline structure surrounded by an electron-lucent halo and bounded by a narrow membrane. In a few vesicles the core is missing, possibly owing to the recent discharge of insulin (the central core is thought to be composed of insulin complexed with zinc). The peptide amylin is thought to modulate the action of insulin.

Fig. 14.30 Glucagon-Secreting Cells. Glucagon-secreting cells are located mainly at the periphery of the pancreatic islets, as shown in this micrograph of a section stained to show glucagon by an immunohisto-chemical technique. Glucagon-secreting cells possess similar ultrastructural features to those of insulin-secreting cells, except that the secretory vesicles are smaller and have a more spherical electron-dense core, which is usually eccentrically located.

Fig. 14.31 Somatostatin-Secreting Cells. Somatostatin-secreting cells are a minority population and, in humans, are scattered apparently randomly throughout the pancreatic islets, as shown in this micrograph stained to show somatostatin by an immunohistochemical technique. Some islets contain substantial numbers of these cells, whereas others contain none at all. Somatostatin-secreting cells contain larger neurosecretory vesicles than insulin-secreting and glucagon-secreting cells, being up to 35 nm in diameter, and their core is much less electron-dense.

Their neurosecretory vacuoles are spherical, with a central electron-dense core surrounded by a wide electron-lucent area.

The minor cell types are:

- VIP-secreting cells (D-1 or type IV cells)
- Ghrelin-secreting cells (ε cells)
- Mixed secretion cells (EC or enterochromaffin cells)

Minor cell types are present in small numbers in the islets and scattered in the exocrine and ductular components. The mixed secretion cells have been reported to produce a number of active peptides, including serotonin, motilin and substance P.

> **The islets contain a complex network of capillaries with fenestrated endothelium.**

These capillaries arise from small arterioles outside the islet and, after penetrating the islet, merge with capillaries supplying the exocrine component of the pancreas. Fenestrated capillary endothelium is a common feature in endocrine tissue.

> **Pancreatic islets are innervated by the autonomic nervous system.**

There are both sympathetic and parasympathetic twigs contacting the surfaces of about 10% of all the cells directly. There are well-developed gap junctions between adjacent islet cells, which may provide the mechanism whereby the neural stimulus is passed to all cells. The autonomic nervous system also innervates the blood vessels and possibly affects perfusion.

Parasympathetic stimulation increases insulin and glucagon output, whereas sympathetic stimulation inhibits insulin release.

OVARY AND TESTIS

Although their main function is to produce female and male gametes, the testis and ovary also act as endocrine organs (see Chapters 16 and 17).

DIFFUSE NEUROENDOCRINE SYSTEM

Introduction

So far, only those neuroendocrine cells that are gathered together to form distinct endocrine glands have been discussed. There is, however, an extensive system of scattered neuroendocrine cells producing hormones and active peptides, many of which act on the local environment, rather than having a distant systemic impact. Many of these cells belong to the so-called *APUD* or *diffuse neuroendocrine system* and have the following common characteristics:

- Uptake and decarboxylation of amine precursor compounds, producing active amines, peptides and hormones (APUD cells)
- Possession of characteristic cytoplasmic organelles, known as *dense-core granules, neurosecretory vesicles* or *rimmed vacuoles*

These have a common basic structure of a variably electron-dense core (usually spherical, but occasionally angulated), a clear electron-lucent halo around the dense core, a thin distinct membrane surrounding the halo and, irrespective of the shape of the central dense core, the entire vesicle is usually spherical or oval. The vesicles vary in size (usually 100–600 nm in diameter), shape (spherical or oval), width of electron-lucent halo and electron density of the central core, depending on the nature of the amine, peptide or hormone produced. In some cases, their secretion is under neural control.

Examples of neuroendocrine cells have already been described in this chapter, for example, adrenal medullary cells (see p. 284), calcitonin-secreting C cells (see p. 279) and pancreatic islet cells (see p. 285). Further examples occur in other chapters, for example, renin-producing juxtaglomerular cells (see p. 319).

The important cells of the diffuse neuroendocrine system are gut-associated endocrine cells and respiratory-associated endocrine cells.

> **Gut-associated endocrine cells are seen throughout the intestinal tract.**

Throughout the alimentary tract, the lining epithelium contains scattered endocrine cells termed *gut-associated endocrine cells* or *enteroendocrine cells*. Enteroendocrine cells are mainly concentrated in the stomach and small intestine (see Figs. 11.32 and 11.41). They are also present in the lower oesophagus and large intestine and in the ducts of organs draining into the gut (i.e. the bile and pancreatic ducts).

In general, enteroendocrine cells are small, with a spherical nucleus and pale-staining cytoplasm, and lie in contact with the basement membrane on which the mucosal epithelial cells sit (Fig. 14.32); many are not in contact with the lumen. Neurosecretory vesicles are concentrated mainly in the basal portion of these cells.

Enteroendocrine cells are difficult to identify by routine H&E staining but can be highlighted by certain silver stains, which is why they were formerly termed *argentaffin* or *argyrophil cells*. Another old synonym, *enterochromaffin cells*, is based on their reaction with potassium dichromate to produce a brown pigment. Immunocytochemical methods have demonstrated many more enteroendocrine cells than are visible by silver methods; they also indicate the cells' main secretion. These methods therefore have effectively replaced silver staining methods for demonstrating such cells.

The ultrastructural features of enteroendocrine cells, particularly the size, shape and number of neurosecretory vesicles, vary according to the amine or peptide hormone produced, and more than 20 such products have been identified. Most of these hormones cannot be accurately matched with an ultrastructurally characteristic cell type, and it is likely that some or all of the cells can produce more than one active secretion.

Fig. 14.32 Enteroendocrine Cell. (a) Micrograph showing enteroendocrine cells *(brown)* in the crypts of colonic mucosal glands demonstrated by an immunohistochemical method to detect chromogranin A, a protein found in neurosecretory granules. **(b)** Low-power electron micrograph showing enteroendocrine cells (E) in the base of a small bowel gland. This contrasts with a Paneth cell (P) (see also Fig. 11.41). **(c)** High-power electron micrograph showing neuroendocrine vesicles facing the basement membrane (BM) of the gland and an adjacent capillary vessel (C) (Image (a) used under Creative Commons License. https://creativecommons.org/licenses/by-sa/3.0/. From the Human Protein Atlas. Antibody to chromogranin A CAB058688. https://www.proteinatlas.org/ENSG00000100604-CHGA/tissue/colon#img.)

Tumours of the gut-associated endocrine cells occur but are rare; for historical reasons they are given the uninformative and unsatisfactory name of **carcinoid tumours**. They are most often seen in the small intestine and are malignant but grow for a long time before spreading to different sites.

> Respiratory-associated endocrine cells are seen throughout the respiratory tract.

Pulmonary neuroendocrine cells in humans exist in two forms: scattered and aggregated.

Individual neuroendocrine cells are scattered throughout the trachea, the intrapulmonary airways and occasionally in the alveolar wall. These cells are pale when stained by H&E and are difficult to distinguish without the aid of special methods such as immunocytochemical techniques. Most of the cell sits on the epithelial basement membrane in a manner similar to that of enteroendocrine cells (see Fig. 14.32b), but a cytoplasmic process extends toward the lumen between adjacent epithelial cells.

Small aggregates of neuroendocrine cells form small mounds protruding into the airway lumen or alveoli. These aggregates, which are particularly prominent where airways branch, receive unmyelinated axons from peribronchial and peribronchiolar nerves and have been called *neuroepithelial bodies*.

The cytoplasm of both individual and clumped pulmonary neuroendocrine cells contains numerous neurosecretory vesicles. Serotonin, calcitonin gene–related peptide and bombesin have all been demonstrated within these cells.

In humans, respiratory-associated neuroendocrine cells are most numerous and prominent at birth, where they secrete factors involved in lung development, decreasing rapidly thereafter.

A malignant tumour of neuroendocrine cells in the bronchial mucosa (called a *small cell undifferentiated carcinoma*) is one of the most common and important types of 'lung cancer'. It is highly malignant and spreads rapidly and widely (see p. 187).

PARAGANGLIA

> The paraganglia are specialized neuroendocrine glands associated with the autonomic nervous system.

Paraganglia consist of prominent neuroendocrine cells containing neurosecretory vesicles. They contain active amine or peptide hormones and are therefore regarded as part of the neuroendocrine system.

In some cases, their precise function and the nature of their secretions is not clear, but it is known that some of the larger paraganglia in the thorax and neck (e.g. aortic body and carotid body) act as chemoreceptors.

Paraganglia vary in size from clumps of a few cells associated with nerves, visible only with microscopy, to structures up to 3 mm in diameter, which are anatomically distinct. The largest are the intercarotid paraganglia (carotid bodies) and the aortic sympathetic paraganglia (organ of Zuckerkandl).

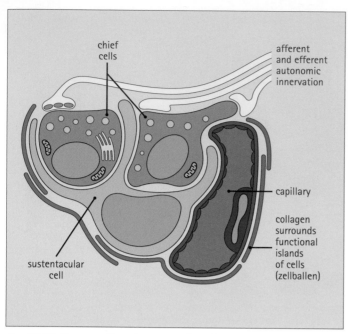

Fig. 14.33 Paraganglion. A paraganglion, showing that it is composed of chief cells arranged into clumps surrounded by sustentacular cells and capillaries.

Paraganglia are composed of type I (glomus or chief) cells, type II (sustentacular) cells and blood vessels.

Type I (chief or glomus) cells are neuroendocrine cells containing neurosecretory vesicles arranged into roughly round clumps or nests (zellballen). Each clump is surrounded by an intimate network of capillaries with fenestrated endothelium and a basement membrane. The neuroendocrine cells are of two types.

Most are termed *light cells* and have pale vacuolated cytoplasm containing moderate numbers of spherical electron-dense neurosecretory vesicles about 100–150 nm in diameter.

A small proportion are termed *dark cells* and have darker-staining cytoplasm containing large numbers of pleomorphic, often angulated, neurosecretory vesicles 50–250 nm in diameter.

Between the neuroendocrine cells and the capillaries are occasional flattened support cells, the type II (sustentacular) cells (Fig. 14.33).

Type II (sustentacular) cells, which account for 20%–30% of paraganglion cells, have elongated spindle-shaped nuclei and pale-staining cytoplasm that envelops nests or clumps of type I cells. Concentrated at the periphery of the clumps of

neuroendocrine cells, they send cytoplasmic processes into the clumps and also around nerve axons. Type II cells are thought to be modified Schwann cells, because they are S-100 positive and they behave like and resemble them both histologically and ultrastructurally.

Paraganglia are richly innervated by both the sympathetic and parasympathetic nervous systems.

▶▶ KEY FACTS

Carotid Body Function

The human carotid body contains a mixture of peptides, particularly acetylcholine, methionine enkephalin and leucine enkephalin. In addition, some of the neurosecretory vacuoles contain active amines, including epinephrine (adrenaline), norepinephrine (noradrenaline), serotonin and dopamine.

The carotid body acts as a peripheral chemoreceptor, responding to significant alterations in arterial blood gas tensions and blood pH. Acute hypoxia is countered by an increase in the respiratory rate; this is thought to be mediated by the release of some of the previous noted transmitters together with cytokines, which in turn stimulate afferent nerve terminals.

Chronic hypoxia (such as that seen physiologically in people living at high altitude and pathologically in patients with chronic lung disease, cyanotic congenital heart disease or sleep apnoea) leads to persistent enlargement of the carotid bodies, up to two or three times the normal size, because of hyperplasia of both type I and type II cells.

With old age, the carotid bodies may show progressive lymphocytic infiltration and fibrosis.

The carotid and aortic bodies are important paraganglia.

A single oval carotid body lies in the fibrocollagenous support tissue between the bifurcation of each common carotid artery into internal and external branches. Each carotid body measures about 3 × 2 × 2 mm and weighs 5–15 mg.

Carotid bodies are most prominent in children and teenagers, becoming progressively less obvious with increasing age, except in people with chronic hypoxia caused by lung disease or those living in low oxygen tension at high altitudes; in these people, the carotid bodies increase in size as a result of hyperplasia (an increase in cell numbers) and may reach 40 mg in weight.

The carotid body has the general structure of all paraganglia (see Fig. 14.33), and in humans the main peptides identified in it are enkephalins. Similar in structure to the carotid bodies, but smaller, are the aortic pulmonary paraganglia (aortic bodies), located on the concave surface of the arch of the aorta, close to where the right pulmonary artery passes beneath.

The carotid and aortic bodies act as chemoreceptors, monitoring the arterial oxygen tension by cellular systems involving mitochondrial proteins and membrane K^+ channels.

> **Numerous aortic sympathetic paraganglia lie around the abdominal aorta.**

Aortic sympathetic paraganglia are mainly situated around the abdominal aorta from above the level of origin of the renal arteries to the iliac bifurcation and beyond. On the anterior surface of the aorta they are particularly numerous around the coeliac axis and around the origin of the inferior mesenteric artery. Although prominent in infants, they are much less obvious in adults and are rarely discernible with the naked eye. Collectively, they are known as *the organs of Zuckerkandl,* particularly the cluster around the origin of the inferior mesenteric artery.

Histologically, aortic sympathetic paraganglia have the same general structure of paraganglia, but the neuroendocrine cells have larger neurosecretory granules than those in the carotid body and more closely resemble those of the adrenal medulla (Fig. 14.34).

For online review questions, please visit https://studentconsult. inkling.com.

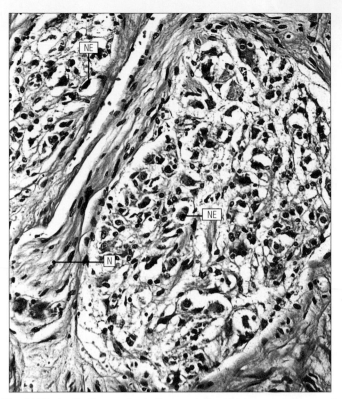

Fig. 14.34 Aortic Sympathetic Paraganglion. Low-power micrograph showing a small aortic sympathetic-type paraganglion. Note the afferent nerve fibres (N) and the nests of neuroendocrine cells (NE).

Urinary System

INTRODUCTION

The main function of the urinary system is the production, storage and voiding of urine.

- Urine production and the control of its composition are the responsibility of the kidneys.
- The pelvicalyceal systems and ureters transfer urine from the kidneys to the bladder, and the urethra is the channel through which stored urine is voided from the bladder.

The pelvicalyceal systems, ureters, bladder and urethra have a relatively uncomplicated structure (see p. 323). The kidney, however, performs a wide range of endocrine, biochemical and physiological tasks during the production of urine, and its structure is accordingly intricate.

The functions of the kidney are closely aligned to its different structural components.

- Renal function is based on specializations of microscopic vascular anatomy within the kidney which allow filtering, ion exchange and fluid absorption. A knowledge of the micro-anatomy of renal blood vessels is an essential part of understanding normal and renal function and the effects of disease.
- Filtration of blood in the first phase of production of urine takes place in a structure called the **glomerulus** which produces a filtrate.
- Modification of the filtrate to form urine takes place in an epithelial-lined **tubule** which is continuous with each glomerulus. The tubule is made up of several named parts, each with a different function linked to each length, being lined by specialized types of epithelium.

The basic functional unit of the kidney, composed of a glomerulus and its attached tubule, is called a **nephron**. Each nephron produces urine at a concentration which is appropriate for metabolic needs. The output of multiple nephrons drains into collecting ducts within the kidney, eventually draining into the renal pelvis and moving onwards through the renal pelvis and ureters to the urinary bladder.

KIDNEY STRUCTURE

> The kidney is divided into the cortex and medulla.

Each kidney has two distinct zones: an outer cortex and an inner medulla (Fig. 15.1).

The cortex forms an outer shell and also forms columns (the so-called *columns of Bertin*) that lie between the individual units of the medulla.

The medulla is composed of a series of conical structures (medullary pyramids), the base of each cone being continuous with the inner limit of the cortex and the pointed peak of the pyramid protruding into part of the urine collecting system (the calyceal system) toward the hilum of the kidney. This pointed tip of the medullary pyramid is known as the *papilla*.

Each human kidney contains 10–18 medullary pyramids; thus 10–18 papillae protrude into the collecting calyces.

Each medullary pyramid, with its associated shell of cortex, comprises a functional and structural lobe of the kidney.

KIDNEY FUNCTION

> The kidney is essential for fluid, electrolyte and acid–base balance and also has an endocrine function.

Urine is produced in the kidney by the selective removal of substances from the blood plasma. Subsequent controlled reabsorption of water, ions, salts, sugars and small molecular weight proteins results in urine, the composition of which is appropriate to the body's internal environment and requirements at the time.

An inability to produce concentrated or dilute urine is an important feature of kidney failure, which is also associated with inadequate excretion of nitrogenous waste products and other substances, for example, potassium ions (see p. 318).

It is important to realize that the kidneys (and the lungs) differ from most other organs in a common, important respect. In most organs, the vascular supply is the servant of the parenchymal tissues, providing them with oxygen and other raw materials required for the tissue's metabolic processes and carrying synthesized cell products and waste materials away from the organ. In the kidney, however, the parenchymatous components of the organ are the servants of the blood supply, as the function of the kidney, in broad terms, is the filtration and cleansing of the blood.

Thus the parenchymal unit of the kidney, the **nephron**, which is composed of the glomerulus and cortical and medullary tubular systems, can be regarded as an appendage of the renal blood vascular system, attached to it for servicing purposes. It is not surprising therefore that the blood vascular system of the kidney is both substantial and structurally unusual, reflecting its central role. The two kidneys receive 25% of the total cardiac output. Consequently, many of the important and common diseases of the kidney result from abnormality in the blood vascular component (see p. 294).

In addition to its role in producing urine, the kidney produces the hormones erythropoietin and renin.

Fig. 15.1 Anatomy of Adult Kidney. (a) Sectioned adult kidney, which has been fixed in formalin and the near-natural colour restored in alcohol. Note the cortex (C) and the medullary pyramid (M) culminating in the papillary tip (P), which protrudes into the lumen of a calyx (Ca). Interlobar arteries (IA) and arcuate arteries (ArcA) can also be seen. Little detail of cortical structure is visible with the naked eye, but the vertical linearity of the components of the medulla is highlighted by clusters of prominent blood vessels (vasa recta). **(b)** In this very low-magnification H&E-stained paraffin section the distinction between cortex (C) and medulla (M) is easily seen. This section also shows the vertical linearity of the components of the medulla, both tubules and vessels. At this magnification, glomeruli can just be seen as small dots in the cortex. Note that some areas of the cortex are free of glomeruli but contain vertically running duct systems; these areas are known as *medullary rays* and represent the sites where cortical tubules drain into the collecting ducts. **(c)** In this micrograph of cortex at a higher magnification than in **(b)** it can be seen that the medullary ray (MR) area is devoid of glomeruli and that the interlobular arteries (ILA) run in the glomeruli-rich area. **(d)** Renal cortex – glomerulus (G) and cortical tubules (T).

KIDNEY VASCULATURE

> **Arteries supplying the kidney branch within the renal substance to supply distinct regions.**

In most cases, the arterial supply to each kidney comes from a single renal artery, which is a substantial, direct lateral branch of the abdominal aorta. A common variant is the presence of a separate artery arising directly from the aorta and supplying one or the other pole.

The renal artery runs toward the concave hilum of the kidney and divides into two main branches, one anterior and one posterior, each of which divides into a number of interlobar arteries that run between the medullary pyramids, one branch to each developmental lobe.

At about the midpoint of the thickness of the kidney parenchyma, where the cortex abuts on the broad base of the medullary pyramid (the corticomedullary junction), the interlobar artery divides into several arcuate arteries, which make a right angle turn and run laterally along the corticomedullary junction.

The arcuate arteries then give rise to a series of side branches (interlobular arteries), which again make a right angle turn and run vertically upward into the cortex.

Interlobular arteries give rise laterally to a series of arterioles, called **afferent arterioles**, usually directly, but sometimes via a short intralobular artery. These arteries terminate at the periphery of the kidney, just beneath the capsule, supplying a stellate subcapsular arteriolar and capillary plexus.

So far, the arterial supply has been anatomically unremarkable. From the afferent arterioles onward, however, the renal vascular system becomes unique.

RENAL MICROCIRCULATION

> **The renal microcirculation contains two capillary systems.**

In almost every other organ, the capillary network lies between the terminal part of the arterial/arteriolar system and the proximal part of the venular/venous system and is the major site of oxygen/carbon dioxide exchange. The renal vascular system, in contrast, has a highly specialized preliminary capillary network, the **glomerular tuft**, which receives blood from an afferent arteriole and which is the site of filtration of waste products from plasma, together with a second capillary system arising from the efferent arteriole, which varies in structure and function according to its location within the kidney (Fig. 15.2).

In most cases, after leaving the glomerulus, the efferent arteriole divides into a complex capillary system, which runs in the interstitial spaces between the components of the system of cortical tubules. Each capillary is in intimate contact with these tubules and is thus ideally placed to take up any substances reabsorbed from the glomerular filtrate by tubular epithelial cells (see p. 307).

However, the capillary system originating from efferent arterioles leaving glomeruli situated deep in the cortex, close to the corticomedullary junction (juxtamedullary glomeruli), is different (see Fig. 15.2). These efferent arterioles divide into a series of long, thin-walled vessels, the **vasa recta**, which run straight down into the medulla alongside the medullary components of the tubular systems. These vessels play an important role in the ionic and fluid exchanges occurring in the medulla (see p. 311). Some vasa recta arise as direct, vertically running side branches of the arcuate artery.

The first capillary system, the glomerular tuft, does not transfer its contained oxygen to the tissues, nor does it take up a significant amount of carbon dioxide. The major exchange of dissolved gases takes place in the second capillary system. Oxygen is supplied to the cortical and medullary parts of the renal parenchyma, which have the highest demand because of their high metabolic activity.

> **The venous drainage of the kidney mirrors the arterial supply.**

In general, the renal venous drainage mirrors the arterial supply, except that there is no venous equivalent of the glomerular capillary tuft. The subcapsular arteriolar and capillary plexuses drain into a subcapsular venular and venous plexus of stellate veins that forms the origin of the interlobular veins. As they proceed toward the corticomedullary junction, the interlobular veins receive venous tributaries from the peritubular capillary network and, as the juxtamedullary zone is approached, from some of the venous tributaries from the medulla, which are the venous equivalent of the arterial vasa recta.

Many of the medullary venous vessels drain directly into the arcuate veins, which run laterally with the equivalent artery at the corticomedullary junction. These in turn drain into large interlobular veins lying between adjacent medullary pyramids, and then into the major vein tributaries at the renal hilum. The major renal vein opens end-to-side into the inferior vena cava.

NEPHRON

> **The functional unit of the kidney parenchyma that serves the blood supply is called the nephron.**

The nephron has two main components:
- The glomerulus, which is associated with the first capillary system
- The cortical and medullary tubular systems, which are associated with the second capillary system

The glomerulus is the site of initial blood filtration, and the tubular systems are the site where the concentration and chemical content of blood returned to the general systemic circulation, and hence the concentration and content of the urine to be voided from the body, are controlled.

Fig. 15.2 Renal Microcirculation. (a) The principles of renal microcirculation. The afferent arteriole, which is a branch of the interlobular artery, enters the glomerular capillary tuft at the vascular hilum. The emerging vessel, the efferent arteriole, normally divides into a complex system of capillaries: the peritubular capillary network, which surrounds the cortical tubules. The venous tributaries arising from the peritubular capillary network drain into small veins opening into the interlobular vein, which runs vertically alongside the interlobular artery and drains into the arcuate vein, running alongside the arcuate artery at the corticomedullary junction. Close to the corticomedullary junction, some of the efferent arterioles give rise to vertically running vessels, the vasa recta, which pass down into the medulla alongside the medullary duct and tubular systems. Some vasa recta arise as direct branches of the arcuate artery and drain directly into the arcuate vein. **(b)** A carmine–gelatine injection specimen, showing a vertically running interlobular artery (ILA) in the renal cortex, with glomerular capillary tufts (G) arising from lateral branches of the artery and the afferent arterioles (AA). Some peritubular capillary networks (PCN) can also be seen. **(c)** A carmine–gelatine injection specimen showing the interlobular artery (ILA), the afferent (AA) and efferent arterioles (EA), the glomerular tuft (G) and the PCN. **(d)** PAS-stained section showing interlobular artery (ILA) giving rise to an afferent arteriole (AA), which leads into a glomerular capillary bed (G). (Micrograph from digital pathology whole slide image provided by the University of Leeds Virtual Pathology Project https://www.virtualpathology.leeds.ac.uk. Reproduced with permission.)

Fig. 15.3 shows the structure of a nephron and its relationship to its microcirculation. The simplified overview of the various homeostatic functions of the tubular component of the nephron will be dealt with in greater detail later in the chapter.

> **Within the renal cortex, the nephrons are organized into a distinct repeated lobular pattern.**

The glomeruli and proximal and distal tubules are aligned mainly on either side of the interlobular arteries that supply them with blood (see Fig. 15.2).

At the midpoint between adjacent interlobular arteries is a vertically running arrangement of tubules and ducts known as the *medullary ray* (see Fig. 15.1c), at the centre of which is a main collecting duct that collects all of the largely unconcentrated urine from the nephrons on either side. The other tubular components of the medullary ray are the straight collecting tubules carrying urine from the end of the distal tubule to the main cortical collecting duct. The duct systems of the medullary ray run vertically downward into the medulla.

The subunit of the cortex, comprising a centrally placed medullary ray and the nephrons on either side of it, is called the *renal lobule,* and each interlobular artery runs upward in the cortex between adjacent lobules. This lobular arrangement and the medullary ray system can be seen in Fig. 15.1.

GLOMERULUS

The first functional component of the nephron encountered by the microcirculation is the **glomerulus**, which is the site of initial filtration of the blood arriving by the afferent arterioles. Three main cell types are crucial to the specialized function of the renal glomerulus: endothelial cells, podocytes and mesangial cells. The function of the glomerulus depends on the microanatomical arrangement of these cells and the associated specialized extracellular matrix.

> **The afferent arteriole enters the glomerulus at the vascular pole.**

The afferent arteriole, which enters the glomerulus immediately, splits up into about five main branches. Each branch then subdivides into its own capillary network (see Fig. 15.2), with the short main branch and its capillaries being supported by its own strip or stalk of mesangium (see p. 304).

The division of the glomerular capillary network into about five independent segments gives the glomerular tuft an implicit lobulation, which is rarely apparent by routine light microscopy in health but which becomes evident in some forms of primary glomerular disease, particularly when the mesangial component of each segment is enlarged (see Fig. 15.18). The independence of each glomerular segment is also demonstrated by disease affecting only one segment (e.g. focal segmental glomerulonephritis).

The glomerular capillaries converge to form a single efferent arteriole, which leaves the glomerulus at the same vascular pole as the afferent arteriole enters.

> **The glomerulus is an intricate structure in which capillaries are in intimate contact with a specialized epithelium.**

In simple terms, the structure of the glomerulus is best conceived as a globular capillary network intruding into a hollow sphere of epithelial cells called *Bowman's capsule,* which represents the bulbous, distended closed end of a long hollow tubular system (Fig. 15.4). This means that the glomerular capillary system, which is lined internally by endothelial cells, acquires an outer layer of epithelial cells that is continuous at the vascular pole, with the cells lining Bowman's capsule. The structure of the glomerulus is shown in Fig. 15.5, and the diagram in Fig. 15.6 summarizes the fine detail of the structural relationship between key components of the glomerulus.

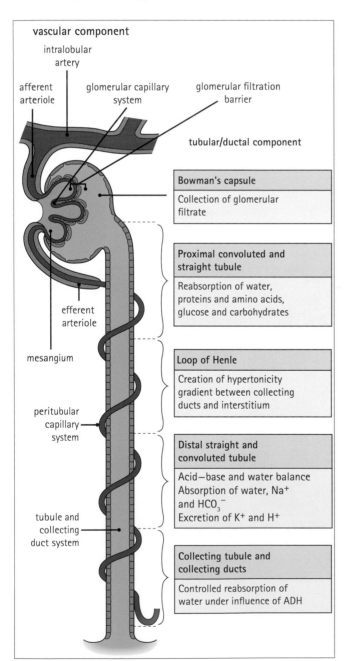

vascular component
intralobular artery
afferent arteriole
glomerular capillary system
glomerular filtration barrier
tubular/ductal component

Bowman's capsule
Collection of glomerular filtrate

Proximal convoluted and straight tubule
Reabsorption of water, proteins and amino acids, glucose and carbohydrates

efferent arteriole

mesangium

Loop of Henle
Creation of hypertonicity gradient between collecting ducts and interstitium

peritubular capillary system

Distal straight and convoluted tubule
Acid–base and water balance
Absorption of water, Na^+ and HCO_3^-
Excretion of K^+ and H^+

tubule and collecting duct system

Collecting tubule and collecting ducts
Controlled reabsorption of water under influence of ADH

Fig. 15.3 The Nephron. A simple diagram to show different parts of the nephron and associated blood vessels.

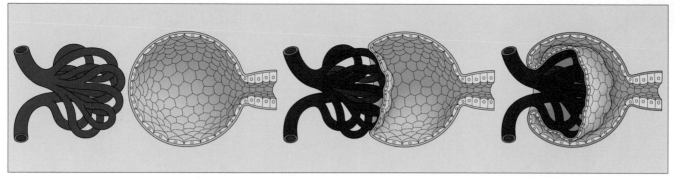

Fig. 15.4 Relationship Between the Glomerular Capillary Tuft and Bowman's Capsule. Although the glomerulus and Bowman's capsule do not in fact develop in this way, the relationships between the two are best conceived by imagining the intrusion of the glomerular tuft into the spherical, distended and closed end of the tubular system. This is particularly helpful in conceptualizing the glomerular tuft with its outer coating of epithelial cells, which is continuous with the cells lining Bowman's capsule.

The epithelial cells of Bowman's capsule are flat and simple, except near the opening of the tubular system, where they become more cuboidal and acquire some of the cytoplasmic organelles of the proximal convoluted tubule epithelial cells (see p. 307).

In contrast, the epithelial cells coating the glomerular capillary tuft are larger and have a highly specialized and unusual structure characterized by multiple cell processes, which has led to their being named **podocytes** (see p. 301).

The epithelium-lined space between the coated glomerular capillary network and the parietal shell of Bowman's capsule is called the *urinary space* and is continuous with the lumen of the long tubular system of the nephron.

In addition to the outer epithelial (podocyte) coating, the glomerular capillary network has other unusual features, including the possession of a thick basement membrane derived from the fusion of basement membranes originating from both the podocyte and endothelial cell (the glomerular basement membrane) and the presence of a supporting strip or stalk, analogous to the mesentery of the small bowel, called the *mesangium* (see Fig. 15.6).

Blood enters the glomerular capillary network from the afferent arteriole. Ultrafiltration of the blood then occurs in the glomerular capillary network, and the filtrate passes into the urinary space before passing down the tubular system. The partly filtered blood leaves the glomerulus via the efferent arteriole and flows onward to provide an oxygenated blood supply to the tubular systems.

GLOMERULAR FILTRATION BARRIER

The barrier between circulating blood and the urinary space is the glomerular filtration barrier (Fig. 15.7). It has five components:

- The glycocalyx associated with the surface of capillary endothelial cells
- Capillary endothelial cells
- The unusually thick glomerular capillary basement membrane
- The podocyte (the outer epithelial) layer
- Filtration slits between adjacent podocytes

An additional component of the functional barrier is a high polyanionic charge associated with the endothelial glycocalyx and basement membrane.

> **Glomerular capillary endothelial cells are attenuated and fenestrated.**

A diagrammatic representation, illustrating the structure of the endothelium and its relationships with other glomerular components, is shown in Fig. 15.6.

The endothelial cells which line the capillaries of renal glomeruli are adapted for specialized function. The cytoplasm forms a thin sheet broken by numerous small circular pores, or fenestrations, each about 70 nm in diameter. Their nuclei are usually located near the mesangium (see Fig. 15.5e).

An important functional component of the glomerular endothelium is the presence of a glycocalyx layer which maintains a charge barrier to the passage of certain materials, for example, proteins. The endothelial glycocalyx may be disrupted in some disease states, and this leads to a change in permeability of the glomerular filtration barrier.

> **The glomerular basement membrane is divided into three distinct layers.**

The basic structure of the basement membrane is presented in Chapter 4. The glomerular basement membrane can be specially stained using silver-staining techniques, and this is used in routine examination of biopsies of the kidney in clinical work (Fig. 15.8a). Immunostaining for basement membrane components shows the extended and convoluted profile of the basement membrane (see Fig. 15.8b). The main components of the glomerular basement membrane are type IV collagen, laminin, agrin and nidogen. Distinguishing this structure from other types of basement membrane, specific isoforms are present (laminin-521 [α5β2γ1] and the α3α4α5 chain of type IV collagen).

As illustrated in Fig. 15.6 and shown by electron microscopy in Fig. 15.9a, the glomerular basement membrane supports both podocytes and capillary endothelial cells.

Fig. 15.5 Normal Glomerulus. (a) An H&E paraffin section of normal human kidney, which has been inflation fixed to distend the blood vessels. Note the afferent arteriole (AA) and efferent arteriole (EA) at the vascular pole. Opposite the vascular pole is the tubular pole (TP), where the urinary space (US) empties into the first part of the tubular system. Although fine details of the glomerular structure are not apparent in this micrograph, the suggestion of glomerular lobulation is evident. The flattened epithelial lining of Bowman's capsule (BC) is easily seen. **(b)** PAS staining enhances the contrast of structures containing glycoproteins. The basement membrane (BM) can be seen as magenta rings around the empty lumen of capillaries (C). The mesangium (M) is also shown as magenta-stained material within the glomerulus. **(c)** Glomerulus immunostained with an endothelial marker CD34 *(brown)* which highlights the capillary vessels. The blue nuclei outside the capillaries are mainly podocytes wrapped around the capillaries with a small number of mesangial cells. **(d)** Thin epoxy-resin section stained with toluidine blue. This technique permits greater resolution of the glomerular structure. The capillary loops contain red blood cells (RBC) and are supported by the darkly stained mesangium (M). **(e)** Higher-power micrograph of the epoxy-resin section. Details of the glomerular capillary wall, endothelial and epithelial cells and mesangium become apparent. The capillary loops are supported by darkly stained mesangial stalks, comprising acellular matrix (Mx) and nucleated mesangial cells (Mc). The capillary basement membrane is lined internally by endothelial cytoplasm, and endothelial cell nuclei € are apparent. External to the glomerular basement membrane are the epithelial podocytes (P). [Image (b) used under Creative Commons License https://creativecommons.org/licenses/by-sa/3.0/ from the Human Protein Atlas. Antibody to CD34 HPA036722 https://www.proteinatlas.org/ENSG00000174059-CD34/tissue/kidney#img.]

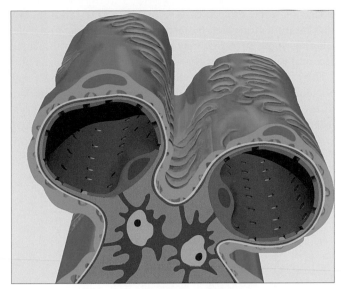

Fig. 15.6 Structural Relationships in the Glomerulus. This diagram shows two glomerular capillaries supported by mesangium and covered by a layer of podocytes. The podocytes with their ramified, interdigitating processes *(green)* are separated from the fenestrated capillary endothelium *(red)* by the glomerular basement membrane. Note the supporting role of the mesangium *(matrix beige, cytoplasm brown).* The lamina densa *(purple)* and lamina rara externa *(blue)* of the basement membrane are not continuous around the capillary, but are reflected over the mesangial surface to the next capillary. The lamina rara interna *(beige)* appears to blend with the mesangial matrix where the capillary is attached to the mesangium.

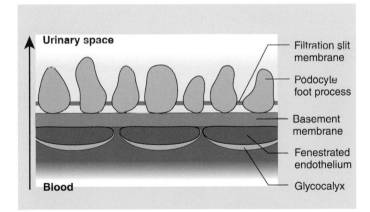

Fig. 15.7 The Blood Filtration Barrier. There are five main components of the glomerular blood filtration barrier. Podocytes form foot processes which interdigitate and are separated by filtration slits associated with filtration slit membranes.

The glomerular basement membrane is much thicker than normal capillary basement membranes elsewhere. It measures approximately 310–350 nm in healthy young adults, being slightly thicker in males. Both the inner endothelial and outer epithelial cell (podocytes) populations contribute to its production as a double basement membrane (see Fig. 4.14). It has three layers:

- A central electron-dense lamina densa
- Electron-lucent lamina rara interna on the endothelial or capillary lumen side
- Electron-lucent lamina rara externa on the epithelial podocyte, or urinary space, side

Fig. 15.8 Glomerular Basement Membrane. (a) Jones methenamine silver stain is used as a routine stain in clinical work. The black silver staining highlights the basement membrane, which can be seen looping around capillary lumina (C) as a thin line in addition to staining ribbons of mesangial matrix material within the glomerular structure (M). **(b)** The contour of the basement membrane can be seen in this micrograph immunostained for one of its laminin components (γ1 chain). The plane of section allows loops of basement membrane to be seen, especially at the periphery of the glomerulus, corresponding to the contour around individual capillaries. Refer back to Fig. 15.4 to understand how the 3D sheet of basement membrane investing the glomerular tuft has a convoluted profile when seen in a single plane of cut. (Micrograph (a) from digital pathology whole slide image provided by the University of Leeds Virtual Pathology Project https://www.virtual-pathology.leeds.ac.uk. Reproduced with permission. Image (b) used under Creative Commons License https://creativecommons.org/licenses/by-sa/3.0/ from the Human Protein Atlas. Antibody to lamininC1 γ1 chain CAB004486 https://www.proteinatlas.org/ENSG00000135862-LAMC1/tissue/kidney#img.]

This layered structure becomes less apparent in most adults (see Fig. 15.9b).

The lamina densa is partly composed of type IV collagen (see Chapter 4).

The lamina rara layers contain fixed negatively charged (polyanionic) sites composed of glycosaminoglycans. In the basement membrane, this is mainly heparan sulphate. These polyanionic sites act as a charge barrier, preventing the passage of cationic molecules.

The combination of layers in the glomerular basement membrane produces both a physical and a charge barrier to the passage of large molecules (i.e. over 70 kDa) and to even small cationic molecules. Nevertheless, certain large molecules, including some proteins, may pass through into the urinary space and require reabsorption in the tubular system.

The full glomerular basement membrane is partly deficient at the site of the attachment of the capillary to the mesangium. The lamina rara interna continues as an ill-defined layer between the endothelial cytoplasm and the cytoplasmic and matrix components of the mesangium (see Fig. 15.6).

Fig. 15.9 Glomerular Structure. (a) Electron micrograph showing the relationship between the glomerular basement membrane (GBM), capillary lumen (L), endothelial cytoplasm (EnC) and epithelial podocyte (EP), with its primary (P1) and secondary (P2) foot process system. **(b)** High-power electron micrograph of the glomerular filtration barrier comprising fenestrated EnC, glomerular basement membrane and podocyte foot processes. Note the filtration slit diaphragm membrane (FSM, see p. 302). In this high-magnification electron micrograph, the three layers of the basement membrane can be seen, although they are indistinct in adult humans (as here). The layers are lamina densa (LD) and, on either side of it, lamina rara interna (LRI) and lamina rara externa (LRE).

CLINICAL EXAMPLE

Basement Membrane Abnormalities in Glomerular Disease

Abnormalities in the structure of the glomerular basement membrane are responsible for some important kidney diseases, which are characterized by an excessive loss of protein in urine (proteinuria). Sometimes so much is lost in the urine that the capacity of the liver to synthesize fresh protein (particularly albumin) is outstripped. The patient then develops a low blood albumin (hypoalbuminaemia) and oedema because of the low oncotic pressure of the blood.

The combination of proteinuria, hypoalbuminaemia and oedema is called **nephrotic syndrome**.

There are rare genetic disorders in which mutations in genes coding for basement membrane components result in an abnormal basement membrane structure and associated functional impairment. Examples include:

- Alport syndrome, linked to mutations in the genes *COL4A3*, *COL4A4*, and *COL4A5*, which code for α3, α4, and α5 chains, respectively, of type IV collagen. Alport syndrome presents with renal dysfunction, which starts with red blood cells leaking into the urine. Many of those affected develop hearing loss, and over time there is progressive renal dysfunction.
- Pierson syndrome is linked to mutations in the *LAMB2* gene leading to formation of abnormal laminin β2. Those affected present in childhood with protein loss in the urine. Over time there is progression to chronic kidney disease and renal failure.

Many cause of nephrotic syndrome are related to a structural abnormality of the glomerular basement membrane. Diseases in which the abnormality is structural include diabetes mellitus and membranous nephropathy.

In nephrotic syndrome associated with diabetes mellitus, the glomerular basement is thickened three- to five-fold, and the demarcation into three laminae is lost (Fig. 15.10a). In membranous nephropathy, the basement membrane is thickened and damaged by the deposition of antigen–antibody complexes (see Fig. 15.10b).

Although in these examples the basement membrane is physically thickened, and one might instinctively associate thickening of a barrier with a reduction in permeability, this is not the case. The abnormal basement membrane leads to functional impairment of podocytes and an overall failure of the glomerular filtration barrier (increased permeability) such that many large molecules pass into the urinary space, including large molecular weight proteins.

Fig. 15.10 Patterns of Basement Membrane Thickening in Disease. (a) Electron micrograph of a uniformly thickened basement membrane from a patient with diabetes mellitus who presented with nephrotic syndrome. Photographed at the same magnification as Fig. 15.9a. **(b)** Electron micrograph of a basement membrane thickened by deposition of antigen–antibody complexes on the epithelial side. It was taken from a patient with membranous nephropathy who presented with nephrotic syndrome. Photographed at same magnification as Fig. 15.9a.

The podocyte layer lies on the outer surface of the glomerular capillaries.

The podocyte layer is composed of specialized epithelium, which is continuous at the vascular hilum with the flat, relatively inert epithelium lining Bowman's capsule. It is highly specialized in structure and function, being so named because of its ramified structure and having numerous foot processes. Although podocytes can be readily seen in thin resin sections and by electron microscopy, they are difficult to pick out from the other cells in the glomerulus using conventional stains in wax-embedded sections. Immunostaining with a variety of podocyte markers is possible, but these tend to highlight the extended network of foot processes and effectively create a map of the contour of the basement membrane without showing much detail of the cell body (see Figs. 15.13b and 15.13c). In contrast, immunostaining for the intermediate filament of podocytes (vimentin), which is mainly located in the cell body, gives a better appreciation of the distribution of this cell type in the glomerulus. Immunostaining for another form of intermediate filament, nestin, allows detail of podocyte morphology to be appreciated by conventional light microscopy (Fig. 15.11).

Fig. 15.11 Podocytes immunostained for nestin *(brown)* show the distribution of podocytes within the glomerulus. **(a)** Note the layer of podocytes surrounding the outer surface of the glomerular capillaries. Inspecting the detail of the staining pattern shows a podocyte (P) with a cell body giving rise to primary processes. Where the plane of section has fortuitously passed just above the edge of a capillary, interdigitating, fine secondary podocyte foot processes can be seen (F) as an array of parallel linear bands. **(b)** This is a tangential section from the very edge of a glomerulus and shows the podocyte cell bodies giving rise to primary foot processes. The micrograph is at the limits of resolution of the digital system used and has been edge-enhanced to better show the cellular detail and demonstrate the multiprocessed, ramified shape. (Images used under Creative Commons License https://creativecommons.org/licenses/by-sa/3.0/ from the Human Protein Atlas. Antibody to nestin CAB058692 https://www.proteinatlas.org/ENSG00000132688-NES/tissue/kidney#img.)

Podocytes have a negatively charged (polyanionic) glycocalyx composed of glycosaminoglycans, including the sialomucin podocalyxin, which has an important role in maintaining the structure of the foot processes.

The podocyte main cell body is located above the external surface of the glomerular capillary and sends down cytoplasmic extensions (foot processes) that make contact with the glomerular basement membrane (Fig. 15.12 but also see Figs. 15.9 and 15.11). A mental image that helps to understand the structure of a podocyte is to imagine the cell body of the podocyte as the body of a microscopic octopus, with its tentacles wrapped around the adjacent capillaries. From each podocyte a small number of main, primary podocyte processes (the tentacles) give rise to a large number of finer secondary foot processes, which interdigitate and are adherent to the glomerular basement membrane.

The primary, main processes have a cytoskeleton composed of microtubules and intermediate filaments. The secondary peripheral foot processes have a cytoskeleton based on both nestin and actin and are in turn tethered by linking proteins to the basement membrane.

Between adjacent foot processes adherent to the glomerular basement membrane is a fairly consistent gap of 60 nm, the **filtration slit**. A thin membrane, the **filtration slit diaphragm**, bridges the gap between adjacent foot processes. This filtration slit diaphragm is responsible for cell:cell adhesion between adjacent foot processes and for maintaining a selective filtration function in this part of the glomerular filtration barrier (see the Advanced Concept box).

If podocytes are damaged or lost, some functional adaptation can be achieved by enlargement (hypertrophy) of the remaining podocytes. Progenitor cells are also present, derived

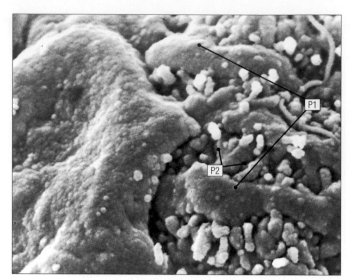

Fig. 15.12 Podocyte. Scanning electron micrograph of the epithelial podocyte and its foot processes in a healthy human adult. Arising from the main cell body of each epithelial cell are a number of broad cytoplasmic processes, the primary processes (P1), which extend along and wrap around the capillary, giving rise at regular intervals to a series of smaller processes, the secondary processes (P2), which rest on the glomerular basement membrane. There is interdigitation of secondary processes so that adjacent foot processes may be derived from different podocytes.

from the epithelial cells lining Bowman's capsule, and these may give rise to new podocytes.

Loss of the normal podocyte foot process pattern in some renal diseases is associated with such excessive protein loss (mainly albumin) that the affected patient develops nephrotic syndrome (see later).

◎ ADVANCED CONCEPT

Podocyte Slit Diaphragm
The slit diaphragm is shown diagrammatically (Fig. 15.13a).

Foot Processes Are Tightly Anchored in Place by Cell Adhesion Mechanisms
- Foot processes are tightly attached to the glomerular basement membrane by dystroglycans and $\alpha_3\beta_1$ integrin. This attachment is essential to prevent damage being caused by the shear stresses imposed on foot processes by the hydrostatic pressure and flow of the ultrafiltrate.
- Foot processes contain an actin cytoskeleton, which maintains the overall architecture of the cell process.
- Adjacent foot processes are joined together by interactions between proteins around the slit diaphragm. The protein **nephrin** spans the cell membrane and, through several other interacting and adaptor proteins including **podocin**,

anchors internally to the actin cytoskeleton of the foot process. In this way, the cytoskeleton of foot processes are anchored together to form a large structural unit.

The Slit Diaphragm Is a Selectively Permeable Barrier
- The podocyte filtration slit diaphragm sits between adjacent foot processes. Its constituent transmembrane proteins interact together such that the slit and slit diaphragm do not permit passage of material above ~60 kDa in size. Glucose and electrolytes can pass through the barrier, but proteins such as albumen are prevented from passing into the urinary space.

The Proteins in the Foot Process Act as Signal Transducers
- Several of the proteins located within the foot processes are part of signal transduction systems which are involved in cell signalling.

Fig. 15.13 Podocyte Slit Diaphragm Membrane. (a) Adjacent foot processes are anchored together by transmembrane proteins that include nephrin, neph 1 and neph 2. These proteins form the slit diaphragm in between adjacent processes. Inside the cytoplasm, these transmembrane complexes link to adaptor proteins within the foot process, including podocin, to bind with actin filaments. Each foot process is also tightly adherent to the basement membrane. **(b)** Immunofluorescent micrograph of a glomerulus stained to show nephrin *(green)* endothelium in capillaries *(pink)* and nuclei *(blue)*. Nephrin is an abundant protein in podocyte foot processes located in the slit diaphragm membrane, and the green staining tracks the outer contour of the glomerular basement membrane. Note the relationship between capillaries and the podocyte layer. **(c)** Micrograph of a glomerulus immunostained to show podocin *(brown)*. As another abundant protein in podocytes, the pattern of staining also tracks the contour of the outer side of the glomerular basement membrane. [Images used under Creative Commons License https://creativecommons.org/licenses/by-sa/3.0/ from the Human Protein Atlas. (b) Antibody to nephrin CAB035555 https://www.proteinatlas.org/ENSG00000161270-NPHS1/tissue/kidney#img and (c) Antibody to podocin CAB037267 https://www.proteinatlas.org/ENSG00000116218-NPHS2/tissue/kidney#img.]

Podocyte Abnormalities in Glomerular Disease

The loss of protein in the urine (proteinuria) is the main clinical presentation of renal disease, and in most cases, such protein loss is related to damage to podocytes. These conditions have been grouped together under the term *podocytopathies*.

Damage to podocytes can be caused by haemodynamic, metabolic, immune-mediated, toxic and genetic factors.

- Hypertension is an important cause of renal damage. Dilatation and expansion of glomerular capillaries are understood to cause stress to podocyte foot processes, as they respond to covering what is effectively an increasing area of the expanded, dilated capillary wall. Such stress leads to podocyte damage. Over time, adaptive systems fail and reactive changes develop in the glomerulus leading to glomerular scarring and failure of the nephron.
- Metabolic factors are also important causes of podocyte damage. A high body mass index is a risk factor for podocyte damage because it can lead to so-called *hyperfiltration* whereby individual glomeruli experience an abnormally high filtration rate with consequential physical shear stress, damaging podocytes. This mechanism is also understood to occur in diabetes mellitus.
- Immune complexes may form in the blood in response to infection or autoimmune conditions. These may become deposited in the glomerulus and lead to so-called *immune-complex glomerulonephritis*. Direct and indirect damage to podocytes leads to proteinuria as a component of disease.
- Important toxic causes include side effects of certain drugs and environmental exposure to heavy metals.
- There are also several genetic susceptibility factors that may predispose to podocyte damage, the best characterized of which is with the apolipoprotein variant L1. In addition, mutations in over 40 genes coding for proteins involved in structure or signalling in podocyte foot processes can lead to impaired podocyte structure and function. For example, mutation in the gene coding for nephrin leads to impaired or absent function of the slit diaphragm and congenital nephrotic syndrome.

In renal biopsy, damage to podocytes is first evident by detachment and loss of foot processes, a condition known as *foot process effacement*. Further damage to podocytes can give rise to several secondary reactive changes within the glomerulus, including mesangial cell reactive changes leading to scarring of the glomerulus (mesangial sclerosis), which may affect the whole glomerulus (global sclerosis) or be limited to segments (focal segmental sclerosis)

In children, the most common cause of nephrotic syndrome is *minimal change nephropathy*. By light microscopy, the glomerulus appears normal, but electron microscopy reveals loss of the normal foot process pattern, with the outer surface of the glomerular capillaries being covered by an almost continuous sheet of podocyte cytoplasm (Fig. 15.14).

Fig. 15.14 Foot Process Effacement. Compare the foot process arrangement with that seen normally (see Fig. 15.9). In this kidney the complex secondary foot process arrangement is lost and the primary foot processes (P1) lie directly on the basement membrane (BM). This loss of foot processes is termed *foot process efface-ment* and is an early stage in the response of podocytes to injury. Minimal change nephropathy is the most common cause of ne-phrotic syndrome in childhood and resolves spontaneously with no long-term renal impairment.

MESANGIUM

The mesangial support to the glomerular capillary network has two components:, mesangial cells and extracellular mesangial matrix. The role of the mesangium as a support for the glomerular capillary system can be seen by electron microscopy in Fig. 15.15 and diagrammatically in Fig. 15.6, which illustrates the details of the structure of the mesangium and its relationship to the glomerular capillary and the glomerular basement membrane. Note that in terms of cell:cell signalling, mesangial cells are in close contact with endothelial cells, being only separated by basement membrane. They have no close contact with podocytes.

> **Mesangial cells are irregular in shape, have a number of cytoplasmic processes and produce the mesangial matrix.**

Mesangial cells are present within the support tissues of the glomerulus (see Fig. 15.6) and have been regarded as a type of mesenchymal stromal cell, similar to pericytes (see p. 93). They account for about a third of all cells present in the glomerulus.

Mesangial cells are surrounded by an extracellular matrix, the **mesangial matrix**. The combination of mesangial cells and mesangial matrix is referred to as the **mesangium**.

Fig. 15.15 Mesangial Cells. Electron micrograph of mesangium (M) and its relationship with the glomerular capillary (GC). The capillary wall is deficient in basement membrane (BM) at the site of attachment to the mesangium, the wall being composed of endothelial cell cytoplasm (EnC) lying directly on mesangial matrix (MM). The basement membrane continues over the surface of the mesangium to the next capillary loop.

Mesangial cell processes run in an apparently haphazard fashion through the extracellular mesangial matrix. The mesangial cell nucleus is round or oval and is larger than the endothelial cell nucleus (see Fig. 15.5e). There is a dense rim of nuclear chromatin inside the nuclear membrane, and numerous small chromatin clumps are scattered throughout the nucleoplasm (see Fig. 15.15).

The application of single-cell RNA sequencing has identified mesangial cells as distinct from other cell types. Mesangial cells express some markers similar to those of vascular smooth muscle cells (Fig. 15.16a) in addition to some markers of myofibroblasts (see Fig.15.16b). Mesangial cells also express markers of phagocytic cells, for example, the low-density lipoprotein receptor-related protein 1 (LRP1) is a receptor involved in phagocytosis of a wide range of extracellular material and is expressed in mesangial cells (see Fig. 15.16c).

Fig. 15.16 Mesangial Cells. (a) A contractile function can be identified using immunostaining with an antibody to smooth muscle actin *(brown)*, which also shows the distribution of mesangial cells (M) located in between the glomerular capillary loops. Note an afferent arteriole (AA) is also stained because of the smooth muscle in its wall. **(b)** Mesangial cells (M) can also be identified using immunostaining for PDFGRA, which is expressed in myofibroblastic cells and acts as a growth factor receptor that is important in renal development and is also involved in mesangial cell responses in disease. **(c)** The phagocytic capability of mesangial cells *(brown)* is illustrated by immunostaining for LRP1, which is a scavenger receptor involved in phagocytosis of a wide range of targets. [Images used under Creative Commons License https://creativecommons.org/licenses/by-sa/3.0/ from the Human Protein Atlas. (a) Antibody to ACTA2 CAB000002 https://www.proteinatlas.org/ENSG00000107796-ACTA2/tissue/kidney#im; (b) Antibody to PGFGFRA CAB018143 https://www.proteinatlas.org/ENSG00000134853-PDGFRA/tissue/kidney#img; and (c) Antibody to LRP1 HPA022903 https://www.proteinatlas.org/ENSG00000123384-LRP1/tissue/kidney#img.]

The mesangial matrix is an acellular material produced by the mesangial cell.

The mesangial matrix is a form of extracellular matrix composed of collagens, laminin, fibronectin and proteoglycans (see Chapter 4). The matrix largely encloses the mesangial cells and is also permeated by mesangial cell cytoplasmic processes. Ultrastructurally, it is of variable electron density, with the more electron-lucent parts closely resembling the lamina rara interna of the glomerular basement membrane, with which it is in continuity where the glomerular capillary and mesangium meet.

Mesangium can be seen in special stains such as periodic acid–Schiff (PAS) (see Fig. 15.5b) and Jones methenamine silver (see Fig. 15.8a) and by using immunohistochemical techniques (Fig. 15.17).

Fig. 15.17 Mesangial Matrix. Immunohistochemistry to detect collagen 6 highlights the distribution of mesangial matrix in the glomerulus *(brown)*. (Image used under Creative Commons License https://creativecommons.org/licenses/by-sa/3.0/ from the Human Protein Atlas Antibody to COL6A1 HPA019142 https://www.proteinatlas.org/ENSG00000142156-COL6A1/tissue/kidney#img.)

The mesangium has roles in structural support, modulating blood flow, cell signalling, phagocytosis and responses to stimuli in disease.

The precise mechanisms of action of the mesangium in humans are not fully understood. It has several known functions:

- Structural support of the glomerular capillary loop system. The intricate microanatomical alignment of all the structures involved in the glomerular filtration barrier is supported by the mesangium.
- Modulation of glomerular blood flow is achieved through the contractile properties of mesangial cells, which can respond to vasoactive substances, including angiotensin II (AngII). Any increase in glomerular capillary pressure would lead to increasing tensile stress in the capillary wall and increased individual glomerular filtration rate (hyperfiltration), which can be potentially damaging. This is countered and stabilized by mesangial cell contraction, thus preventing hyperfiltration at an individual glomerular level.
- Maintenance of the mesangial matrix by production and secretion of matrix components.
- Cell signalling through the production of several cytokines and growth factors.
- Phagocytic functions allow mesangial cells to remove material from the glomerular environment. This includes removal of immune complexes and other material that may gain access to the glomerular tuft from the blood.
- Reactive responses in disease are important functions of mesangial cells. In many conditions proliferation of mesangial cells, secretion of excess matrix and consequential sclerosis (scarring) of the glomerulus are central for disease onset and progression and lead to a reduction or cessation of function in individual glomeruli so affected.

▶▶ KEY FACTS

The Glomerulus

- The glomerulus is the site of ultrafiltration of blood.
- Filtration occurs across the highly specialized glomerular capillary wall, with filtrate entering the urinary space enclosed by Bowman's capsule.
- The filtration barrier comprises the glomerular capillary glycocalyx and endothelium, glomerular basement membrane and epithelial podocyte attached to the outer surface of the glomerular basement membrane.
- A further physicochemical barrier is the high polyanionic charge on the outer surface of the glomerular basement membrane and podocyte surface, preventing passage of cationic molecules.
- Initially, glomerular filtrate passes down the tubular and collecting duct systems, where controlled reabsorption and further excretion of small molecules (including water) occur.
- Filtered blood leaving the glomerulus via efferent arterioles enters a second capillary system around the tubules.

Mesangial Abnormalities

Abnormalities of the mesangium are an important component of many glomerular diseases.

In some forms of damage to the glomerulus, there is a proliferation of mesangial cells and production of a mesangial matrix, which lead to a reduction or cessation of capillary blood flow in the affected areas. This is a feature of several disorders, including some with a genetic cause and others caused by deposition of immune complexes in the glomerulus, which stimulate reactive or inflammatory responses termed *glomerulonephritis*.

Focal segmental glomerulosclerosis (FSGS) is a term used to describe findings on renal biopsy where one or more segments of glomeruli show mesangial proliferation and loss of capillary lumina. There are several causes, including genetic, autoimmune and a set of idiopathic cases (Fig. 15.18).

Diabetes mellitus is a common cause of glomerular pathology. As glomerular damage progresses, the mesangial cells of one or more of the glomerular segments produce excessive amounts of acellular matrix to form spherical nodules known as *Kimmelstiel–Wilson nodules* (Fig. 15.19). Such deposition effaces capillary lumina and causes reduced glomerular filtration.

In permanently damaged glomeruli, whatever the cause, excessive formation of mesangial matrix in all segments eventually converts the glomerular tuft into an acellular spherical mass (hyalinization and end-stage kidney disease; see Fig. 15.36).

Fig. 15.18 Focal Segmental Glomerulosclerosis. This PAS-stained micrograph is from a renal biopsy taken from a middle-aged adult who presented with nephrotic syndrome. One glomerulus has a normal mesangium. The other shows one segment replaced by expansion of the mesangium composed of mesangial cells and pink-staining matrix (FSS) with no capillaries seen in the affected segment. Investigations found no cause, and a diagnosis of primary focal segmental glomerulosclerosis was made. (Micrograph from digital pathology whole slide image provided by the University of Leeds Virtual Pathology Project https://www.virtualpathology.leeds.ac.uk. Reproduced with permission.)

Fig. 15.19 Kimmelstiel–Wilson Nodule. A PAS-stained paraffin section of kidney from a patient with diabetes mellitus showing localized nodules of mesangial matrix (Kimmelstiel–Wilson nodule, [K] in several of the glomerular lobules. (Micrograph from digital pathology whole slide image provided by the University of Leeds Virtual Pathology Project https://www.virtualpathology.leeds.ac.uk. Reproduced with permission.)

TUBULAR AND COLLECTING SYSTEM

Introduction

The glomerular filtrate leaves the urinary space at the tubular pole of the glomerulus and enters a tubule, which modifies its composition. The names of the different parts of this tubule and the course of the glomerular filtrate after leaving the glomerulus on its way to being excreted are illustrated in Fig. 15.20a.

The convoluted parts of both proximal and distal tubules are found close to the glomeruli, which are usually clustered around the ascending interlobular arteries from which their afferent arterioles are derived (see Fig. 15.20b).

In contrast, the straight parts of the tubular system and the cortical parts of the collecting duct system are concentrated together in the segments of cortex virtually devoid of glomeruli; these segments are inaccurately called *medullary rays*.

Such zoning divides the cortex into lobules. Each lobule is the segment of cortex between adjacent interlobular arteries and has a medullary ray at its centre.

The proximal tubule is vital for reabsorption of glomerular filtrate.

In the proximal tubule, there is extensive reabsorption of various components of the glomerular filtrate (Fig. 15.21a).

The cells that line the proximal tubule are continuous with the cells lining Bowman's capsule, and there is an abrupt transition of cell form at the tubular pole of the glomerulus.

The apical microvilli of the proximal tubule cells provide an immense surface area for absorption and the mitochondria, which are particularly numerous and prominent in the convoluted portion and provide the energy for the active transport of various components against gradients. In the brush border,

Fig. 15.20 Tubular and Collecting System of the Nephron. (a) The first part of the tubular system is the proximal tubule, which is a continuation of Bowman's capsule and initially pursues a convoluted course (the proximal convoluted tubule), remaining close to the glomerulus from which it arises. The proximal tubule then straightens and descends toward the medulla (proximal straight tubule, or the thick descending limb of the loop of Henle), merging with a thin-walled part of the tubular system (thin limb of the loop of Henle). This runs down in the cortex, and then in the medulla, toward the papillary tip (descending thin limb). It then loops back on itself (ascending thin limb) and re-enters the cortex. The wall then becomes thicker, forming the straight segment of the distal tubule (the thick ascending limb of the loop of Henle or the distal straight tubule). In the cortex, close to the glomeruli, the distal tubule becomes convoluted (distal convoluted tubule) and empties into a collecting tubule, which in turn empties into a collecting duct lying within the medullary ray. The collecting ducts descend into the medulla, where a number converge to produce large-diameter ducts in the papillae (papillary ducts or ducts of Bellini). These ducts open into the calyces at the tips of the papillae, with the concentration of the openings producing a sieve-like surface appearance to the papillary tip (the area cribrosa). The lengths of the various components of the tubular system vary, mainly according to the location of the glomerulus from which each is derived. The main variation in length occurs in the thin ascending and descending limbs of the loop of Henle. The proximal convoluted tubule is longer than the distal convoluted tubule. **(b)** Cortical tubules. H&E micrograph of cortical tubules. The proximal tubules (PT) are most numerous and prominent, having tall epithelium and small lumina. Distal tubules (DT) are smaller and have a cuboidal epithelium and proportionately larger lumina. Note the intimate capillary network (CN). Collecting ducts on their way to the medullary ray and thick and thin loops of Henle are also visible.

membrane ion pumps (ATPases) bring Na$^+$ ions into the cell from the glomerular filtrate passing through the tubular lumen. Other ions (e.g. H$^+$ and K$^+$) may be exchanged and pass into the lumen from the cell. Once in the cell, further membrane pumps in the basolateral membranes push Na$^+$ into the intercellular space, where their presence creates a high osmotic force. This force pulls water and Cl$^-$ ions from the lumen, past the tight junctions and into the intercellular space (paracellular route). From here, water and Cl$^-$ ions pass through the basement membrane into the interstitium, where hydrostatic pressure forces them into the adjacent peritubular capillaries.

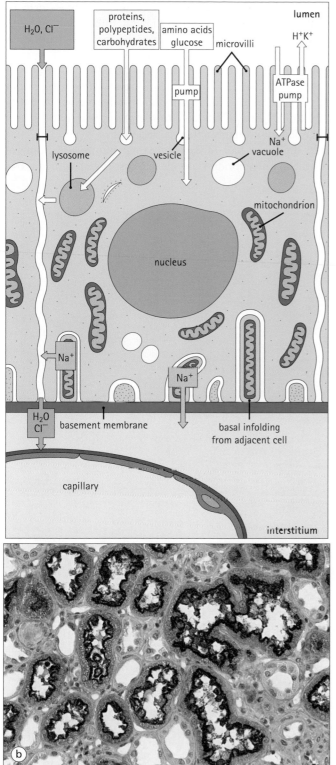

Fig. 15.21 Functional Aspects of Proximal Convoluted Tubule Cells.
(a) Apical microvilli of the proximal tubule cells express ion pumps, glucose transporter and membrane involved in receptor-mediated endocytosis to recycle substances from the passing filtrate. Cell function is energy-intensive, and mitochondria are located in basal membrane infoldings. The basolateral membrane is the site of the transport of Na^+ into the intercellular space, and this drives gradients that are used in fluid and ion exchange. **(b)** The transport function is seen in this micrograph of immunostained renal cortex using an antibody to cubilin *(brown)*, which is expressed in the apical cell membrane (brush border) of the proximal tubule and is involved in the endocytic uptake of many substances. Distal tubules seen in the micrograph do not express the receptor. Other transporters and receptors are also located in the apical membrane and transport and recover material back from the ultrafiltrate. (Image used under Creative Commons License https://creativecommons.org/licenses/by-sa/3.0/ from the Human Protein Atlas Antibody to cubilin HPA043854 https://www.proteinatlas.org/ENSG00000107611-CUBN/tissue/kidney#img.)

Proteins, polypeptides and some carbohydrates are also reabsorbed into the cell by endocytosis to enter the endosome–lysosome pathway and then pass into the intercellular space and thence into the interstitium and capillaries.

Glucose and certain amino acids in the tubular lumen are transported into the cell by specific transport systems at the microvillar surface. The majority of the small proteins that pass through the glomerular filtration barrier are reabsorbed in the proximal tubule through receptor-mediated endocytosis by binding to the megalin–cubilin receptor expressed on the brush border membrane (see Fig. 15.21b), including albumin, transferrin and vitamin D–binding protein.

The cells lining the proximal tubule are adapted for endocytosis, fluid and ion exchange.

Proximal tubule cells are cuboidal or columnar and have a centrally placed nucleus and a well-developed luminal brush border. The brush border is composed of numerous closely packed microvilli about 1 μm in length. At the base of the microvilli brush border are endocytic and pinocytotic vesicles that lie close to lysosomes. Each cell rests on a basement membrane, which is continuous with the basement membrane of Bowman's capsule.

The basal membrane of each tubule cell shows extensive basal interdigitation and some lateral interdigitation, which makes the lateral borders irregular and difficult to define except apically, where the intercellular space is sealed off from the tubule lumen by a tight junction (Fig. 15.22).

Although the lateral intercellular space of proximal tubule cells is narrow and difficult to define throughout its length from apex to base, it is often easy to see places where the space is distended into roughly spherical saccules.

In the lower half of each proximal tubule cell, numerous elongated mitochondria are closely associated with the basal

Fig. 15.22 Proximal Convoluted Tubule. (a) The microvillous surface, the complex basal interdigitations and the lateral interdigitations of proximal convoluted tubule cells. **(b)** High-power micrograph showing the microvillus brush border (MV) lining the lumen of the azan-stained proximal tubule. **(c)** High-power electron micrograph of the microvillus brush border (MV) and the system of pinocytotic vesicles (PV). Note the tight junction (TJ) joining adjacent cells near the base of the brush border. **(d)** Electron micrograph showing the system of basal interdigitations (BI) at the site of attachment of the proximal convoluted tubule cell to its basement membrane (BM). Note the abundant large mitochondria (M) and the proximity of an interstitial capillary (C). **(e)** Scanning electron micrograph of the lumen of a proximal convoluted tubule showing the complex system of microvilli.

interdigitations from adjacent cells and are arranged in parallel with the interdigitating basal cytoplasmic membranes.

The membrane and cytoplasmic specializations are most developed in the convoluted part of the proximal tubule. In the straight descending portion, as the thin loop of Henle is approached, the microvilli become smaller and less numerous, the degree of basal and lateral interdigitation less marked and mitochondria and lysosomes fewer. The cells also become more cuboidal.

The loop of Henle is divided into thick and thin parts.

Traditionally, the loop of Henle is regarded as having thick descending and ascending components and a thin-walled section in between. It is better, however, to regard the thin-walled part as a distinct functional and structural entity for the following two reasons. First, the thick descending and ascending components are ultrastructurally closely identifiable with the proximal and distal convoluted tubules. Second, the transitions between thick and thin tubules are abrupt, whereas the thick ascending and descending parts merge gradually with the proximal and distal convoluted tubules.

The thin limbs of the loop of Henle are lined by a flat epithelium and vary in length.

The thin limbs of the loop of Henle vary in length. Those associated with juxtamedullary glomeruli are long and extend deep into the medulla towards the papillary tip (long-loop nephrons), whereas those associated with mid-cortical or subcapsular glomeruli extend only partway into the medulla (short-loop nephrons).

The thin limbs, both ascending and descending, have flat lining epithelium showing very little cytoplasmic specialization (Fig. 15.23). At its simplest, the thin loop resembles a dilated capillary by light microscopy and can be difficult to distinguish in routine paraffin sections.

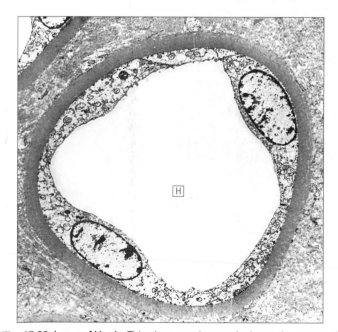

Fig. 15.23 Loop of Henle. This electron micrograph shows the structural simplicity of the thin loops of Henle (H) in the medulla.

In other areas, however, the epithelium, although flat, is rather more prominent and ultrastructurally has short microvilli and some of the basal and lateral interdigitations seen to a greater degree in proximal tubules.

The thin limb of the loop of Henle maintains an osmotic gradient in the renal parenchyma.

The thin limb of the loop of Henle creates a gradient of hypertonicity. The gradient is from the corticomedullary junction to the tip of the renal papilla and is affected by the variable passage of sodium and chloride ions between the lumen of the loop of Henle and the interstitium. This gradient allows concentration of the urine in the collecting duct system as it passes through the medulla. The widely accepted explanation of this mechanism is called the *countercurrent multiplier hypothesis* (Fig. 15.24).

Fig. 15.24 Countercurrent Multiplier Hypothesis. The descending thin limb of the loop of Henle is freely permeable to water and Na$^+$ and Cl$^-$ ions, whereas the ascending thin limb, which is impermeable to water, actively pumps Cl$^-$ ions out of the lumen into the interstitium, whereupon Na$^+$ ions follow to maintain ionic neutrality. Thus the ascending limb discharges Na$^+$ and Cl$^-$ ions into the interstitium but retains water within its lumen. Some of the Na$^+$ and Cl$^-$ ions diffuse back into the tubular lumen at the descending thin limb but are pushed out again when they reach the ascending limb. This produces the multiplier effect and leads to hypertonicity of the interstitial tissue in relation to the fluid in the tubular lumen, particularly near the papillary tip. The fluid emerging from the end of the ascending limb of the loop of Henle into the distal tubule system is hypotonic.

The distal tubule starts after the loop of Henle.

The ascending thin limb of the loop of Henle opens into the short straight part of the distal tubule, which passes into the cortex running in a medullary ray and then becomes convoluted before opening into the collecting tubule. At about the junction between the straight and convoluted parts, the distal tubule runs close to the glomerular hilum to form a specialized segment called the *macula densa* (see p. 319).

◎ ADVANCED CONCEPT

The Cells Lining the Distal Nephron Are Adapted for Fluid and Ion Exchange

The distal nephron is lined by cuboidal epithelial cells with extensive basal and lateral interdigitations. These are similar to those seen in the proximal tubule, but the microvilli on the luminal surface are less well formed and comparatively scanty (Fig. 15.25a). Mitochondria are numerous and mainly situated close to the lateral and basal interdigitations. There are none of the luminal invaginations and vesicles seen close to the microvillus border in the proximal convoluted tubule. The apical membrane of distal tubule cells is the location of transporter proteins (see Fig. 15.25b).

The structure of the distal tubule is virtually identical in the convoluted and straight segments (ascending thick limb of loop of Henle), but the macula densa (see p. 319) shows a local variation in structure.

Beyond the macula densa, the distal convoluted tubule, connecting segment and collecting duct are lined by two types of cells which regulate salt and acid–base balance through several transport proteins differentially present in the different cell types: the **principal** and **intercalated** cells.

The proportion of each cell type varies between different regions of the distal nephron:

- Principal cells are mainly involved in fluid–electrolyte regulation. They express the water-permeability channel aquaporin-2, which is under the control of antidiuretic hormone (ADH). They respond to aldosterone and absorb sodium and excrete potassium in accordance with metabolic needs.
- Intercalated cells are mainly involved in acid–base regulation.

Functional studies have identified subtypes of intercalated cells according to the pattern of expression of different transport systems:

- Types involved mainly in hydrogen ion transport expressing H+-ATPase
- A type also expressing the chloride/bicarbonate exchanger pendrin responsible for bicarbonate exchange

In conventionally stained sections it is not possible to discriminate between the different cell types. Electron microscopy can broadly distinguish between principal and intercalated cells. Immunohistochemistry for the different transport proteins can separate subtypes of intercalated cells (Fig. 15.26c and d).

Fig. 15.25 Distal Tubule. (a) Electron micrograph showing the features of a distal convoluted tubule cell. Note that it shows similar basal interdigitations (BI) to those of the proximal convoluted tubule cell, but the luminal microvilli (MV) are scanty and less well formed. **(b)** The transport function is shown in this micrograph immunostained to show the location of a potassium exchange transporter located in the apical membrane of the distal tubular epithelial cells *(brown)*. (Image used under Creative Commons License https://creativecommons.org/licenses/by-sa/3.0/ from the Human Protein Atlas Antibody to Potassium inwardly rectifying channel subfamily J member 1 ROMK1 HPA026962 https://www.proteinatlas.org/ENSG00000151704-KCNJ1/tissue/kidney#img.)

The Cells Lining the Distal Nephron Are Adapted for Fluid and Ion Exchange

Fig. 15.26 Collecting Tubule. (a) Electron micrograph of the collecting tubule, which connects the end of the distal convoluted tubule and the collecting duct in the medullary ray of the cortex. Note the darkly stained intercalated cell (IC), which is rich in mitochondria, and the sparse, short microvilli (MV) of the clearer-stained principal cells (PC). **(b)** Micrograph of a collecting duct stained to show aquaporin-2 *(brown)*. Principal cells (PC) show apical staining indicating permeability of cells to water. There is also faint granular staining of cytoplasm corresponding to storage vesicles containing aquaporin. A small number of cells do not show an apical membrane or cytoplasmic staining and correspond to intercalated cells (IC) whose role is in acid–base balance rather than electrolyte–fluid balance. **(c)** Micrograph showing collecting ducts stained to show an anion exchange protein. Strong expression in some cells and absent expression in other cells serve to emphasis the mosaic-like population of epithelial cells within the collecting tubules and ducts, each with a specialized function. **(d)** Micrograph immunostained for pendrin *(brown)*. This transport protein is expressed in intercalated cells of the collecting tubules. Cells lining the tubule that do not express this transporter correspond to principal cells [Images used under Creative Commons License https://creativecommons.org/licenses/by-sa/3.0/ from the Human Protein Atlas. (b) Antibody to aquaporin2 AQP2 HPA046834 https://www.proteinatlas.org/ENSG00000167580-AQP2/tissue/kidney#img; (c) Antibody to Solute carrier family 4 member 1 AE1 HPA015584 https://www.proteinatlas.org/ENSG00000004939-SLC4A1/tissue/kidney#img; (d) Antibody to Solute carrier family 26 member 4 (pendrin) HPA042860 https://www.proteinatlas.org/ENSG00000091137-SLC26A4/tissue/kidney#img.]

> **The distal tubule is crucial to the control of acid–base balance and is also important in urine concentration.**

The epithelial cells in the distal tubule have the ability to pump ions against concentration gradients. This part of the nephron is crucial for acid–base regulation and also for sodium/potassium exchange as part of maintaining fluid and electrolyte balance.

- Sodium ions can be reabsorbed from the dilute urine in the lumen, and potassium ions are excreted as required.
- Bicarbonate ions can be reabsorbed and hydrogen ions excreted, thus rendering the urine acidic as required.

These functions are dependent on the presence of the hormone aldosterone, a mineralocorticoid secreted by the adrenal cortex (see p. 283).

> **Antidiuretic hormone (ADH) controls the permeability of the distal tubular epithelium to water.**

ADH secreted by the posterior pituitary acts on the last part of the distal convoluted tubule. Its effect is to increase the permeability of the tubule, thus permitting the absorption of water to produce a more concentrated urine.

ADH also acts on the collecting ducts in a similar manner, permitting the absorption of water from the duct lumen into the hypertonic interstitium, and thence into the blood system (vasa recta). This movement of water is dependent on the countercurrent exchanger system (see Fig. 15.30).

◎ ADVANCED CONCEPT

ADH Changes the Permeability of Epithelium by Controlling the Location of Aquaporin

Aquaporins are a family of integral membrane proteins which function as water channels, allowing passage of water (permeability) through a cell membrane. Several different aquaporins are present in different locations in the nephron, and they permit the passage of water through cell membranes as part of the mechanisms in the kidney used to maintain homeostasis. One member of the family, aquaporin-2 (AQP2), is expressed in principal cells of the distal nephron, and, importantly, its location in the cell membrane is controlled by ADH (see Fig. 15.26b). Principal cells express AQP3 and AQP4 in the basal cell membrane (not in contact with urine). The apical membrane of principal cells does not normally contain aquaporins, and so the tubule lining is normally impermeable to water. AQP2, however, is present in principal cells but is stored in intracellular vesicles, not in the surface membrane. After stimulation of collecting duct principal cells by ADH, vesicles dock with the cell membrane, and AQP2 is transferred to the apical cell surface. With aquaporin in this location, water can enter the cell, pass through the basal membrane using AQP3 and AQP4 and so be resorbed from the filtrate. With cessation of ADH stimulation, endosomal vesicles form and AQP2 is removed from the apical cell membrane, restoring impermeability of the tubular epithelium to water.

🐾 CLINICAL EXAMPLE

Diabetes Insipidus

In the permanent absence of ADH, as occurs in diabetes insipidus, vast quantities of dilute urine are formed because of the failure of water reabsorption at the distal convoluted tubule and collecting ducts.

Fatal body water depletion is only prevented by drinking large quantities of water, which is stimulated by a constant feeling of thirst.

> **The collecting tubules and ducts start after the distal tubule.**

The convoluted segment of the distal tubule opens into the collecting system of tubules and ducts. This transition is not abrupt, as there is a variable segment ('connecting segment'), where the epithelial lining contains both distal tubule and collecting tubule cell types.

> **The collecting tubules are lined by two cell types.**

The collecting tubule (see Fig. 15.26) is lined by two types of cells: principal cells (clear cells) and intercalated cells (dark cells). Principal cells form the majority within this part of the tubule and regulate electrolyte–fluid balance. Intercalated cells are fewer in number and regulate acid–base balance.

The principal cells are cuboidal in the proximal part of the collecting system; they have light, poorly staining cytoplasm, which contains few cytoplasmic organelles (mainly randomly arranged, small, round mitochondria). Basal membrane infoldings are present in the proximal part of the collecting system but become less apparent farther along. Cells have short, stubby surface microvilli, and vesicles are present in the cytoplasm at the base of the microvilli. Ultrastructurally, cells have a surface mechanoreceptor primary cilium (see Chapter 2).

The intercalated or dark cells are richer in cytoplasmic organelles, possessing numerous mitochondria. Their luminal surface has microvilli, with a pattern depending on the subtype of intercalated cell. Normally, there are few basal infoldings. These cells do not bear a surface primary cilium.

> **The collecting tubules in the cortex pass toward the medullary rays and open into collecting ducts.**

The collecting ducts run vertically within the rays into the medulla. All of the medullary collecting ducts merge near the papilla to form large straight papillary ducts that run to the tip of papilla, where they open out into the pelvicalyceal system (see Fig. 15.29).

The collecting ducts are lined initially by epithelium that is similar in pattern to that of the collecting tubules. As they pass down the medullary rays and into the medulla, however, the number of intercalated cells decreases and the principal cells become progressively taller and more prominent, so that, as the papilla is approached, the ducts are lined by regular, straight-sided columnar cells (Fig. 15.27).

In humans, the basement membrane of the collecting duct system becomes progressively thicker as it nears the papillary tip. This feature becomes exaggerated with age.

Fig. 15.27 Collecting Duct. Electron micrograph of a large collecting duct in the medulla. Note the lining of regular cuboidal or columnar clear cells and the sparse organelles.

PRACTICAL HISTOLOGY

Haemoxylin and eosin (H&E) micrographs of the renal medulla showing morphology of renal tubular system (Figs. 15.28 and 15.29).

Fig. 15.28 Histology of Tubules in the Medulla. In the medulla, all the various tubules, ducts and vessels run in the same direction: towards the papillary tip. The appearance on histological examination depends on whether the section has been cut longitudinally to the axis of the tubules (in which case the tubules and ducts are cut in longitudinal section) or transversely. In most randomly selected tissue blocks, the section is usually oblique to the longitudinal plane of the medulla to a greater or lesser extent. **(a)** In this micrograph of the outer medulla, just below the corticomedullary junction, the tubules and ducts are seen in transverse section. The outer medulla contains a mixture of thick descending and ascending portions of loops of Henle (HT), which are histologically similar to proximal and distal convoluted tubule; thin loops of Henle (HL); small collecting ducts (CD); and vasa recta (VR). In this region, there is a small amount of interstitium in which a few interstitial cells (IC) can be seen. **(b)** Micrograph of the same area of outer medulla shown sectioned almost longitudinally.

Continued

Fig. 15.28, cont'd (c) In this micrograph of the lower medulla note the difference in the content of tubules and ducts from that of the outer medulla shown in **(a)** and **(b)**. There are now no thick portions of loops of Henle, but thin Henle loops (HL) are numerous, as are thin-walled capillaries (C). The collecting ducts (CD) are larger and lined by distinct, clear-celled cuboidal epithelium. The pale-staining interstitium now forms a substantial part of the tissue, and scattered small stellate and spindle-shaped interstitial cells (IC) are numerous. In this micrograph, the loops of Henle, vessels and collecting ducts are in transverse section. **(d)** Micrograph of same area of lower medulla shown in **(c)** sectioned longitudinally. Note the prominent straight collecting ducts running down towards the papilla; the nearer the tip of the papilla, the larger the ducts become. The intricate functionality is belied by the apparent structural simplicity.

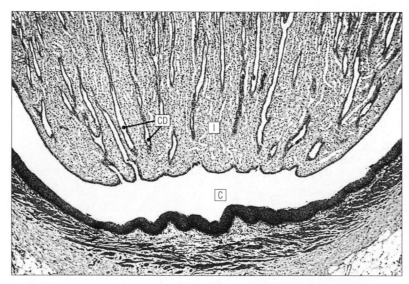

Fig. 15.29 Papilla. The large collecting ducts (CD) are few in number as a result of fusion; they open into the calyx (C) at the papillary tip. At the papilla, the distal medulla consists almost entirely of large collecting ducts embedded in bulky interstitium (I), with very few thin Henle loops and a number of vasa recta vessels. Interstitial cells are numerous.

The collecting tubules and ducts play an important role in the final concentration of urine.

The collecting tubules and ducts are instrumental in concentrating urine to a degree appropriate to the level of blood hydration. This is achieved by interplay between the collecting tubules and ducts, the interstitium and the vasa recta to produce a countercurrent exchanger system (Fig. 15.30). Controlled water transport is made possible by the variable permeability of the collecting duct under the influence of ADH (see p. 314). The amount of ADH released depends on the body's requirement for water excretion or retention.

In the presence of high levels of ADH, water is resorbed from the collecting duct lumen into the interstitium, from where it passes into the blood circulation via the ascending vasa recta. This results in the production of a small amount of highly concentrated urine. When low levels of ADH are present, water remains within the collecting duct lumen and is lost in the form of copious dilute urine.

KEY FACTS
Tubular and Collecting Duct System Functions

- Proximal convoluted tubule – reabsorption of water, glucose and amino acid by the Na^+/K^+/ATPase pump, whereas larger molecules such as proteins are reabsorbed by endocytosis
- Thin loop of Henle – creates a gradient of hypertonicity to allow concentration of urine in collecting duct system
- Distal tubule – Na^+ and HCO_3^- ions reabsorbed from urine in exchange for K^+ and H^+, which are excreted, dependent on aldosterone
- Collecting tubules and ducts – control final concentration of urine by regulated reabsorption of water from urine under influence of hypertonicity gradient and ADH

The vascular networks of the vasa recta also play a role in the concentration of urine in the medulla.

On the descending (arterial) side of the looped vessels, the walls are permeable to water and salts; water passes out into the interstitium and sodium and chloride ions pass in. Thus blood in the vasa recta is more or less in equilibrium with the hypertonic medullary interstitium.

On the ascending (venous) side of the vascular loop, sodium and chloride ions pass from the vessel lumen to the interstitium, and water is reabsorbed into the venous blood from the interstitium.

Fig. 15.30 Countercurrent Exchanger System. Dilute urine in the collecting tubule and duct system is progressively concentrated by the osmotic transfer of water from the lumen into the hypertonic medullary interstitial tissue, whence it is reabsorbed into the vasa recta. The hypertonicity is caused by the high concentration of Na^+ and Cl^- ions in the medulla, resulting from the countercurrent multiplier activity of the loops of Henle. Thus an increasingly concentrated urine is produced.

Acute Kidney Injury

Failure of tubular function because of poor oxygenation can also occur in the absence of any significant disease of arteries or glomeruli. The most common cause is a central failure of blood circulation owing to poor cardiac output, which in turn is usually either the result of low blood volume (hypovolaemia), for example, in severe sepsis or after massive blood loss through haemorrhage, or the result of low blood pressure (hypotension), for example, after a myocardial infarction.

Poor perfusion through the peritubular capillary network leads to inadequate oxygen supplies for the tubular epithelial cells, and this leads to failure of the enzyme systems and pump mechanisms, with consequent biochemical abnormalities, particularly acidosis and hyperkalaemia. Because the glomeruli are not being perfused with arterial blood at an adequate pressure, little filtration takes place, so the production of urine falls or may even cease. Acute kidney injury leads to the syndrome of acute renal failure:

- Oliguria or anuria (partial or total cessation of urine production)
- Hyperkalaemia (elevated K^+ level in the blood)
- Acidosis (elevated H^+ level in the blood)

When the tubular failure is the result of a central cause such as hypovolaemia or hypotension, the tubular epithelial cells degenerate (Fig. 15.31). Their histological appearance is caused by the accumulation of water within the cytosol.

If hypovolaemia or hypotension is treated promptly, tubular epithelial cells can recover; otherwise, the cells die (acute tubular necrosis).

Fig. 15.31 Acute Kidney Injury. H&E micrograph of kidney from a patient with early acute renal failure caused by hypovolaemic shock. Part of a glomerulus (G) and numerous tubules are seen. One relatively normal tubule is present (T) in which the normal nuclei are pale-stained and the cytoplasm has some faint basophilia. Many other tubules are damaged (D), and epithelial cells have dense-stained contracted nuclei and eosinophilic cytoplasm. In other tubules (B) epithelial cells are swollen and pale-stained, an appearance called *ballooning*. The interstitium between the tubules (I) contains fluid (oedema) pushing the tubules apart. With failure of energy-dependent ion pumps, cells accumulate fluid and become swollen. More severe damage leads to cell death, seen as small, dense-stained nuclei and eosinophilic cytoplasm. This type of damage to tubules is typical in acute kidney injury caused by poor renal perfusion. Compare with Fig. 15.19. (Micrograph from digital pathology whole slide image provided by the University of Leeds Virtual Pathology Project https://www.virtualpathology.leeds.ac.uk. Reproduced with permission.)

RENAL INTERSTITIUM

> The renal interstitium is an extracellular matrix which supports all kidney structures and contains a population of specialized interstitial cells.

The renal interstitium is filled with a specialized extracellular matrix which supports all structures of the renal parenchyma. Specialized **renal interstitial cells** are resident within the interstitium.

In the cortex of the human kidney, the interstitial space is small and largely occupied by small blood vessels, lymphatics and sparse interstitial cells all set in an extracellular matrix. The basement membrane of tubules and capillaries is adherent to this extracellular matrix (see Chapter 4). In the medulla, the interstitium becomes a significant component, both in bulk and in function. The interstitium increases in both size and importance as the tip of the papilla is neared (see Fig. 15.29).

Ultrastructurally, the interstitium is an extracellular matrix composed largely of loose electron-lucent acellular material, partly protein and partly glycosaminoglycans, in which collagen fibres, lipid droplets and basal lamina–like material are scattered.

Fig. 15.32 Medullary Interstitial Cell and Matrix. Electron micrograph showing a typical human medullary interstitial cell (IC) located in the loose matrix near the loop of Henle (H). The characteristic cytoplasmic feature is the presence of electron-dense spherical lipid droplets (LD); there is abundant rough endoplasmic reticulum and a few mitochondria.

Variable numbers of interstitial cells are also present (Fig. 15.32). There are two cell types:

- Fibroblasts which are linked by junctions to vessels and basement membranes of tubules and produce erythropoietin in the renal cortex. Fibroblasts also produce the proteins of the interstitial extracellular matrix.
- Dendritic cells (see Chapter 8), which act as tissue resident immune cells and can respond by recruiting other immune effector cells.

In renal disease, activation of interstitial cells leads to fibroblasts developing a myofibroblast phenotype, and it is this cell that can produce collagen and lead to interstitial scarring.

JUXTAGLOMERULAR APPARATUS

The juxtaglomerular apparatus is involved in maintaining blood pressure and volume by the production of the hormone renin. It is a specialized adaptation of vascular and tubular tissues that allows blood flow to affect renin output. The juxtaglomerular apparatus comprises:

- Juxtaglomerular cells, which are renin-producing cells located in the walls of the afferent and efferent arterioles at the vascular hilum of the glomerulus
- Lacis or extraglomerular mesangial cells
- The macula densa area of distal tubule (Fig. 15.33)

> **Juxtaglomerular cells contain neuroendocrine granules.**

Juxtaglomerular renin-producing cells are concentrated mainly in the walls of the afferent arteriole, although small numbers are present in the efferent arteriole.

Juxtaglomerular cells have the ultrastructural features of highly specialized myoepithelial cells, with some contractile filaments. They also contain neuroendocrine granules of many shapes and sizes, although two distinct types can be recognized.

Type I granules are irregular in shape and contain rhomboidal crystalline bodies (protogranules), which are believed to be the precursors of the other types of granules.

Type II granules are larger, spherical, uniformly electron dense and have an ill-defined membrane; they are thought to represent the mature renin-secreting granules.

> **The lacis or extraglomerular mesangial cells resemble mesangial cells.**

Lacis cells have a network (lacis) of thin interwoven processes, which are separated by an acellular matrix of basement membrane–like material. Lacis cells occupy the triangular region bordered by the macula densa at the base and the afferent and efferent arterioles at the sides; the apex is formed by the base of the glomerular mesangium.

Their function is not definitively known, but they have numerous processes containing gap junctions and are thought to provide electrical coupling among themselves and to the mesangium and glomerular arterioles.

> **The macula densa is a specialized adaptation of distal tubular epithelium.**

The macula densa is a specialized zone of the distal tubule where it is in close contact with the vascular hilum of the glomerulus.

In this region, the epithelial cells of the distal tubule are taller and more tightly packed than elsewhere in the tubule and the nuclei lie closer to the luminal surface; the Golgi is located between the nucleus and the basement membrane. Cells are anchored together with tight junctions located close to the apical end, and each has a primary cilium extending into the tubular lumen which can act as a sensor (see Chapter 2). Single-cell RNA studies have identified markers of epithelial cells of the macula densa that distinguish them from other tubular cell types (Fig. 15.34).

> **Renin converts angiotensinogen to active angiotensin, which then causes the adrenals to secrete aldosterone.**

Renin produced in the juxtaglomerular apparatus catalyses the conversion of inactive angiotensinogen. Angiotensinogen is an α_2-globulin produced in the liver, converted by renin to the decapeptide angiotensin I. Angiotensin I is then converted to angiotensin II, which stimulates the secretion of aldosterone by the zona glomerulosa of the adrenal cortex (see p. 283).

Aldosterone is a mineralocorticoid hormone that regulates body sodium and potassium ion levels through its effect on the sodium pump mechanism at the cell membranes.

Fig. 15.33 Juxtaglomerular Apparatus. (a) The juxtaglomerular apparatus, which consists of the macula densa, lacis cells, and the afferent and efferent arterioles. Within the walls of the arterioles are granular renin-secreting cells. **(b)** Masson's trichrome stain showing the macula densa (MD) and afferent arteriole (AA) with prominent muscle cells (M) containing renin granules. The efferent vessel and lacis cells are not visible in this section. **(c)** Electron micrograph of human juxtaglomerular apparatus. Note the macula densa (MD), renin-producing cells (R), lacis cells (L), glomerular mesangial cells (G) and urinary space (US). **(d)** High-power electron micrograph of the renin-secreting granular cells in the afferent arteriole wall. Note the protogranules (PG) (type I) and mature granules (MG) (type II).

Fig. 15.34 Macula Densa. Micrograph immunostained for cytosolic 5′-nucleotidase, an enzyme involved in nucleoside metabolism. This highlights the cells of the macula densa as part of the juxtaglomerular apparatus. (Image used under Creative Commons License https://creativecommons.org/licenses/by-sa/3.0/ from the Human Protein Atlas. Antibody to cytosolic 5′-nucleotidase IA [cN-IA] HPA054158 https://www.proteinatlas.org/ENSG00000116981-NT5C1A/tissue/kidney#img.)

Fig. 15.35 Renin–Angiotensin–Aldosterone System. **(a)** Renin secreted by the juxtaglomerular apparatus (JGA) catalyses the production of angiotensin I from its inactive precursor, angiotensinogen. Angiotensin I is then converted in the lung into the active octapeptide angiotensin II, which stimulates the release of aldosterone from the adrenal cortex. Aldosterone mediates the absorption of sodium and water from the glomerular filtrate at the distal tubule. **(b)** Immunohistochemical staining for renin *(brown)* showing its location in relation to the afferent arteriole (R) at the hilum of the glomerulus (G). Note the macula densa (M). See also Fig. 15.33a. [Image (b) used under Creative Commons License https://creativecommons.org/licenses/by-sa/3.0/ from the Human Protein Atlas Antibody to Renin HPA005131 https://www.proteinatlas.org/ENSG00000143839-REN/tissue/kidney#img.]

In the distal tubule of the kidney, aldosterone promotes the reabsorption of sodium ions and water from the glomerular filtrate (Fig. 15.35) and thereby contributes to the maintenance of plasma volume and blood pressure.

> **Renin synthesis may be modulated by sodium concentration or blood pressure.**

Macula densa cells monitor the sodium concentration in the distal tubule lumen contents and signal renin release by the juxtaglomerular cells in the arteriole walls via production of prostaglandins (PGI_2 and PGE_2) and nitric oxide. Renal renin release is inversely related to renal perfusion pressure such that a drop in perfusion pressure stimulates renin secretion, whereas an increase in perfusion pressure inhibits it. This is the so-called *renal baroreceptor mechanism*. It is now widely accepted that blood pressure changes are detected within the afferent arteriole itself, and pressure-dependent regulation of renin release is not absolutely dependent on macula densa function.

ERYTHROPOIETIN SYNTHESIS

> **The kidney is the main source of erythropoietin (EPO) in adults.**

EPO acts as a major regulator of erythropoiesis by promoting the survival, proliferation and differentiation of erythroid progenitor cells and by regulating the number of erythrocytes in peripheral blood.

In adults, about 90% of EPO is produced by renal interstitial cortical and outer medullary fibroblasts, whereas 10% is contributed by extrarenal sources, primarily liver cells. In the fetus, the liver is the primary site of EPO production, especially in the hepatocytes surrounding central veins.

CLINICAL EXAMPLE

Kidney Failure

Because the blood circulatory system in the kidney is its most important component, it is not surprising that many renal diseases are the result of vascular pathology. Common vascular diseases, such as systemic hypertension, diabetes mellitus and atherosclerosis, frequently damage the kidney, leading to impaired excretory and homeostatic functions.

Chronic Kidney Disease

Decreased blood flow through the glomerular capillary system can occur because of many causes, a common factor being damage to podocytes (see p. 301).

Hypertension can lead to thickening of arteriolar walls and damage to the glomerular structure through excessive shear stress on podocytes. Mesangial cells react by proliferation and production of a mesangial matrix, which causes effacement of the glomerular capillary lumen and a reduction in glomerular filtration.

Diabetes mellitus leads to thickening of the glomerular basement membrane and reactive changes in mesangial cells that efface the capillary vessels in the glomerular tuft (see Fig. 15.19).

Immune-mediated damage caused by deposition of immune complexes (glomerulonephritis) induces changes in the glomerular basement membrane together with reactive changes in mesangial cells, leading to mesangial sclerosis and effacement of glomerular capillary vessels (see Fig. 15.18).

When disease is prolonged, this leads to the glomerulus being gradually replaced by mesangial matrix and mesangial cells, followed by further collagen deposition (glomerular hyalinization). Each nephron is a single functional entity, and once the glomerulus is devoid of blood flow, the associated tubule undergoes atrophy and is lost (Fig. 15.36). When these changes affect most of the glomeruli and their associated tubular systems, all of the functions of the kidney are impaired, and the patient develops features of chronic kidney disease leading to end-stage kidney disease with the clinical pattern of chronic renal failure.

Failure of the kidney's excretory function leads to retention in the blood of toxic metabolic waste materials, particularly urea and creatinine, from the endogenous breakdown of body protein. This is called **uraemia**; the accumulation of urea and creatinine can be measured in blood tests. Eventually, without treatment such intoxication leads to coma, seizures and death. Failure of homeostatic functions carried out by the renal tubules leads to a loss of control of the body's water and electrolyte concentration; hydrogen and potassium ions accumulate in the blood, producing acidosis and hyperkalaemia.

The kidneys are unable to produce urine with a concentration or dilution commensurate with the body's needs. Instead, urine of constant specific gravity is produced, irrespective of the degree of haemoconcentration or haemodilution.

These biochemical disorders are the result of inexorable destruction of all of the activities of all nephrons. Chronic renal failure is irreversible.

Acute Renal Failure (Acute Kidney Injury)

In acute renal failure, there is a sudden transient cessation of all nephron activity, which is usually the result of damage to all tubules, or all glomeruli, or both linked to acute kidney injury. Depending on the cause, some recovery is usually possible if the patient can be sustained by haemodialysis through the period of intense metabolic upset while the nephrons are non-functional and until regeneration can occur.

Fig. 15.36 End-Stage Kidney Disease. This H&E section shows the kidney from a patient with long-standing chronic kidney disease caused by progressive disease of the renal arterial supply as a result of hypertension. Little remains of the normal structure of the nephron. The glomeruli have been converted into acellular spheres of collagen containing no capillary network, and remaining tubules have atrophied, with the epithelial cells being flattened or cuboidal. There is fibrosis in the interstitium.

LYMPHATIC DRAINAGE AND NERVE SUPPLY OF THE KIDNEY

The importance of the lymphatic drainage of the kidney in normal function is probably minimal, as this is effaced during renal transplantation with no obvious serious side effects. Renal autonomic innervation influences blood pressure through the innervation of blood vessels. Sympathetic denervation is used as a medical procedure in the management of some patients who have hypertension resistant to drug treatment.

> **Lymphatics in the kidney run with blood vessels.**

The lymphatic drainage of the cortex of the kidney is mainly by a series of lymphatics that run in parallel with the cortical blood vessels. The main channels follow the interlobular, arcuate and interlobar blood vessels and emerge from the kidney at the renal hilum. A minor lymphatic system runs in the renal capsule and receives small tributaries from the outer cortex. There is some communication between these two systems within the cortex.

> **The kidney is supplied by autonomic innervation.**

The nerve supply to the kidney arises mainly from the coeliac plexus. Both adrenergic and cholinergic fibres have been demonstrated. In general, these nerves have been seen to follow the course of blood vessels throughout the cortex and the outer medulla.

CLINICAL EXAMPLE
Important Tumours of the Kidney

The most common tumour arising from the kidney parenchyma (renal cell carcinoma) is malignant and is derived from the glandular cells lining the tubules and is therefore an **adenocarcinoma**. It occurs in the middle-aged and elderly and can spread extensively to other sites of the body via the bloodstream. The other important type occurs only in young children, and the cell of origin is a multipotential stem cell called the *nephroblast,* which, during embryonic life, differentiates to produce all the specific cells of the kidney. Rarely, some of these persist after birth and can give rise to rapidly growing malignant tumours called **nephroblastomas**.

LOWER URINARY TRACT

> **The lower urinary tract is a series of conduits and reservoirs for urine.**

The lower urinary tract is a functional rather than geographical entity, as it extends from an intrarenal component high in the abdominal cavity to the tip of the urethra. It comprises:
- The calyceal collecting system, into which the large collecting ducts of Bellini in the medullary papillae discharge the urine.
- The renal pelvis, which is the reservoir at the hilum of the kidney into which the various calyces pass the urine.
- The ureter, which is a long muscular tube that conducts urine down to the bladder.
- The bladder, which acts as a major reservoir, holding the urine until it can be voided.
- The urethra, through which the urine stored in the bladder is voided to the exterior.

At various points, there are sphincters capable of closing off parts of the lower urinary tract so that it can act as a reservoir. The most important of these muscular sphincters is located at the junction between the bladder and urethra and is under voluntary control.

These excretory passages are essentially hollow tubes with muscular walls. Except for part of the urethra, they are lined by a specialized epithelium that is capable of withstanding contact with urine, a fluid of variable concentration containing a number of toxic substances. This specialized lining is a form of stratified epithelium, known as *transitional epithelium,* or, in this site, the *urothelium* (Fig. 15.37).

> **The lower urinary tract is lined by specialized transitional epithelium termed *urothelium*.**

The urothelium is a multilayered epithelium that varies in thickness at various sites in the lower urinary tract. In the small calyces, it is only two to three cell layers thick, but in the empty bladder, it may contain up to five or six layers; presumably this reflects the different degrees of distension to which the two components are usually subjected. As these epithelial cells have the ability to stretch, shift on each other and flatten, a distended bladder may appear to be lined by only a two- to three-cell layer of stretched, flat cells.

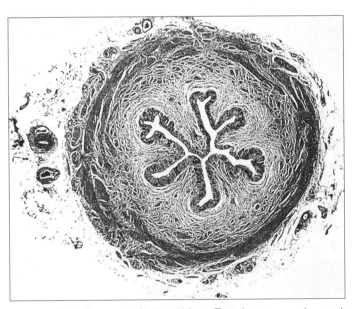

Fig. 15.37 Basic Structure of Lower Urinary Tract. Low-power micrograph of a transverse section of human ureter showing the basic structure of the lower urinary tract. The walls are muscular, and there is an internal lining of specialized urothelium.

In the non-distended state, urothelium has a rather compact, cuboidal basal layer; polygonal-celled middle layers; and a surface layer composed of tall, rather columnar cells, which are often binucleate, with a convex luminal surface bulging into the lumen (sometimes referred to as *umbrella cells*).

By light microscopy, the luminal surface of urothelium often appears fuzzy in the undistended bladder owing to the relaxation of the complex and convoluted cell surface membrane (Fig. 15.38). This appearance in the surface cells is related to the presence of special membrane proteins termed *uroplakins*, which function to provide an impermeable barrier to back-diffusion of substances in the urine (urine–blood barrier).

> **Urothelial cells have specialized plaques in the apical cell membrane containing uroplakin.**

Ultrastructurally, the surface layer of urothelium is highly specialized. The luminal aspect of each cell is convoluted, with deep clefts running down into the cytoplasm, which also contains fusiform vesicles lined by cell membrane, identical to that seen on the luminal surface (Fig. 15.39). These plaques are composed of membrane proteins called *uroplakins* (see Fig. 15.38c).

In conditions of distension, the tall cells of the surface layer become flattened and lose their convex apical bulge, whereas ultrastructurally the deep clefts and multilaminate vesicles largely disappear. Throughout most of the lower urinary tract the urothelium stands on a thin, indistinct basement membrane supported by a variable layer of dense subepithelial support tissue, which is mainly collagen (the lamina propria).

> **The lamina propria and muscle layers are external to the urothelium.**

The urothelium is supported by a vascular lamina propria. Beneath the lamina propria are the layers of smooth muscle which, in the pelvicalyceal system and ureters, are responsible for the peristaltic contractions forcing urine down into the bladder in one direction only.

> **The ureter has a spiral arrangement of smooth muscle in its wall.**

In the simple tubular ureter, there appears to be two distinct layers of muscle: an inner longitudinal layer and an outer circular layer (see Fig. 15.37). However, three-dimensional studies suggest that both muscle layers are in fact helical arrangements,

Fig. 15.38 Urothelium. (a) High-power micrograph showing the characteristic appearance of the H&E-stained urothelium in the non-distended state. The dome-shaped appearance of surface cells has led to them being referred to as *umbrella cells.* When the lumen is distended with urine, the cells flatten and form a thinner layer. Note the five to six layers, the occasional binucleate surface cell and the indistinct luminal surface (LS). **(b)** Masson's trichrome stain showing the lateral cell borders of urothelium and its stratified nature. Note the indistinct luminal surface membrane (LS). **(c)** Micrograph immunostained to detect uroplakin *(brown),* which is expressed in the surface epithelial cells and correlates with membrane plaques. There are several forms of uroplakin, some expressed throughout urothelial layers and others in surface layers. (Image used under Creative Commons License https://creativecommons.org/licenses/by-sa/3.0/ from the Human Protein Atlas Antibody to uroplakin3A HPA018407 https://www.proteinatlas.org/ENSG00000100373-UPK3A/tissue/urinary+bladder.)

Fig. 15.39 Urothelial Cell Surface. Electron micrograph of a non-distended human bladder postmortem, showing something of the unique structure of the surface of the urothelial cell. The luminal surface shows areas of a three-layered cell membrane (asymmetric membrane), most clearly seen in the invagination forming membrane plaques. The membrane has a central lucent lamina between a thick, electron-dense outer lamina and a thinner, dense inner lamina. Immediately beneath the surface the cytoplasm contains numerous round or oval vesicles (multilaminate vesicles) lined by identical trilaminar membrane. These vesicles become incorporated into the luminal surface by fusing with the frequent invaginations as the bladder fills and the surface urothelium stretches. The distinct appearance of the membrane is related to the presence of uroplakin membrane proteins.

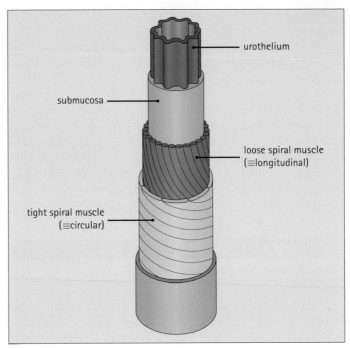

Fig. 15.40 Musculature of the Lower Urinary Tract. The arrangement of the muscle layers in the ureter is shown, emphasizing that the muscles are not truly circular and longitudinal, but rather are tight spirals and loose spirals.

Fig. 15.41 Bladder Wall. Beneath the urothelium is a fibrocollagenous submucosal region. The bulk of the wall is composed of smooth muscle, which is loosely organized into three layers. This arrangement is most clearly seen at the bladder neck, as in this micrograph.

with a loosely spiralled internal helix and a more tightly spiralled outer helix (Fig. 15.40), which appear to be, respectively, longitudinal and circular when the ureter is sectioned transversely.

In the architecturally more complex pelvicalyceal system and in the virtually spherical bladder, the arrangement of the muscle layers is less clearly defined.

The urinary bladder has three layers of smooth muscle.

The bladder has three muscle layers:
- An inner layer continuous with the inner longitudinal layer of the ureter
- A middle layer continuous with the outer circular layer of the ureter
- An additional outer layer in which the fibres run in approximately the same direction as the innermost layer (i.e. approximately longitudinal)

Because the bladder is roughly spherical instead of cylindrical and the bladder musculature is, in any case, a distorted continuation of the helical arrangement seen in the ureter, the terms *longitudinal* and *circular* have little meaning.

The arrangement of muscle often appears rather haphazard in histological sections, except at the narrow bladder neck, where the layers again become more distinct (Fig. 15.41).

A functional 'valve' prevents urine reflux during micturition.

In the normal ureter, which is a narrow-bore tube, urine is forced downward by peristalsis to prevent reflux back toward the kidney. In the larger spherical bladder, however, this cannot be achieved, as the lumen of the fully distended reservoir is too large for a segment of it to be closed off by muscle contraction; thus when the bladder musculature contracts during micturition, urine could reflux back up the open ureters and damage the kidney.

Although there are no anatomical valves at the junction of the ureters and bladder, potentially damaging reflux is prevented by a physiological valve, which results from the oblique path by which the ureters enter the posterolateral bladder wall musculature.

As the bladder distends and enlarges, the ureteric openings close, partly because of compression of the ureter lumen by extrinsic pressure from the musculature of the bladder wall and partly by acute angulation at the site of opening produced by bladder distension. At the junction between the bladder and the urethra is a muscular sphincter, the internal sphincter, which when closed permits the bladder to act as a reservoir of urine. When this sphincter relaxes, micturition occurs.

CLINICAL EXAMPLE

Tumours of the Bladder

The most common tumour of the bladder is derived from the epithelium that lines the organ internally, the urothelium, which is a specialized type of transitional cell epithelium. The tumours range in behaviour from virtually benign to aggressively malignant, but all are called **urothelial (transitional cell) carcinomas** (Fig. 15.42). This tumour can affect any part of the lower urinary tract, which is lined by urothelium, and can also occur in the ureters and in the pelvicalyceal epithelium within the kidney. Most tumours grow as a frond-like papillae into the bladder lumen. These papillae are fragile and are easily traumatized by the normal micturition cycle, leading to bleeding from the tumour. A common presentation is therefore with blood in the urine (haematuria)

Fig. 15.42 Low-Magnification Micrograph Showing a Transitional Cell Carcinoma of the Bladder. The tumour has a papillary growth pattern with frond-like growth composed of cores of lamina propria covered by neoplastic urothelium (P). Beneath the tumour is the muscle of the bladder wall (M).

The bladder is supplied by autonomic innervation.

The bladder nerve supply is from the autonomic nervous system, and both sympathetic and parasympathetic nerves are found.

Sensory fibres from the bladder transmit signals as to the degree of bladder distension to the sacral spinal cord.

Parasympathetic fibres ending in the muscles and adventitia of the bladder act as the effector nerves for micturition.

Sympathetic nerves innervate the blood vessels to the bladder.

The urethra conducts urine from the bladder to be voided.

The urethra is the final conduit through which urine passes to the exterior. The anatomy of the urethra differs in the male and female.

The human female urethra is short, being approximately 5 cm long. It runs from the bladder and opens to the exterior in the midline of the genital vestibule just between the clitoris and the superior border of the vaginal introitus.

The urethra is lined mainly by stratified squamous epithelium, and its lamina propria contains many vascular channels and a few small mucus-secreting glands.

Although the urethral muscular wall is a continuation of the involuntary smooth muscle of the bladder, there is a sphincter: the external sphincter. This is composed of striated muscle and is under voluntary control; it is found around the midportion of the urethra, where it passes through the striated muscles of the pelvic floor.

The male urethra is 20–25 cm long and is more complex than the female urethra, as it serves two purposes. Not only is it the final conduit of the urinary system but it is also the terminal conduit of the male reproductive system (see Fig. 16.1). It can be divided into three segments: the prostatic urethra, the membranous urethra and the penile urethra.

The prostatic urethra begins at the bladder neck and runs through the prostate gland, from which many periurethral glands open into it through short ducts. It also receives the openings of the ejaculatory ducts.

The membranous urethra is the short segment (i.e. approximately 1 cm long) which runs through the pelvic floor muscles. This is the site of voluntary control of micturition, as it is here that the external sphincter of striated muscle surrounds the urethra.

The penile urethra is the distal part of the urethra and runs through the corpus spongiosum of the penis, opening to the exterior at the external meatus of the glans penis; small mucous glands, analogous to those in the female, open into the penile urethra.

The male urethra is lined proximally by transitional epithelium similar to that in the remainder of the lower urinary tract, but this becomes progressively less urothelial in character in the membranous and penile segments, where it changes to a rather non-specialized, pseudostratified columnar epithelium. This finally changes to a stratified squamous epithelium at the distal penile urethra close to the external urinary meatus, where the epithelium merges with the stratified squamous epithelium of the glans penis.

For online review questions, please visit https://studentconsult.inkling.com.

Male Reproductive System

INTRODUCTION

The male reproductive system is responsible for:
- Production, nourishment and temporary storage of the haploid male gametes (spermatozoa)
- Intromission of a suspension of spermatozoa (semen) into the female genital system
- Production of male sex hormones (androgens)

Whereas the first two functions are important only during the years of sexual maturity, hormone production is required throughout life, even in utero.

The male genital system (Fig. 16.1) comprises:
- Testes, which produce spermatozoa, and synthesize and secrete androgens
- Epididymis, vas deferens, ejaculatory duct and part of the male urethra, which form the ductal system responsible for the carriage of spermatozoa to the exterior
- Seminal vesicles, the prostate gland and the bulbourethral glands (of Cowper), which are secretory glands providing fluid and nutrients to support and nourish the spermatozoa and forming the bulk of the semen
- Penis, which is an organ capable of becoming erect for insertion into the female vagina during sexual intercourse

The testes, epididymis and vas deferens are located in the scrotal sac (Fig. 16.2), which is a skin-covered pouch enclosing a mesothelium-lined cavity continuous with the peritoneal cavity at the inguinal canal.

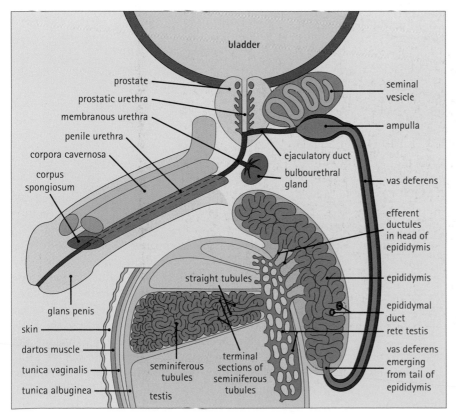

Fig. 16.1 The Male Genital System. Spermatogenesis occurs in the seminiferous tubules; the resulting spermatozoa pass into the rete testis at the hilum (mediastinum) of the testis. From the rete testis, spermatozoa are transported by about a dozen efferent ductules into the head of the epididymis, where the ductules fuse to form the single highly coiled epididymal duct. Within this duct the sperm acquire their motility. The spermatozoa then pass into a long straight tube, the vas deferens, which travels via the spermatic cord, transporting them from the scrotal sac into the short ejaculatory duct, receiving abundant secretions from the seminal vesicles. The ejaculatory ducts from the right and left sides run through the tissue of the prostate gland and open into the prostatic urethra. Prostatic secretions and the secretions of the bulbourethral glands accompany or precede the semen along the penile urethra.

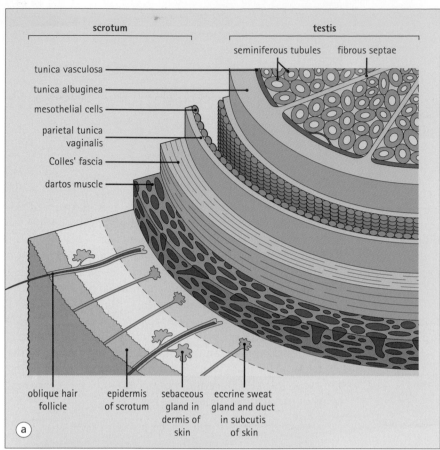

seminiferous tubules   fibrous septae

tunica vasculosa
tunica albuginea
mesothelial cells
parietal tunica vaginalis
Colles' fascia
dartos muscle

oblique hair follicle | epidermis of scrotum | sebaceous gland in dermis of skin | eccrine sweat gland and duct in subcutis of skin

a

Fig. 16.2 Scrotum and Tunica Vaginalis. **(a)** The scrotum is covered externally by skin (epidermis, dermis and subcutis) with oblique hair follicles (producing curly hair) and numerous eccrine sweat glands. In the deeper layers of the skin, smooth muscle fibres, arranged in a rather haphazard manner, form the poorly defined dartos muscle, contraction of which produces wrinkling of the scrotal skin. Beneath the dartos muscle lies fibrocollagenous fascia (Colles' fascia), the deepest layer being compacted to form the dense parietal layer of the tunica vaginalis, which is lined internally by flattened mesothelial cells similar to those lining the peritoneal cavity, with which it is continuous. This smooth mesothelial-coated parietal tunica vaginalis forms the inner layer of the scrotal sac and is separated from the external surface of the testis by a potential space containing a watery fluid. This fluid acts as a lubricant, allowing the testis to move smoothly within the scrotal sac without friction. The testis is covered externally by a thick collagenous capsule, the visceral layer of the tunica vaginalis (the tunica albuginea), with the outer surface being coated with flattened mesothelial cells. Beneath the tunica albuginea lies a narrow variable layer of loosely arranged collagen containing superficial blood vessels; internal to this are the seminiferous tubules. **(b)** Micrograph of the tunica albuginea of the testis. Note the scrotal cavity (C), the collagenous tunica albuginea (T) covered externally by small mesothelial cells, the narrow vascular layer (V), which is sometimes called the *tunica vasculosa*, and the seminiferous tubules (S).

b

TESTES

Anatomy and Development

> The testes are paired organs located outside the body cavity in the scrotum.

The location of the testes in the scrotum means that they are maintained at a temperature approximately 2–3°C below body temperature; this is essential for normal spermatogenesis.

Embryologically, the testes develop high on the posterior abdominal wall and migrate to the scrotum, usually arriving there in the seventh month of intrauterine life.

Sometimes a testis fails to migrate from the posterior abdominal wall and does not arrive in the scrotum. It may stay on the posterior abdominal wall at its site of original development, or it may become stuck on its way down to the scrotum, the common site being within the inguinal canal. This is called *undescended testis* or *maldescent of the testis*. Because the testis does not arrive in the cooler environment of the scrotal sac, the germ cells in the seminiferous tubules degenerate and die without ever producing spermatozoa. This is called **cryptorchidism**, and the testis remains small and non-functional throughout life, although the testosterone-producing Leydig cells (see p. 336) remain undamaged and functional. Undescended testes have a high risk of developing malignant tumours.

Each mature adult testis is a solid ovoid organ approximately 4–5 cm long, 3 cm deep and 2.5 cm wide and usually weighs 11–17 g. The right testis is commonly slightly larger and heavier than the left.

Each testis has an epididymis (see p. 337) attached to its posterior surface and is suspended in the scrotal sac by the spermatic cord. The spermatic cord contains the vas deferens (see p. 338), the arterial supply and the venous and lymphatic drainage and is enclosed by an extension of the pelvic peritoneum, the tunica vaginalis.

The testis is completely enclosed by a fibrous connective tissue layer with a white appearance resulting from plentiful collagen, the **tunica albuginea**. This is thickened posteriorly to form the mediastinum of the testis, projecting some way into the body of the testis (Fig. 16.3). Blood and lymphatic vessels, and the channels carrying spermatozoa, pass through this area (rete testis, see p. 336). Fibrous septa from the mediastinum divide the body of the testis into 250–350 lobules, each lobule containing one to four seminiferous tubules.

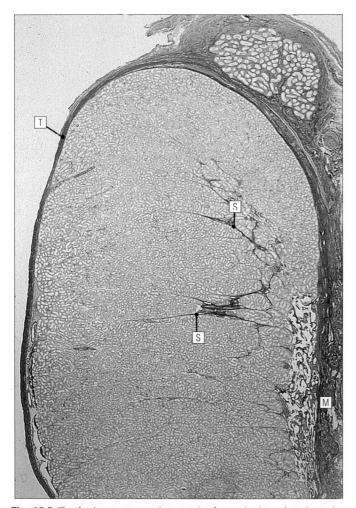

Fig. 16.3 Testis. Low-power micrograph of a sagittal section through a testis stained by the van Gieson method, which colours collagen *red*. Note the tunica albuginea (T), which is thickened posteriorly to form the mediastinum testis (M). From the mediastinum, fibrous septa (S) enter the testis, separating it into lobules.

CLINICAL EXAMPLE
Scrotal Swellings

Common causes of scrotal swelling are hydrocele, haematocele and inguinal hernia.
1. A **hydrocele** results when excessive fluid forms or accumulates within the scrotal cavity.
2. After trauma, bleeding into the scrotal cavity may produce a **haematocele**.
3. An **inguinal hernia** occurs when loops of intestine pass into the sac through the inguinal canal.

Less common, but more important, are tumours of the testis, which present as a solid scrotal mass. Most testicular tumours arise from germ cells, and there are two main types. **Seminoma** affects older males; tumour cells resemble spermatocytes (see Fig. 16.6). **Teratoma** affects younger males; tumour cells resemble structures seen in the developing embryo and can be well differentiated, resembling mature tissues from all embryological lineages such as hair, fat and cartilage.

Seminiferous Tubules

> A seminiferous tubule is a coiled, non-branching closed loop, both ends of which open into the rete testis.

The rete testis is a system of channels located at the posterior hilum of the testis, close to the mediastinum.

Each seminiferous tubule is approximately 150 μm in diameter and 80 cm long. It has been calculated that the combined total length of all the seminiferous tubules in each testis is 300–900 m.

In a sexually mature adult, each seminiferous tubule has a central lumen lined by an actively replicating epithelium, the seminiferous or germinal epithelium, mixed with a population of supporting cells, the Sertoli cells. Blood vessels and clusters of hormone-producing interstitial (Leydig) cells are found between adjacent seminiferous tubules (Fig. 16.4a and b).

The lining cells sit on a well-defined basement membrane lying inside a collagenous layer containing fibroblasts and other spindle-shaped cells. These are also contractile myoid cells similar to smooth muscle containing desmin (see Fig. 16.4c). In some animals, these myoid cells form a continuous peritubular layer and contract rhythmically, possibly propelling the non-motile spermatozoa toward the rete testis (spermatozoa only acquire their motility after they have passed through the epididymis). In human testis, the myoid cells form a less distinct layer and are not usually circumferential.

The outer wall of the tubule, comprising the basal lamina, collagen layer and myoid cell layer, is sometimes called the *tunica propria*.

Fig. 16.4 Seminiferous Tubules and Interstitium. (a) Micrograph showing seminiferous tubules (T) cut in transverse, longitudinal and oblique section, lined by germinal epithelium and enclosed by tunica propria. In the interstices are blood vessels and clumps of Leydig (interstitial) cells (L). **(b)** Van Gieson stain of a seminiferous tubule showing mature spermatids. **(c)** Immunostained to show desmin, highlighting the peritubular myoid cells *(brown)* [Image (c) used under Creative Commons License https://creativecommons.org/licenses/by-sa/3.0/ from the Human Protein Atlas Antibody to desmin HPA054158 https://www.proteinatlas.org/ENSG00000175084-DES/tissue/testis#img.]

Germinal epithelium produces spermatozoa

The germinal epithelium lining the seminiferous tubules produces the haploid male gametes (spermatozoa) by a series of steps called, in sequence, *spermatocytogenesis, meiosis and spermiogenesis* (Fig. 16.5).

In spermatocytogenesis, the stem cells (spermatogonia) undergo mitosis.

Spermatogonia undergo mitotic division which not only maintains them as a population of stem cells but also results in cells which differentiate into primary spermatocytes (Fig. 16.6).

In man, spermatogonia can be morphologically divided into three groups according to their nuclear appearances: type A-dark (Ad) cells, type A-pale (Ap) cell and type B cells. It is thought that type Ad spermatogonia are the reserve stem cells of the system, with their infrequent mitotic division producing more type Ad cells and new type Ap cells. The type Ap spermatogonia are committed stem cells that divide and mature into type B cells, which further divide mitotically to produce further type B cells; these cells then divide and mature in a cluster to produce primary spermatocytes. Immunohistochemical studies using markers of spermatogonia, mostly transcription factors located within the nuclei, do not show consistent expression of markers according to the morphological classification, suggesting a discordance between functional and morphological classifications (see Fig. 16.6d)

Primary spermatocytes replicate their DNA shortly after their formation (i.e. they are 4n). Primary spermatocyte formation marks the end of spermatocytogenesis.

Meiotic division occurs at the spermatocyte stages.

Primary spermatocytes pass through a long prophase lasting about 22 days, during which changing patterns of nuclear chromatin enable preleptotene, leptotene, zygotene, pachytene and diplotene stages to be identified (see Fig. 16.5). Meiosis is described on page 42.

The first meiotic division occurs after the late pachytene/diplotene stages, with the formation of diploid secondary spermatocytes, which rapidly (i.e. within a few hours) undergo the second meiotic division to produce haploid spermatids.

Spermiogenesis is the process by which haploid spermatids are transformed into spermatozoa.

Spermiogenesis can be divided into four phases, all of which occur while the spermatids are embedded in small hollows in the free luminal surface of the Sertoli cells (see p. 334) (Fig. 16.7):

- The Golgi phase
- The cap phase
- The acrosome phase
- The maturation phase

Mature spermatozoon. The mature spermatozoon comprises a head and a tail region, the latter being composed of a neck, a middle piece, a principal piece and an end piece (Fig. 16.8).

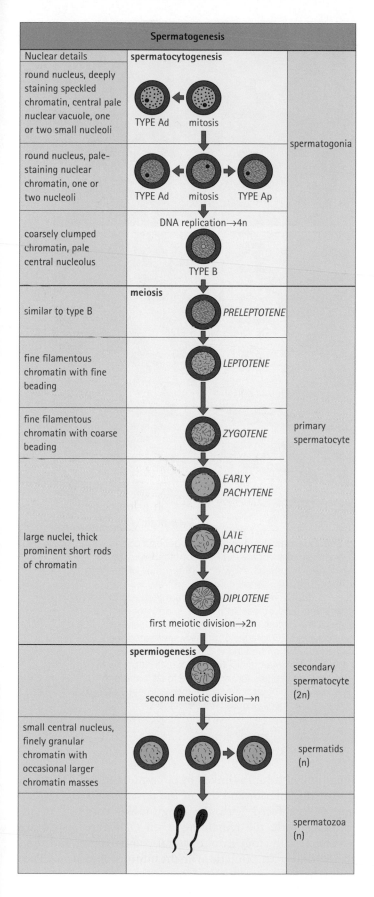

Spermatogenesis		
Nuclear details	**spermatocytogenesis**	
round nucleus, deeply staining speckled chromatin, central pale nuclear vacuole, one or two small nucleoli	TYPE Ad ← mitosis	spermatogonia
round nucleus, pale-staining nuclear chromatin, one or two nucleoli	TYPE Ad ← mitosis → TYPE Ap	
coarsely clumped chromatin, pale central nucleolus	DNA replication→4n TYPE B	
similar to type B	**meiosis** PRELEPTOTENE	
fine filamentous chromatin with fine beading	LEPTOTENE	
fine filamentous chromatin with coarse beading	ZYGOTENE	primary spermatocyte
	EARLY PACHYTENE	
large nuclei, thick prominent short rods of chromatin	LATE PACHYTENE	
	DIPLOTENE first meiotic division→2n	
	spermiogenesis second meiotic division→n	secondary spermatocyte (2n)
small central nucleus, finely granular chromatin with occasional larger chromatin masses		spermatids (n)
		spermatozoa (n)

Fig. 16.5 Spermatocytogenesis, Meiosis and Spermiogenesis. Spermatocytogenesis begins with the development of spermatogonia, of which three types are recognized: the type A-dark (Ad) cell, the type A-pale (Ap) cell and the type B cell. It is thought that the Ad cells are reserve stem cells that divide to produce Ap cells; the latter act as a committed stem cell pool and give rise to type B cells, which subsequently pass through a meiotic phase to produce spermatocytes. The B cells pass through several stages of maturation before the first meiotic division, and in these early stages are known as *primary spermatocytes*. The preleptotene cell is similar to the type B cell but is not in contact with the basement membrane of the seminiferous tubule. After maturation, at the diplotene stage, the cell then undergoes its first meiotic division to produce a secondary spermatocyte, which is smaller than its parent primary spermatocyte and has fine granular chromatin. This immediately undergoes a second meiotic division to produce the haploid spermatids from which the spermatozoa will develop. The spermatids are located toward the lumen of the seminiferous tubule and have spherical central nuclei with finely granular chromatin and occasional larger chromatin masses. Their nuclear diameter is about half that of the primary spermatocytes from which they are derived.

> **The head of a mature spermatozoon is composed of the nucleus covered by the acrosomal cap.**

The spermatozoon head is flattened and pointed, and the chromatin of the nucleus is condensed and broken only by occasional clear nuclear vacuoles.

The acrosomal cap covers the anterior two-thirds to three quarters of the nucleus; it is a glycoprotein containing numerous enzymes, including a protease, acid phosphatase, neuraminidase and hyaluronidase, and can be regarded as a specialized giant lysosome.

The acrosomal enzymes are released when the spermatozoon contacts the ovum; they facilitate penetration of the corona radiata and zona pellucida of the ovum (see Chapter 17) by the spermatozoal nuclear head.

> **The tail region of a mature spermatozoon is composed of the neck region and middle, principal and end pieces.**

Running throughout the tail is the axoneme, which is responsible for spermatozoon motility; it is essentially a long, specialized cilium, with nine outer doublet tubules around a central tubule pair (see Fig. 3.11).

The proximal part of the tail is the neck. This is a short narrow segment containing the pair of centrioles and a connecting piece that forms nine fibrous rings surrounding the axoneme. These are the outer dense fibres (ODFs), formed of cytoskeletal proteins and providing protection and elasticity to the sperm tail. The ODFs are present throughout the entirety of middle and principal pieces of the tail.

Fig. 16.6 Spermatocytogenesis and Spermiogenesis in Seminiferous Tubules. Spermatogenesis occurs in waves along the length of the seminiferous tubules (ST), and thus adjacent areas of the same tubule show spermatocytogenesis and spermiogenesis at various stages. **(a)** Micrograph showing further detail of the seminiferous tubules (ST), interstitial Leydig cells (L) and tunica propria. Sertoli calls (SC) can be seen as tall, ghost-like cells in the periphery of the seminiferous tubules. **(b)** Micrograph showing spermatogonia of various types, including Ad and B types, and zygotene/pachytene (Z/P) stages of primary spermatocytes. Some spermatids (St) are also present. **(c)** Micrograph showing a later stage in which there is spermiogenesis and spermatocytogenesis. Ad spermatogonia and zygotene/pachytene (Z/P) stages of primary spermatocytes and spermatids (St) are shown, along with developing spermatozoa (Sz) embedded in Sertoli cell cytoplasm. Sertoli cells are poorly defined in routine light microscopic sections of human testis. **(d)** Immunostaining for a transcription factor regulator involved in spermatocytogenesis showing staining *(brown)* limited to a proportion of spermatogonia adjacent to the basal lamina of tubules. The expression of such functional markers does not always correlate with morphological type. (Image used under Creative Commons License https://creativecommons.org/licenses/by-sa/3.0/ from the Human Protein Atlas Antibody to Zinc finger protein 654 HPA036173 https://www.proteinatlas.org/ENSG00000175105-ZNF654/tissue/testis#img.)

The axoneme runs through the centre of the middle piece and is surrounded by the ODFs from the connecting piece in the neck and an outer zone of tightly packed, elongated, spiral mitochondria. The lower limit of the middle piece is marked by a sudden narrowing, sometimes associated with an annular thickening of the cell membrane, the annulus.

The principal piece is the longest part of the tail and comprises the axoneme surrounded by the nine ODFs, which are in turn enclosed by a fibrous sheath. There are no mitochondria in this region. The fibrous sheath consists of two longitudinal columns linked by circumferential ribs. Because one of the anterior and one of the posterior ODFs (ODFs 3 and 8) are fused with the longitudinal columns of the fibrous sheath, the remaining seven ODFs are distributed asymmetrically, four in one lateral compartment and three in the other. The function of the fibrous sheath has been linked to sperm motility and flexibility in addition to acting as a scaffold for a variety of proteins involved in sperm function. Malfunctions of the ODFs and/or fibrous sheath are linked to subfertility.

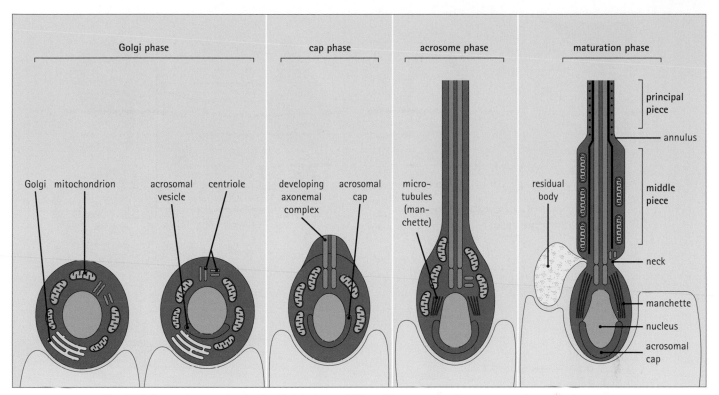

Fig. 16.7 Spermiogenesis. In the Golgi phase, PAS-positive granules (pre-acrosomal granules) appear in the Golgi apparatus and fuse to form a membrane-bound acrosomal vesicle close to the nuclear membrane. This vesicle enlarges, and its location marks what will be the anterior pole of the spermatozoon. The two centrioles migrate to the opposite (posterior) pole of the spermatid, with the distal centriole becoming aligned at right angles to the cell membrane. It then begins the formation of the axoneme complex of the sperm tail. In the cap phase, the acrosomal vesicle changes shape to enclose the anterior half of the nucleus and become the acrosomal cap. The nuclear membrane beneath the acrosomal cap thickens and loses its pores, and the nuclear chromatin becomes more condensed. In the acrosome phase, the increasingly dense nucleus flattens and elongates; an anterior pole, capped by the acrosomal cap, and a posterior pole closely related to the developing axonemal complex, can be identified. With the changed shape of the nucleus, the cytoplasm between the acrosomal cap and the anterior cell membrane migrates to the posterior part of the cell. The entire cell orients itself so that the anterior pole is embedded in the luminal surface of the Sertoli cell, pointing down toward the base of the seminiferous tubule; the cytoplasm-rich posterior pole of the spermatid protrudes into the tubule lumen. At the same time, a sheath of microtubules, called the *manchette,* extends from the posterior part of the acrosomal cap toward the developing tail. The centrioles (see Fig. 2.29) have migrated posteriorly from the neck of the developing spermatozoon, which is the connecting piece between the head (containing the nucleus and acrosomal cap) and the developing tail. One centriole continues to synthesize the axonemal complex of the sperm tail, producing a regular tubular complex comprising two central microtubules surrounded by a ring of nine peripheral doublets. In the neck region, nine coarse fibres are produced which extend down into the tail around the microtubules of the axonemal complex. Prominent mitochondria aggregate in and below the neck to surround the nine coarse fibres; this forms the segment known as the *middle piece.* The mitochondria finish abruptly at a ring (annulus) demarcating the middle piece from the main parts of the tail (the principal piece and end piece). The maturation phase is characterized by the pinching-off of surplus cytoplasm, particularly from the neck and middle piece regions, and its phagocytosis by Sertoli cells. The immature spermatozoa then become disconnected from the Sertoli cell surface and lie free in the seminiferous tubule lumen, marking the end of spermiogenesis. The immature male gametes are later modified in the ductular systems leading to the penis. The duration of spermatocytogenesis from spermatogonium type Ad to released immature spermatozoon is about 70 days.

Fig. 16.8 Mature Human Spermatozoon. A mature spermatozoon accompanied by electron micrographs confirming its structure in longitudinal *(left side)* and transverse *(right side)* orientations.

At the junction between the principal piece and the short end piece, the longitudinal and circumferential fibres cease. Thus the end piece is composed of axoneme only.

Sertoli Cells

> **The Sertoli cell sits on a basement membrane with its irregular apex extending into the lumen of the seminiferous tubule.**

Sertoli cells are tall, columnar cells (Fig. 16.9a and b) and are the main cell type until puberty, after which they comprise only about 10% of the cells lining the seminiferous tubules. In elderly men, however, a decrease in the number of germinal epithelial cells is common, so Sertoli cells again become a significant component of the tubule cell population.

Sertoli cells are not affected by any of the factors that injure the sensitive germinal epithelium. For example, they do not degenerate when exposed to normal body temperature and can therefore survive in the undescended testis.

The cell nucleus is irregular with deep folds, but tends toward an oval shape, with the long axis at right angles to the basement membrane. The nucleus has a vesicular chromatin pattern and a prominent nucleolus.

The Sertoli cell outline is irregular, with many ramifying cytoplasmic extensions that make contact with those from neighbouring Sertoli cells to form a meshwork of cytoplasm. This encloses the developing cells of the germinal epithelium and forms occluding junctions (see Fig. 3.3), which divide the seminiferous tubule lining into basal and adluminal compartments. These occluding junctions between Sertoli cells form the **blood–testis barrier**, which isolates the adluminal compartment of the seminiferous tubules from the blood and lymphatic systems. Functionally this barrier allows for a highly specialized microenvironment to be maintained within the lumen of the seminiferous tubule that facilitates maturation of sperm. In addition, this barrier is thought to prevent antigens from germ cells being exposed to the immune system and causing an autoimmune response.

Fig. 16.9 Sertoli Cells. (a) With H&E, Sertoli cells (SC) are not clearly identifiable in the lining of seminiferous tubules in which active spermatogenesis is occurring (see Fig. 16.6a). However, they form the entire lining of the tubule (S) for a short distance at its distal end shortly before it drains into the rete testis system (R) at the mediastinum testis. This micrograph is taken from such an area. **(b)** Immunohistochemical staining for vimentin *(brown)* highlights Sertoli cells in a normal seminiferous tubule. Cells extend from the margin of the tubule up to the luminal surface with processes surrounding spermatogonia (Image used under Creative Commons License https://creativecommons.org/licenses/by-sa/3.0/ from the Human Protein Atlas Antibody to vimentin CAB058687 https://www.proteinatlas.org/ENSG00000026025-VIM/tissue/testis#img.)

Other forms of intercellular junctions (see Chapter 3) between Sertoli cells, including gap junctions and (occasionally) desmosomes, have been described, and intercellular junction–like structures have been seen between Sertoli cells and developing germinal epithelial cells.

Sertoli cell cytoplasm is eosinophilic and finely granular; it may contain lipid vacuoles. Ultrastructurally, it has abundant endoplasmic reticulum, often arranged as flat-stacked cisternae (annulate lamellae) with associated ribosomes. The lipid vacuoles are usually found close to the larger cisternae.

Endoplasmic reticulum is also prominent in the cytoplasmic processes interdigitating between the developing germ cells, and clusters of free ribosomes are numerous at the base of the cell. Microfibrils and microtubules are common in areas of cytoplasm close to the developing spermatids.

Spermatogonia and preleptotene spermatocytes occupy the basal compartment, whereas the remaining primary spermatocytes, secondary spermatocytes and spermatids are located in the adluminal compartment. These compartments are clearly distinguishable in some animal species, including primates, but not in humans.

> **Sertoli cells have supportive, phagocytic and secretory functions.**

Sertoli cells form a vital function as part of the stem cell niche in which spermiogenesis takes place. Although originally thought to be merely sustentacular cells with a primary purpose to support and sustain sperm in various stages of spermiogenesis, they are now known to be multifunctional with additional endocrine roles.

Supportive functions include the provision of nutrients to developing germinal cells, which dock into Sertoli cells via cytoplasmic processes and junctions, and the transport of waste materials from spermiogenesis to blood and lymph vascular systems surrounding seminiferous tubules.

Sertoli cells phagocytose any residual cytoplasm (residual bodies) shed by maturing spermatids during spermiogenesis and may also phagocytose any effete cellular material derived from degenerate germinal cells that fail to complete spermatogenesis.

Secretory functions vary with sexual maturity. In the male embryo at about the eighth or ninth week of fetal development, Sertoli cells secrete anti-müllerian hormone (AMH), a glycoprotein from the transforming growth factor beta (TGF-β) family that further suppresses development of the müllerian duct system in men. In the prepubertal testis they may secrete a substance preventing meiotic division of the germinal epithelial cells. At puberty, AMH levels are reduced as the gene expression is inhibited by testosterone.

◎ ADVANCED CONCEPT

Sertoli Cells

In the mature testis, Sertoli cells secrete androgen-binding protein (ABP), which binds testosterone and hydroxytestosterone produced outside the seminiferous tubule in the Leydig cells of the interstitium. High concentrations of these hormones are required within the germinal epithelium and tubule lumen for normal germ cell maturation; ABP enables concentrations of these androgens far higher than their normal solubility should allow to accumulate in the lumen of the seminiferous tubule.

ABP secretion is dependent on follicle-stimulating hormone (FSH) secretion by the pituitary, and FSH receptors are present on Sertoli cells. FSH promotes spermatogenesis, probably by inducing Sertoli cells to produce varying amounts of ABP.

Sertoli cells also express and secrete the hormone inhibin A, a glycoprotein from the TGF-β family, which inhibits the secretion of FSH by the pituitary gland and therefore plays an important feedback role in controlling the rate of spermatogenesis. Sertoli cells can be stained for inhibin-A using immunohistochemistry.

The testicular interstitium contains hormone-secreting Leydig (interstitial) cells.

The interstitial tissue lying between the seminiferous tubules is a loose network of fibrocollagenous tissue composed of:

- Fibroblasts
- Collagen, in which occasional macrophages and mast cells are present
- Blood and lymphatic vessels
- Clumps of interstitial or Leydig cells

Leydig cells synthesize testosterone, and although they are most common in the tubular interstitium (Fig. 16.10a), they can occasionally be found in the mediastinum of the testis, in the epididymis or even in the spermatic cord. They are often closely related to nerves, like their female equivalent, the hilus cells of the ovary (see Chapter 17).

Leydig cells have granular eosinophilic cytoplasm containing lipases, oxidative enzymes, esterases and a number of steroid dehydrogenases. They have round vesicular nuclei with prominent nuclear membranes and one or two nucleoli. Some of the cells are small and spindle shaped and are thought to be immature forms, but most are round or polygonal (see Fig. 16.10b). Yellow-brown lipofuscin pigment is present in most Leydig cells.

A characteristic feature of Leydig cells is Reinke's crystalloid, which is an intracytoplasmic, eosinophilic, elongated, rectangular or rhomboid mass, approximately 3 μm thick and up to 20 μm long (see Fig. 16.10b). Reinke's crystalloids are not seen before puberty. They increase in number during the years of sexual maturity, becoming most common in old age.

The rete testis is a complex arrangement of interconnecting channels located at the mediastinum of the testis.

Spermatozoa formed in the seminiferous tubule loops pass to the terminal portions, which are lined entirely by Sertoli cells (see Fig. 16.9a), and thence via the short straight tubules into the rete testis (Fig. 16.11) embedded in a fibrous stroma continuous with the tunica albuginea.

Fig. 16.10 Leydig (Interstitial) Cells. (a) The distribution of Leydig cells can be seen in this section immunostained to show an enzyme involved in the biosynthesis of testosterone *(black)* highlighting islands of Leydig cells (L) in the interstitial between seminiferous tubules (ST). **(b)** H&E micrograph showing a cluster of Leydig cells (L) in the interstitium with adjacent seminiferous tubules (ST). They have abundant eosinophilic cytoplasm, and some of the cells contain Reinke's crystalloids (RC). [Image (a) used under Creative Commons License https://creativecommons.org/licenses/by-sa/3.0/ from the Human Protein Atlas. Antibody to Aldo-keto reductase family 1 member C3 CAB010874 https://www.proteinatlas.org/ENSG00000196139-AKR1C3/tissue/testis#img.]

Both straight tubules and rete testis are lined by a simple epithelium of cuboidal or low columnar cells bearing microvilli on their luminal surface. Most of the rete testis epithelial cells bear a single, long central flagellum.

Channels of the rete testis fuse to form about a dozen efferent ductules.

These emerge from the upper end of the mediastinum of the testis, penetrating the tunica albuginea (see Fig. 16.1) and entering the head of the epididymis. Here, they gradually merge to become a single tube, the epididymal duct.

The efferent ductules are lined by a mixed epithelium of tall ciliated columnar cells and non-ciliated cuboidal or low columnar cells with microvilli on their luminal surface (Fig. 16.12). The cilia beat toward the epididymis and propel the spermatozoa onward, whereas the non-ciliated cells absorb some of the testicular fluid, which is the transport medium for the immature and still immotile spermatozoa.

Fig. 16.11 Rete Testis. The rete testis is a network of interconnecting channels (C) into which the seminiferous tubules (T) empty. Spermatozoa are transferred from the rete testis to the epididymis via the efferent ductules.

Fig. 16.12 Efferent Ductules. Note the mixed columnar and cuboidal epithelium (E), the typical fringed internal lumen and the circumferential ring of smooth muscle (SM) fibres.

The efferent ductules are highly convoluted and have a narrow sheath of circumferential smooth muscle cells interspersed with elastic fibres; peristaltic contractions of this muscle enhance the progression of the spermatozoa.

EPIDIDYMIS

> **The epididymal duct (ductus epididymis) is formed by the fusion of the efferent ductules.**

The epididymal duct is a single highly convoluted tube embedded in a loose vascular supporting stroma of fibroblasts, collagen and glycosaminoglycan matrix and is surrounded by a dense fibrocollagenous capsule to form the comma-shaped body called the *epididymis*.

The epididymis can be divided into head, body and tail regions, with the efferent ductules entering the head and the distal end of the epididymal duct emerging at the tail to become the vas deferens.

The human epididymis is usually 5 cm long and 1 cm wide, and, as the entire 5 m of epididymal duct is contained within it, the duct is enormously convoluted.

> **The epididymal duct provides a highly specialized microenvironment essential for sperm maturation.**

It is only while moving through the epididymis that spermatozoa mature and develop motility and finally the capability to fertilize an ovum. During the process of maturation proteins produced by cells lining the epididymis are transferred to the maturing sperm, and there are modifications to sperm membrane such that the final function of the sperm is dependent on successful interaction with these proteins.

The epididymis is lined by a pseudostratified epithelium with several cell types described: principal, basal, clear, narrow, apical and halo cells.

These principal cells represent over 80% of the total and are tall, columnar cells that carry large microvilli and are largely responsible for maintaining a highly specialized microenvironment within the lumen of the epididymis. It has been noted that the fluid in the epididymal lumen is the most complex produced by any glandular epithelium. The secreted proteins coat the sperm, and some are taken up by the sperm. The ability of sperm to respond to calcium signalling, which is necessary for hypermobility once within the female reproductive tract, depends on proteins provided to the spermatozoa in the lumen of the epididymis. The ability of a spermatozoa to recognize, adhere and penetrate the outer ovum depends on the proteins coating the sperm from the lumen of the epididymis.

The giant apical microvilli (Fig. 16.13) are largely immotile and termed *stereocilia;* they neither contain the internal microtubular structures of cilia (see Fig. 3.11) nor function like cilia. They are about 80 μm long in the epididymal head and 40 μm long in the tail. The function of the stereocilia is to maintain the microenvironment by modifying the fluid secreted into the lumen. The cells also possess coated vesicles and lysosomes, rough endoplasmic reticulum and a prominent Golgi related to a secretory role. Tight junctions between principal cells maintain a blood–epididymis barrier, similar in concept to the blood–testis barrier described earlier.

The function of principal cells in humans varies only slightly between the different anatomical sections of the epididymis, unlike in rodents where there are significant differences. As a whole, principal cells exhibit expression of a distinct set of genes that relate to secretion of the proteins required for normal sperm function. Adjacent cells may show differences between their neighbours. Some products are put into the lumen by principal cells using apocrine secretion and give rise to membrane-bound vesicles within the fluid termed *epididymosomes.*

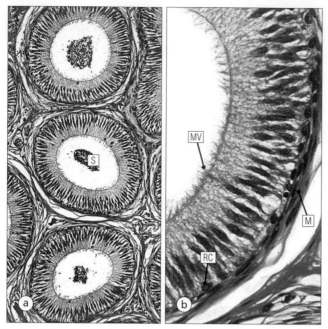

Fig. 16.13 Epididymal Duct. (a) Micrograph of epididymal duct lined by tall columnar epithelium composed of principal cells with basal nuclei; the lumina contain clumps of spermatozoa (S). **(b)** High-power micrograph showing a single duct. Note the unusually tall microvilli (MV) forming stereocilia, the scattered small round cells at the base of the columnar epithelium representing basal cells (RC) and the narrow band of circular muscle fibres (M).

The other cell types within the epididymal lining epithelium have the following functions:

- **Basal cells** are restricted to the basement membrane zone and lie beneath and partly surround overlying principal cells, where they are understood to have a signalling and support cell function.
- **Apical** and clear cells contain an H^+-ATPase and secrete hydrogen ions into the lumen to lower the pH and maintain an acid environment.

- **Clear cells** and **apical cells** show endocytic activity and are thought to remove material from the epididymal lumen.
- **Halo cells** appear to be the main immune effector cell in the epididymis and consist of helper T lymphocytes, cytotoxic T lymphocytes and monocytes.

The entire epididymal duct is surrounded by a narrow sheath of circular smooth muscle similar to that in the efferent ductules, but in the tail there is also a longitudinal layer internal to the circular layer and an outer longitudinal layer. These muscle layers allow for peristaltic propulsion of the contents.

All of the muscle layers thicken within the epididymal tail, becoming significant layers where the duct emerges to become the vas deferens.

VAS DEFERENS

> The ductus (vas) deferens is a tube emerging from the epididymis and running vertically upward behind the epididymis within the spermatic cord.

The spermatic cord also contains arteries, veins, lymphatics and nerves. The veins form a complex anastomotic plexus called the *pampiniform plexus*. Externally, the spermatic cord contains longitudinal fibres of voluntary striated muscle, the cremaster muscle.

The vas deferens has a thick, muscular wall composed of a middle circular and outer and inner longitudinal layers. Internal to the inner layer is a fibroelastic lamina propria covered with a tall columnar epithelium almost identical to that of the epididymis but thrown up into longitudinal folds by the lamina propria; this produces a small stellate lumen (Fig. 16.14). Peristalsis of the thick muscular wall propels spermatozoa forward during emission.

Each vas deferens enters the pelvic cavity via the inguinal canal and then passes downward and medially to the base of the bladder. Near its distal end, close to the base of the bladder, each

Fig. 16.14 Vas Deferens. (a) Low-power micrograph showing the three muscle layers (a central circular [C] layer between the outer [OL] and inner longitudinal [IL] layers) and the stellate lumen (SL). **(b)** High-power micrograph showing the tall ciliated columnar epithelium (E), the basal layer of small regular round cells (RC) and the pattern of folds.

vas deferens has a dilatation (the ampulla) where the muscle layer becomes thinner; the mucosal layer in the ampulla appears thicker because the folds, some of which are branched, are taller.

At the distal end of the ampulla, the vas deferens is joined by a short duct from the seminal vesicles.

SEMINAL VESICLES

Each seminal vesicle is a highly convoluted, unbranched tubular diverticulum of the vas deferens, the lumen of which contains no sperm.

The seminal vesicle is 15 cm long but is coiled on itself to form a body about 5–6 cm long. This tube is surrounded by an inner circular and an outer longitudinal smooth muscle layer, with an external layer of fibrocollagenous tissue containing many elastic fibres.

Seminal vesicle mucosa is composed of a fibroelastic lamina propria thrown up into tall, narrow complicated folds (Fig. 16.15) covered by non-ciliated, tall columnar epithelial cells and a population of non-specialized basal round cells similar to those seen in the proximal ducts and ductules. The tall cells have the characteristics of secretory cells, with large secretory vacuoles near their luminal surface and abundant rough endoplasmic reticulum; they may also contain small, yellow-brown lipofuscin granules.

The complexity of the mucosal folding produces a vast surface area for secretion, and 70%–80% of the human ejaculate is a thick, creamy-yellow secretion of the seminal vesicles. This secretion contains abundant fructose and other sugars, prostaglandins, proteins, amino acids, citric acid and ascorbic acid. Fructose is a major nutrient of spermatozoa.

> **Contraction of the seminal vesicle smooth muscle propels accumulated secretion into the ejaculatory duct.**

The ejaculatory duct is formed by the merging of the short duct from the seminal vesicle with the vas deferens distal to the ampulla.

Each ejaculatory duct is only 1 cm long and is lined by an epithelium of tall columnar and small round cells identical to that of the ampulla; there is no smooth muscle in its wall. The right and left ejaculatory ducts run through the prostate gland and open into the prostatic urethra at the prostatic utricle.

PROSTATE

Introduction

The function of the prostate is to produce an alkaline fluid that makes up around 30% of the volume of ejaculated semen. The prostate is composed of secreting glands that open into the urethra. These prostatic glands and ducts are embedded in a supporting stroma of fibroblasts, collagen and smooth muscle.

The entire prostate gland is surrounded by a fibrocollagenous capsule from which septa extend partway into its body, dividing it into ill-defined lobes. Grossly, these are described as transitional, central and peripheral lobes.

> **The prostatic glands are arranged in three concentric groups.**

A small group of mucosal glands open directly into the urethra; a larger group of submucosal glands open into the urethra via short ducts – these are equivalent to the transitional and central zones. A substantial outer group of so-called *main prostatic glands* open into the urethra via long ducts, and these are equivalent to the peripheral zones (Fig. 16.16).

Fig. 16.15 Seminal Vesicle. (a) Micrograph of seminal vesicle showing part of the surrounding muscle (M) and the pattern of tall mucosal folds. The lumen contains blobs of eosinophilic secretion (ES). **(b)** Micrograph showing the tall columnar secretory epithelium at high magnification.

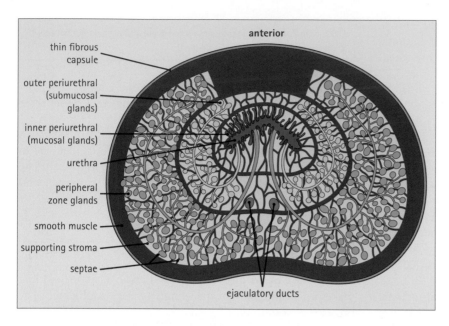

anterior

thin fibrous capsule

outer periurethral (submucosal glands)

inner periurethral (mucosal glands)

urethra

peripheral zone glands

smooth muscle

supporting stroma

septae

ejaculatory ducts

Fig. 16.16 Prostate. The prostate is surrounded by a thin fibrous capsule internal to which is a substantial layer of smooth muscle giving rise to septa (mainly muscular but with a fine fibrocollagenous components) that penetrate the organ to provide an intimate stroma supporting and demarcating the glandular elements. Division into central and peripheral zones is indistinct. The inner periurethral (mucosal) glands are small and open directly into the urethra around its entire surface; the outer periurethral glands are more numerous and open into the urethra through short ducts that enter the posterolateral urethral sinuses on their posterior surface on either side of the central ridge, the urethral crest. These two groups of glands comprise the central zone. The glands of the peripheral zone empty their secretions into the urethra by way of long ducts opening alongside the urethral crest.

Fig. 16.17 Prostatic Glands. (a) Micrograph of prostatic mucosal glands (M) opening directly into the urethra (U). **(b)** Micrograph showing the general architecture of a typical prostatic gland with its papillary pattern of ingrowths. Note the smooth muscular and fibrocollagenous stroma (S). **(c)** Micrograph showing the cytological detail of prostatic gland lining epithelium. It is composed of tall, pale-staining columnar cells (C) and occasional small basal cells (B) with darker-staining nuclei. Note the delicate supporting stroma of the papillary ingrowth (P) and the narrow periglandular layer of smooth muscle fibres (SM). The lumen contains an uncalcified, concentrically laminated corpus amylacea (CA).

The ducts of the submucosal and main prostatic glands open posteriorly into the urethral sinuses on either side of a longitudinal ridge called the *urethral crest*.

The epithelium lining of the prostate glands is thrown up into complex folds accompanied by a narrow supporting lamina propria (Fig. 16.17a and b). There are two types of epithelial cells:

- Tall columnar or cuboidal secretory cells with pale foamy cytoplasm and basal pale-staining nuclei

- Scanty flat basal cells with small dark-staining nuclei in contact with the basement membrane acting as myoepithelial cells (see Fig. 16.17c).

Ultrastructurally, the tall columnar cells have a prominent Golgi located between the basal nucleus and the luminal surface; lysosomes, secretory granules and rough endoplasmic reticulum are numerous.

The secretory products of these cells include prostate-specific acid phosphatase, prostate-specific antigen, β-microseminoprotein (prostate secretory protein 94) and simple sugars. The gland lumina usually contain some stored secretions; in older men, small spherical corpora amylacea, which are mainly condensed glycoprotein secretions, often calcified, are found.

The ducts of the prostate gland may also be lined by tall columnar epithelium, but as they near the urethra, this becomes progressively more cuboidal, and even transitional, like that of the urethra itself.

CLINICAL EXAMPLE

Benign Prostatic Hyperplasia

The most common disorder of the prostate is benign prostatic hyperplasia (BPH) and occurs in elderly men. This is characterized by considerable enlargement of the prostatic glands in the mucous and submucosal gland groups owing to an increase in the number and size of the cells of the glands and ducts (hyperplasia) and an increase in the bulk of the supporting fibromuscular stroma. Many glands are overdistended with secretion (Fig. 16.18). Because the enlarged glands are in the central and transitional zones, in proximity to the urethra, BPH leads to compression of the urethra, causing urinary retention and lower urinary tract symptoms such as hesitancy and increased frequency (including nocturia). Options for relief of these common symptoms are α_1-blockers (adrenoceptor antagonists) to relax the smooth muscle in the wall of the urethra relieving pressure, reduction of available testosterone via 5α-reductase inhibitors or transurethral surgery.

Fig. 16.18 Benign Prostatic Hyperplasia. Gross photograph of the cut surface of a prostate removed at autopsy showing the typical appearance of benign prostatic hyperplasia. There is nodular overgrowth of the periurethral glands (PUG), which is causing compression and distortion of the urethra (U). Note that the peripheral zone glands (PZG) are not involved.

CLINICAL EXAMPLE

Carcinoma of the Prostate

Cancer in the prostate gland almost always originates in the main glands arranged around the periphery. This peripheral presentation, away from the urethra, means it does not lead to urinary symptoms and is therefore often advanced before symptoms arise (Fig. 16.19). Again, because of its initial peripheral location, adenocarcinoma of the prostate may be detected by digital rectal examination (DRE) as a fixed, hard prostate, in contrast to BPH, which reveals a smooth, rubbery enlarged prostate. Transrectal ultrasound-guided needle biopsy provides cores of tissue for histological diagnosis and grading.

Fig. 16.19 Adenocarcinoma of the Prostate. Micrograph showing cancerous transformation of the prostatic glands. Those on the *left* are normal with regular, tall, columnar epithelium. The cancerous prostatic glands on the *right* have lost their tall columnar pattern and their regular architecture.

The bulbourethral glands are lined by tall mucus-secreting epithelium.

BULBOURETHRAL GLANDS

Seminal fluid enters the prostatic urethra from the right and left ejaculatory ducts, passing through the short membranous urethra and the penile urethra, before entering the vagina during sexual intercourse. Opening into the membranous urethra are the long narrow ducts from the paired small bulbourethral glands.

The bulbourethral glands are about 5 mm in diameter, and the epithelium produces a watery, slightly mucoid fluid containing abundant sugars (mainly galactose) and some sialic acid. This fluid precedes the thicker semen along the penile urethra during emission and may have a lubricating function.

PENIS

The penis is composed of erectile tissue and contains part of the male urethra.

The erectile tissue is arranged into two dorsal cylinders (corpora cavernosa) and a smaller central ventral cylinder (corpus spongiosum) through which the penile urethra runs. The cylinders are each surrounded by a dense fibrocollagenous sheath, the tunica albuginea, which also holds them together (Fig. 16.20).

The erectile tissues are essentially interconnecting vascular spaces, which are empty when the penis is flaccid (Figs. 16.21 and 16.22) but which fill with blood during erection to form an enlarged, rigid organ.

Fig. 16.21 Corpus Spongiosum. Micrograph of corpus spongiosum showing large, irregular interconnecting vascular channels (C) lined by flat endothelium and separated by a fibrocollagenous stroma (S) containing some smooth muscle bundles.

Fig. 16.20 Penis. Transverse section of penis showing the arrangement of the vascular erectile tissue into two dorsal corpora cavernosa (CC) and a single ventral corpus spongiosum (CS) through which the penile urethra (U) runs. Small mucous glands in the corpus spongiosum are particularly concentrated around the penile urethra into which they open. The corpora are enclosed within and divided by a broad fibrocollagenous capsule (C). The erectile core is surrounded by a sheath of skin to which it is connected by a very loose subcutis containing a number of blood vessels, including the small paired dorsal arteries and the midline superficial and deep dorsal veins.

The blood supply to the penis is provided by the dorsal and the deep arteries. From the deep arteries arise arteries supplying the tunica albuginea and the helicine arteries, which supply the erectile tissue. The helicine arteries are so named because they are spiral in the flaccid penis but during erection they straighten and dilate, filling the corpora with blood.

These helicine arteries contain an intimal cushion composed of smooth muscle, which is normally in a contracted state, maintaining a low flow and allowing blood to instead flow to the deep dorsal vein of the penis. This maintains a flaccid state. During arousal, parasympathetic stimulation causes relaxation of smooth muscle in artery and erectile tissues, leading to vasodilation and allowing blood flow into the cavernous spaces.

After ejaculation the parasympathetic stimulation ceases, smooth muscle returns to a contracted state and blood is shunted directly to the dorsal vein, leading to loss of the erectile state.

Fig. 16.22 Corpora Cavernosa. (a) Micrograph of part of the corpora cavernosa (CC) with the central deep artery (A). **(b)** Micrograph showing the system of interconnecting vascular channels (V) of the corpora cavernosa in the non-erectile state.

During erection, the two corpora cavernosa become more turgid than the corpus spongiosum. The pressure exerted by the corpus spongiosum on the urethra running through it is not sufficient to prevent passage of the semen, which is forcibly ejected by contraction of the smooth muscle, but is usually sufficient to prevent successful unrestricted micturition.

The erectile component of the penis is surrounded by skin, which has a very loose subcutis, permitting it to move considerably during intercourse.

At the distal end of the penis the corpus spongiosum terminates on the glans penis, which is covered with non-keratinizing squamous epithelium containing sebaceous glands.

CLINICAL EXAMPLE

Drugs to Treat Erectile Dysfunction Maintain Relaxation of Smooth Muscle

This relaxation in smooth muscle leading to diversion of blood to erectile tissues is brought about by the release of nitric oxide (NO). This binds to an enzyme, guanylate cyclase, which increases levels of cyclic guanosine monophosphate (cGMP) that then mediates the relaxation of smooth muscle and allows blood to flow into the erectile tissues of the penis. However, once formed, cGMP is broken down by an enzyme, cGMP-specific phosphodiesterase type 5 (PDE5), resulting in the return of contraction of the smooth muscle, shunting of blood and loss of the erectile state. Drugs such as sildenafil, tadalafil and vardenafil inhibit PDE5 from breaking down cGMP, thereby prolonging relaxation of smooth muscle, maintaining vasodilation and blood flow through the helicine arteries to the corpora cavernosa and maintaining penile erection.

The penile urethra opens to the exterior at the meatus at the centre of the glans penis.

For most of its length the penile urethra is lined by non-secreting columnar epithelium into which small mucous glands embedded in the corpus spongiosum drain. Within the glans penis, however, the urethra dilates (navicular fossa) and becomes lined by nonkeratinizing stratified squamous epithelium identical to that covering the glans.

The end of the penis is normally covered by an overlap of penile skin (the prepuce), which is rich in elastic fibres, permitting it to retract over the glans penis during erection.

ENDOCRINE CONTROL

> The male sex hormone testosterone is essential for the male reproductive system to function successfully.

In the embryo, testosterone and other androgens produced by the immature testes are responsible for the development of the penis and accessory sex glands, such as the prostate and epididymis.

With the onset of puberty, male secondary sexual characteristics develop under the influence of testosterone (Fig. 16.23). This hormone also induces maturation and division of spermatogonia in the seminiferous tubules, leading eventually to full spermatogenesis with the production of mature spermatozoa.

In addition, testosterone is responsible for the maturation of the characteristic epithelia of the male genital ducts and the accessory glands that discharge secretions into them.

In the adult male, continued production of spermatozoa, and maintenance of the normal structure and function of the ducts and accessory glands, is dependent on continued testosterone production.

Failing testosterone production in old age leads to partial or complete cessation of spermatogenesis and alteration of the specialized secretory, absorptive and microvillus epithelium of the ducts and accessory glands to a more simplified cuboidal or squamous epithelium, which is unable to perform its previous functions.

Thus testosterone is the hub of the structure and function of the male genital system. It is produced by Leydig (interstitial) cells from cholesterol under the influence of luteinizing hormone secreted by the gonadotroph cells of the pituitary (see p. 274).

Fig. 16.23 Hormonal Control of the Male Reproductive System. Testosterone stimulates spermatogenesis in seminiferous tubules (A), maintains the structure and function of the ducts and accessory glands (B), stimulates and maintains secondary sexual characteristics (C) and provides a feedback mechanism (D) controlling pituitary output of luteinizing hormone (LH). Secretion of testosterone by Leydig cells is stimulated by LH. Sertoli cells secrete androgen-binding protein under the influence of follicle-stimulating hormone (FSH) from the pituitary and also produce inhibin, which is responsible for feedback control.

For online review questions, please visit https://studentconsult.inkling.com.

Female Reproductive System

INTRODUCTION

The female reproductive system:
- Produces haploid female gametes (ova)
- Receives haploid male gametes (spermatozoa) before fertilization
- Provides a suitable environment for fertilization of ova by spermatozoa
- Provides a suitable physical and hormonal environment for implantation of the embryo
- Accommodates and nourishes the embryo and fetus during pregnancy
- Expels the mature fetus at the end of pregnancy

The structure of the human female reproductive system changes considerably from childhood into reproductive maturity, and later menopause, under the control of tropic hormones.

Unlike many other mammals, the human female ovulates at regular intervals (approximately every 28 days) throughout the year and undergoes structural and functional modification at different stages in the monthly cycle.

The system (Figs. 17.1 and 17.2) comprises the ovaries, uterine tubes, uterus and vagina (collectively referred to as the **internal genitalia**), together with the mons pubis, vulva (labia majora and labia minora) and clitoris (referred to as the **external genitalia**).

MONS PUBIS, LABIA MAJORA AND LABIA MINORA

The mons pubis, labia majora and labia minora all consist of modified skin (see Chapter 18) as described next.

> **The mons pubis (mons veneris) is skin superimposed on a substantial pad of subcutaneous fat.**

The mons pubis is the area overlying the symphysis pubis. It is characterized by the presence of unusually oblique hair follicles, which produce the coarse, curly pubic hair common to most races. Underneath the skin is a pad of fat.

> **The labia majora are posterolateral extensions of the mons pubis on either side of the vaginal introitus.**

The labia majora are similarly richly endowed with subcutaneous fat and oblique hair follicles (see Fig. 17.1c). There are smooth muscle fibres in the subcutaneous fat.

The accumulation of subcutaneous fat and the development of the oblique hair follicles and pubic hair is hormone dependent and begins with the onset of sexual maturity, usually between the ages of 10 and 13 years.

This area is also rich in apocrine glands and prominent sebaceous glands, both of which mature and become active at the onset of sexual maturity, but eccrine sweat glands, which are present from birth, show no change.

> **The labia minora are thin flaps of skin devoid of adipose tissue and with abundant blood vessels, nerve endings and elastic fibres.**

Although hair follicles are absent, there are many sebaceous glands that open directly on to the epidermal surface (see Fig. 17.1d).

The epidermis of both the labia majora and minora becomes pigmented by melanin with the onset of puberty. The outer, lateral aspect of the labia minora is usually more pigmented than the inner medial aspect, and the epidermis has a well-developed rete ridge system, as this is an area subject to friction during coitus and childbirth.

On the inner aspect, the melanin pigmentation becomes progressively reduced as the vaginal introitus is approached and the keratinized, stratified, squamous epithelium becomes thinner, with flattening of the rete ridges and thinning of the keratin layer.

This keratinized epithelium extends into the vaginal vestibule as far as the hymen, which is a thin fibrous membrane that is rarely completely intact and usually appears as an irregular 'frill' in the lining of the lower vagina, the hymeneal tegmentum. On its exterior (vulval) surface the hymen is covered with the keratinized, stratified, squamous epithelium, whereas the inner (vaginal) surface is covered with non-keratinized, stratified, squamous epithelium, rich in glycogen, which is similar to that lining the vagina (Fig. 17.3).

The hymen can be regarded as the junction between the internal and external genitalia.

CLITORIS

> **The clitoris, a wishbone-shaped organ, is the female counterpart of the penis.**

The full extent of the human clitoris was mapped in 1998, and it consists of a small external part, the glans and hood, and a more extensive internal body. The pea-sized glans lies at the apex of the labia minora and above the opening of the urethra.

Fig. 17.1 Internal and External Genitalia. (a) The relationship between the external and internal genitalia. **(b)** Micrograph of glans of clitoris; note the two corpora cavernosa (CC) arranged side by side and engorged with blood, the incomplete central septum (S) and the fibrocollagenous sheath (F), outside of which are prominent nerve endings (mainly Pacinian touch corpuscles [PC]; see also Chapter 18). **(c)** Micrograph of labia majora. The skin contains many oblique hair follicles (HF), sebaceous glands (SG) and eccrine sweat glands and ducts. **(d)** Micrograph of labia minora. The skin is devoid of hair follicles but is rich in sebaceous glands (SG), which open directly on to the surface. Note that the dermis is highly vascular. **(e)** Figure showing the extent and location of the clitoris in relation to the external genitalia.

It is composed of two corpora cavernosa of erectile vascular tissue that lie side by side surrounded by a fibrocollagenous sheath; an incomplete central septum partly separates the two corpora (see Fig. 17.1b).

The glans of the clitoris is covered by thin epidermis that is devoid of hair follicles, sebaceous glands and eccrine and apocrine glands. The function of the clitoris in humans is uniquely for sexual pleasure, being richly equipped with sensory nerves and a variety of receptors and surrounded by Pacinian nerve endings, sensitive to deep pressure and vibration.

Externally, the skin forms an incomplete hood (the clitoral prepuce), with a thin midline frenulum inferiorly. Internally, at the base of the body of the clitoris, the corpora cavernosa diverge to lie along the pubic rami, where they contain fibres of the ischiocavernosus muscle and terminate as the crura. Also considered as part of the clitoris, because of being composed of erectile tissue, the vestibular bulbs lie deep to the labia majora. The structure of the clitoris is shown in Fig. 17.1e.

The clitoris is small before puberty and enlarges with the onset of sexual maturity. During sexual arousal, the erectile tissue becomes engorged.

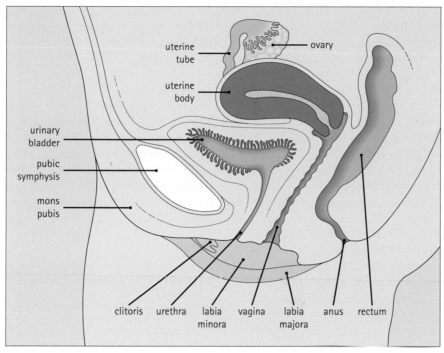

Fig. 17.2 Lateral View of Female Genitalia. Note the angle of insertion of the uterus into the vagina.

Fig. 17.3 Vagina. Micrograph of vaginal wall showing glycogen-rich, stratified, squamous epithelial mucosa (M), a highly vascular submucosa (S) and irregular smooth muscle (SM).

> **The urethral meatus opens to the exterior in the midline below the clitoris.**

On either side of the meatus are the openings of the paraurethral glands (of Skene). These glands are located around the urethra, mainly posteriorly and laterally, and are lined by pseudostratified columnar epithelium. Although their function is uncertain, they are now regarded as homologues of the male prostate gland. They are capable of secretion and may lubricate the area around the urethra; however, their secretion contains many components similar in nature to prostatic secretions, including prostate-specific antigen (PSA), and may contribute to female ejaculate.

VAGINA

> **The vagina is a fibromuscular tube extending from the vestibule to the uterus.**

In the mature female, the vagina is 7–9 cm long, but is capable of both marked distension and elongation (see Fig. 17.1). It forms an angle of more than 90 degrees with the normal anteverted uterus (see Fig. 17.2).

At its inner end, the vagina forms a cuff around the protruding cervix of the uterus, forming anterior, posterior and lateral pouches known as the *fornices*.

The vagina has four layers (see Fig. 17.3) as follows:
- Stratified, squamous, epithelial mucosa
- Lamina propria (subepithelial region), which is rich in elastic fibres and thin-walled blood vessels, mainly veins and venules
- A fibromuscular layer containing ill-defined bundles of circularly arranged smooth muscle and a more prominent outer layer of longitudinally arranged smooth muscle
- Adventitia, which is composed of fibrocollagenous tissue containing numerous thick elastic fibres, large blood vessels, nerves and clumps of ganglion cells. At the lower end, the fibromuscular layer also contains some skeletal muscle, which is found mainly around the vaginal introitus in the hymeneal region

The rich meshwork of elastic fibres in the vaginal wall is responsible for its elasticity and permits the great temporary distension required during parturition. The extensive submucosal plexus of thin-walled blood vessels is thought to permit the diffusion of watery fluid across the epithelium and to contribute to vaginal fluid.

Although structurally a tube, at rest, the vagina is collapsed so that the anterior wall is in contact with the posterior wall, and for much of its length there are shallow longitudinal grooves in the midline of both these walls. In addition, the vaginal mucosa is rugose, being thrown up into a series of closely packed transverse mucosal folds or ridges.

> **The structure of the vagina varies with age and hormonal activity.**

Changes occur in the non-keratinizing, stratified, squamous epithelium which lines the vagina.

Before puberty, the epithelium is thin, a state to which it reverts after menopause, but during the reproductive years the epithelium responds to the activity of oestrogens and thickens. The basal cells and the distinct parabasal layer show increased mitotic activity, and the more superficial cells increase not only in number but also in size as a result of the accumulation of stored glycogen and some lipid within the cytoplasm.

Glycogen content is maximal at the time of ovulation, and some glycogen-rich surface squames are shed into the vaginal cavity after ovulation, during the secretory phase of the menstrual cycle.

Breakdown of the glycogen by commensal lactobacilli in the vaginal cavity produces lactic acid, resulting in an acid pH. This restricts the vaginal bacterial flora to acid-loving commensals and deters invasion by bacterial pathogens and fungi, such as *Candida albicans*, which is the cause of vaginal 'thrush'.

> **Bartholin's (vulvovaginal) glands are located around the lower vagina.**

Bartholin's glands are composed of acini lined by tall, columnar, mucus-secreting cells with pale cytoplasm and small basal nuclei. They are considered homologous to the bulbourethral glands in the male.

These glands open into the vagina posterolaterally at the level of the hymeneal remnants through a duct lined by a transitional epithelium with a surface mucin-secreting layer for lubrication.

UTERUS

The uterus is a muscular organ and receives the right and left uterine (fallopian) tubes. It is lined by columnar epithelium and, at its lower end, it opens into the vagina.

The uterus can be divided into three parts: the fundus, the body and the cervix (Fig. 17.4). Whereas the fundus and body have the same histological structure (see p. 352), that of the cervix is different.

Cervix

> **The cervix is the lower part of the uterus, part of which protrudes into the vagina.**

The junction between the cervix and the uterine body is the internal os, and at this point the nature of the lining epithelium and the uterine wall changes (Fig. 17.5).

The cervical lumen opens into the vaginal cavity at the external os, where again there is an important change in the nature of the lining epithelium. This zone is the site of many important pathological changes (see Figs. 17.8 and 17.9).

Fig. 17.4 Uterus. Section through the uterus of a 35-year-old woman showing the fundus (F), body (B) and cervix (Cx). Note the endometrial cavity (EMC), endocervical canal (ECC) and ectocervix (ECx). The smooth muscle of the body contains a small tumour, a leiomyoma (L) (see also Fig. 17.11).

Fig. 17.5 Cervix. Low-power micrograph of the cervix. The stroma (S) is composed of smooth muscle fibres embedded in collagen, with the proportions of muscle and fibrous tissue varying according to age and parity; blood and lymphatic vessels are prominent and numerous. The ectocervix (ECx) is covered with stratified squamous epithelium (see detail in Fig. 17.6), and the endocervical canal (ECC) is lined by tall columnar epithelium (see detail in Fig. 17.7). The junction between the squamous and columnar epithelium is located in the region of the external os. In this example there is a transformation zone (TZ) (see p. 350) of squamous epithelium, which has extended into the endocervical canal; note the Nabothian follicles (NF) (see Fig. 17.8c). The areas shown in boxes (EC and ECx) are also shown in Fig. 17.6 and Fig. 17.7 at higher magnification.

The cervix is cylindrical and symmetrical, being about 3 cm long and 2–2.5 cm in diameter, but it becomes more barrel-shaped after pregnancy and parturition. After childbirth, the external os becomes a transverse slit dividing the distal end of the cervix into anterior and posterior lips, whereas the external os of the nulliparous cervix is circular.

> **The cervical stroma is important in childbirth.**

The cervical stroma is composed of smooth muscle fibres embedded in collagen, with the proportions of the two components varying with age and parity. Normally, the cervix is firm and rubbery and the cervical lumen is a narrow channel, but the cervix can be dilated under some circumstances, a fact which is used in investigative gynaecological practice to obtain samples of the uterine lining epithelium for histological examination. A measure of the capacity of the cervix for dilatation is the fact that a cervical lumen, which is normally a narrow canal around the diameter of a small pencil, becomes, at childbirth, capable of allowing the passage of a baby. Furthermore, after delivery, the cervix reverts to normal in a very short time.

This capacity depends on radical alterations in the nature of the cervical stroma, attended by a change in texture ('cervical softening').

ADVANCED CONCEPT

The Cervix in Childbirth

The normally firm and rubbery uterine cervix with a narrow lumen of less than 1 cm in diameter dilates to approximately 10 cm during labour. This is achieved by softening and increased elasticity in the cervical stroma. The changes in the cervix in late pregnancy are complex.

In the glycosaminoglycan matrix, hyaluronic acid concentration between collagen fibres increases, drawing in water molecules, which increase the bulk and softness of the matrix and separate the collagen fibres of the cervical stroma. Dermatan sulphate concentration decreases, leading to weakening of the dermatan sulphate bridges holding adjacent collagen and elastin fibres together. This further contributes to the separation of collagen fibres.

There are also changes in collagen and elastin fibres. Type I and type II collagen fibres become separated from each other, lose their strong parallel alignment and become shorter. The separation of collagen fibres, their rearrangement from a compact parallel pattern to a more haphazard arrangement and the shortening of individual fibres all lead to a reduction in tensile strength and a decreased resistance to the pressure exerted by the presenting part of the fetus being expelled from the uterine body. Similar changes probably occur in elastin fibres.

The Epithelial Content of the Cervix

The external surface of the part of the cervix that protrudes into the vagina is the ectocervix, and the lining of the lumen is the endocervix.

> **The ectocervix is covered by epithelium continuous with that of the vagina at the vaginal fornices.**

The ectocervical epithelium is non-keratinizing, stratified, squamous and rich in glycogen in the sexually mature period (Fig. 17.6).

Fig. 17.6 Ectocervix. This micrograph is from the box area labelled (ECx) shown in Fig. 17.5. Stratified squamous epithelium covers the ectocervix. Like those of the vagina, the cells are rich in glycogen during the period of sexual maturity, giving the middle and upper layers a vacuolated appearance.

Before menarche and after menopause, the epithelium is much thinner, with fewer layers and smaller cells.

> **The endocervical canal runs between the uterine and vaginal cavities.**

The canal is lined by a single layer of tall, columnar, mucus-secreting epithelium, the endocervical epithelium (Fig. 17.7a).

Longitudinal or transverse histological sections of the cervix have given the impression that there are glandular structures (endocervical mucous glands) extending into the underlying stroma. Three-dimensional studies, however, indicate that the structures are in fact deep, slit-like invaginations of the surface epithelium, with blind-ended tubules arising from the clefts (see Fig. 17.7b). Thus there is a large surface area for the production of cervical mucus, which fills the endocervical canal. Before puberty and after menopause, the amount of cervical mucus is greatly reduced.

The mucin in the endocervical canal acts as a protective barrier, preventing bacterial ascent into the endometrial cavity.

Movement of endocervical mucus into the vaginal canal is facilitated by ciliated columnar epithelial cells scattered among the mucus-secreting endocervical cells.

Both the mucin-secreting and ciliated cells have fine microvilli, which are only visible ultrastructurally.

> **The columnar epithelium of the endocervical canal and the squamous epithelium of the ectocervix meet at the squamocolumnar junction of the cervix.**

This is the most likely area of the cervical epithelium to be affected by disease.

The original squamocolumnar junction is usually located in the region of the external os, but its precise location at birth is influenced by maternal hormone exposure in utero.

At about puberty, hormonal influences lead to extension of the columnar epithelium onto the ectocervix, forming an ectropion or cervical erosion (Fig. 17.8), which is augmented by a first pregnancy, particularly when this occurs shortly after menarche.

Before puberty, the pH of the vagina and cervix is alkaline, but afterwards, bacterial breakdown of the glycogen in the vaginal and cervical squamous epithelium renders an acidic environment, with a pH of about 3.

Exposure of the sensitive columnar epithelium of the ectropion to the postpubertal acidic environment of the vagina induces a change in the type of epithelium to stratified squamous (termed *squamous metaplasia*) and a transformation zone between the endocervical columnar epithelium and the ectocervical squamous epithelium.

Thus the squamocolumnar junction is of variable size, but its site always approximates to the external os. In older women, it may retreat into the endocervical canal.

The transformation zone is composed of new squamous epithelium in an area previously occupied by columnar epithelium.

Fig. 17.7 Endocervix. These micrographs are from the box area labelled (EC) shown in Fig. 17.5. **(a)** The endocervical canal is lined by a single layer of tall, columnar, mucus-secreting epithelium (E). **(b)** Numerous deep invaginations (I) of the mucus-secreting epithelium extend into the pink-stained cervical stroma and greatly increase the surface for mucus production. A small amount of cervical mucus (Mu) is present within the endocervical canal (EC).

Fig. 17.8 Squamocolumnar Junction of the Cervix. The mobility of the squamocolumnar junction, the development of ectropion and the formation of the transformation zone. **(a)** The squamocolumnar junction is originally situated in the region of the external os. **(b)** At puberty, the endocervical epithelium extends distally into the acid environment of the vagina and forms an ectropion. **(c)** A transformation zone forms as squamous epithelium regrows over the ectropion. The openings of the crypts may be obliterated in the process, resulting in the formation of mucus-filled Nabothian follicles (see Fig. 17.5).

CLINICAL EXAMPLE

Carcinoma of the Cervix

The transformation zone of the cervical epithelium is the most common site of origin of carcinoma of the cervix. Current research suggests that the vast majority of cervical cancers are caused by infection with 'high-risk' cancer-inducing human papillomaviruses (HPV), and a vaccine against harmful HPV subtypes has been developed. The development of cervical cancer is usually preceded by histological abnormality of the squamous epithelial cells in this transformation zone. The abnormal cells:

- Lose their regular stratified pattern
- Have a high nucleus-to-cytoplasm ratio
- Show variation in shape and size and increased mitotic activity

These cytological features are characteristic of malignant tumour cells and are usually associated with evidence of invasive behaviour. However, in the cervix, the cytological changes of malignancy may be present for years before the abnormal epithelium begins to invade the underlying stroma; they are referred to as *carcinoma in situ* or *cervical intra-epithelial neoplasia* (CIN) (Fig. 17.9a). Cytological examination of squames of surface epithelium for dysplastic changes forms the basis of the cervical smear screening programme.

Eventually, the abnormal epithelial cells breach the basement membrane and invade the cervical stroma (see Fig. 17.9b), gaining access to blood and lymphatic vessels, which are their route for spread to other sites, such as the lymph nodes around the iliac arteries. This is invasive carcinoma. Early diagnosis of CIN can be obtained by cervical cytology (cervical smear); cells are scraped from the epithelial surface in the region of the cervical os and examined microscopically for abnormal cells. Abnormal areas can then be treated, usually by surgical removal, thus preventing the future development of invasive cancer.

Fig. 17.9 Carcinoma of the Cervix. (a) The cervical epithelial cells (E) have lost their regular stratified pattern, have high nucleus-to-cytoplasm ratios and show increased mitotic activity (compare with Fig. 17.6). As the basement membrane (BM) between the epithelium and underlying stroma (S) is intact, this is carcinoma in situ or cervical intra-epithelial neoplasia. **(b)** Some of the abnormal epithelial cells have breached the basement membrane and invaded the cervical stroma *(arrows)*; this is invasive carcinoma.

One almost invariable consequence of squamous metaplasia near the external os is that the openings of some of the deep crypts of previously everted endocervical mucous glands become obliterated so that mucin produced deep in the crypts cannot be excreted into the endocervical lumen or vagina. Instead, it accumulates within the blocked clefts and produces spherical cystic masses of inspissated mucus lined by flattened endocervical mucus-secreting epithelium; these are called **Nabothian follicles**.

KEY FACTS

Uterine Cervix

- Lower part of uterus, protruding into the vagina
- Canal is lined by tall, columnar, mucin-secreting epithelium
- Surface protruding into vagina is covered by stratified squamous epithelium
- Squamocolumnar junction is an important site of disease (transformation zone)
- Has a stroma of smooth muscle fibres embedded in collagen; proportions of each vary according to age and parity

Uterine Body

> **The body and fundus of the uterus have thick walls composed of smooth muscle (myometrium).**

The myometrial smooth muscle is arranged into three ill-defined layers.

Myometrium is hormone sensitive and undergoes both hypertrophy (an increase in cell size) and hyperplasia (an increase in cell numbers) during pregnancy (Fig. 17.10), progressively returning to its normal size (involution) in the weeks after delivery.

Within the myometrium are prominent blood vessels, both arterial and venous, which undergo marked dilation and thickening of their walls during pregnancy. Abundant gap junctions are seen between myometrial cells to facilitate coordinated contraction of the muscle wall for parturition.

With cessation of hormonal stimulation after menopause, the myometrial cells atrophy and the uterus shrinks. The fibrocollagenous tissue between the muscle bundles becomes more prominent.

Fig. 17.10 Myometrium. (a) Normal myometrium from a non-pregnant 35-year-old woman. The muscle cells are small and tightly packed. **(b)** Myometrium from a 28-year-old woman in the eighth month of pregnancy, photographed at the same magnification as **(a)**. Note the enormous increase in size of the individual muscle fibres, caused almost entirely by an increase in cytoplasm. This is an example of physiological hypertrophy and is a common response of muscle cells to an increased workload, in this case the need to increase the propulsive power of the uterus to expel the childbirth.

CLINICAL EXAMPLE

Leiomyoma

The myometrium is the site of one of the most common benign tumours: the leiomyoma or fibroid (Fig. 17.11, see also Fig. 17.4), which is derived from smooth muscle of the uterine wall. These tumours are well demarcated from the surrounding normal tissue, often by fibrous tissue, and contain stromal elements, giving the tumour a rubbery consistency.

Like normal uterine smooth muscle, leiomyomas are hormone dependent and progressively enlarge until menopause, after which time they regress.

Fig. 17.11 Leiomyoma. Micrograph of a typical small leiomyoma surrounded by the myometrium in which it has developed,

> **The body of the uterus is lined by the endometrium, which is composed of glands and supporting stroma.**

Before puberty, the endometrium is simple and composed of low cuboidal epithelium supported by a scanty spindle-celled stroma. Downgrowths of epithelium into the stroma produce a small number of rudimentary tubular glands.

Between menarche (the first menstrual period) and menopause, the function of the endometrium is to produce a welcome environment into which a fertilized egg can implant. It therefore goes through a monthly cycle of expansion to form abundant nutrient-rich glands and extensive vascular supply. If fertilization does not occur, the lining is shed as menses. During reproductive life, the endometrium is differentiated into two layers: a deep basal layer at the junction with the myometrium and a superficial functional layer lining the lumen. The functional layer is hormone responsive and undergoes the **menstrual cycle**. The relationships between histological changes and hormone secretions are discussed in Fig. 17.24 (see p. 362).

If fertilization and successful implantation of an ovum occur, the endometrium remains unshed and forms the decidua (see p. 368).

The basal layer, which is not shed at menstruation, provides a cellular reserve from which a new functional layer develops after menstrual shedding. The endometrium does not respond evenly to ovarian hormonal stimulation: functional endometrium in the lower segment close to the junction with the cervix and patches around the entrances of the uterine tubes may show little proliferative or secretory activity and often resemble the basal layer.

Uterine Tubes

> The uterine (fallopian) tubes convey ova from the ovary to the lumen of the body of the uterus (endometrial cavity).

The uterine tubes are also the site of fertilization of the ovum by spermatozoa. After fertilization, the tube transmits the fertilized ovum to the endometrial cavity, where implantation can take place.

Each uterine tube is 10–12 cm long and extends from a dilated open end close to the ovary to a narrow portion that passes through the myometrial wall of the uterus before opening into the uterine cavity. There are four recognizable tubal segments (Fig. 17.12), each differing histologically, particularly in their proportions of muscle and epithelium and the degree of convolution of their epithelium.

The infundibulum is surrounded by a fringe of epithelial-coated **fimbriae**, some of which may become adherent to the nearby ovary. Medial to the infundibulum is a thin-walled zone called the *ampulla*, where ovum fertilization usually takes place.

The ampulla leads into a narrower, thick-walled segment called the *isthmus*. In turn, the isthmus is continuous with the short intramural segment, which opens into the uterus.

Fig. 17.12 Uterine (Fallopian) Tube. (a) The uterine tube, ovary and uterus. **(b)** Low-power micrograph of the ampulla showing its thin muscular wall and large lumen with markedly papillary mucosa. **(c)** High-power micrograph of tubal epithelium at the ampulla showing a high proportion of ciliated cells (CC), thin delicate stroma (S) and an occasional intra-epithelial lymphocyte (IEL). **(d)** Scanning electron micrograph of tubal mucosa at the ampulla, showing numerous ciliated cells (CC) and relatively scanty secretory cells (SC). **(e)** Low-power micrograph of the isthmus, showing its thick muscular wall and small lumen with simpler, non-papillary mucosa. **(f)** Scanning electron micrograph of tubal mucosa at the isthmus, showing few ciliated cells (CC) and many secretory cells (SC) with abundant microvilli.

The uterine tube is a muscular tube lined by epithelium, differing in appearance at different sites.

> **The smooth muscle wall of the uterine tube is composed of two layers.**

The inner layer of smooth muscle appears to be circular and the outer longitudinal in sections. They are actually spirals (tight circular and loose longitudinal), similar to the ureter (see Fig. 15.40). Close to the uterus is a third muscular layer. Internally, a thin vascular lamina propria supports the tubal epithelium.

> **There are two types of epithelial cells lining the uterine tube: ciliated cells and secretory cells.**

The ciliated cells are particularly numerous near the ovarian end of the tube, where they form the majority population (about 60%–80%), but close to the uterus they are the minority population (about 25%) and secretory cells predominate (see Fig. 17.12).

> **The ciliated tubal epithelial cell is a columnar cell, the height of which varies during the menstrual cycle.**

The ciliated tubal epithelial cell is responsive to oestrogen and is at its tallest and most ciliated at about the time of ovulation, after which it progressively shortens and loses some cilia until menstruation. The decrease in height and ciliation also occurs and persists throughout the duration of a pregnancy, presumably because of the dominance of progesterone. With the resumption of oestrogen secretion after menstruation or delivery, the cells again lengthen and become more ciliated.

The ciliated cells may be responsible for movement of the ovum through the infundibulum and ampulla, although tubal peristalsis probably plays a greater role. They may also have a role in propelling the spermatozoa in the opposite direction.

> **The secretory cells are columnar cells with surface microvilli.**

The secretory cells produce a watery tubal fluid (see Fig. 17.12), which is rich in potassium and chloride ions and also contains normal serum proteins, including immunoglobulins.

The tubal fluid is assumed to have a nutritive function for spermatozoa and fertilized or unfertilized ova.

Two other cell types have been described in the tubal epithelium: the peg cell and the reserve basal cell. The peg cell has been considered to be an effete secretory cell, but recent evidence suggests that it has stem cell–like functions. The reserve basal cells have been shown to be intraepithelial cells of the lymphoid series.

CLINICAL EXAMPLE

Disorders of the Fallopian Tube

Tubal Ectopic Pregnancy

Occasionally, the fertilized ovum is held up in the tubal lumen and implants in the wall of the uterine tube, producing a tubal ectopic pregnancy.

Partial development of the embryo and placenta proceeds for a time, but the thin-walled uterine tube is an unsatisfactory site for implantation, and the embryo cannot survive. The vascular placental tissues penetrate into the thin tubal wall (Fig. 17.13a) and often perforate through, producing brisk bleeding into the lumen of the tube and into the peritoneal cavity. This produces lower abdominal pain and, if the blood loss is severe, shock.

Acute and Chronic Salpingitis

Bacterial infection of the tube (e.g. by gonococcus) produces acute inflammation in the papillary folds and muscular wall and pus formation in the lumen (see Fig. 17.13b).

Such infections may persist, with abscess formation and chronic inflammation, or may heal with scarring, leaving a blocked or distorted lumen, which may obstruct the passage of the fertilized ovum and predispose to tubal ectopic pregnancy or infertility.

Fig. 17.13 Disorders of the Fallopian Tube. (a) Micrograph of a tubal ectopic pregnancy; chorionic villi (CV) are developing in the lumen of the tube, and a trophoblast (T) is eroding into the tubal wall, producing bleeding (B). **(b)** In this section from an infected tube, the papillary folds and muscular wall are infiltrated by neutrophils and there is pus (P) in the lumen.

OVARY

Introduction

The paired ovaries are small, flattened ovoid organs lying in the right and left lateral pelvic cavities. They have two major functions:

- They are the source of mature ova.
- They are endocrine organs, producing the steroid hormones that prepare the endometrium for conception and maintain pregnancy should fertilization occur.

> **The surface of the ovary is covered by a single layer of epithelium.**

This surface layer is usually cuboidal or low columnar in type (see Fig. 17.16), but commonly flattens with increasing age and when the ovary is enlarged.

The epithelium is continuous with the pelvic peritoneum at the hilum of the ovary (although the cells differ structurally from the peritoneal mesothelial cells). It is called the *germinal epithelium*, which is, however, a misnomer because the epithelial cells are not the source of the female gametes.

The surface epithelial cells have prominent surface microvilli and occasional cilia; mitochondria are abundant, and small pinocytotic vesicles are associated with the base of some microvilli.

The ovarian surface is usually irregularly fissured, and the fissures are also lined by the surface epithelium. The necks of the fissures may seal over, leaving islands of surface epithelium within the ovarian cortex. Fluid secretion by the cells then converts these islands into cysts (germinal inclusion cysts), which are common.

The surface epithelial cells show little alteration during the menstrual cycle but usually lengthen during pregnancy. The most prevalent types of ovarian tumours originate from these cells.

A substantial basement membrane (the tunica albuginea) separates the surface cells from the underlying ovarian tissue in the mature ovary.

> **The ovary can be divided into three components: hilum, medulla and outer cortex.**

The ovarian **hilum** is the route whereby blood vessels, lymphatics and nerves enter and leave the ovary and is continuous with the medulla, the central core of the ovary (Fig. 17.14).

In addition to the vessels and lymphatics, the medulla and hilum also contain vestigial remnants of the embryonic Wolffian duct and clusters of hilus or hilar cells.

The Wolffian duct remnants persist as irregular tubules lined by flat or cuboidal epithelium (rete ovarii).

The **hilus cells** are histologically identical to the interstitial (Leydig) cells of the testis (see Fig. 16.10) and are round or oval, with eosinophilic granular or foamy cytoplasm containing brown lipofuscin-like pigment. They are closely packed in clusters (Fig. 17.15). Occasional hilus cells contain Reinke's

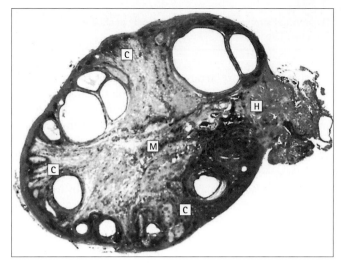

Fig. 17.14 Ovary. Micrograph of ovary showing the hilum (H), medulla (M) and cortex (C). Gamete formation and maturation occur in the cortex and are responsible for the cystic spaces seen here.

Fig. 17.15 Ovary – Hilus Cells. H&E micrograph showing clusters of hilus cells (H) in loose connective tissue at the ovarian hilum, the characteristic location. These cells have ill-defined borders, slightly granular eosinophilic cytoplasm and granules of lipofuscin pigment giving a faint *yellow* colour to a few cells.

crystalloids (see p. 336), and some also contain round eosinophilic hyaline bodies. The small clumps of hilus cells are often found close to nerves and blood vessels. They are steroid-producing cells, mainly androstenedione, and in keeping with being a steroid-secreting cell, their mitochondria have tubular cristae.

The ovarian **medulla** often contains clusters of stromal cells identical to those occupying the bulk of the cortex.

The ovarian **cortex** has two components:

- A supporting stroma
- Gamete-producing structures and their derivatives

The proportions and appearances of these two components in any individual ovary will depend on both age and hormonal stimulation.

The cortical stroma is composed of closely packed, spindle-shaped, fibroblast-like cells.

The stromal cells are arranged haphazardly or in a variable whorled pattern (Fig. 17.16). The cytoplasm of these cells is rich in ribosomes and microfilaments; mitochondria are also numerous. Micropinocytotic vesicles are found in association with the cell surface, with small numbers of lipid droplets.

Reticulin and collagen fibres are prominent in the outer cortex. Progressive collagenization begins early in reproductive life and becomes more marked with time, so that by menopause it is almost universal.

The cellularity of the ovarian stroma, and the amount of lipid the cells contain, is dependent on hormonal stimulation. An increase in lipid accumulation in the stromal cells is called **luteinization of stromal cells** and is particularly prominent during pregnancy.

The ovarian stroma has three main functions:
· It provides structural support for the developing ova.
· It gives rise to the theca interna and theca externa around the developing follicle (see Fig. 17.19b).
· It secretes steroid hormones.

Although it is probable that all stromal cells have the potential to produce steroid hormones under appropriate circumstances, three types of steroid-secreting stromal cells are recognized:
· The cells that surround the follicle (i.e. theca layers, see Figs. 17.19b and 17.21b)
· The scattered lipid-rich luteinized stromal cells
· A population of stromal cells, called *enzymically active stromal cells* (EASCs), which exhibit marked oxidative and other enzyme activity. They are particularly numerous in postmenopausal women, disseminated in clusters in the cortex and medulla and secrete androgenic steroids.

Gamete Production and Maturation in the Ovary

The number of gametes in an ovary, and their appearance, varies with age. Embryologically, they are derived from primordial germ cells, which develop in the yolk sac and migrate to the developing ovary (Fig. 17.17).

Mitotic divisions of primordial germ cells produce small oogonia.

Oogonia multiply within the developing fetal ovary.

During the second trimester of pregnancy, divisions cease and the oogonia increase in size (**primary oocytes**), but many degenerate, so that by birth, each ovary contains about 1 million oocytes.

Oocytes continue to degenerate, and at puberty oocyte numbers are a quarter of a million or so.

Fig. 17.17 Ovary in Embryo. (a) The developing ovary (O) in a 9-week-old embryo is shown close to the developing kidney (K). **(b)** At this stage of development, the columns of primordial germ cells (G) are embedded in a mesenchymal stroma (S) covered by a layer of cuboidal surface cells (E).

Fig. 17.16 Ovarian Cortical Stroma and Surface Epithelium. Note the whorled pattern of the spindle-shaped ovarian stromal cells (S) and the single layer of cuboidal surface epithelial cells (E).

The primary oocytes that survive degeneration in the second trimester enter the prophase of the first meiotic division.

Primary oocytes remain in this phase for many years and acquire a single layer of flat surrounding cells (granulosa cells); these structures are called **primordial follicles** (Fig. 17.18a). At birth, the ovarian cortex is packed with large numbers of primordial follicles embedded in the cellular cortical stroma, and some of these persist in the ovarian cortex throughout the period of sexual maturity (see Fig. 17.18b).

Some primordial follicles develop further at puberty to produce primary follicles.

At puberty, the cyclical secretion of follicle-stimulating hormone (FSH) from the pituitary stimulates the further development of a small number (probably 30–40) of the primordial follicles.

The first step is enlargement of the oocyte, which is associated with an increase in size of the surrounding granulosa cells, so that they become cuboidal or columnar; at this stage, the structure is called a **unilaminar primary follicle**.

Continuing FSH secretion then induces the granulosa cells to divide to produce a multilayered surround to the enlarging oocyte, and a distinct glycoprotein layer of eosinophilic (PAS-positive) material forms between the oocyte and these cells (Fig. 17.19a). This layer is called the **zona pellucida** and is traversed by microvilli protruding outward from the oocyte and by thin cytoplasmic processes from the inner layer of the granulosa cells. The follicle is now known as a **multilaminar primary follicle**.

Fig. 17.18 Primordial Follicles. (a) Ovarian cortex from a 32-week-old fetus; it is packed with primordial follicles, each comprising a large primary oocyte (O) with a single surrounding layer of flat granulosa cells (G). Most primordial follicles undergo continuing atresia throughout infancy, childhood and the years of sexual maturity. **(b)** Ovarian cortex from a 25-year-old woman showing persistence of some primordial follicles (F).

Fig. 17.19 Follicle Maturation. (a) Micrograph of a multilaminar primary follicle. The granulosa cells (G) have divided to produce a layer 3–5 cells thick, and the *pink-staining* zona pellucida (ZP) becomes apparent between the oocyte (O) and the granulosa cells. **(b)** Further maturation to a secondary follicle occurs by continuing proliferation of the granulosa cells (G), the appearance of a fluid-filled cavity (C) within them and condensation of stromal cells around the follicle to form an inner layer of plump cells (theca interna, TI) and an outer layer of smaller spindle-shaped cells (theca externa, TE). O, oocyte.

Meanwhile, ovarian stromal cells come to lie in roughly concentric layers around the enlarging follicle to form a capsule-like arrangement. At about this stage, most follicles then degenerate by a process called **atresia** (see p. 360).

A small number of follicles, however, continue to develop, although atretic degeneration still occurs at all subsequent stages; thus only a few follicles reach full maturity.

Continuing maturation leads to the formation of secondary follicles.

With continuing follicle maturation, the granulosa cell layers increase in thickness and the outer capsule of ovarian stromal cells begins to differentiate into two layers.

The inner layer of stromal cells (the **theca interna**) increases in size as the cells develop prominent smooth endoplasmic reticulum and mitochondria with tubular cristae (features characteristic of cells producing steroid hormones) and begin to secrete oestrogens; this layer also acquires a prominent capillary network.

The outer layer of stromal cells (the **theca externa**) remains small and compact and has no known secretory function. The follicle is now known as a **secondary follicle** (see Fig. 17.19b).

The fully mature follicle is called the *tertiary (Graafian) follicle* and is ready for ovulation.

A small fluid-filled split appears in the layers of granulosa cells surrounding the oocyte. It enlarges to form a fluid-filled cavity (the **antrum**) that progressively increases in size; the fluid is slightly viscous and is rich in hyaluronic acid.

The oocyte lies to one side of the by-now large follicle and is separated from the follicle fluid by a coat of granulosa cells called the *cumulus oophorus*. The follicle is now known as a **tertiary** or **Graafian follicle** and is ripe for ovulation (Fig. 17.20).

The first stage of meiosis is then completed to produce a haploid gamete and a small polar body, which can sometimes be seen attached to the oocyte (now called a **secondary oocyte**). Follicle maturation takes approximately 15 days, by which time the mature follicle is ready for ovulation.

The theca interna secretes increasing amounts of oestrogen to stimulate proliferation of the endometrium (see Fig. 17.24) in preparation for possible implantation of a fertilized ovum.

Ovulation is stimulated by luteinizing hormone from the anterior pituitary.

At ovulation, the Graafian follicle is usually so large that it distorts the surface of the ovary; it appears to the naked eye as a small cystic mass bulging from the ovarian surface, covered only by a thin layer of germinal epithelium and membrane and an attenuated zone of cortical stromal cells.

The stimulus to ovulation is probably a surge of luteinizing hormone (LH) from the pituitary, which induces completion of

Fig. 17.20 Tertiary (Graafian) Follicle. **(a)** A mature tertiary follicle. Note the fluid-filled antrum (A), the eccentrically located oocyte (O) and the cumulus oophorus (C) of granulosa cells around the oocyte. **(b)** Micrograph of the oocyte (O), cumulus oophorus (C) and granulosa cell layer (G) at higher magnification. The theca layer (T) is highly vascular.

the first stage of meiosis and probably leads to disruption of the structure of the follicle as well.

Before leaving the ovary, the oocyte may break free from its attachment in the follicle wall and float freely in the follicle fluid, surrounded by an irregular ring of granulosa cells, which remain attached to it (the **corona radiata**).

The area of follicle wall in intimate contact with the germinal epithelial covering of the ovarian surface breaks down, and the follicular fluid containing the oocyte is disgorged into the peritoneal cavity.

The oocyte with its surrounding corona radiata is then drawn into the infundibular opening of the uterine tube, possibly by the waving action of the fimbriae at the infundibular margin.

With rupture of the follicle, there is bleeding from the decompressed lining (particularly from the highly vascular theca interna), filling the follicle antrum with a blood clot. Small quantities of blood may pass into the peritoneal cavity.

The disgorgement of blood and follicular fluid onto the pain-sensitive peritoneal surface is thought to be responsible for the transient midcycle (days 14–16) lower abdominal pain experienced by some women.

The ruptured follicle becomes a corpus luteum after ovulation.

After ovulation, the remains of the follicle change under the influence of continuing LH secretion by the pituitary gland. The clot-filled lumen of the follicle (corpus haemorrhagicum) undergoes progressive organization and fibrosis over the following weeks.

The main changes occur in the granulosa and theca interna cells. In these cells, LH induces changes (luteinization) that convert the follicle remnants into an endocrine structure known as the *corpus luteum.*

Thus the granulosa cells enlarge, acquire a substantial network of smooth endoplasmic reticulum, become distended with lipid (granulosa lutein cells) and secrete progesterone (Fig. 17.21).

Some of the theca interna cells, already well equipped with smooth endoplasmic reticulum, also accumulate lipid and persist as theca lutein or paralutein cells, continuing to secrete oestrogens as they did before ovulation. However, many theca interna and externa cells involute, becoming small, compact and spindle-shaped.

The formed corpus luteum therefore has a central area of fibrosing blood clot surrounded by a broad zone of yellow, lipid-rich granulosa lutein cells, with scantier collections of smaller theca lutein cells scattered around the periphery.

Fibrous septa partly separate the granulosa lutein masses, and clusters of theca lutein cells are particularly prominent in the regions of these septa (see Fig. 17.21b).

At its maximum size (usually on about day 20 of the menstrual cycle), a corpus luteum is commonly an ovoid structure up to 2 cm long and 1.5 cm wide; it then begins to involute, unless the cycle has been interrupted by fertilization of the oocyte in the uterine tube (see p. 365).

The corpus luteum changes into a corpus albicans.

Normally, involution of the corpus luteum begins by a decrease in the size of the granulosa and theca lutein cells with the appearance of vacuoles in their previously uniformly eosinophilic cytoplasm. Progression of this change leads to reduced secretion of progesterone and oestrogen by the two cell types.

At the same time, the spindle-shaped cells of the theca externa and the spindle-shaped fibroblasts forming the fibrous septa rapidly produce collagen, which replaces the involuting lutein cells.

Fig. 17.21 Corpus Luteum. (a) Micrograph of an ovary containing two corpora lutea (CL), two follicles having ripened to maturity in the same ovary in the same menstrual cycle, providing the potential for non-identical twins. Each corpus luteum shows a central blood clot (BC) surrounded by a thick layer of lipid-rich granulosa lutein cells (GL). **(b)** Micrograph of the large, pale-staining granulosa lutein (GL) cells and the small, compact theca lutein (TL) cells, which are mainly concentrated along fibrous septa at the periphery of the corpus luteum.

By about the 26th day of the cycle, the hormone-secreting cells are completely eliminated and the progesterone and oestrogen levels fall dramatically, with a significant impact on the endometrium (see Fig. 17.24g).

The end result of corpus luteum involution is a small ovoid mass of relatively acellular (hyaline) collagenous tissue with the general physical configuration of the corpus luteum. This structure is a corpus albicans (Fig. 17.22) and remains in the ovary, decreasing in size with the passing years but never disappearing.

Fig. 17.22 Corpus Albicans. The corpus luteum involutes to form a shrunken mass of collagenous tissue, the corpus albicans (CA), which maintains approximately the shape of the original corpus luteum. Incomplete involution of a corpus luteum may produce a luteal cyst, which is a cyst lined by attenuated granulosa and theca lutein cells.

Most female gametes do not grow to maturity, but undergo atresia.

Of the vast number of oogonia formed in utero by mitotic division of primitive germ cells, only about 500–600 reach full maturity and ovulation during a woman's reproductive life. Some fail to develop, and others undergo a process called **atresia.**

Atresia can occur at any stage but is most marked during intrauterine life, when primary oocyte numbers are enormously reduced. As atresia continues throughout infancy, childhood and the reproductive years, degenerating primary and secondary oocytes can be seen on histological examination of any ovary.

Atresia can supervene at any stage of follicle development. When the follicles are small (primary and secondary stages), the components of the follicle undergo cellular degeneration and complete resorption, leaving no scar (Fig. 17.23a).

Fig. 17.23 Follicle Atresia. (a) Micrograph showing a cluster of four primordial follicles, of which three are undergoing atresia (A); they will leave no scar. **(b)** Micrograph showing a primary follicle undergoing atresia, which is mainly manifest by a degenerate oocyte (O) and a collapsing zona pellucida (ZP).

However, larger follicles (tertiary stage) with a substantial cellular component undergo gradual disintegration and replacement by hyaline fibrous tissue (see Fig. 17.23b). The oocyte disintegrates and the granulosa cells separate and degenerate, whereas the zona pellucida collapses and wrinkles but remains identifiable.

Often a glassy membrane develops between the degenerating granulosa cells and the outer thecal layers; this may proliferate transiently, perhaps providing the source of the fibrocollagenous fibrous tissue that ultimately replaces the atretic follicle.

When a large follicle has undergone atresia, a substantial collagenous scar may form, a **corpus fibrosum**, which resembles a small corpus albicans in shape.

MENSTRUAL CYCLE

Introduction

During the reproductive years, the histological appearance of the superficial functional zone of the endometrial lining varies from day to day on a regular cyclical basis, the **menstrual cycle**.

A complete cycle normally takes about 28 days, but there is considerable variation between women and also some variation in individual women at different times. For example, the first few cycles after menarche and after a pregnancy tend to be irregular, and increasing irregularity of the cycle is common before menopause.

At the end of every cycle the superficial functional endometrium undergoes necrosis and is shed via the cervix and vagina with bleeding (**menstruation**), leaving only the basal endometrium to act as a reservoir for the development of a new functional layer during the next cycle.

Menstruation lasts for about 4 days, and the day it starts is taken as the first day of the menstrual cycle.

The cyclical changes in the functional endometrium are governed by the changing pattern of hormone secretion by the ovaries, which in turn is influenced by the cyclical secretion of hormones (FSH and LH) by the pituitary gland. The secretion of the gonadotropic hormones is in turn controlled by the secretion of gonadotropin-releasing hormones by the hypothalamus. Thus the histological appearance of endometrial curettings can be used to stage (within a few days on either side) the endometrial cycle.

The sequence of changes in the menstrual cycle is repeated throughout the period of sexual maturity, from menarche to menopause, and is interrupted only by pregnancy or hormone therapy: for example, oestrogen and progesterone given as a contraceptive.

The proliferative (oestrin or follicular) phase of the menstrual cycle lasts from day 4 to about day 14 or 16.

During menstruation, the entire superficial functional zone of endometrium is shed (days 1–4), leaving the compact basal endometrium behind.

At the same time, a new cycle of ovarian follicle maturation begins, resulting in an increase of oestrogen secretion by the developing follicle stimulating mitotic activity in the basal endometrial glands and stroma (Fig. 17.24a and b).

Continued proliferation of these cells over 10–12 days re-establishes a substantial functional endometrial layer comprising straight tubular endometrial glands embedded in stroma rich in hormone-sensitive spiral arterioles.

As the levels of oestrogen continue to rise in the latter stages of this phase, the glands usually become slightly tortuous and their lumina may distend, and continued mitotic proliferation of endometrial gland columnar cells may produce some heaping up of cells, and therefore a pseudostratified appearance.

> **Ovulation occurs at about days 14–16.**

Ovulation is accompanied by the development of subnuclear vacuolation in the endometrial glands (see Fig. 17.24c), which coincides with peak levels of LH secretion by the pituitary gland. Eventually all of the glands show this change.

> **The secretory (luteal) phase lasts from about day 16 to day 25.**

The onset of the next (secretory or luteal) phase in the menstrual cycle is marked by the appearance of supranuclear secretory vacuoles at the apical poles of the endometrial gland cells. Secretory material is shed into the gland lumen by the apocrine method (see Fig. 3.15), and the luminal surfaces of the gland cells become irregular and ill-defined. The glands themselves become tortuous (see Fig. 17.24d), and their lumina distend with secretion (see Fig. 17.24e). The spiral arterioles in the stroma are extensive and more coiled.

This phase of gland secretion occurs in response to progesterone secreted by the corpus luteum.

> **The premenstrual phase lasts from about day 25 to menstruation at day 28.**

At about day 22, the secretory activity of the endometrial glands declines and they begin to show involutional changes; the luminal secretion diminishes and that which remains becomes inspissated. The glands become irregular and begin to collapse, and there are significant changes in the stroma (see Fig. 17.24f and g) and swelling of the stromal cells, particularly around the spiral arterioles.

> **At menstruation, the superficial functional layer of the endometrium undergoes necrosis and is shed.**

The changes noted earlier are precipitated by the sudden fall in progesterone and oestrogen secretion caused by involution of the corpus luteum. This is associated with a prostaglandin-mediated constriction of the spiral arterioles, leading to ischaemic necrosis of the functional endometrium. This, combined with dilatation of deeper vessels, leads to haemorrhage into the stroma.

The necrotic endometrial glands and stroma, together with the stromal accumulations of blood, are then shed as menstrual debris, usually piecemeal, with the most superficial endometrium shed first; the deeper layers are lost over the next 4–5 days until only basal endometrium remains to regenerate the functional layer as the next cycle begins.

> **The end of reproductive life is marked by menopause and results in cessation of menstruation and endometrial changes.**

As menopause approaches, more and more of the endometrium may fail to respond fully to the hormonal stimulus, showing little proliferative or secretory activity.

At menopause, when hormonal stimulation ceases, the endometrium reverts to a simple inactive pattern. The menopausal endometrium shows no proliferative activity, some glands may undergo cystic distension and the stroma become compact, described as a menopausal endometrial atrophic pattern (see Fig. 17.25).

> **The changes in the menstrual cycle are suspended during pregnancy.**

The cyclical changes in the ovary and endometrium described earlier are seen either when fertilization of the ovum does not occur or if fertilization is followed by death of the zygote or failure of implantation into the endometrium.

In the event of successful fertilization and implantation, the cyclical changes are suspended until sometime after childbirth, and almost all of the tissues of the female genital tract undergo structural changes.

The structural changes in the cervix, myometrium and uterine tube have been described on pp. 349, 352 and 354.

CLINICAL EXAMPLE
Menstrual Irregularities

Irregularity and abnormality of menstruation are common and important complaints in women of reproductive age. There is a normal tendency for menstrual periods to be irregular in interval, duration and intensity at three times in a woman's life: for the first few cycles after puberty, for the first one or two cycles after pregnancy and for a variable number of cycles before menopause. The following clinical features imply some form of pathology.

Amenorrhoea (absence of menstruation) is complete absence of menstruation after puberty, which is termed *primary amenorrhoea,* and the cause is usually an endocrine abnormality. Amenorrhoea where there has previously been normal menstruation is termed *secondary amenorrhoea.*

Menorrhagia describes excessive bleeding at menstruation in both intensity and duration of blood loss. There is often an underlying endometrial or myometrial abnormality.

Dysmenorrhoea is excessively painful menstruation often caused by an endometrial or myometrial disorder.

Intermenstrual bleeding is usually caused by an abnormality in the cervix, vagina or vulva.

Postmenopausal bleeding is a most important symptom, as it is the way in which most malignant tumours of the uterus present.

hypothalamus

pituitary

FSH stimulates maturation of one or more follicles

continuing FSH stimulation of ripening Graafian follicle

surge of LH initiates ovulation

continuing LH secretion induces luteinization of granulosa and theca cells of ruptured follicle

LH and FSH secretion ceases, corpus luteum begins to involute

changes in spiral arterioles in stroma produce ischaemic necrosis of functional endometrium which is shed (menstruation)

oestrogen secretion from follicle granulosa cells initiates proliferation of endometrium

endometrial proliferation maintained by increasing oestrogen secretion from enlarging follicle

early progesterone secretion by luteinizing follicle stimulates early secretory changes in endometrium

continued progesterone secretion from granuloma lutein cells maintains secretory change in endometrium; some oestrogen from theca lutein cells

involuting granulosa and theca lutein cells suddenly cease to produce progesterone and oestrogen; secretory endometrial glands degenerate

Day 1–4   Day 4–14   Day 14–16   Day 16–28

Fig. 17.24 Menstrual Cycle. The interrelationships between pituitary hormones and ovary and ovarian hormones and the endometrium in the menstrual cycle. The cycle starts on the first day of menstruation, when the functional endometrium from the previous cycle is shed, with bleeding (days 1–4). Release of pituitary follicle-stimulating hormone (FSH) stimulates the maturation of an ovarian follicle, some of the cells of which secrete oestrogen, which initiates and maintains the proliferation of new functional endometrium. **(a)** A new layer of functional endometrium (F) in the early proliferative stage arising from the compact basal endometrium (B). **(b)** High-power detail of one of the proliferating endometrial glands. Nuclei are prominent, and some cells are in mitosis *(arrow)*. The proliferative stage lasts from day 4 to day 14, at which time a surge of pituitary luteinizing hormone initiates ovulation (days 14–16) and luteinization of the wall of the ovarian follicle. The luteinized cells of the follicle begin to secrete progesterone, which initiates early secretory changes in the endometrium. **(c)** The earliest changes of secretory activity in the endometrial glands. They develop subnuclear vacuoles (V), and the previously straight tubular glands begin to become convoluted. Continuing secretion of progesterone by the corpus luteum produces further convolution of the endometrial glands, increase in bulk of the stroma and increasing secretory activity of the gland epithelium. **(d)** A low-power photomicrograph of the endometrium at about day 22 of the cycle. The glands (G) are markedly convoluted and distended by secretion. **(e)** High-power detail of a late secretory endometrium with secretory vacuoles (V) now in a supranuclear position and secretion (S) in the lumen of the convoluted gland. At about day 25 of the cycle, the secretion of LH and FSH by the pituitary ceases, causing involution of the corpus luteum in the ovary with consequent abrupt reduction in progesterone and oestrogen secretion. This reduction in hormones leads to ischaemic necrosis of the late secretory endometrium, initiating menstruation. Just before undergoing necrosis, the endometrium is very bulky, with early decidual change in the stroma and prominent spiral arterioles. **(f)** Part of the premenstrual endometrium at low magnification. Note the highly convoluted glands and the very bulky decidualized endometrial stroma (DC), particularly near the surface. **(g)** A high-power photomicrograph showing the thick-walled and contorted spiral arterioles (SA).

Fig 17.25 Endometrium Menopausal Pattern. H&E micrograph showing postmenopausal endometrium (E) with underlying myometrium (M). The endometrial stroma has a denser cellularity adjacent to the myometrium, and inactive basal glands are present in this area. The superficial endometrium has very few glands, and some are cystically dilated (CG). There is no evidence of proliferative activity. This inactive pattern with few glands is termed a *menopausal endometrial atrophic pattern.*

⊚ ADVANCED CONCEPT

The Endometrium May Be Stimulated to Grow After Menopause by Other Sources of Endogenous Oestrogen

Before puberty, the endometrium consists of simple tubular glands in a fibroelastic stroma with thin blood vessels. At puberty, each of these elements undergoes cyclical change in response to the sex steroid hormones secreted from the ovary (Fig. 17.24). After menopause, the cessation of ovulation withdraws progesterone, preventing the secretory phase. Lack of stimulation from oestrogen and progesterone causes atrophy of the endometrium with low cuboidal epithelium overlying a fibrous stroma (see Fig. 17.25).

It is possible for non-ovarian sources of oestrogen to continue to stimulate endometrial proliferation and cause postmenopausal endometrial growth (hyperplasia). This extragonadal endogenous oestrogen arises because of conversion of circulating steroid precursors from the ovaries or adrenal glands. This conversion (aromatization) takes place in adipose tissue and is enhanced in metabolic disorders such as diabetes or obesity. After menopause, adipose tissue is the main source of oestrogen production, and in the presence of obesity the levels rise in proportion to the body mass index.

Unopposed oestrogen drives endometrial proliferation and can lead to endometrial hyperplasia, which is a risk factor for the development of neoplastic change (Fig. 17.26). For this reason, postmenopausal bleeding should always be investigated.

👥 CLINICAL EXAMPLE

Exogenous Hormones Are Given for the Purpose of Manipulating Reproductive Hormones

Exogenous hormone therapy may be given for contraceptive family planning, hormone replacement therapy (HRT) after menopause or in fertility treatment. These result in a wide range of structural changes to the endometrium that do not replicate stages of the normal cyclical changes. The appearance of the endometrium and stroma varies in the individual and with dose and duration of treatment.

In general, the endometrium is thinned using most forms of birth control and HRT.

Contraceptive family planning: Many oral contraceptives contain progesterone, which is used to inhibit the proliferative changes associated with unopposed oestrogen. These generally result in a thin atrophic endometrium with glandular atrophy and pseudodecidualization of stroma. **Intrauterine devices** (IUDs) also suppress endometrial growth. There may also be mechanical effects of the IUD, including erosion of epithelium and activation of inflammatory cells. Some IUDs contain progestins used to treat menorrhagia, to balance HRT and to protect the endometrium in patients receiving the anti-oestrogen drug tamoxifen for breast cancer.

HRT can be given during menopause to counter the impacts of reduced oestrogen. It generally consists of a combination of oestrogen and progesterone and results in atrophic endometrium.

⧁ KEY FACTS

Endometrial Changes in Normal (28-Day) Menstrual Cycle

- Days 1–4: menstrual phase – necrotic endometrium from previous cycle shed
- Days 4–14: proliferative phase – new straight tubular endometrial glands and stroma grow from residual basal endometrium; much mitotic activity
- Days 14–16: ovulatory phase – earliest sign of secretory activity in endometrial glands in subnuclear vacuolation
- Days 16–25: secretory phase – endometrial glands become tortuous, and lumina fill with secretion
- Days 25–28: premenstrual phase – spiral arterioles prominent in stroma; ischaemia leads to degeneration, then necrosis, of secretory endometrium

CLINICAL EXAMPLE

Endometrial Disorders

Many abnormalities can occur in the endometrium, most resulting from inappropriate ovarian hormone stimulation and causing abnormal patterns of menstruation.

Because the endometrium is largely shed once a month, many abnormalities are transient, but persisting endometrial abnormalities are important.

Benign cystic hyperplasia (see Fig. 17.26a) of the endometrium is the result of unopposed oestrogen secretion and may occur in the presence of an oestrogen-secreting ovarian tumour.

Atypical endometrial hyperplasia is marked by hyperplastic endometrial glands, which show disorganization of architectural arrangement, whereas the epithelial cells show atypical dysplastic features similar to those seen in malignant tumours of endometrial glands. This condition (see Fig. 17.26b) is considered capable of conversion into an invasive endometrial tumour.

The typical malignant tumour of the endometrium, the **endometrial adenocarcinoma** (see Fig. 17.26c), occurs mainly in postmenopausal women and presents as postmenopausal bleeding.

Fig. 17.26 Important Endometrial Growth Disorders. (a) Simple cystic hyperplasia of the endometrial glands. Note the cystically dilated glands. **(b)** Atypical complex hyperplasia. Note the crowded irregular glands composed of tall epithelial cells, in which some dysplastic features will be present, typically abnormally large and darkly stained nuclei. **(c)** Invasive endometrial adenocarcinoma (C) fills the endometrial cavity and is invading into the myometrium (M) and part of the way down the endocervical cavity (EC). Note that near the fundus *(arrowhead)* the malignant tumour has almost infiltrated through the myometrium to the serosal surface of the uterus.

CLINICAL EXAMPLE

Endometriosis

Endometriosis describes the presence of endometrial tissue which has spread and is implanted outside of the uterus, commonly associated with the uterine tubes, ovary and pelvic peritoneum. Because the ectopic endometrium is still responsive to hormones, it undergoes cyclical changes, including bleeding and proliferation, and often appears as brown-coloured areas because of accumulated iron pigment from breakdown of repeated bleeding events. The cyclical pattern causes an inflammatory response, and associated healing and scarring can cause fibrous adhesions. These cause pelvic pain as adjacent organs become attached. Adhesions also adversely affect fertility, for example, by affecting patency of the uterine tubes or disrupting the relationship of the ovary to the uterine tube.

PREGNANCY

> **Fertilization of the ovum usually occurs in the uterine tube (oviduct).**

When the ovum is disgorged from the ovary at ovulation, it enters the open infundibular end of the uterine tube and passes into the dilated ampullary portion, which is the most common site for its fertilization (Fig. 17.27).

The second meiotic division of the ovum is only completed once the ovum has been successfully penetrated by a spermatozoon. The nuclear material of the penetrating haploid spermatozoon then joins with that of the haploid ovum, forming a diploid zygote, which immediately begins a series of mitotic divisions to produce a solid ball of cells, the **morula**.

> **The morula migrates down the uterine tube and enters the endometrial cavity about 4–5 days after fertilization.**

In the endometrial cavity, further cell divisions of the morula rapidly produce a cystic mass called the **blastocyst**, comprising a fluid-filled cavity (the **blastocoele**) surrounded by a cellular wall (the **trophoblast**). A solid collection of cells, internal to the trophoblast at one pole of the blastocyst, is called the **inner cell mass** and gives rise to the embryo.

After a day or so floating free in the endometrial cavity, the blastocyst must implant in the secretory endometrium if the pregnancy is to continue.

> **Attempts at implantation begin about 6 days after fertilization.**

Implantation is usually 7–8 days after ovulation and on days 21–22 of the menstrual cycle. If unsuccessful, the blastocyst degenerates and is expelled with the degenerate endometrium and blood with the onset of menstruation at 28 days.

Sometimes implantation occurs but cannot be maintained; menstruation eventually supervenes, often after some delay, and the menstrual loss may be greater than usual.

When implantation is successful, the blastocyst gains access to the endometrial stroma, probably directly across the endometrial surface, and by about 11 days after fertilization (i.e. day 27 of the cycle) is completely embedded in endometrial stroma.

> **After implantation, the pregnancy is initially maintained by progesterone secreted by the persisting corpus luteum.**

From about the time of ovulation, the corpus luteum secretes progesterone. If fertilization and implantation occur, it increases in size up to 3–4 cm in diameter (the **corpus luteum of pregnancy**). This persists throughout the first trimester of pregnancy and produces progesterone; thereafter the placenta takes over this function, and the corpus luteum of pregnancy involutes.

At the time of implantation, the endometrium is in its late secretory phase (see Fig. 17.24e and f). Implantation stimulates the development of true decidual change under the influence of the continuing progesterone secretion.

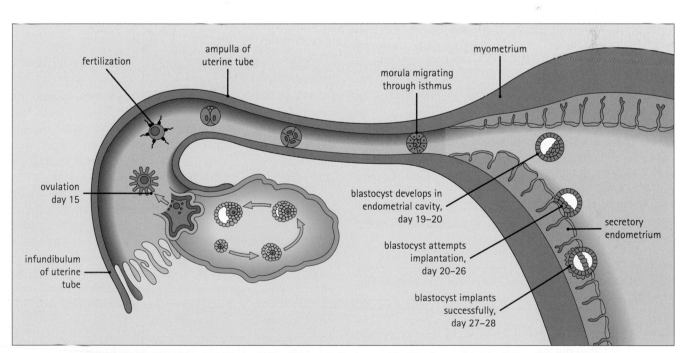

Fig. 17.27 Fertilization and Implantation. The main features of fertilization and implantation. The timing is from the onset of the last menstrual period and is approximate, there being great individual variation between women and from cycle to cycle.

Because of the progesterone secretion, the endometrial glands develop exaggerated secretory appearances which, with the stromal decidual change, produce the appearance known as **pregnancy pattern endometrium**.

> Further development of the trophoblast and some of the decidual endometrial stroma produce the placenta.

The placenta is responsible for nourishment of the developing embryo and secretion of hormones for maintaining the pregnancy. Further development of the embryo from the inner cell mass is beyond the scope of this book.

TROPHOBLAST AND PLACENTA

Introduction

On implantation, the single layer of the trophoblast, which forms the outer wall of the blastocyst, becomes a double layer.

The outer layer is characterized by the loss of its lateral cell margins so that it forms a thin syncytial layer, the **syncytiotrophoblast**. The inner layer begins as a continuous monolayer of cuboidal cells with pale-staining cytoplasm, the **cytotrophoblast**.

> The syncytiotrophoblast has numerous surface microvilli and the ability to erode or invade adjacent tissue.

This syncytiotrophoblast ensures successful erosion of the endometrial tissues at implantation. The blastocyst initially attaches to the surface epithelium of the endometrium. Individual trophoblast cells then intrude between epithelial cells so that the blastocyst can insinuate itself into the endometrial stroma, where erosion of an endometrial capillary ensures a blood supply (Fig. 17.28a). The breach in the endometrial surface is quickly re-epithelialized.

The presence of the blastocyst within the endometrial stroma induces early decidualization of the stromal cells and leads to marked endometrial thickening. Once the blastocyst is embedded in the endometrial stroma, the trophoblast proliferates and the outer syncytial layer extends as irregular protrusions into surrounding stroma, eroding the walls of small blood vessels.

Lakes of maternal blood form between the protrusions (see Fig. 17.28b), and the surface microvilli of the syncytiotrophoblast assist in transferring oxygen and nutrients from the maternal blood to the developing blastocyst.

> The cytotrophoblast grows into the syncytial protrusions as finger-like extensions.

The solid masses of cytotrophoblast covered by syncytium form the **primary** or **stem chorionic villi**.

With the development of a loose mesenchymal core, the villi are known as **secondary villi** and soon acquire a system of capillaries that become part of the blood circulatory system of the embryo.

Fig. 17.28 Implantation Site. (a) Low-power micrograph showing an early human implantation site. The blastocyst has infiltrated the superficial endometrium, and the trophoblast (T) is beginning to infiltrate the endometrial stroma. Part of the inner cell mass (M) can be seen. **(b)** High-power micrograph from the area of trophoblast infiltration. Cords of syncytiotrophoblast (S) have eroded blood vessels and produced lakes of maternal blood (L). Islands of cytotrophoblast (C) are extending into the syncytial masses.

Fully vascularized villi are referred to as **tertiary villi** (see Fig. 17.30).

As the placental villi mature, the mesenchymal core contains interlacing vascular channels, fibroblasts, some smooth muscle cells and large pleomorphic cells with vacuolated cytoplasm (**Hofbauer cells**) which are placental macrophages of fetal origin (see Fig. 17.30d) involved in placental development, angiogenesis and maintaining placental homeostasis.

The early chorionic villi subdivide in an arborizing pattern to form a complex system that provides an immense surface area for exchange between the maternal and fetal circulations.

After the complex branching of the villi, the terminal villi contain small, thin-walled capillaries, all of which connect with larger vessels in the larger 'twigs', 'branches' and 'trunks' of the tree-like proliferation; these vessels ultimately combine to form the two arteries and single vein that run in the umbilicus to the blood circulation of the embryo (Fig. 17.29).

> The appearance of the chorionic villi changes with time.

In early pregnancy, the villi contain central capillaries embedded in bulky mesenchyme, but later, the capillaries proliferate and come to lie close to the trophoblast surface.

As the capillaries become more numerous and dilated, the mesenchyme is reduced in bulk and its cellular component is reduced; in particular, Hofbauer cells become scarce.

Initially, the cytotrophoblast cells predominate and the syncytiotrophoblast is a thin layer (Fig. 17.30a). Division of the cytotrophoblast probably maintains the syncytial cell mass throughout gestation. As the pregnancy progresses, the syncytiotrophoblast becomes the predominant layer (see Fig. 17.30b) and the cytotrophoblast appears to partly regress, becoming a discontinuous layer and then collections of scattered cells beneath the syncytiotrophoblast.

At term, the villi show increasing hyalinization of the mesenchymal stroma, and fibrin is deposited in the blood-filled intervillous spaces, often coating the outer surface of the villi.

The arrangement of complex chorionic villi of fetal origin intruding into a constantly blood-filled intervillous space of maternal origin provides an efficient means of transferring oxygen, nutrients, maternal antibodies and hormones from the mother to the fetus and waste metabolites from the fetus to the mother (see Fig. 17.29).

Fig. 17.29 Placental Structure. The basic structure of the placenta and the relationship between the fetal and maternal blood.

Fig. 17.30 Chorionic Villi. (a) Micrograph showing part of an early chorionic villus, which is covered by a layer of cuboidal cytotrophoblast (C) and an outer layer of syncytiotrophoblast (S). Note the villus capillaries (VC) filled with nucleated fetal red cells (FRC). **(b)** Low magnification micrograph of placenta close to term. Large villi (LV) give rise to smaller villi, eventually forming small terminal villi (TV). Maternal blood is present in the intervillous space (IVS). Dark-staining clumps of nuclei are seen at the edge of several villi, which are termed *syncytial knots* (SK). In the mature placenta they usually reflect oblique sectioning of areas of cellular syncytiotrophoblast.

Continued

Fig. 17.30, cont'd (c) Micrograph of tertiary chorionic villi close to the end of pregnancy; note the prominent heaped-up syncytiotrophoblast (S), maternal blood in the intervillous space (IVS) and fetal blood in the villous capillaries (VC). **(d)** Micrograph of chorionic villi from early in pregnancy immunostained to show a marker of macrophages *(brown)*, which highlights the **Hofbauer cells** within the core of placental villi. Note the trophoblast covering the villi still showing two distinct layers as in **(a)** consistent with early villi. Later more mature villi have fewer Hofbauer cells (Image (d) used under Creative Commons License https://creativecommons. org/licenses/by-sa/3.0/ from the Human Protein Atlas Antibody to macrophage marker CD163 CAB002432 https://www.proteinatlas.org/ENSG00000177575-CD163/tissue/placenta#img. Micrograph (b) and (c) from digital pathology whole slide image provided by the University of Leeds Virtual Pathology Project https://www. virtualpathology.leeds.ac.uk. Reproduced with permission.)

◎ ADVANCED CONCEPT

Endocrine Functions of the Placenta

In addition to being a site of exchange, the placenta also acts as an endocrine organ.

- The syncytiotrophoblast secretes human chorionic gonadotropin (hCG) (Fig. 17.31), which is responsible for maintaining the corpus luteum of pregnancy (see p. 365) after cessation of the LH stimulus from the pituitary gland.
- The syncytiotrophoblast secretes human chorionic somatomammotropin (hCS) (human placental lactogen [hPL]), which is involved in regulating a range of metabolic pathways to ensure nutrition from maternal resources is provided to the fetus even in the presence of maternal malnutrition.
- The placenta secretes progesterone and oestrogens; oestrogen precursors produced by the adrenal cortex and liver of the fetus are converted into active oestrogens in the placenta.

Fig. 17.31 Chorionic Villi and hCG. Micrograph showing chorionic villi from a term placenta demonstrating localization of human chorionic gonadotropin (hCG), stained *brown,* to the syncytiotrophoblast covering each villus. (Image used under Creative Commons License https:// creativecommons.org/licenses/by-sa/3.0/ from the Human Protein Atlas Antibody to Glycoprotein hormones, alpha polypeptide HPA029698 https:// www.proteinatlas.org/ENSG00000135346-CGA/tissue/placenta#img.)

Decidua

> After implantation, the endometrial stroma undergoes decidualization.

The normally small, compact cells of the endometrial stroma undergo remarkable enlargement; this process is known as **decidualization**.

Decidualization begins in the stromal cells around the implanted blastocyst, but soon spreads to involve the rest of the pregnancy endometrium. As the stromal cells enlarge, they dominate the endometrium, and the glandular component becomes insignificant. The thickened, superficial endometrial layers become the decidua, as follows (Fig. 17.32):

- The endometrium immediately beneath the implantation site, into which the major trophoblast growth occurs, becomes the **decidua basalis**.
- The thin rim of endometrial stroma overlying the blastocyst becomes the **decidua capsularis**.
- The endometrium lining the rest of the uterine cavity is called the **decidua parietalis**.

Of the decidua, the decidua basalis is the most important, as the vessels in this part of the modified endometrium supply maternal arterial blood to the lacunae between the fetal chorionic villi and receive venous blood from the lacunae. The villous trophoblast (from the fetus) and the decidua basalis (from the mother), and the intervillous spaces between them, comprise the placenta.

Decidual stromal cells have prominent, pale-staining, round or ovoid nuclei, often with finely granular chromatin and one or two nucleoli; their cytoplasm is bulky, and usually eosinophilic, and granular or slightly foamy, although some cells may have a basophilic tinge (see Fig. 17.32c).

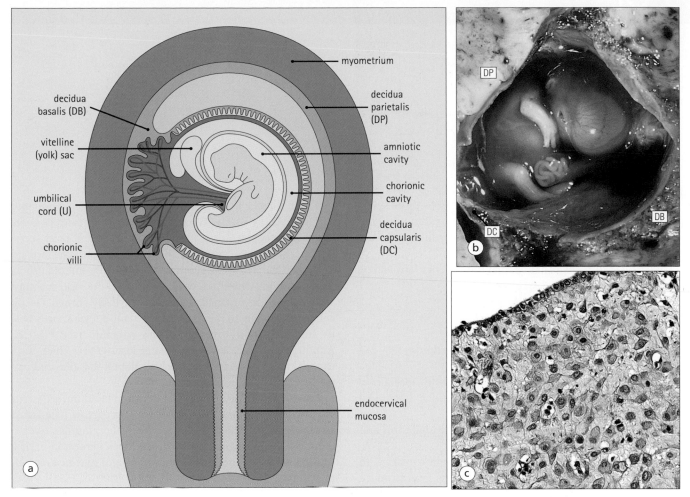

Fig. 17.32 Decidua. (a) The decidua and their relationships with the developing fetus and placenta. **(b)** The decidua defined in **(a)**. Note the decidua parietalis (DP), decidua capsularis (DC) and decidua basalis (DB). **(c)** Micrograph of decidual cells. They are large and polygonal with a granular eosinophilic cytoplasm. Nuclei have an open chromatin pattern. Note surface endometrial epithelium. (Micrograph (c) from digital pathology whole slide image provided by the University of Leeds Virtual Pathology Project https://www.virtualpathology.leeds.ac.uk. Reproduced with permission.)

Ultrastructurally, the decidualized stromal cells contain prominent, often long mitochondria, together with variable amounts of rough endoplasmic reticulum.

The eosinophilia or basophilia of the cytoplasm in individual cells depends on the relative proportions of mitochondria (eosinophilic) and rough endoplasmic reticulum (basophilic).

⚕ CLINICAL EXAMPLE

Placental Insufficiency

The placenta is essential for growth of the fetus, and any abnormality can lead to problems in growth and development. If this happens early in pregnancy, there may be a reduction in growth of the fetus, termed *intrauterine growth restriction (IUGR)*. This problem develops in about 5% of all pregnancies. It can be suspected if the size of the uterus is smaller than that which would be expected for the stage of pregnancy.

Several conditions are recognized as being associated with placental insufficiency and IUGR:
- Poor maternal nutrition
- Maternal diabetes
- Alcohol abuse
- Heavy smoking
- Twin or triplet pregnancies
- Pre-eclampsia or eclampsia, both of which are conditions associated with elevated maternal blood pressure
- Infection with cytomegalovirus, toxoplasmosis, rubella or syphilis, known collectively as *TORCH infections*
- Structural defects of the placental membranes or the umbilical cord
- Abnormal implantation of the placenta in the uterus

One of the functions of regular examinations in pregnancy is to check that the growth of the fetus and placenta is satisfactory.

Babies born after IUGR and placental insufficiency are recognized to be physically small with risks for neurological problems.

For online review questions, please visit https://studentconsult.inkling.com.

Skin and Breast

INTRODUCTION

The skin is an extensive organ covering the exterior of the body. It varies in structure from site to site according to specific functions, which include:

- Protection from external damaging agents (infective, mechanical, thermal)
- Prevention of loss of water
- Thermoregulation
- Sensation (touch, heat, pressure, pain)
- Secretion of sebum, composed of protective lipids
- Vitamin D production

The breast is a highly modified area of skin with specialized glands to produce nutritious secretions under hormonal influences.

The skin is composed of two main layers, the epidermis and dermis, and a variable third layer, the subcutis.

The **epidermis** is the surface epithelial layer in contact with the external environment. Downgrowths of this layer produce sweat glands, hair follicles and other epidermal appendages.

The epidermis is firmly adhered to the underlying support tissue of the dermis by its **basement membrane** and other specializations (see p. 375).

The **dermis** is a middle supporting layer containing the epidermal appendages, blood vessels, nerves and nerve endings, which are embedded in an elastocollagenous stroma produced by fibroblasts.

The **subcutis** (sometimes referred to as the *hypodermis*) is the deepest layer and varies in size and content but is usually composed mainly of adipose tissue (Fig. 18.1).

EPIDERMIS

> **The epidermis is the protective epithelium of skin in contact with the external environment.**

The epithelium of skin is a stratified squamous keratinizing epithelium called the *epidermis* with the predominant cell type being the *keratinocyte*. The epidermis is divided into several layers according to cell structure (Fig. 18.2). Keratinocytes divide from the basal layer to produce the upper layers, which become more specialized and mature and produce a substance called **keratin**. The outer layers are the prickle cell, granular and keratin layers. The basal and prickle layers are cuboidal/polyhedral in shape, while the granular and keratin layers become progressively flatter in shape, in common with other stratified squamous epithelia. At the surface of the epithelium, flat plates of keratin, called **corneocytes**, form a tough, water-repellent layer (keratin layer). The corneocytes that form the keratin layer are non-living and derived from keratinocytes by cross-linking proteins, forming a protein–lipid envelope inside the cell membrane and the loss of organelles and nuclei. Each corneocyte plate conforms roughly to the shape of the keratinocyte shortly before its transformation to a non-living structure (see Fig. 18.2). Although normally thin, the keratin layer is very thick in skin exposed to constant trauma, such as that on the soles and palms (see p. 387 for the different types of skin).

In addition, a further layer, the stratum lucidum, is described in the thick skin of the sole. This refers to a narrow, pale-staining layer of compact keratin seen between the granular layer and the more deeply staining bulk of the thick keratin layer. It has no structural or functional significance and may be an artefact of staining.

> ### KEY FACTS
> #### Nomenclature of the Epidermal Layers
> In this book, we use the English nomenclature for the layers of the epidermis, rather than their Latin equivalents:
> - Basal layer ≡ stratum basale or stratum germinativum
> - Prickle cell layer ≡ stratum spinosum
> - Granular layer ≡ stratum granulosum
> - Keratin layer ≡ stratum corneum

> **The basal layer is the deepest cell layer of the epidermis and is responsible for the constant production of keratinocytes.**

The basal layer cells are cuboidal or low columnar in shape and are attached to the basement membrane, which separates it from the underlying dermis, by hemidesmosomes and to adjacent basal cells by true desmosomes.

Basal cells have round or oval nuclei (see Fig. 18.2c) with prominent nucleoli, and their cytoplasm is rich in ribosomes and mitochondria; tonofilaments are present in small numbers. In pigmented skin the cytoplasm also contains melanin granules and lysosomes.

It is in the basal layer that cells in mitosis are seen, in addition to scattered non-keratinocyte cells, melanocytes and Merkel cells (see p. 377).

Fig. 18.1 Architecture of the Skin. Schematic representations and micrographs of thick **(a, c)** and thin **(b, d)** skin. The most superficial layer of the skin is the epidermis (E). This varies in thickness from site to site and is covered by acellular keratin (K), which is mainly thin but is thick in special sites, for example, the sole. Beneath the epidermis is the dermis (D), which has two components: a more superficial loose papillary dermis (PD) and a denser reticular dermis (RD), which comprises the bulk of the layer. The dermis is composed mainly of collagen, with some elastic fibres, and contains the downgrowths from the epithelium such as hair follicles (H) and associated sebaceous glands (SG), eccrine sweat glands (EG) and ducts (ED). Beneath the dermis is subcutaneous tissue composed of adipose and collagenous tissue (S). Interdigitations between the epidermis and dermis in thick skin **(a, c)** called *rete ridges* (RR) provide a bigger surface area for attachment. The deepest layer of the skin, the subcutis, has a variable structure; when prominent, it is composed largely of adipose tissue intersected by fibrocollagenous septa. The subcutis contains the main subcutaneous network of arteries and veins from which vessels extend upward and form a network (the cutaneous plexus) at the dermosubcutaneous junction. From here, smaller vessels penetrate the dermis (BV), giving branches to the skin appendages and culminating in a superficial network of small venules and arterioles (the subpapillary plexus). Capillary loops from this plexus extend upward into the dermal papillae to lie close to the dermoepidermal junction. Blood vessels do not penetrate the epidermis.

Fig. 18.2 Structure of the Epidermis. (a) The basal layer (B) (stratum basale) sits on the basement membrane and is covered by the prickle cell layer (P) (stratum spinosum) and then the granular layer (G) (stratum granulosum), which contains dark-staining keratohyaline granules. The surface layer is pink-staining acellular keratin (K) composed of non-living corneocytes (stratum corneum). The keratin layer has an outer basket-weave texture which lies above a compact layer. Two non-keratinocyte cells of the epidermis, a melanocyte (M) and a Langerhans' cell (L) (see p. 51), are also evident. **(b)** A thin H&E section of skin showing the basal layer (B) and the prickle cell layer (P) above it. The characteristic intercellular bridges to which the prickle cells owe their name are seen and are the site of desmosomal attachments between adjacent cells. **(c)** The basal cells (B) are smaller than the other keratinocytes and may show a regular, regimented arrangement (palisading). They have rounded or oval nuclei and rest on the basement membrane, marking the junction between epidermis and dermis. **(d)** Micrograph showing the granular layer (G) of the epidermis with pink-staining acellular keratin (K) above it. The cytoplasm becomes progressively darker-staining near the surface owing to its increasing content of keratohyaline granules. The most superficial cells have lost their nuclei and are flat plates of keratohyaline and keratin (KK) forming corneocytes **(e)** in thick skin. A layer between the granular and keratin layers may be present called the **stratum lucidum**, so named because it does not stain with H&E and appears translucent

The keratinocytes above the basal cells form the prickle cell layers.

The prickle cells form a layer of variable thickness. The cells are polyhedral with central round nuclei and pinkish-staining cytoplasm.

Prickle cells are in contact and strongly adherent with each other by a system of intercellular bridges, formed from small cytoplasmic projections from the cell surface terminating in desmosomal junctions (see Fig. 18.2b and Fig. 3.5).

The cytoplasm of the prickle cells contains many bundles of cytokeratin intermediate filaments called *tonofilaments,* which are particularly concentrated in the cytoplasmic projections leading into the desmosomes and are more numerous in the cell layers closest to the granular layer (Fig. 18.3).

The cells of the upper prickle cell layer are flatter than the polyhedral cells of the deeper layers. The narrow intercellular spaces between the prickle cells contain lipid material extruded from keratinocytes, which contributes to the barrier function of the epidermis. The space also contains cytoplasmic projections of melanocytes and Langerhans' cells.

The granular cell layer transforms into surface corneocytes by cross-linking of proteins.

In the process of transforming into a non-living keratinized cell termed a **corneocyte**, the keratinocyte in the granule cell layer cross-links proteins, and the desmosomes of the prickle cell layer are transformed into a derivative called **corneodesmosomes**. In addition to desmosomes, cells of the granular cell layer also have occluding (tight) junctions which form a barrier to loss of proteins and other substances from the intercellular space of the epidermis and act as a barrier to the entry of allergens or harmful substances from the environment.

The keratinocytes of the granular layer contain several subcellular structures (see Fig. 18.3).

Tonofibrils are intermediate filaments composed of cyto-keratins, which become complexed and cross-linked with other proteins in the process of forming keratinized cells.

Keratohyaline granules are small, round or oval haematoxy-philic structures (see Fig 18.2d) composed of several aggregating proteins, including cytokeratin, loricrin, and profilaggrin, which are involved in the process of keratinization.

Lamellar bodies (also called *keratinosomes* or *Odland bodies*) contain the precursors and enzymes for the formation of the barrier lipids, which are present in the intercellular space between keratinocytes, in addition to the protein corneodesmosin.

It is believed that compaction and cross-linking of cytokeratin filaments drive the change in the shape of cells to become plate-like and flat (squames). The secretion of the protein corneodesmosin converts desmosomes in the living keratinocytes to corneodesmosomes, which bind the non-living corneocytes together and ensure a tough cohesive outer layer to the skin.

Progressive protein cross-linking, flattening of the cell and loss of organelles and nucleus lead to adjacent corneocytes bound together as the acellular surface layer, the keratin layer (see Fig. 18.3).

The protein **profilaggrin** is a main protein in keratohyaline granules and is processed to form filaggrin, a vital component of the barrier function provided by the epidermis. Its presence stabilizes the lipid–protein envelope that has replaced the cell membrane and minimizes water loss from the skin. It functions as a barrier to the entry of allergens that might otherwise cause dermatitis (eczema). The amino acid composition of filaggrin is also thought to contribute to creating a low pH in the keratin layer, sometimes called an *acid mantle,* which is believed to contribute to inhibiting bacterial growth. Other keratin filament–associated proteins include involucrin (see Fig. 18.3) and loricrin, a protein that interacts with filaggrin.

The keratin cell layer functions as a barrier resistant to environmental stresses and microbiological agents.

In skin covering the majority of the body, the terminal differ-entiation of the epithelium to form corneocytes results in a keratin layer composed of non-living superficial cells which are flat, tile-like overlapping plates of keratohyaline devoid of nuclei and organelles. The adjacent 'tiles' remain tightly bonded to each other by modifications of the original desmosomal junctions of the prickle cell layer, the corneodesmosomes, and the gap between them is filled with a protective lipid-rich material that contributes to forming an impervious barrier (see Fig. 18.2d and 18.2e). The structure of the outer layers of the epidermis contributes to its function as a barrier to infective agents, the entry of allergens and its integrity in response to friction or trauma. The extracellular lipid component also prevents loss of water through the skin.

In thin skin the keratin layer is composed of 2–3 corneocyte layers, whereas in thick skin the keratin layer can be 20–30 corneocyte layers deep. Typically, there is a compact layer of keratin immediately above the granular cell layer, which gives way to a so-called *'basket weave' layer* with a partially open lamellar pattern (see Fig. 18.2a). The functional significance of the basket weave layer is unclear.

Fig. 18.3 Keratinization. (a) Basal cells of keratinizing squamous epithelium are anchored by hemidesmosomes and desmosomes to basement membrane and adjacent cells and contain abundant cytokeratin intermediate filaments (tonofibrils). As the cells differentiate and move up the stratified epithelium, they remain tightly bound by desmosomal junctions, but the cytokeratin proteins expressed change to higher molecular weight forms and the cells develop lamellar bodies (keratinosomes). Lamellar bodies are membrane-bound vesicles containing phospholipids, which are secreted by exocytosis into the extracellular space and form a protective lamellar sheet composed of ceramides, cholesterol and fatty acids between cells in the upper epithelium. Cells in the upper part of the epithelium express genes encoding a variety of specialized proteins, which interact with the cytokeratin filaments to produce a resilient and mechanically robust compact mass (keratin). Other proteins aggregate around the inner face of the cell membrane as a protein–lipid envelope. Desmosomes are converted into **corneodesmosomes** that bind the devitalized keratinized cells together. After loss of nuclei and organelles, the surface keratinized cells are termed **corneocytes. (b)** H&E section of keratinized squamous epithelium. Note the purplish keratohyaline granules (KHG) and the absence of nuclei in the surface keratin layer (K) composed of corneocytes. **(c)** Keratinizing squamous epithelium stained to show involucrin *(brown)*, which is present only in the upper part of the epithelium as keratinization takes place. This protein forms part of a lamellar envelope beneath the cell membrane in keratinized cells in their transformation into corneocytes.

In areas of thick skin (mainly the palms of the hands and soles of the feet) the keratin layer is much thicker as part of the regional modifications in withstanding shear stress and trauma. Histologically, thick skin may have an additional layer between the granular cell layer and the keratin layer called the *stratum lucidum* (see Fig. 18.2e). The reason for this staining property is uncertain.

CLINICAL EXAMPLE

Scaling Skin and Eczema Linked to Mutations in the Profilaggrin Gene

Filaggrin, as discussed earlier, is found in the keratohyaline of the granule cell layer and is important for maintaining the epidermal barrier function. Mutation in the gene encoding its precursor, profilaggrin, is linked to the condition of **ichthyosis vulgaris** in which those affected have thick, scaly skin. Mutations causing filaggrin haploinsufficiency, leading to reduced amounts of filaggrin protein, are linked to a predisposition to eczema (atopic dermatitis). These insights have been described as the single most significant development in understanding the mechanisms of atopic allergic skin disease.

CLINICAL EXAMPLE

Tumours of the Epidermal Cells

Tumours of the epidermal cells in skin are quite common, and most are associated with prolonged exposure of the skin to ultraviolet light. They are therefore most common in sun-exposed areas of skin such as the face and the backs of the hands, and particularly in the elderly or those who have had excessive sun exposure at an early age through their lifestyle or occupation.

The most common tumour histologically resembles the basal cells of the epidermis and is called **basal cell carcinoma**. These tumours are malignant and, unless treated by complete excision when they are first noticed, may continue to grow slowly and locally destroy skin and deep tissues; it is extremely rare that they metastasize to distant sites. Slightly less common are tumours derived from the keratinocytes from the prickle cell layer. These are called **squamous cell carcinomas** and, like basal cell carcinomas, are locally invasive and destructive, but these tumours can also spread to distant sites via lymphatics.

> Surface keratin is constantly lost because of normal wear and tear from surface friction, washing and scrubbing.

Loss of surface corneocytes (desquamation) takes place when proteolytic degradation of the extracellular component of corneodesmosomes occurs.

Surface keratin needs to be constantly replenished from the granular layer, which in turn is constantly repopulated by cells from the prickle layer. The prickle cells are produced by proliferation of cells in the basal layer.

Turnover, from basal cell to desquamated corneocyte, varies from site to site, being faster (i.e. 25–30 days) in areas subject to friction (e.g. soles); slow turnover ranges from 40 to 50 days. The turnover period is considerably shortened in some skin diseases, particularly psoriasis.

> Keratinocytes are separated from the underlying support tissues of the dermis by a basement membrane.

The junction between the dermis and epidermis is an important area, tethering the two layers together (Fig. 18.4) and structured to minimize the risk of dermoepidermal separation by shearing forces as follows:

- Tethering fibres connect the dermis and epidermis to the intervening basement membrane.
- The basal cell membrane of individual basal cells and the underlying basement membrane are convoluted (see Fig. 18.2b).
- There is a system of **rete ridges** (i.e. downgrowths of epidermis into dermis), which varies markedly from site to site. In protected areas, where the skin is not normally subjected to shearing stress (e.g. the trunk), rete ridges are barely evident and the dermoepidermal junction appears flat (see Fig. 18.2b and 18.2e), but in areas constantly exposed to shearing stress (e.g. tips of fingers, palms and soles), the rete ridge system is highly developed (see Fig. 18.1a and 18.1c).

The basement membrane at the dermoepidermal junction can be seen to consist of three main layers, specifically:

- An electron-lucent lamina lucida on the epidermal side
- An electron-dense lamina densa in the middle
- An ill-defined fibroreticular lamina, which contains abundant fibronectin, on the dermal side

The basal cells are tethered to the lamina densa by hemidesmosomes from which anchoring proteins cross the lamina lucida. On the dermal aspect, fine anchoring fibrils of type VII collagen attach the lower surface of the lamina densa to collagen fibres in the papillary dermis, whereas fibrillin microfibrils attach it to upper dermal elastic fibres. In addition, the zone immediately beneath the lamina densa contains abundant fibronectin (see p. 69 and Fig. 18.4).

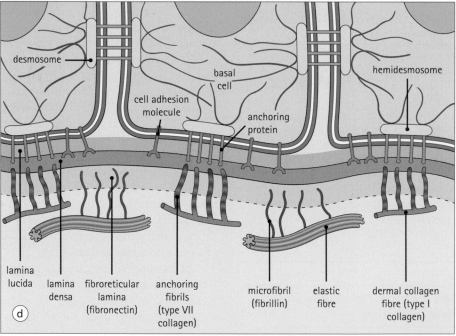

Fig. 18.4 Dermoepidermal Junction. (a) In this paraffin section, the basement membrane (BM) at the dermoepidermal junction is demonstrated by the PAS stain. **(b)** Dermoepidermal junction stained to show type VII collagen which forms anchoring fibrils. This is part of the basement membrane (BM) seen by light microscopy. **(c)** In this electron micrograph of the dermoepidermal junction, the basement membrane can be seen to consist of three main layers: a superficial electron-lucent lamina lucida (L), an electron-dense lamina densa (D) and an ill-defined fibroreticular lamina. The basal cells are tethered to the lamina densa by hemidesmosomes (Hd), from which anchoring proteins (A) cross the lamina lucida. On the dermal aspect, fine anchoring fibrils (F) of type VII collagen attach the lower surface of the lamina densa to collagen fibres (C) in the papillary dermis, and fibrillin microfibrils attach it to elastic fibres. In addition, the zone immediately beneath the lamina densa contains abundant fibronectin (see p. 69). **(d)** The dermoepidermal junction showing the components of the basement membrane and its attachments to basal cells and dermal fibres. [Image (b) used under Creative Commons License https://creativecommons.org/licenses/by-sa/3.0/ from the Human Protein Atlas Antibody to COL7A1 HPA042420 https://www.proteinatlas.org/ENSG00000114270-COL7A1/tissue/skin#img.]

Blisters

A blister forms when fluid accumulates in the region of the epidermis. This can result from:

- Excessive shearing force
- Structural abnormality (Fig. 18.5)

Excessive shearing forces are the most common cause and are usually the result of constant shearing friction, such as occurs with tight-fitting shoes.

Structural abnormalities may be primary or secondary, and the most important primary cause is the rare inherited skin disease **epidermolysis bullosa**, in which mutations in genes coding for structural proteins in skin lead to fragility such that it is unable to resist even minimal shearing trauma, leading to blistering. There are a number of different types of epidermolysis bullosa, depending on the site of separation, which can be ascertained by electron microscopy and genetic testing.

There are several secondary disorders which result in blisters. In such cases, histology may be needed to investigate the cause. Different diseases cause blisters to form at different levels in the epidermis. Some blisters develop because of separation of the basal layer from the dermis, whereas others develop because of separation within the cells of the epidermis (suprabasal blisters). Pemphigus vulgaris is an autoimmune condition caused by antibodies to the so-called *pemphigus antigen*. These autoantibodies bind to desmogleins, the transmembrane glycoproteins forming desmosomes, which mediate cell-cell adhesion within the epidermis. Epidermal cells lose adhesion to each other, allowing a fluid-filled blister to form. Patients develop blisters in the mouth and on the skin, which are usually painful and can become secondarily infected (see Fig. 18.5).

Fig. 18.5 Pemphigus Vulgaris. Histology of a fluid-filled blister **(a)** shows that the roof of the blister (R) is formed from the keratin layer and upper epidermis, with the split being within the prickle cell layer. The blister is filled with pink-staining fluid (F). **(b)** This micrograph is from the edge of the blister, as outlined in the box. The basal cells (R) remain attached to the basement membrane and the dermis. The blister has developed as separation (S) in the layers above the basal layer. Direct immunofluorescence showed intercellular positivity with IgG and C3 in the epidermis, confirming a diagnosis of pemphigus vulgaris. (Micrograph from digital pathology whole slide image provided by the University of Leeds Virtual Pathology Project https://www.virtualpathology.leeds.ac.uk. Reproduced with permission.)

Non-keratinizing Epidermal Cells

In addition to keratinocytes, the epidermis also contains melanocytes, Langerhans' cells and Merkel cells.

> **Melanocytes produce the protective pigment melanin.**

Melanin, produced by melanocytes, minimizes skin damage by ultraviolet radiation. Because melanin is pigmented (eumelanin = brown-black; pheomelanin = yellow-red), the type, quantity and distribution of melanin result in a wide variation in skin colour.

Melanocytes are derived from neuroectoderm and are located in the basal layer of keratinocytes in contact with the basement membrane. They are pale staining, with large ovoid nuclei (Fig. 18.6a) and abundant cytoplasm, from which numerous long cytoplasmic processes (dendrites) extend into the spaces between the keratinocytes.

Melanocyte cytoplasm contains characteristic membrane-bound ovoid granules (**premelanosomes** and **melanosomes**), which have a striated electron-dense core and produce melanin (see Fig. 18.6c). Melanocytes synthesise melanin from tyrosine in lysosome-like cellular compartments called *melanosomes*. In the production of melanin, tyrosine is converted into an intermediate pigment, which polymerizes into melanin. Melanin binds to proteins to form the active melanoprotein complex, which appears ultrastructurally as spherical masses of homogeneous electron-dense material and often obscures the premelanosomes.

Fig. 18.6 Melanocyte. (a) Micrograph showing a melanocyte (M) with its pale-staining cytoplasm. In this section of black skin, it can be seen clearly against the pigment-laden basal cells. **(b)** Ultrastructurally, melanocytes contain premelanosomes (PM) and melanosomes, and their cytoplasmic processes (CP) extend between keratinocytes of the basal and lower prickle cell layers. **(c)** High-magnification electron micrograph showing the characteristic boat shape of premelanosomes; both coarse longitudinal and fine transverse striations can be seen. **(d)** H&E micrograph of skin showing melanocytes with surrounding artefactual vacuolation (M) and some melanin pigment in some basal epidermal cells (P). **(e)** H&E micrograph of skin showing melanocytes with surrounding artefactual vacuolation (M) and heavy melanin pigment in most basal epidermal cells (P).

Melanoprotein complexes pass along the cytoplasmic processes of the melanocyte and are transferred into the cytoplasm of basal and prickle cell layer keratinocytes; each melanocyte can supply up to 40 keratinocytes with melanin. Keratinocytes store the melanin in a supranuclear area, which protects their nucleus from ultraviolet radiation damage. The highest concentration of melanin is in the basal layer. It is thought that melanin retained in the upper keratinocyte layers is correlated with darker skin tone. It is also hypothesized that different mechanisms may operate in the transfer of melanin to keratinocytes under different circumstances. For example, tanning requires rapid transfer mechanisms to transfer melanin to keratinocytes and possibly between keratinocytes.

Melanocyte numbers remain more or less constant, accounting for approximately one in six cells in the basal layer. Variation in skin pigmentation is therefore not a function of increased melanocyte number, but their degree of activity is genetically variable, accounting for racial and individual variation in skin colour. Increased melanocyte activity leads to increased size and type of melanin clusters present, leading to skin tone variation among individuals and in different parts of the same individual. The ratio of eumelanin to pheomelanin pigments also plays a part. Fig. 18.6d shows a section of skin from an individual with a paler skin tone compared with Fig. 18.6e from an individual with darker skin. In both images the number of melanocytes remains similar but the amount of pigment seen is much greater in Fig. 18.6e, reflecting the increased melanocyte activity.

CLINICAL EXAMPLE

Tumours of Melanocytes

Moles or nevi are local aggregations of melanocytes in the epidermis and dermis, producing the familiar regular, slightly raised, pigmented skin lesions. These are local developmental abnormalities and are not true tumours. Malignant melanocytic tumours can develop in normal skin or occasionally develop within an existing mole, with the early indications that this is about to happen being changes in the shape (seen as asymmetry, change in or irregular/indistinct border), size and pigmentation of a nevus, which had previously been unchanged for many years.

Malignant tumours of melanocytes are called **malignant melanomas** (Fig. 18.7). If recognized and excised at an early stage, malignant melanomas are curable, but once they reach a certain size and depth of invasion into the dermis, they begin to spread away from the site of origin (metastasize), initially by lymphatic channels to regional lymph nodes, and eventually by the bloodstream to many different sites, such as the liver, lungs and brain, leading to a poorer prognosis.

Fig. 18.7 Malignant Melanoma. This tumour was removed from the back of a young adult. The low-magnification image **(a)** shows the tumour (T) arising from the skin and extending into the dermis. There is ulceration of the overlying epidermis (U), and this fits with the clinical history that the lesion was black in colour and had started bleeding. Adjacent epidermis (E), including a hair follicle (F), are included for scale, so the mass of tumour is around 3 mm thick. **(b)** The high-magnification image shows pleomorphic cells with large nuclei and very large nucleoli. Dark-brown melanin pigment can be seen in some cells. This is a malignant melanoma. Despite excision, this tumour spread to the lymph nodes and lung as metastatic malignant melanoma. (Micrograph from digital pathology whole slide image provided by the University of Leeds Virtual Pathology Project https://www.virtualpathology.leeds.ac.uk. Reproduced with permission.)

Langerhans' cells are antigen recognition cells.

Langerhans' cells are located in all layers of the epidermis but are most easily seen in the prickle cell layer (Fig. 18.8a). They recognize and can present antigen to lymphocytes and are an important component of the immune system (see p. 141).

Similar to the haematoxylin and eosin (H&E) appearance of melanocytes, Langerhans' cells have an ovoid, pale-staining nucleus surrounded by pale-staining cytoplasm from which cytoplasmic (dendritic) processes extend between the keratinocytes. Langerhans' cell cytoplasm contains scattered characteristic **Birbeck granules**, which are rod-like structures with periodic cross-striations and are most numerous near the Golgi. Sometimes one end of the rod is distended to form a spherical saccule, giving the appearance of a tennis racket (see Fig. 18.8d). The granules contain the CD1a protein and CD207 (Langerin).

Although present in small numbers in healthy skin, Langerhans' cells are increased both in number and in the extent and complexity of their dendritic processes in many chronic inflammatory skin disorders, particularly those with an allergic or immune causation, such as chronic atopic dermatitis.

Merkel cells are sensory receptors in the epidermis.

Merkel cells are a type of neuroendocrine cell and are difficult to see in routine H&E preparations, where they are found in the basal layer and look like pale-stained cells resembling melanocytes. Immunohistochemistry can be used to identify them and confirms that they are rare cells, widely scattered (Fig. 18.9a). Electron microscopy reveals rounded, membrane-bound cytoplasmic neuroendocrine-type granules (see Fig. 18.9b).

Fig. 18.8 Langerhans' Cells. (a) In paraffin or resin sections stained with H&E, Langerhans' cells (L) are irregular, pale-staining cells in the prickle cell layer with pale-staining oval or reniform nuclei, which are often cleft. Their numerous cytoplasmic processes (CP) pass between the keratinocytes. **(b)** Langerhans' cells (L) carry CD1 marker and can be clearly visualized by immunoperoxidase techniques. **(c)** Ultrastructurally, Langerhans' cells have an irregular cleft nucleus and are devoid of tonofilaments. They have prominent mitochondria (M), lysosomes and rough endoplasmic reticulum (RER). Birbeck granules are not seen at this magnification. **(d)** High-magnification electron micrograph showing characteristic Birbeck granules, one with a distended vesicle (V) at one end. [Image (b) used under Creative Commons License https://creativecommons.org/licenses/by-sa/3.0/ from the Human Protein Atlas Antibody to CD1A HPA010734 https://www.proteinatlas.org/ENSG00000158477-CD1A/tissue/skin#img.]

Fig. 18.9 Merkel Cells. (a) Micrograph of skin stained to show the neuroendocrine marker chromogranin. A single brown-stained cell is seen in the basal layer, corresponding to a Merkel cell. They are few and far between. **(b)** Merkel cells can be distinguished from melanocytes by their ultrastructural features (compare with Fig. 18.8c and 18.8d). They have a convoluted nucleus, which occupies much of the cell, and no cytoplasmic processes insinuating between keratinocytes, but may have short protrusions, which contact adjacent keratinocytes at occasional desmosomes (D). Round neuroendocrine vesicles (EV) are present in the cytoplasm, particularly at the base of the cell, close to the basal nerve terminal, which communicate with the underlying nerve disc (not shown here). [Image (a) used under Creative Commons License https://creativecommons.org/licenses/by-sa/3.0/ from the Human Protein Atlas Antibody to chromogranin-A CAB058688 https://www.proteinatlas.org/ENSG00000100604-CHGA/tissue/skin#img.]

Merkel cells form synaptic junctions with peripheral nerve endings at the base of the cell and also scanty desmosomal attachments to adjacent keratinocytes (see Fig. 18.9b). They occur either as scattered solitary cells or as aggregates, when they are associated with a so-called *hair disc,* located immediately beneath the basement membrane. Such aggregates are thought to be touch receptors and are sometimes called *tactile corpuscles.*

CLINICAL EXAMPLE

Dermatitis (Inflammation of Skin)

The skin is exposed to many damaging agents, such as chemicals and ultraviolet irradiation, which produce a wide variety of common rashes. Dermatitis affects both the dermis and epidermis and can be chronic, for example, psoriasis or associated with allergen influx if the barrier fails (eczema).

In addition, the skin reacts to internal abnormalities and produces rashes in response to disorders, such as viral infections (e.g. measles).

Drug eruptions are common and present as skin rashes, which are typically red and itchy. Whereas most are diagnosed on the basis of clinical appearance and history of taking a drug, some are diagnosed using a skin biopsy. Several different patterns of inflammation can be associated with drug-induced skin disease (Fig. 18.10).

Fig. 18.10 Spongiform Dermatitis Caused by Drugs. This micrograph is from a biopsy performed to establish the diagnosis in a patient who presented with a widespread, red and itchy rash. There are two areas of the epidermis (S) which show separation of cells and infiltration by dark-stained inflammatory cells. The separation of cells is associated with fluid accumulation, and the term *spongiosis* is used to describe this appearance. In the dermis, dark-staining areas (D) are composed of inflammatory cells mainly centred on blood vessels. The suggested diagnosis of a drug-related dermatitis led to a detailed review of the patient's clinical history, and it turned out that, in an attempt to treat a cold, they had taken antibiotics prescribed to another member of the family. (Micrograph from digital pathology whole slide image provided by the University of Leeds Virtual Pathology Project https://www.virtualpathology.leeds.ac.uk. Reproduced with permission.)

SKIN APPENDAGES

The skin appendages are the pilosebaceous apparatus, isolated sebaceous glands, eccrine sweat glands and ducts and apocrine sweat glands and ducts.

The pilosebaceous apparatus produces hair and sebum, which is a non-wettable secretion that protects the hair and augments the non-wettable characteristics of the keratin.

The components of a pilosebaceous apparatus are hair follicle, hair shaft, sebaceous glands and erector pili muscle.

Pilosebaceous Apparatus

> **Hair is derived from the epithelium of the follicle.**

The **hair follicle** is a tubular epithelial structure opening onto the epidermal surface. At its lower end, a bulbous expansion (the **hair bulb**) with a concave lower surface contains a specialized area of dermis called the **hair papilla**. This is richly supplied with myelinated and non-myelinated nerve endings and abundant small blood vessels.

In the hair bulb, numerous small, actively proliferating germinative cells produce the hair shaft and the internal root sheath, which lie within the external root sheath.

Germinative hair bulb cells have dark basophilic cytoplasm with a scattering of melanocytes.

The internal root sheath of the hair follicle is composed of three layers:
- Henle's layer, which is a single cell layer
- A thicker layer characterized by the presence of large eosinophilic trichohyalin granules
- The cuticle, which consists of overlapping keratin plates

The cuticle is continuous with the cuticle of the hair shaft (see later) in the lower regions of the hair follicle.

The internal root sheath undergoes keratinization to produce the hair shaft. It extends up from the hair bulb to about the level of the insertion of the sebaceous glands, where it disintegrates, leaving a potential space around the hair shaft into which the sebaceous gland products are secreted.

> **The external root sheath of the follicle is modified epidermis.**

Near the opening of the follicle onto the skin surface, it consists of all three epidermal layers (basal, prickle cell and granular). In the deeper parts of the hair follicle, below the point of insertion of the sebaceous glands, it is composed of highly modified prickle cells, with large, pale-staining cells rich in glycogen.

Outside the external root sheath is a thick basement membrane, which is strongly eosinophilic and is known as the *glassy membrane* (Fig. 18.11).

Fig. 18.11 Pilosebaceous Apparatus. (a) The general architecture of the pilosebaceous apparatus. The hair bulb is a collection of compact epithelial cells surrounding a vascularized fibrocollagenous dermal papilla and produces the various components of the hair shaft (i.e. medulla, cortex and cuticle). In dark-haired people, abundant active melanocytes in the basal layer of the hair bulb supply melanin to the precortex cells; the medulla and cuticle are not pigmented. The outer cells of the hair bulb epithelium produce the internal root sheath, the middle layer of which contains numerous red-staining trichohyalin granules. The external root sheath is derived from the epidermis by downgrowth and is bound externally by a distinct homogeneous membrane: the glassy membrane. This separates it from the fibrocollagenous follicle sheath, which surrounds the entire follicle and also encloses the sebaceous glands as a thin, variably distinct layer. Attached to the fibrocollagenous follicle sheath at, or just below, the level of the sebaceous glands is the erector pili muscle, which extends obliquely upward from this lower attachment to its upper attachment in the papillary dermis. The lower parts of the hair shaft consist of partly keratinized cells in which the nuclei of the progenitor epithelium can still be seen, but higher up the hair is composed of anuclear hard compact keratin, which does not stain with eosin. **(b)** Transverse section through a hair follicle just below the sebaceous glands. The hair shaft (H) is anuclear and composed of non-staining hard keratin; a central medullary remnant (M) can be seen. The outer fibrocollagenous root sheath (F) and glassy membrane (G) around the external root sheath (E) are well formed, but the internal root sheath (I) is acellular and degenerate. **(c)** Transverse section through a hair follicle just above the hair bulb. The hair shaft (H) contains nuclear remnants and is strongly eosinophilic. The cellular internal root sheath (I) is well formed and contains eosinophilic trichohyalin granules. Note the external root sheath (E) and the outer fibrocollagenous root sheath (F). **(d)** Transverse section through a hair bulb showing melanocytes (M) supplying melanin to the precortex epithelium. **(e)** Longitudinal section through a hair bulb. There are no active melanocytes in this example.

> **Each hair shaft is composed of two or three layers of highly organized keratin.**

Each hair can be divided into an inner medulla, an outer cortex and a superficial cuticle.

The **medulla** is a variable component and is not present in the finer vellus and lanugo hairs. When present, it is composed of layers of tightly packed polyhedral cells. The **cortex** is composed of tightly packed keratin, which is produced without the incorporation of keratohyaline granules; it is 'hard' keratin and differs in composition from the soft keratin of the epidermal surface. The **cuticle** consists of a single layer of flat keratinous scales, which overlap in a highly organized manner.

Hair shafts contain variable amounts of melanin, depending on melanocyte activity in the germinative cells of the hair bulb.

> **The erector pili muscle positions the hair follicle and hair shaft.**

A further component of the pilosebaceous apparatus is a narrow band of smooth muscle, the **erector pili**, which originates in the fibrocollagenous sheath surrounding the hair follicle and runs obliquely upward into the upper dermis (Fig. 18.12). Its contraction makes the hair follicle and shaft more vertical, so that the hair appears to stand on end.

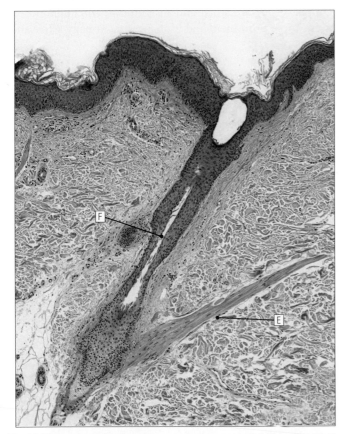

Fig 18.12 Erector Pili. This micrograph shows a hair follicle (F) with the erector pili (E) seen as a pink-stained bundle of smooth muscle attached to the base. In most histological sections only parts of the erector pili are seen, and it is seldom that one encounters such an exact plane of cut as shown here.

> **Sebaceous glands develop as lateral outgrowths of the external root sheath.**

Sebaceous glands secrete a mixture of lipids called *sebum*. They are largely inactive until puberty, after which they enlarge and become secretory.

Sebaceous glands are composed of lobules of large polyhedral, pale-staining cells containing abundant lipid droplets and small, dark-staining central nuclei. There is a single layer of cuboidal or flattened precursor cells between the basement membrane of each lobule and the central mass of cells. The sebaceous gland lobules are connected to the hair follicle, usually about two-thirds to three-quarters of the way up from the hair bulb, by short ducts lined by stratified squamous epithelium, showing all the layers seen in the normal epidermis.

> **Sebum is a lipid mixture that includes triglycerides and various complex waxes.**

Sebum is produced by programmed cell death of sebaceous cells, resulting in the release of their lipid content into the ducts (Fig. 18.13), and thus into the space between the formed hair shaft and the external root sheath, after degeneration of the internal root sheath. This pattern of secretion is called *holocrine secretion* (see Fig. 3.15).

> **The number, size and activity of sebaceous glands vary from site to site within the skin.**

Sebaceous glands are particularly abundant on the face, scalp, ears, nostrils and vulva and around the anus, but are absent from the soles and palms.

In certain areas of the body, the sebaceous glands do not empty into hair follicles, but open directly onto the epidermal surface. This occurs in:

- The labia minora (see p. 345)
- Areolar skin around the nipple, where they are known as *Montgomery's tubercles* (see p. 389)
- The eyelids, where they are known as *meibomian glands* (see p. 414)
- The lips and buccal mucosa (Fordyce spots)

Eccrine Sweat Glands and Ducts

> **Eccrine glands produce sweat and are controlled by the autonomic nervous system.**

Sweat is a hypotonic watery solution with a neutral or slightly acid pH that contains various ions, particularly sodium, potassium and chloride ions.

Fig. 18.13 Sebaceous Gland. (a) Micrograph showing a sebaceous gland (G) opening through a narrow duct (D) into the hair follicle (HF). The sebum is formed by programmed cell death (N) of the lipid-packed cells of the gland. **(b)** A sebaceous gland at higher magnification showing the single layer of cuboidal or flat precursor cells (P) and the large sebaceous cells (S) distended with lipid droplets.

> **Eccrine sweat glands and ducts are found everywhere in the skin.**

Eccrine glands are particularly numerous on the forehead, scalp, axillae, palms and soles. They arise as downgrowths of the epidermis at about the 16th week of intrauterine life.

The secretory gland component, which is situated deep in the dermis or in the upper subcutis near the dermosubcutaneous junction, communicates with the exterior by a duct. Proximal to the gland the duct is coiled, but thereafter it proceeds in a single direction up to the dermoepidermal junction. Within the epidermis, it again becomes coiled, but this is only seen to any extent where the epidermis is thick, for example, in the soles of the feet.

Eccrine sweat glands are composed of two layers of cells: an inner layer of secretory cells and an outer, flat layer of contractile myoepithelial cells, which is bounded by a distinct, sometimes thick membrane. The dermal ducts consist of two layers of dark-staining cuboidal cells surrounding a distinct lumen, the surface of which is often strongly eosinophilic (Fig. 18.14).

Apocrine Glands

> **Apocrine glands produce a viscid, slightly milky secretion.**

External stimuli, such as fear and sexual excitement, cause secretion from apocrine glands, the function of which is not known in humans; similar glands in mammals act as scent organs and produce pheromones for the delineation of territory and sexual attraction.

Apocrine glands develop as downgrowths of the epidermis and are scanty in humans but well developed in many other mammals. They are small and insignificant in childhood but become more prominent and probably functionally active after puberty.

In humans, apocrine glands are concentrated mainly in the perineal region, around the anus and genitalia, and in the axillae. Modified apocrine glands are found in the eyelids (**Moll's glands**), in the areolar skin around the nipple and in the external auditory canal, where they form the **ceruminous glands** responsible for the production of ear wax.

Apocrine glands are composed of:
- A secretory glandular unit situated, like the eccrine gland, in the lower dermis or at the dermosubcutaneous junction
- A more or less straight duct, which opens into a pilosebaceous unit near the surface, usually above the entrance of the sebaceous duct

The secretory unit of an apocrine gland is composed of an inner layer of cuboidal epithelial cells and an outer layer of discontinuous flat cells surrounded by basement membrane. It has a large lumen (Fig. 18.15). The duct resembles the eccrine duct (see Fig. 18.14), having a double layer of cuboidal epithelium.

Fig. 18.14 Eccrine Gland and Duct. (a) Micrograph showing eccrine glands (G) and ducts (D) in the deep dermis at low magnification. **(b)** High-power micrograph showing that the glands (G) are composed of pale-staining secretory cells (S) with an outer layer of indistinct myoepithelial cells (M). The ducts (D) have a more distinct double layer of dark-staining cells. **(c)** Thin epoxy resin section stained with *toluidine blue* showing that the gland (G) is composed of large, pale-staining glycogen-rich cells, some of which contain dark secretory granules (SG) and a smaller number of narrow darker-staining cells (DC) that secrete sialomucins. Eccrine glands are surrounded by a thick amorphous membrane (M), and their ducts (D) are lined internally by a homogeneous cuticle, which is composed of microvilli covered by an amorphous glycocalyx. **(d)** Micrograph showing intra-epidermal portion of eccrine duct, which is spiral and is sometimes called the *acrosyringium*. There is a single layer of cells lining the lumen and two or three layers of outer cells. The lining cells develop small keratohyaline granules (K) and become keratinized where they emerge through the granular layer of the epidermis. The spiral course continues through the keratin layer and is most clearly seen in skin with a thick epidermis.

Fig. 18.15 Apocrine Gland. **(a)** Axillary skin. Micrograph showing the abundant apocrine glands (AG), oblique hair follicles (HF) and thin epidermis (E) of axillary skin. **(b)** Micrograph showing part of an actively secreting apocrine gland (A) from axillary skin, with part of an eccrine gland (E) for comparison. The apocrine gland has an inner layer of cuboidal epithelial cells (C) with markedly eosinophilic cytoplasm and an outer layer of discontinuous flat cells, which are thought to be myoepithelial. It is surrounded by a prominent eosinophilic basement membrane. **(c)** High-power view showing the roughly cuboidal eosinophilic lining cells (C) and the irregular luminal surface resulting from the apocrine secretory process, in which fragments of secretion-containing cytoplasm are 'pinched off' into the lumen. Flat myoepithelial cells (M) are present but inconspicuous.

DERMIS

> **The dermis is the supporting tissue on which epidermis sits.**

In the dermis are located the epidermal appendages, blood supply, nerve supply and lymphatic drainage (Fig. 18.16). It is composed of:

- Fibroblasts, fibrocytes and their extracellular products (see p. 73)
- Collagen and elastic fibres
- Glycosaminoglycan-containing matrix
- Blood vessels and nerves
- Small numbers of macrophages, lymphocytes and mast cells

Two distinct zones of dermis can usually be identified: an upper, narrow papillary dermis, which is close to the dermoepidermal junction, and a thicker reticular dermis, between the papillary dermis and the subcutaneous adipose tissue.

Papillary dermis is paler than reticular dermis and contains less collagen and elastin but more matrix. The thin collagen and elastin fibres are more randomly arranged, with a high proportion perpendicular to the skin surface. It contains small blood vessels of capillary size, fine nerve twigs and nerve endings (see Fig. 18.16a).

Reticular dermis forms the bulk of the dermis. It is composed of prominent broad bands of dense collagen with intervening long, thick fibres of elastin, which usually run parallel to the skin surface. Within this tissue are the blood vessels, lymphatics and nerves of the skin.

> **The dermis contains two vascular plexuses.**

The main blood supply to the skin is located within the dermis and arises from larger vessels in the subcutaneous fat. Two distinct plexuses can be identified (see Fig. 18.1):

- A deep vascular plexus in the lower reticular dermis close to its border with the subcutis
- A superficial vascular plexus in the upper reticular dermis close to its junction with the papillary dermis

Loops of small vessels from the superficial vascular plexus run up into the papillary dermis, with small capillaries lying close to the epidermal basement membrane. No blood vessels penetrate the epidermis.

The dermis contains many arteriovenous anastomotic channels, including highly specialized shunts (**glomus bodies**), which are found mainly in the fingertips. Blood flow variation within the dermis is important to the skin's function as a thermoregulatory organ.

The skin appendages are supplied by branches from vessels connecting the deep and superficial vascular plexuses.

Fig. 18.16 Dermis. (a) Low-power view of dermis stained with H&E. It is eosinophilic because of its high collagen content; the papillary dermis (PD), which contains less collagen, is paler. An eccrine unit (E) can be seen in the deeper part of the reticular dermis (RD). Note the concentration of small blood vessels (BV) at the junction between the papillary dermis and the densely collagenous reticular dermis. **(b)** High-power micrograph showing the different natures of the loose, pale-staining papillary dermis (PD) and the more densely collagenous reticular dermis (RD). **(c)** Elastic van Gieson–stained section of upper dermis demonstrating elastic *(black)* and collagen *(red)* fibres, showing the difference between papillary dermis (PD) in which both collagen and elastin are fine and vertically orientated, and reticular dermis (RD) in which the collagen and elastin fibres are thicker and coarser and are mainly arranged horizontally.

> **The dermis contains numerous nerves and nerve endings.**

The nerve supply of the skin is located in the dermis and comprises:

- A rich, non-myelinated supply derived from the sympathetic autonomic nervous system, which controls the skin appendages and vascular flow
- An afferent myelinated and non-myelinated system, which detects cutaneous sensation

In addition to cutaneous free nerve endings, which detect pain, itch and temperature cutaneous, sensation is also served by nerve endings which form part of **cutaneous end-organ complexes** (CEOCs) (Fig. 18.17), the most important of which are:

- **Pacinian corpuscles** – encapsulated nerve endings with a characteristic lamellar structure; they detect pressure and vibration as part of proprioception and are found in the deep dermis or subcutaneous fat of the palms and soles
- **Meissner's corpuscles** – structured nerve endings confined to the dermal papillae; they are most numerous on the feet and hands and detect fine touch, vibration and fine movements
- **Merkel cells** and their nerve attachments (see Fig. 18.9) – slowly adapting touch receptors

SUBCUTANEOUS TISSUE

> **Subcutaneous tissue is composed largely of adipose tissue.**

The adipose tissue in subcutaneous tissue is separated by fibrocollagenous septa and contains the main blood vessels and nerves from which the overlying dermis is supplied (Fig. 18.18). It acts as an effective heat insulator, food store and shock absorber.

Subcutaneous tissue may contain extensions of skin structures, for example:

- In the scalp it contains the lower parts of the long hair follicles
- Some apocrine and eccrine glands

Subcutaneous injections are administered to vessels and nerves in this area, also called the *hypodermis* (hence the term *hypodermic needle*).

FEATURES OF SKIN IN DIFFERENT SITES

> **The skin shows marked variation in structure at different sites.**

Most of the skin covering the body is protected by clothing and is not excessively traumatized; it is not particularly specialized. Thus **skin on the back, abdomen, thighs and arms** has:

- A thin epidermis producing only small amounts of loosely packed keratin
- A poorly formed rete ridge system
- A thin epidermis producing only small amounts of loosely packed keratin
- Small numbers of hair follicles producing fine hairs (large follicles and coarser hairs in men)
- Variable numbers of eccrine glands
- No stratum lucidum

Fig. 18.17 Cutaneous End-Organ Complexes. These structures consist of an axon surrounded by specialized cells called *terminal glial cells* or *skin end-organ glia*, which are derived from Schwann cells or perineurial cells (see Chapter 6). **(a)** Skin section stained with H&E showing a Meissner's corpuscle, which is an elongated oval body. Meissner's corpuscles are arranged vertically in the dermal papillae of hairless skin, particularly in fingers and toes, but also around lips and nipples. Internally, Meissner's corpuscles are composed of spirally arranged cells surrounded by a thin fibrocollagenous capsule. In H&E sections, the most commonly seen cells are non-myelinated glial cells (see p. 114), the axons not being easily visible. **(b)** Meissner's corpuscle stained by an immunoperoxidase method for neurofilament protein (NFP) to demonstrate the spirally arranged axon (A). **(c)** Micrograph showing a Pacinian corpuscle in subcutaneous fat from the fingertip demonstrated by an immunoperoxidase method for NFP. It is a large, loosely laminated structure with a central core (axon, A) surrounded by concentrically arranged lamellae (L) of non-myelinated glial cells separated from each other by fluid-filled spaces. There are three regions separated into the inner core, with partial lamellae; outer core with complete lamellae; and a dense pseudocapsule (P) formed from fibroblastic cells. **(d)** Pacinian corpuscles are usually encountered in sections as incomplete structures identifiable by the concentric lamellar arrangement of cells. In addition to the hands and feet, it is common to find them in the genital skin, including the male foreskin, as shown here where three can be seen.

Thick skin is present on the palms of the hands and soles of the feet. It has:

- Been modified for its function in withstanding shear stress and trauma by having a thick epidermis, where prickle, granular and keratin layers have more layers compared with thin skin
- No pilosebaceous units but has eccrine glands linked to an ability to have sweaty palms and sweaty feet

Sole. The skin of the sole is modified to withstand constant trauma. It has:

- A well-developed rete ridge system to prevent epidermal separation from shearing stress
- Abundant eccrine glands and ducts but no apocrine sweat glands

Fingertip. Fingertip skin shows two structural modifications: one to minimize damage from shearing stress, the other because of its role as a tactile sensory organ (see Fig. 18.1a). Thus the skin in this region is characterized by:

- A well-developed rete ridge system
- Numerous Meissner's corpuscles in the dermal papillae
- Pacinian corpuscles in the dermis and subcutis
- Specialized arteriovenous shunts (glomus bodies)
- Abundant eccrine sweat glands and ducts but no apocrine sweat glands

Scalp. The characteristic feature of the scalp is the presence of tightly packed hair follicles with their associated sebaceous glands (see Fig. 18.1b). In straight-haired people, the follicles are almost vertical, but in curly-haired people they are oblique, with the degree of curliness depending on the degree of obliquity.

Fig. 18.18 Subcutaneous Tissue. Micrograph of subcutaneous tissue from the scalp. It is composed largely of adipose tissue (A) intersected by vertically running bands of fibrocollagenous tissue (F) that extend down from the deep dermis. In this example, the fibrous septa extend through the full thickness of subcutaneous tissues to join the dense fibrocollagenous layer (DF) covering the periosteum of the underlying skull. Subcutaneous tissue contains the major blood vessels (BV) from which the blood supply of the dermis arises.

Axilla and groin. The skin in the axilla and groin is similar, possibly because of our quadruped origins. Its most important features are:

- An abundance of highly active apocrine glands
- Numerous oblique hair follicles
- Numerous eccrine glands
- Thin epidermis

BREAST

Breasts first develop as early as the fourth week of gestation as thickenings known as the *mammary crest* or *milk lines*, which run from the axilla to the upper inguinal area. Most of the mammary crest atrophies, except in the region of the fourth

intercostal space, where mammary buds are formed, which then grow into the dermis. In humans, normally only one breast develops on each side; however, occasionally accessory breast tissue can be identified along the milk line and particularly in the axilla. Accessory breast tissue can develop any pathology seen in normally located breast tissue. The most common alterations of mammary development are supernumerary nipples, usually placed in an inframammary location.

Nipple

> Breast secretions and, during lactation, milk emerge to the surface at the nipple.

At the tip of the nipple are the 15–20 small openings of the large nipple ducts arranged in a ring (Fig 18.19a). These opening are lined by keratinizing, stratified squamous epithelium and plugged with keratin in the resting, non-lactating state. There is a sharp transition from the squamous epithelium of the nipple ducts to the bilayer columnar cuboidal epithelium of the draining ducts.

The nipple is a circular, raised area of modified skin with a slightly convoluted epidermis. The nipple is surrounded by the **areola**, which is modified skin containing large sebaceous units that form small nodular elevations called **Montgomery's tubercles**. The nipple and the areola show increased melanin pigmentation after the first pregnancy.

Breast Structure: Lobes and Lobules

> The parenchyma of the breast is composed of 15–20 distinct lobes.

The breast is composed of 15–20 distinct lobes arranged in a segmental pattern similar to an orange (see Fig. 18.19b). Prominent collagenous bands termed the *suspensory ligaments of Cooper* separate the lobes and tether the skin to the fascia overlying the pectoralis major at the deep aspect.

Each lobe has a draining duct, which has its own separate opening at the nipple (see Fig. 18.19a), via a channel called the *lactiferous duct* (see Fig 18.19d). Each lobe consists of multiple **lobules** composed of secretory glandular tissue (see Fig. 18.19c), each with an intralobular terminal duct and extralobular terminal duct. This arrangement forms the basic functional unit of the breast termed the **terminal duct lobular unit (TDLU)**, which will be described in more detail later (Fig. 18.20).

The secretory tissues of the breast are surrounded by fibrocollagenous support tissue intermingled with adipose tissue (see Fig. 18.19c).

The resting-state breast (non-pregnant, non-lactating) has a relatively small volume fraction of ducts and breast glandular parenchyma (lobules). The breast parenchyma expands and develops during pregnancy and lactation. Most disease processes of the breast arise from the TDLU (see later).

Fig. 18.19 Breast Structure. (a) There are 15–20 openings arranged in a ring on the surface of the nipple, each being lined by keratinized, stratified squamous epithelium. In the inactive, non-lactating breast they are normally plugged by keratin. Each opening is the site of emergence of a single lactiferous duct, which is lined by a two-layered epithelium, the basal layer being myoepithelial cells. Each lactiferous duct receives large mammary ducts, and there is a dilation, the lactiferous sinus, shortly afterward. The support tissue consists of fibroadipose tissue containing numerous longitudinal and circular smooth muscle bundles. **(b)** Mammary lobes and ducts. Each lactiferous sinus leads to a segmental mammary duct and its associated secretory unit called a *lobe*. The breast comprises 15-20 lobes separated by fibrocollagenous interlobar septa and adipose tissue. Within each lobe are clusters of secretory units called *lobules*. **(c)** This is a low-magnification micrograph to show the architecture of a breast lobe. The secretory tissue of the breast is arranged in lobules of glandular acini (L), each of which is surrounded by collagenous tissues. Each lobule drains into a terminal duct and in turn into small ducts (SD) that lead to larger subsegmental ducts (SSD) before joining a main segmental lactiferous duct. **(d)** Micrograph showing lactiferous sinuses with a characteristic undulated profile, which can distend to accommodate milk in lactation. The sinuses and the large mammary ducts leading into them are lined by an epithelial bilayer with inner luminal epithelial cells and an outer layer of myoepithelial cells. (Micrograph (c) from digital pathology whole slide image provided by the University of Leeds Virtual Pathology Project https://www.virtualpathology.leeds.ac.uk. Reproduced with permission.)

> **The ducts of the breast have a two-layered structure and express oestrogen receptor.**

The breast parenchymal tree, from ducts to lobules, consists of an epithelial bilayer. The inner luminal epithelium consists of cuboidal to low columnar epithelial cells (see Fig. 18.20a and 18.20c), which in normal breast tissue shows heterogenous staining with oestrogen receptor (see Fig. 18.20d). The outer layer is the basal or myoepithelial cell layer (see Fig. 18.20b), which lies beneath the luminal epithelium and sits on the basement membrane.

Fig. 18.20 Bilayer Structure of Breast Ducts. (a) Micrograph showing the epithelium of a terminal duct lined by two cell layers. The luminal inner layer varies between a cuboidal and a low columnar pattern (C), whereas the outer layer consists of prominent myoepithelial cells (M). Note the minute amount of secretion (S) in the lumen of the duct. **(b)** Micrograph of breast lobule stained to show myosin heavy chain 11, which is a marker of myoepithelial cells *(brown)*. Ducts and acini have a two-layered structure, with a brown-stained outer layer of myoepithelial cells beneath a luminal layer of epithelial cells, which only show blue nuclear staining. **(c)** Micrograph of terminal ducts immunostained to show keratin 8, which marks luminal epithelial cells *(brown)*. The outer myoepithelial cell layer (M) shows only nuclear staining by the blue counterstain, The luminal epithelial cells (L) are strongly stained. **(d)** Micrograph immunostained to show oestrogen receptor *(brown)* showing positive staining in the nuclei of epithelial cells. [Images used under Creative Commons License https://creativecommons.org/licenses/by-sa/3.0/ from the Human Protein Atlas; (b) Antibody to Myosin heavy chain 11 HPA015310 https://www.proteinatlas.org/ENSG00000133392-MYH11/tissue/breast#img; (c) Antibody to keratin 8 CAB001696 https://www.proteinatlas.org/ENSG00000170421-KRT8/tissue/breast#img.]

> **The duct system terminates in the functional unit of the breast, called the TDLU.**

The peripheral, and hence smallest, part of the branching duct system ends in a cluster of blind-ending terminal ducts and acini, with each cluster and its draining terminal duct comprising a **mammary lobule**. The combined structure of the lobule and its associated terminal duct is called a TDLU (Fig. 18.21a and Fig. 18.21b).

The connective tissue within lobules differs from the general support tissue in the breast, being a hormone-sensitive, intralobular, loose fibrocollagenous stroma rich in capillaries and with scattered lymphoid and plasma cells (see Fig. 18.21c).

The proportion of acini and stroma varies in the adult breast according to age and hormone levels during the menstrual cycle, pregnancy and lactation and menopause.

Breast Development

> **Full development of the female breast occurs at puberty.**

The nipple and its simple system of ducts are present at birth (Fig. 18.22a), but full development does not occur until puberty.

At puberty, and under the influence of increasing oestrogen secretion, the breasts increase in bulk, caused initially by an increase in fibrous and fatty tissue.

After a period of stromal changes, ductal elongation and branching occur (see Fig. 18.22b).

The growth and activity of the female breast are entirely hormone dependent. Continued oestrogen secretion after the onset of puberty leads to progressive enlargement and complexity of the duct system (see Fig. 18.22c). The architecture of lobules changes after pregnancy to form a more extended intralobular duct pattern.

Fig. 18.21 Terminal Duct Lobular Unit (TDLU). (a) Diagram of a TDLU, which consists of a terminal duct (intralobular and extralobular terminal ducts) and the associated ductules and acini within the lobule. The lobule contains hormone-responsive intralobular stroma. **(b)** Terminal ductal lobular unit showing terminal duct (TD) leading into a branched system of ductules and glandular acini (A). Each TDLU has a specialized intralobular stroma (IS) which surrounds the acini. **(c)** This lobule is stained for CD34, which marks the specialized fibroblasts that make up the stroma of the lobules. This stroma is endocrine-responsive and differs from the stroma in support tissues of the breast outside of the lobule, which is not stained.

> **The structure of the mammary lobule undergoes minor transient structural change during the menstrual cycle.**

In the second half of the menstrual cycle, there is gradually increasing progesterone and oestrogen secretion by the corpus luteum produced in the ovary after ovulation (see p. 359). Progesterone stimulates proliferation of the epithelial cells in terminal ductules; these cells also become enlarged and begin to show evidence of early secretory activity. In addition, fluid and glycosaminoglycans accumulate in the loose hormone-responsive intralobular fibrocollagenous stroma. These changes lead to a slight enlargement in the breasts, sometimes accompanied by a feeling of discomfort. If fertilization occurs, the ovarian corpus luteum persists and enlarges, secreting ever-increasing amounts of progesterone, which stimulates the continued proliferation and secretory activity in the terminal ductules of the breast lobule. However, if fertilization does not occur, the progesterone levels fall dramatically at the end of the cycle and the structure of the breast lobule reverts, with cessation of the early secretory activity.

Breast Changes in Pregnancy

> **Breast structure changes early in pregnancy.**

The vascularity and melanin pigmentation of the nipple and areola increase and the mammary lobules enlarge by hyperplastic proliferation of the terminal ductule epithelium, with some vacuolation appearing in the luminal epithelial cells.

By the second trimester, there is evidence of luminal cell secretion, which is copious by the third trimester and accumulates within the hyperplastic terminal ducts (Fig. 18.23).

> **The breast reaches its full functional activity during pregnancy and lactation.**

Functional maturation of the breast in pregnancy is under the influence of pituitary and ovarian hormones, which are secreted in high concentrations during pregnancy and throughout breastfeeding. Lactation may become established if the

Fig. 18.22 Breast Changes Throughout Life. (a) Breast development. Micrograph of breast tissue from a 4-month-old female infant. All that is present is a system of scarcely branching nipple ducts (D) embedded in fibrocollagenous tissue (F). **(b)** Puberty. Micrograph of breast tissue from an 11-year-old girl at the onset of puberty. The ductular system (D) is beginning to proliferate and produce branches, and the surrounding fibrocollagenous supporting tissue (F) is actively increasing in bulk. **(c)** Adult breast. Micrograph showing normal breast tissue from a 23-year-old woman. A breast lobule in which the system of terminal ducts and ductules is embedded in loose intralobular fibrocollagenous stroma (F) is shown. There is a narrow surrounding zone of dense extralobular fibrocollagenous support tissue (DF), outside of which is the soft adipose tissue (A) that forms the bulk of the breast.

infant suckles regularly. In response to stimulation of the nipple by the suckling infant, oxytocin release causes contraction of the myoepithelial cells leading to expression of milk termed *milk let-down* (see Fig. 18.23).

When breastfeeding ceases, the breast returns to its previous, or resting, state by gradual involution over a period of some months. The luminal cells return to their former size without cytoplasmic vacuolation, and the lobular support tissue returns to its previous proportions.

Sometimes there is residual increased collagen in the involuting lobular support tissue, and this can lead to progressive distortion of the mammary lobules and persistent cystic dilation of some of the ducts termed *duct ectasia*.

Pregnancy causes a change in the architecture of lobules, which change from a simple branching pattern seen in the nulliparous individual to a more complex branching pattern, which is consistent with the need for increased secretion during lactation. The glands undergo involution after lactation ceases but retain the complex branching pattern, leaving a persisting sign of a prior pregnancy.

Breast Changes After Menopause

> **Breast parenchyma undergoes involution after menopause.**

With menopause there is involution of the epithelial components, which show an atrophic appearance on histology (Fig. 18.24), and fatty tissue predominates, typically leading to decreased breast density and in a mammography examination a more radiolucent pattern. Breast density is a radiological assessment of the ratio between radio-dense epithelium and stroma to radiolucent fatty tissue, and this has a bearing on the ability of mammography to detect abnormalities.

Collagenous bands (suspensory ligaments of Cooper), which tether the fibrous tissue of the breast to the overlying skin, develop increasing laxity with age and may contribute to breast sagging or ptosis.

Fig 18.23 Breast in Pregnancy. (a) The breast in pregnancy is characterized by greater cellularity of lobules compared with a non-pregnant state (see Fig. 18.19). Gland acini dilated by early secretions can be seen (C). **(b)** In much of the pregnant breast, the cytoplasm and cellular detail of acinar epithelium is partially obscured by non-staining vacuoles composed of secretory material. **(c)** In empty, dilated acinar spaces apical apocrine-type secretory vacuoles containing non-staining lipid can be seen. Once lactation commences, the amount of secretory activity increases and gland spaces distend with milk.

Fig 18.24 Breast After Menopause. (a) Low-power micrograph showing part of a breast lobe with a large duct and adjacent terminal ductal lobular units (TDLUs). Compare with Fig.18.17c and note the reduction in volume of glandular tissue. **(b)** The breast after menopause loses acinar tissue and stroma from the TDLU through a process of involution. There is collagen deposition within the lobule and thickening of the basement membrane around ductules.

The Male Breast

> In the male breast only rudimentary ducts are present.

The male breast is a rudimentary organ with the glandular component limited to ducts located in the retro-areolar region. Proliferation of glandular tissue of the male breast is termed **gynaecomastia**. This may be the result of endogenous causes such as physiological increased circulating oestrogen seen in puberty and in the neonatal period. Gynaecomastia can be caused by a variety of exogenous causes which alter the androgen-to-oestrogen ratio. The male breast can be affected by a variety of benign and malignant conditions.

CLINICAL EXAMPLE

Gynaecomastia

Pronounced development of the male breast (Fig. 18.25) is called *gynaecomastia*. It occurs under the influence of excess oestrogen secretion or exogenous sources, including drugs such as spironolactone or endocrine treatment for prostatic carcinoma. Obesity, alcohol-induced cirrhosis, testicular or adrenal tumours which lead to increased oestrogen in men are other causes of gynaecomastia.

Fig. 18.25 Gynaecomastia. Gynaecomastia is characterized by proliferation and branching of the mammary duct system in the male breast, which often dilates (D), and by an increase in the periductal fibrocollagenous tissue (F).

KEY FACTS

Breast

- The functional unit of the breast is a terminal duct lobular unit surrounded by a specialized stroma which is hormone responsive.
- Lobule epithelium is hormone sensitive and undergoes proliferation in pregnancy.
- Contraction of myoepithelial cells under the influence of oxytocin leads to the expression of milk termed *milk let-down*.
- Milk is transported along duct systems to the nipple.

CLINICAL EXAMPLE

Common Benign Breast Pathology

There are several common causes of benign breast lumps, but all require investigation to rule out the possibility of a malignancy. The two most common causes of a benign well-defined breast lump is a fibroadenoma (a benign tumour) and cysts that occur as part of fibrocystic changes.

Fibrocystic change is a common benign finding and often detected incidentally (Fig. 18.26a). After numerous menstrual cycles, an imbalance between oestrogen and progesterone levels with hyperoestrogenism is the most widely agreed upon cause of fibrocystic change. Excess oestrogen leads to proliferation of epithelium in TDLUs and induces stromal fibrosis. Fibrosis and epithelial proliferation may lead to obstruction of ducts and acini, leading to cyst formation. Some cysts may rupture, causing an adjacent fibroinflammatory stromal reaction.

Fibroadenoma is the most common benign tumour arising in the breast (see Fig. 18.26b) and typically presents as a mobile, well-defined, painless lump with a rubbery texture on palpation, usually less than 3 cm in size.

Fig. 18.26 Benign Breast Disease. (a) Fibrocystic disease showing collagenous fibrosis (F) and development of cystic dilatation of glandular and ductal spaces (C). Some of the cysts (A) are lined by eosinophilic epithelium, which reflects a change to a similar epithelial type as seen in apocrine glands (apocrine metaplasia). **(b)** Micrograph of a fibroadenoma, a benign tumour which has both blue-staining cellular epithelial (E) and pink-staining stromal (S) components arranged in a distinctive pattern in which the epithelial part forms clefts distorted by the stromal part. Note the distinct capsule around the tumour (C) in keeping with a benign (non-invasive) pattern of growth.

CLINICAL EXAMPLE

Carcinoma of the Breast

Breast cancer is the most commonly diagnosed cancer in women, accounting for 24% of all female cancers and the leading cause of female cancer death worldwide. Most carcinomas of the breast are adenocarcinomas, arising from the epithelial component of the breast related to the TDLU (Fig. 18.27).

Invasive breast carcinoma is characterized by the neoplastic epithelial cells invading through the basement membrane and growing into the surrounding stroma (see Fig. 18.27a). Histological features are used to provide a tumour grade, a measure of its malignant potential which considers tubule formation, nuclear pleomorphism and mitotic count. Prognostic scoring systems using histological features such as the Nottingham Prognostic Index (NPI) are used in clinical decision-making and are calculated by the histopathologist using tumour grade, lymph node status and tumour size to give a score. The assessment of tumour biomarkers can also be performed using immunohistochemistry, for example, the expression of oestrogen receptors (Fig. 18.27b).

Fig. 18.27 Carcinoma of the Breast. (a) H&E micrograph from a needle breast biopsy taken under image guidance from a patient with a breast lump. It shows cords and nests of atypical cells infiltrating through pink-staining collagenous stromal tissue. Occasional ill-formed glandular spaces (G) are seen, indicating its origin from breast ducts. This is an invasive ductal adenocarcinoma of the breast. **(b)** Micrograph stained to show oestrogen receptor (ER) expression in the tumour. The brown nuclear staining shows ER positivity, which has both prognostic and therapeutic application. ER assessment is routinely performed as part of establishing a profile of the tumour and used in deciding on appropriate therapy.

For online review questions, please visit https://studentconsult.inkling.com.

Special Senses

INTRODUCTION

> **A vital function of the nervous system is the gathering of sensory information.**

Sensory information is derived from a variety of specialized sensory nerve endings. These include:
- Sensory endings in the skin to detect touch (fine touch, pressure), pain and temperature (see Chapter 18)
- Tendon endings and muscle spindles to detect movement and position of the limbs
- Chemoreceptive organs, such as the carotid body
- Sensory endings on the tongue to detect taste
- Sensory endings in the olfactory mucosa to detect smell

In addition, information is obtained by the specialized sensory organs, the eye and the ear; the ear and the vestibular system detect sound, acceleration and position; and the eye perceives light.

EAR

> **The ear is divided into the external ear, middle ear and inner ear.**

The external ear comprises the **pinna** and **external auditory canal**. The pinna is composed of elastic cartilage covered by hair-bearing skin. The external auditory canal is lined by hair-bearing skin. Within its subcutaneous tissues are wax-secreting **ceruminous glands**, which are modified sebaceous glands. The outer two-thirds of the canal is surrounded by elastic cartilage in continuity with the pinna; the inner third is surrounded by the temporal bone of the skull.

> **The middle ear is separated from the external ear by the tympanic membrane.**

The **tympanic membrane** marks the boundary between the external ear and the cavity of the middle ear, which is also termed the **tympanic cavity** (Fig. 19.1).

The tympanic membrane is a three-layered structure:
- The outer aspect is covered by stratified squamous epithelium.
- The central portion is composed of fibrocollagenous support tissue containing numerous elastic fibres to provide mechanical strength.
- The inner portion is lined by a low cuboidal epithelium, which is continuous with that lining the rest of the middle ear.

> **The middle ear transmits sound vibrations to the inner ear.**

The middle ear cavity is lined by a low cuboidal epithelium and contains three auditory ossicles: the **incus**, **malleus** and **stapes**. These are:
- Composed of compact bone
- Articulated by synovial joints (see Chapter 13)
- Covered externally by the same low cuboidal epithelium that lines the inner ear

Two small skeletal muscles, the stapedius and the tensor tympani, are associated with the ossicles and damp motion between the bones, which occurs in response to loud noise.

The middle ear cavity communicates directly with air-filled spaces in the mastoid bone (**mastoid sinuses**), which are lined by low cuboidal or flattened squamous epithelium.

> **The auditory (Eustachian) tube equalizes pressure in the middle ear cavity.**

The **auditory tube** extends from the middle ear cavity to the nasopharynx and is lined by ciliated epithelium similar to that of the respiratory tract. Its function is to equilibrate pressure between the middle ear cavity and the atmosphere.

Normally, the auditory tube is collapsed, but it is opened by movement of muscles in the nasopharynx, such as occurs with swallowing or yawning.

> **The inner ear is a series of fluid-filled sacs encased in bone.**

The inner ear consists of fluid-filled sacs (membranous labyrinth) that lie in cavities in the temporal bone of the skull (bony or osseous labyrinth).

The membranous labyrinth comprises the cochlear duct, the saccule, the utricle and semicircular canals and the endolymphatic sac and duct, the walls of which are composed of sheets of fibrocollagenous support tissue lined by a flat epithelium. These sacs are filled with a fluid called endolymph and have epithelial and sensory specializations to detect position and sound.

The osseous labyrinth is composed of three cavities – the vestibule, the semicircular canals and the cochlea – which are lined by periosteum and filled with fluid called perilymph.

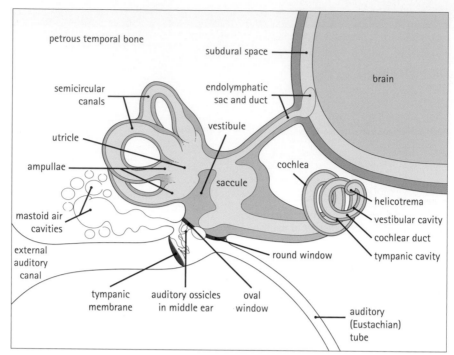

Fig. 19.1 Anatomy of the Ear. The ear consists of the external ear, middle ear and inner ear. The inner third of the external auditory canal of the external ear is surrounded by the temporal bone, and the middle ear and inner ear are contained within cavities in the temporal bone. The middle ear is an air-filled cavity containing the auditory ossicles. It is connected to the nasopharynx by the auditory (Eustachian) tube and is in direct continuity with the mastoid air cells. The inner ear is a fluid-filled cavity divided into three main spaces (semicircular canal space, vestibule and cochlea). Within the inner ear are a series of interconnecting fluid-filled sacs (semicircular canals, utricle, saccule and cochlear duct). The endolymphatic duct runs from the membranous sacs to the subdural space around the brain.

> **Movement is detected by mechanoreceptors in the inner ear.**

Mechanoreceptors, or **hair cells**, are specialized epithelial cells bearing a highly organized system of microvilli (**stereocilia**) on their apical surface. Deflection of the microvilli causes electrical depolarization of the hair cell membrane, which is transmitted to the central nervous system by the connecting axons of sensory nerve cells (Fig. 19.2).

Patches of hair cells are located in three sites:
- Within the vestibular apparatus in the ampullae of the semicircular canals to detect acceleration
- Within the macula of the utricle and saccule to perceive the direction of gravity and static position
- Within the organ of Corti of the cochlea to detect sound vibration

At each site, the hair cell microvilli are embedded in a gelatinous matrix, which moves according to the stimulus it is detecting. Movement of the microvilli toward the tallest row excites (depolarizes) the hair cell membrane, whereas movement toward the shortest row inhibits (hyperpolarizes) it.

Hair cells are arranged in different parts of the membranous labyrinth (Fig. 19.3) in order to sense movement generated by different causes.

Support cells surround the hair cells and are anchored to them at their apex by occluding junctions. These junctions maintain ionic gradients between the endolymph and the extracellular fluid around the cells, with the gradients being reversed on depolarization.

> **Sound is detected in the inner ear by the organ of Corti in the cochlear duct.**

The **cochlear duct** is a blind-ended tubular diverticulum filled with endolymph. It makes two- and three-quarter turns within the spiral-shaped bony cochlea in the temporal bone and is compressed between two other tubular spaces, the **vestibular** and **tympanic cavities**, which are filled with perilymph (Fig. 19.4).

Within the cochlear duct is the **organ of Corti**, which is a special adaptation of the epithelial cells lining the cochlear duct and detects sound vibration (Fig. 19.5).

Fig. 19.2 Hair Cell Microvilli. (a) The apical surface of each hair cell bears a highly organized system of microvilli (stereocilia), which are arranged as three parallel rows in a V- or W-shaped pattern. The height of the microvilli progressively decreases from the back to the front of the hair cell to form a so-called 'organ-pipe' arrangement. Fine filaments link individual microvilli from each row, with the tips of the shorter microvilli being coupled to the shafts of the taller microvilli behind. Whereas the hair cell is rigidly fixed in place by support cells, the tips of the tallest row of microvilli are embedded in a gelatinous extracellular matrix, which is free to move within the fluid cavities of the inner ear or vestibular system. In some hair cells there is a true cilium (kinocilium) at the apex of the stereocilia. **(b)** Hair cells are supported by adjacent cells and are in contact with the axon of a sensory nerve. The support cells are anchored to the hair cells by occluding junctions. The stereocilia are embedded in a gelatinous matrix. **(c)** Movement of the gelatinous matrix deflects the stereocilia, causing membrane depolarization of the hair cell, which is relayed to the central nervous system via the axon of a sensory nerve. Hair cells are arranged in different patterns in the cochlea and vestibular apparatus to detect acceleration (movement), gravity (position) or sound (hearing).

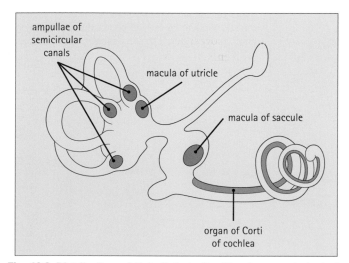

Fig. 19.3 Distribution of Hair Cells in the Membranous Labyrinth. The hair cells are arranged in patches in the ampullae of the semicircular canals to detect acceleration, in the macula of the utricle and saccule to perceive gravity direction and static position and in the organ of Corti of the cochlea to detect sound vibration.

◎ ADVANCED CONCEPT

Detection of Sound in the Inner Ear

Sound waves cause vibration of the tympanic membrane, which is then transmitted to the oval window membrane via the auditory ossicles.

Pressure waves are then transmitted to the perilymph of the vestibular cavity, causing the vestibular and basilar membranes to bow inward toward the tympanic cavity and to the round window, which bows outward.

Because the tectorial membrane remains relatively rigid, bowing of the vestibular and basilar membranes causes relative movement of the hair cell stereocilia, which results in membrane depolarization.

The signal is transmitted to the sensory nerves of the spiral ganglion and then through the cochlear cranial nerve to the brain, where it is perceived as sound.

Low-frequency sound is detected by stereocilia toward the apex of the cochlea, whereas high-frequency sounds are detected at the base.

Fig. 19.4 Cochlea. (a) The cochlea of the osseous labyrinth contains three spaces: the vestibular cavity, the cochlear duct and the tympanic cavity. These spaces are wound in a spiral within the temporal bone. The central spiral of bone within the cochlea is called the *modiolus*. The vestibular cavity and the tympanic cavity contain perilymph continuous with that in the vestibule (see Fig. 19.1), whereas the cochlear duct, which is continuous with and part of the membranous labyrinth, is filled with endolymph. At the apex of the cochlea, the vestibular and tympanic cavities connect at an opening termed the *helicotrema*. The cochlear nerve emerges from the base of the cochlea and carries signals to the brain. **(b)** Shown here is a section through the cochlea. The vestibular membrane (Reissner's membrane) consists of two layers of flattened epithelium separated by a basement membrane, with one cell layer being in continuity with the cells lining the vestibular cavity and the other in continuity with the cells lining the cochlear duct. The cells are held together by well-developed occluding junctions to maintain different electrolyte concentrations between the endolymph and the perilymph. The stria vascularis is a specialized area of epithelium with a rich vascular supply in the lateral wall of the cochlear duct. Many of the cells here have ultrastructural features indicating an ion transport function, and it is thought that they secrete endolymph. The basilar membrane is thicker than the vestibular membrane and consists of collagen fibres and a basement membrane. On one side it is covered by cells lining the tympanic cavity, and on the other by specialized cells lining the cochlear duct. Medially, the basilar membrane is continuous with the organ of Corti, which is a specialized area of support cells and sensory hair cells subserving hearing (see Fig. 19.5). The organ of Corti is supported by a spur of bone called the *osseous spiral lamina*. Laterally, the basilar membrane is attached to the spiral ligament, which is a mass of tissue developed from the endosteum of the surrounding bone. Neurons of the spiral ganglion are present adjacent to the osseous spiral lamina.

Fig. 19.5 Organ of Corti. (a) The organ of Corti is composed of epithelial support cells and sensory hair cells. Medially, it rests on the rigid bony osseous spiral lamina; laterally, it is located on the deformable basilar membrane. There are two groups of hair cells, an inner group and an outer group, which are separated by a small opening at the end of the osseous spiral lamina termed the *inner tunnel* (tunnel of Corti). The inner group are smaller and rounder than the outer group and arranged as a single row along the cochlea. The outer group are tall and thin and arranged in three to five parallel rows, depending on the position in the length of the cochlea. The hair cells are surrounded by epithelial support cells, with the inner hair cells being completely surrounded, whereas the outer hair cells are enclosed only at their extreme apex and basal portions, leaving a bare midzone in contact with extracellular fluid. The microvilli of the outer hair cells are attached to a sheet of gelatinous extracellular matrix braced by filamentous proteins (tectorial membrane), but those of the inner hair cells are free. Axons make synaptic contact with the hair cells and run to the spiral ganglion. The tectorial membrane is secreted by epithelial cells (interdental cells). There are several classes of support cell in the organ of Corti. Pillar cells contain abundant scaffolding microtubules and surround and support the triangular cavity (inner tunnel) at the level of the lip of the osseous spiral lamina. In contrast, phalangeal cells support the hair cells and are attached to them by occluding junctions at their apices, thus isolating the basal membrane of hair cells from the endolymph and maintaining electrochemical gradients. **(b)** Micrograph of the organ of Corti. Note the tectorial membrane (T), the mass of phalangeal cells bearing the hair cells (P), the basilar membrane (B) and the stria vascularis (S) on the spiral ligament (SL) within the cochlear duct (C).

CLINICAL EXAMPLE

Hearing Loss

Many diseases of the ear are associated with temporary or permanent hearing loss. Deafness can be divided into conductive and sensorineural types.

Conductive loss occurs when sound waves cannot be transmitted to the inner ear; common causes include blockage of the external auditory meatus (e.g. wax) or damage to the middle ear by infection ('otitis media').

Sensorineural loss is the result of damage to the inner ear, the nerves linking the cochlea with the brain or in the brain itself. The most common type is called **presbycusis,** which occurs in elderly people; it results from reduction in hair cells, atrophy of the stria vascularis and neuron loss in the spiral ganglia.

Recently, it has been possible to place electronic implants into the cochlea to treat deafness. Sound is detected by an external device, and this causes direct stimulation of the cochlear nerve, allowing hearing.

Gravity and static position are detected by hair cells in the macula of the utricle and the macula of the saccule.

The macula of the utricle lies in the horizontal plane, whereas the macula of the saccule lies in the vertical plane at right angles to the macula of the utricle (see Fig. 19.3).

Each macula is histologically identical and is composed of the following three cell types (Fig. 19.6):

- Support cells (sustentacular cells), which are columnar cells with short apical microvilli
- Type I hair cells, which are polygonal in shape and surrounded by a network of afferent and efferent nerve endings
- Type II hair cells, which are cylindrical in shape, with basal synaptic afferent and efferent nerve endings

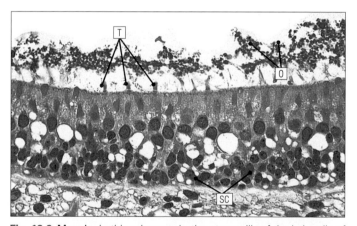

Fig. 19.6 Macula. In this micrograph, the stereocilia of the hair cells of the macula are embedded in the otolithic membrane. The otoconia (O) are visible as numerous purple-stained particles. The stereocilia appear as pink tufts (T) arising from the cell surface, but neither individual microvilli nor type of hair cell can be identified at this magnification. The support cells (SC) appear as an epithelial sheet.

In addition to an organ-pipe arrangement of tall microvilli stereocilia on their apical surface (see Fig. 19.2), these hair cells possess a single true cilium termed a **kinocilium**, which is located just behind the tallest row of stereocilia.

The stereocilia and kinocilium of each new hair cell are embedded in a gelatinous plaque of extracellular matrix called the **otolithic membrane**, which is suspended in the endolymph. This membrane is covered by numerous small particles composed of protein and calcium carbonate, the **otoconia (otoliths)**.

The macula can detect the direction of gravity by sensing the direction of pull of the otolithic membrane and otoconia on the mass of hair cells that results from head movement either backward and forward (macula of utricle) or from side to side (macula of saccule).

> **Acceleration and motion are detected by hair cells in the ampullae at the end of the semicircular canals.**

There are three semicircular canals, which assume posterior, superior and horizontal positions.

Each ampulla is a 1-mm-long dilated region of the membranous labyrinth and contains a patch of hair cells arranged in a tall finger-like structure (an **ampullary crista**). The stereocilia of the sensory hair cells are attached to a dome-shaped gelatinous matrix termed a *cupola* (Fig. 19.7).

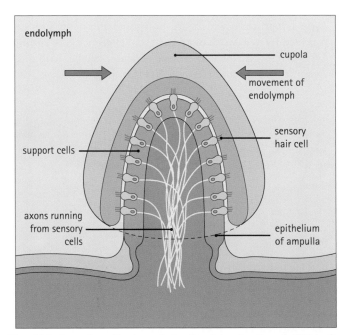

Fig. 19.7 Ampullary Region of the Semicircular Canal. Within the ampullae of the semicircular canals, hair cells are arranged over a finger-like protrusion of the lining called the *ampullary crista*. The hair cells are both type I and type II and are associated with adjacent support cells. The axons innervating the cells emerge from the base of the ampullary crista, being derived from sensory nerve cells in the ganglion of the vestibular nerve (Scarpa's ganglion), which connect with the vestibular nucleus in the brain stem. The hair cell stereocilia and kinocilium are embedded in the gelatinous matrix of the cupola, which, unlike the tectorial membrane of the maculae, does not contain otoconia.

With rotary motion of the head, endolymph moves within the membranous labyrinth because of the static inertia of the fluid relative to the rest of the vestibular apparatus. Such movement causes displacement of the cupola, and the direction of this displacement is detected by the hair cells.

When integrated, perception from the three semicircular canals arranged in planes perpendicular to each other provides information on the direction and rate of acceleration of head movement.

EYE

The eye is designed to focus light onto specialized receptors that respond to light. It is composed of the sclera, cornea, uvea and retina arranged around three chambers (Fig. 19.8).

> **The sclera proper is the outer fibrocollagenous coat of the globe of the eye.**

The sclera varies in thickness from 1 mm posteriorly to 0.5 mm anteriorly and is composed of flat plates of collagen oriented in different directions but parallel to the surface.

The sclera is composed of three layers:
- The episclera, an external layer of loose fibrocollagenous tissue running adjacent to the periorbital fat
- The stroma, the middle layer, which is composed of bundles of collagen thicker than those of the episclera
- The inner part of the sclera, adjacent to the choroid layer

The collagen bundles of the stroma run in sweeping branching patterns, mainly looping from front to back, within the stroma. The lamina fusca contains small numbers of elastic fibres.

The blood vessels and nerves (including the optic nerve) running to and from the eye pass through the periscleral and scleral layers. The scleral stroma itself is avascular. Anteriorly, the sclera blends with the cornea in a transition zone (the limbus), which is 1 mm wide.

> **The cornea is covered on both surfaces by epithelium.**

The cornea is the transparent disc-like anterior portion of the globe, and in the adult, typically measures 10.5 mm from top to bottom and 11.5 mm from side to side. It is more curved than the globe and protrudes anteriorly. The cornea has six layers (Fig. 19.9).

Corneal epithelium. The non-keratinizing, squamous epithelium with a basal cell layer gives rise to five to six superficial layers with a total thickness of about 50 μm. Numerous free nerve endings terminate in this epithelium and are the afferent part of the blink (ciliary) reflex, which is mediated through the sensory part of the fifth cranial nerve.

Bowman's membrane. This is composed of fine collagen fibrils embedded in an extracellular matrix and is 8–10 μm thick. It is limited anteriorly by the basement membrane of the corneal epithelium and blends posteriorly with the corneal stroma.

Fig. 19.8 Anatomy of the Eye. The eye is a spherical structure with a translucent disc-shaped area (cornea) on its anterior surface. This merges at its margins with a tough fibrocollagenous outer coat (sclera) at the limbus. The sclera surrounds the globe and is attached to a series of skeletal muscles (extra-ocular muscles) responsible for eye movement. The choroid is composed of blood vessels, support cells and melanocytes posteriorly and is continuous with the ciliary body and iris anteriorly, the iris being a disc-shaped membrane containing smooth muscle, with a central aperture (the pupil) to allow the passage of light. A special epithelial layer (retinal pigment epithelium) lies inside the choroid and inside this is the receptor and nerve cell layer of the eye (retina). The ora serrata marks the end of the specialized sensory layer of the retina anteriorly. Nerves from the retina emerge from the posterior aspect of the globe in the optic nerve, which is surrounded by a covering layer of fibrocollagenous tissue and cerebrospinal fluid, in continuity with that surrounding the brain. Blood is supplied to the retina by the central artery of the retina, which runs with the optic nerve. The transparent biconvex lens is suspended by a series of fine filaments from the ciliary body. The ciliary body contains smooth muscle, and its contraction regulates the lens shape. The globe is divided into three chambers: the anterior chamber in front of the iris, the posterior chamber behind the iris and the vitreous behind the lens. The anterior and posterior chambers contain a clear fluid called the *aqueous*. The vitreous is a gelatinous, transparent, extracellular matrix material.

Fig. 19.9 Cornea. (a) Micrograph of the six layers of the cornea showing epithelium (E), Bowman's membrane (B), stroma (S), Dua's layer (Du), Descemet's membrane (D) and endothelium (END). Bowman's membrane and Descemet's membrane appear as homogeneous hyaline layers that stain bright pink with H&E. In paraffin-processed material, as here, artefactual splitting of the collagen plates forming the corneal stroma is common and gives rise to small spaces. **(b)** Electron micrograph showing the base of a corneal epithelial basal cell (E) and its basement membrane (BM) resting on Bowman's membrane (B), in which a felt-like arrangement of fine collagen fibrils can just be discerned. Beneath this are the collagen lamellae of the corneal stroma (S) and a corneal fibrocyte (keratocyte, K). **(c)** Electron micrograph showing endothelium (END) resting on Descemet's membrane (D). Above is the acellular Dua's layer (Du), and above this are the collagen lamellae of the corneal stroma (S) and a corneal fibrocyte (keratocyte, K). Below is the anterior chamber (A).

Corneal stroma. The main layer of the cornea is composed of 60–70 broad sheets of tightly bound, parallel collagen fibres (corneal lamellae) embedded in an extracellular matrix composed mainly of sulphated glycosaminoglycans. To provide maximum mechanical strength, the direction of the collagen fibres differs in each layer. Between the lamellae are sparse, inactive, spindle-shaped fibrocytes (**keratocytes**).

Because there are no blood vessels in the cornea, the regular parallel arrangement of the collagen and the paucity of cells render the cornea translucent, and allow it to transmit light.

Dua's layer (pre-Descemet's layer), discovered and characterized in 2014, is a zone composed of collagen lying just in front of Descemet's membrane. Its importance is as a plane of cleavage that is used in corneal surgery.

Descemet's membrane. This 7- to 10-μm thick hyaline layer on the posterior aspect of the corneal stroma is produced by the corneal endothelial cells and is a true basement membrane.

Corneal endothelium. This consists of a single layer of polygonal, plate-like cells that line the inner surface of the cornea. They are adapted for ion pumping and therefore possess numerous mitochondria and are linked together by both desmosomal and occluding junctions.

The corneal endothelial cells pump fluid from the corneal stroma, thereby preventing excessive hydration of the extracellular matrix, which would result in opacification of the cornea.

CLINICAL EXAMPLE

Corneal Disease

The cornea contributes to the refraction of light into the eye, and damage resulting in corneal opacity may impair vision.

Although loss of corneal epithelium (corneal abrasion) is exquisitely painful, it is soon repaired by regeneration of new cells. Damage to Bowman's membrane, however, results in the formation of an opaque corneal scar because repair is by the haphazard deposition of collagen. If such scarring occurs in the visual axis, it causes loss of visual acuity.

The corneal endothelial cells are not replaced during life, and in some instances, become depleted with age. They may also be damaged by disease processes in the anterior chamber of the eye. When the corneal endothelial cells are sufficiently depleted, fluid accumulates in the corneal stroma, which then becomes less transparent. Such waterlogging of the corneal stroma (corneal oedema) may cause the overlying epithelium to separate, and this is intensely painful.

Diseases of the cornea, including endothelial failure, may be treated by corneal transplantation. Increasingly, transplantation involves only part of the corneal structures, either anterior or posterior, performed by lamellar keratoplasty procedures.

The uvea is a specialized support tissue within the globe.

The uvea is an intermediate layer in the eye between the dense support tissue of the sclera and the functional neural tissue of the retina. It contains blood vessels, nerves, support cells, contractile cells and melanocytes and is divided into three specialized areas: the choroid, ciliary body and iris.

The choroid has three layers and supports the retina.

The choroid extends from the ora serrata to the optic nerve and contains the blood vessels and lymphatics supporting the retina (Fig. 19.10). It is a dark brown sheet and blends with the lamina fusca of the sclera in its outer portion, whereas in its inner portion it is attached to the retina. Next to the sclera is the **choroidal stroma**, which is a loose fibrocollagenous support tissue interspersed with melanocytes, lymphocytes and mast cells and through which the main arteries and veins run. Inside this is the **choriocapillary layer**, which is a capillary layer supporting the deep layers of the retina and arises from the larger vessels in the stroma. Finally, at the interface between the choroid and the retinal pigment epithelium is **Bruch's membrane**, which consists of:

- The basement membrane of the choriocapillary endothelial cells
- An outer collagen fibre layer 0.5 μm thick
- An elastic fibre layer 2 μm thick
- An inner collagen fibre layer
- The basement membrane of the retinal pigment epithelium (part of the retina)

CLINICAL EXAMPLE

Uveal Disease

The uvea is the site of several disease processes:

- Inflammation of the uvea is termed *uveitis*. Anterior uveitis, affecting the iris and ciliary body, presents as a painful red eye and reduced visual acuity. Uveitis may be a complication of several systemic inflammatory diseases and infections. Examples include ankylosing spondylitis, rheumatoid arthritis, Behçet's syndrome, syphilis, tuberculosis and inflammatory bowel disease. Uveitis affecting the back of the eye may be caused by direct infection.
- The melanin-containing cells of the uvea give rise to the most common tumour seen in the eye: a malignant melanoma. These tumours have the capacity to spread both locally and to distant organs by metastasis.
- Albinism is a congenital condition characterized by the absence of melanin from the uvea, either alone or from the whole body. Patients have poor vision and may have cerebellar ataxia.

Fig. 19.10 Choroid. Micrograph showing the vascular choroid layer posterior to the retinal pigment epithelium.

The iris is part of the uvea and forms a diaphragm in front of the lens.

The iris delineates the anterior and posterior chambers of the eye. It has a circular aperture (**pupil**) that can be opened and closed by the action of groups of smooth muscle. Contraction of the pupil reduces the amount of light entering the eye and thereby reduces glare from light scattered from the periphery of the lens.

The iris contains pigmented cells and muscle and is composed of four layers: the **anterior limiting membrane**, the **stroma**, the **dilator muscle layer** and the **posterior epithelium** (Fig. 19.11).

The **anterior limiting layer** is an incomplete, fenestrated layer formed from stellate fibroblastic cells and stellate melanocytes.

The **stroma** is a loose fibrocollagenous support tissue associated with spindle-shaped fibroblasts (stromal cells), blood vessels, nerves and macrophages containing phagocytosed melanin pigment; at the pupil margin is the circumferentially arranged smooth muscle of the sphincter muscle of the pupil.

The blood vessels of the iris generally run in a radial direction, with frequent anastomotic channels forming circumferential vascular plexuses.

The **dilator muscle layer** is composed of the contractile processes of the myoepithelial cells of the inner layer of the posterior epithelium; it extends from the base of the iris to the sphincter muscle.

The **posterior epithelium** is composed of two layers of cells which are densely pigmented with melanin. The inner layer of cells is more correctly myoepithelial in type, with a basal zone around the nucleus containing melanin granules, and an apical portion, which is melanin-free, constituting the dilator muscle layer. This inner layer is bound by desmosomal junctions to the outer layer cells, which contain numerous melanin granules and are continuous with the retinal pigment epithelial layer. The pigmented cells eliminate light from the eye and reduce glare.

Eye colour is determined by the relative number of melanocytes in the stroma. Few cells give a blue colour, whereas many melanin-containing cells produce a dark brown colour; grey and green are the intermediate colours.

Fig. 19.11 Iris. (a) The free margin of the iris at the pupil, showing its four constituent layers. An incomplete and fenestrated anterior limiting layer containing stellate fibroblasts and melanocytes lies on a loose fibrocollagenous stroma containing the sphincter muscle of the pupil, in addition to radially orientated collagen fibres that give the iris its ribbed and trabeculated surface. Behind the stroma is the dilator muscle, which is backed posteriorly by two layers of melanin-pigmented cells. **(b)** Micrograph showing the histological appearance of the iris. The four layers are not well defined. The anterior limiting layer (L) merges with the stroma (S). The pigmented posterior epithelium cannot be resolved into two layers because of the density of melanin pigment. The dilator muscle (M) is visible as a pink band.

The **ciliary body** extends from the base of the iris to the ora serrata, where it is continuous with the choroid (see Fig. 19.8). On section (Fig. 19.12), the ciliary body is roughly triangular in shape and is composed of a vascular stroma, smooth muscle and covering epithelium; it has two anatomically recognizable regions: the **pars plica** and the **pars plana**.

The ciliary body contains the **ciliary muscle**, which is a form of smooth muscle. Contraction of the ciliary muscle lessens tension on the suspensory fibres of the lens and allows the lens to assume a more spherical shape.

The pars plica contains the ciliary processes, which are ridges or folds 2 mm long, each with a core of stroma and blood vessels and covered by two layers of columnar epithelium. The outer layer of epithelium is pigmented, but the inner layer, which is in contact with the aqueous, is not.

The non-pigmented epithelial cells in the grooves between the ciliary processes give rise to the suspensory fibres of the lens, which are composed mainly of the protein fibrillin. The ultrastructural features of these non-pigmented cells are those of ion-pumping cells; they secrete the aqueous.

The pars plana is a posterior flat area 4 mm long. Its stroma is continuous with the choroid, whereas the outer pigmented epithelium of the ciliary body is continuous with that of the retina at the ora serrata.

The retina is the innermost layer of the eye and is derived embryonically from an outgrowth of the developing brain (the optic cup). It is composed of pigment epithelial cells, photoreceptor cells, retinal support cells and nerve cells.

The retinal pigment epithelium is a single layer of melanin-containing polygonal cells extending from the optic nerve to the ora serrata. Internally, it lies adjacent to the photoreceptor layer of the retina; externally its basement membrane is a component of Bruch's membrane.

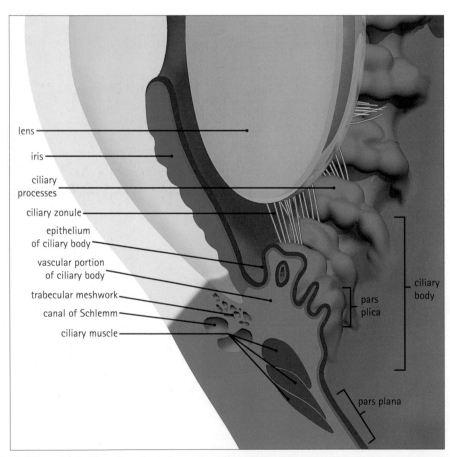

lens
iris
ciliary processes
ciliary zonule
epithelium of ciliary body
vascular portion of ciliary body
trabecular meshwork
canal of Schlemm
ciliary muscle
ciliary body
pars plica
pars plana

Fig. 19.12 Ciliary Body. The ciliary body is continuous with the base of the iris and is divided anatomically into the pars plica and pars plana. The ciliary processes give rise to the suspensory fibres of the lens (ciliary zonule), and the ciliary muscle controls the tension on the suspensory fibres, thereby controlling the shape of the lens. The epithelium of the pars plana secretes the aqueous.

The apical surfaces of the pigmented epithelial cells are covered with large microvilli, which extend upward and surround the photoreceptors of the retina. Retinal pigment epithelial cells phagocytose worn-out components of the photoreceptor cells.

> **The two main types of photoreceptor cells of the retina are termed** *rods* **and** *cones*.

The light-sensitive structures (**photoreceptor discs**) in the photoreceptor cell form huge stacks 600–1000 deep in the outer segment of the cell and originate as deep infolds of the cell membrane (Fig. 19.13).

In rods, photoreceptor discs are formed constantly and pinch off to form free discs, which are shed from the cell when old (Fig. 19.14). In cones, however, photoreceptor discs remain as deep infolds of cell membrane and do not form free discs.

The turnover of cone photoreceptor discs is not clear, but it does not appear to be the same as that of rods.

Rods are about 2 μm thick and an average of 50 μm in length, possessing a roughly cylindrical outer segment. The tips of these cells are embedded in the microvilli of pigment epithelial cells, which phagocytose the old photoreceptor discs.

Cones are thicker and slightly shorter than rods, being 3–5 μm thick and about 40 μm long; their outer segment is conical in shape. Like rods, cones are also located close to the microvilli of the retinal pigment epithelial cells.

The distribution of rods and cones varies within the retina. Cones, which perceive colour, are concentrated in the optical centre of the retina in a small pit (the **fovea**). Rods, which perceive light intensity but not colour, are concentrated at the periphery of the retina.

Between the fovea and the periphery of the retina, there is a mixture of rods and cones (Fig. 19.15).

Fig. 19.13 Photoreceptors. Ultrastructural details of a photoreceptor cell **(a)**. The electron micrographs on the right refer to the areas labelled **(b)**, **(c)**, **(d)** and **(e)** on the artwork. Light is detected by its outer segment (OS), which contains flat plates of membrane (photoreceptor discs, D). The OS is connected to the inner segment (IS) by a connecting cilium (C). The IS contains numerous mitochondria. The cell body (CB) connects to the IS by a microtubule-rich outer fibre (OF). The synaptic body (SB) is cup-shaped and connects to axons (A) from other retinal neurons.

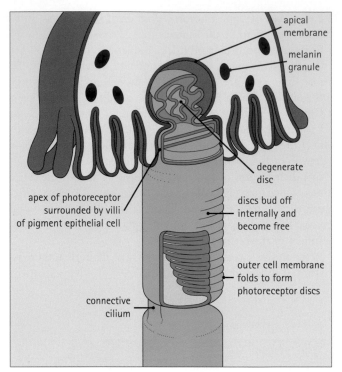

Fig. 19.14 Turnover of Photoreceptor Discs in Rods. In the rod photoreceptor cell, photoreceptor discs originate at the cilial pole of the outer segment as deep infoldings of the cell membrane. These migrate up through the cell and eventually bud off internally to form free discs within the outer segment. At the rod apex, effete and aged discs are eliminated and extruded into the extracellular space, where they are phagocytosed by the retinal pigment epithelial cell into which the rod outer segment is buried. There is a constant flow of new photoreceptor discs along the rod outer segment.

Fig. 19.15 Rods and Cones. Micrograph of a resin section taken tangentially through the retina at the level of the inner segment of the photoreceptors. Rods (R) are identified as thin circular profiles, and cones (C) are larger. There is a mosaic of rods and cones in this retinal area 6 mm temporal to the fovea.

> **The retina contains two main types of support cell: Müller cells and astrocytes.**

Müller cells are tall retinal support cells. They extend from the base of the inner segment of the photoreceptor cells, where they link to each other by adherent junctions (see Fig. 3.9) to form the structure known as the *outer limiting membrane,* up to the retinal surface, where they rest on the internal limiting membrane.

Astrocytes (see p. 106) act as support cells to the nerve cells throughout the retina and are characterized by long dendritic processes that form a scaffold for the delicate processes of nerve cells.

⊚ ADVANCED CONCEPT

Mechanism of Light Detection

In the dark, the photoreceptor cell is strongly depolarized, and this holds voltage-gated Ca^{2+} ion channels open in the synaptic region, resulting in the constant release of an inhibitory transmitter substance at the synaptic terminal. This inhibitor prevents firing of nerve cells connected to the photoreceptor.

When stimulated by light, the photoreceptor becomes hyperpolarized, and release of the inhibitory transmitter substance at the synaptic terminal is reduced. This reduction allows the axons of nerve cells connected to the photoreceptors to fire.

Photoreceptor cells detect light through its interaction with **rhodopsin** molecules. These are membrane-associated glycoproteins in the photoreceptor discs and are composed of a protein (opsin) and a light-sensitive group (*cis*-retinal). The rhodopsin acts as a G protein–coupled receptor.

When *cis*-retinal interacts with a photon, it undergoes a conformational change to the *all-trans*-form (vitamin A), which causes a change in the opsin, leading to a fall in the concentration of a secondary messenger (cyclic guanosine monophosphate [GMP]) within the cytosol of the photoreceptor. This results in closure of sodium channels in the cell membrane and hence hyperpolarization.

> **Nerve cells of the retina interconnect to integrate the signals from photoreceptors.**

The retina contains several classes of nerve cells: bipolar cells, ganglion cells, horizontal cells and amacrine cells. Four phases are involved in light detection in the sensory retina:
1. Photoreception in photoreceptor cells (rods and cones)
2. Synaptic transmission to bipolar cells
3. Synaptic transmission to ganglion cells
4. Transmission along the optic nerve to the brain

At each synaptic stage laterally connecting **horizontal** and **amacrine cells** modulate transmission.

Bipolar cells connect with the synaptic end of the photoreceptor cells and transmit signals to ganglion cells. **Ganglion cells** send axons from the eye to the brain in the optic nerve.

Horizontal cells and **amacrine cells** are neurons that act as 'gates' to modulate the passage of impulses. Their processes interpose the connections between bipolar cells and photoreceptors and between bipolar cells and ganglion cells. This group of gate cells allows the integration of signals from adjacent groups of photoreceptors.

> **Special ganglion cells can detect light and are involved in regulating circadian rhythms.**

A small proportion of retinal ganglion cells are directly able to detect light and are termed *intrinsically photosensitive retinal ganglion cells (ipRGCs).* This understanding has developed after the discovery that individuals with no functioning photoreceptors because of retinal disease were still able to modulate circadian rhythms in response to light. This class of retinal ganglion cell contain the light-sensitive protein melanopsin, which is not expressed by other retinal ganglion cells and is responsive mainly to light in the blue part of the spectrum.

The function of this class of retinal ganglion cells is understood to include:

- Modulating secretion of the hormone melatonin by the pineal gland
- Modulating circadian rhythms through signalling the suprachiasmatic nucleus in the hypothalamus of the brain
- Signalling midbrain nuclei responsible for control of pupillary size in response to light
- Possible roles in mesopic vision

The sensory retina is composed of nine layers made up of different cell types.

- The **photoreceptor layer** of rods and cones, which extends from the retinal pigment epithelium and consists of outer and inner segments of the photoreceptor cells (Fig. 19.16)
- The **external limiting membrane**, which is not a true membrane, but a line marking the zone of adherent junctions between Müller cells
- The **outer nuclear layer**, consisting of the nuclei and cell bodies of the photoreceptor cells, which form eight to nine rows of nuclei

- The **outer plexiform layer**, which contains the cell processes and synaptic connections between the photoreceptor cells, bipolar neurons and horizontal cells
- The **inner nuclear layer**, which is composed of the nuclei and cell bodies of bipolar cells, horizontal cells and amacrine cells, in addition to the nuclei of the Müller cells
- The **inner plexiform layer**, containing the cell processes and synapses of bipolar cells, amacrine cells and ganglion cells
- The **ganglion cell layer**, consisting of a row of ganglion cells which have large nuclei with visible nucleoli, and prominent rough endoplasmic reticulum visible as Nissl substance
- The **nerve fibre layer**, composed of the axons of the ganglion cells en route to the central nervous system via the optic nerve with supporting astrocytic cells
- The **internal limiting membrane**, a barely visible basement membrane at the interface between the vitreous and the retina

The nuclei of rods are small and densely stained, whereas those of cones are larger and pale stained.

In the outer plexiform layer, the synaptic connections to rods are termed *spherals,* whereas those to cones are termed *pedicles.* For both cell types, the terminal of a horizontal cell is interposed between the photoreceptor and the bipolar cell to form a structure termed a *triad.* The horizontal cell can therefore modulate the impulse from the photoreceptors to the bipolar cells and allows integration of signals from adjacent photoreceptors.

Fig. 19.16 Sensory Retina. (a) Micrograph of silver-stained sensory retina showing its nine constituent layers. **(b)** Diagram of the sensory retina showing its nine layers. **(c)** Micrograph of H&E-stained sensory retina.

The amacrine cells of the inner plexiform layer interpose processes between the processes of bipolar cells and ganglion cells and thereby modify the transmission of impulses from the bipolar cells. The ganglion cells of the ganglion layer are separated by the cytoplasm of Müller cells.

CLINICAL EXAMPLE

Diabetic Retinopathy

Ophthalmoscopic examination of the retina (fundoscopy) is an important part of a general medical examination because it provides a direct view of blood vessels in a critical area of the circulation. Retinal blood vessels are frequently affected in disease, particularly diabetes mellitus.

In diabetes mellitus, the basement membrane of small blood vessels in the retina thickens, and the vessels show dilatations termed *microaneurysms*.

The abnormal vessels become leaky and exude fluid into the retina, which is visible as white spots. Haemorrhages may also occur. This particularly affects the macula, leading to loss of visual acuity.

If these changes become severe, the blood supply to the retina is reduced (ischaemia), and this stimulates abnormal growth of new retinal blood vessels (proliferative retinopathy). The newly formed vessels may bleed and also result in retinal detachment.

The severity of diabetic retinopathy, which is the most common cause of blindness in the developed world, is greatly reduced by the careful control of blood sugar levels. Laser coagulation of leaking vessels delays or prevents the development of severe visual loss.

CLINICAL EXAMPLE

Retinal Detachment

The term *retinal detachment* is used to describe splitting of the retina through the photoreceptor layer to leave the attached pigment epithelium. Retinal detachment usually follows a tear in the retina caused either by retinal degeneration or by traction by the vitreous.

The vitreous is normally in contact with the whole of the retina, and rotational shearing forces generated by pulling of the extra-ocular muscles are transmitted uniformly to the whole globe. If the vitreous becomes detached from the retina posteriorly, rotational shearing forces are focally concentrated and cause tearing of the retina.

If the retina does not re-attach, the cell bodies of the rods and cones in the detached area degenerate, with loss of visual function.

The retinal structure is modified in specialized areas.

Optic disc. The axons of the nerve fibre layer converge at the optic disc, which is visible in the retina and gives rise to the optic nerve. This area is devoid of photoreceptors and therefore produces a blind spot in the visual field.

Macula. The macula is a small yellow area located 2.5 mm lateral (temporal) to the optic disc. At its centre, there is a thin zone of retina composed exclusively of cones (the fovea), each cone synapsing with a single bipolar cell and then linking with a single ganglion cell, thus producing a high degree of resolution. This area is at the centre of the visual axis and provides highly detailed colour vision.

The yellow colour of the surrounding macula is caused by the presence of yellow xanthophyll pigment in ganglion cells from the fovea, which are displaced laterally so that light can impinge on the cones of the fovea without being dispersed by an overlying neural layer.

Peripheral retina. In the peripheral retina, many photoreceptors are mapped onto one ganglion cell and form a receptive field with low visual resolution. Electrophysiology has shown that these receptive fields are triggered by different visual stimuli: for example, some ganglion cells only fire in response to a bright light, whereas others respond only to a moving edge.

The retinal blood supply enters with the optic nerve at the back of the globe.

The central artery and vein of the retina enter the back of the eye in the optic nerve and branch in the plane between the vitreous and the inner limiting membrane.

The capillaries, which form a dense plexus within the retina and supply all cells apart from the rods and cones, are characterized by tight junctions between their constituent endothelial cells to prevent diffusion of substances into the neural retina (i.e. they form a **blood–retinal barrier**). The rods and cones are supplied by choroidal vessels.

The retinal vessels are visible by ophthalmoscopic examination and may be damaged in disease: for example, high blood pressure (hypertension) causes visible thickening of the arterial walls.

The optic nerve takes axons from the retina to the brain.

The optic nerve contains the axons from the retinal ganglion cells en route to the central nervous system, in addition to the central artery and vein of the retina.

The optic nerve leaves the retina at the optic disc and penetrates the collagen of the sclera through a sieve-like plate of channels in an area termed the **lamina cribrosa**. Within the orbit, the optic nerve is surrounded by a sheath of dura and an extension of the subarachnoid space (Fig. 19.17).

The optic nerve is invested in the pia arachnoid layers (see Chapter 6), and septa from this layer enter the optic nerve and divide the axons into fascicles.

Fig. 19.17 Optic Nerve and Retina. Micrograph showing the optic nerve (N) in longitudinal section. The central artery and vein of the retina run along its centre. The optic nerve leaves the retina (R) at the optic disc and penetrates the sclera through the lamina cribrosa *(arrow)*. Around the optic nerve is the optic nerve sheath, which is composed of an extension of the dura (D) and subarachnoid space (S) and is filled with cerebrospinal fluid.

CLINICAL EXAMPLE

Papilloedema

If pressure of the cerebrospinal fluid (CSF) within the skull increases (raised intracranial pressure), pressure of the CSF around the optic nerve increases. Initially, this impairs cytoplasmic flow along the optic nerve axons, which swell and cause engorgement of the central artery and vein.

Ophthalmoscopic examination of a normal optic disc reveals that it is a cup-shaped depression, but in cases of raised intracranial pressure, the disc is swollen (papilloedema), with loss of the cup-shaped depression.

Papilloedema is an important physical sign and usually denotes abnormal brain swelling caused by disease.

The lens, a soft transparent biconvex structure composed of crystallin, is encased in a capsule.

In the adult, the lens is 9 mm in diameter and 3.5 mm thick. It has:

- An outer capsule 10–20 μm thick of hyaline material containing type IV collagen
- A layer of large cuboidal epithelial cells (the lens epithelium) beneath the capsule
- A centre composed of tightly packed cells, which have lost their nuclei and become packed by special transparent proteins (crystallin) to form so-called *lens fibres* (Fig. 19.18)

Fig. 19.18 Lens. Micrograph showing the lens capsule (C) as a pink-staining hyaline layer and the subcapsular lens epithelium (E). The centre of the lens (L) is composed of cells devoid of organelles (lens fibres) packed with crystallin proteins.

New lens cells are added to the margin of the lens throughout life from the lens epithelium, but the cells at the centre of the lens do not undergo turnover or replacement and are therefore the oldest cells in the body of an adult.

The lens is avascular and is nourished by diffusion from the aqueous and vitreous.

The lens is suspended by suspensory fibres to the ciliary body, the radial arrangement of suspensory fibres being termed the **ciliary zonule**. These fibres are composed mainly of the fibrillar protein fibrillin (see Chapter 4).

The eye is divided into three chambers.

The **vitreous body** is a transparent gelatinous structure located behind the lens and occupying the space bounded by the inner surface of the retina. The vitreous has a volume of 4 mL and is a specialized support tissue, being composed of a few scattered spindle-shaped cells (hyalocytes); fine, highly dispersed collagen fibres; and an abundant extracellular matrix rich in hyaluronic acid.

The **anterior** and **posterior aqueous chambers** lie anterior to the lens, are delineated by the iris and communicate with each other via the aperture of the pupil (see Fig. 19.8).

The **aqueous humour** is a watery fluid resembling CSF and is secreted at a rate of about 2 mL/min by the epithelial cells of the ciliary body in the posterior chamber. It provides nutrients to the structures it bathes and flows from the posterior chamber through the pupil into the anterior chamber.

Cataracts are areas of opacification in the lens that cause loss of lens transparency and so impair vision. The areas of opacification are caused by degradation of crystallin proteins in the lens fibres. There are three types depending on location within the lens: nuclear, cortical and posterior subcapsular cataracts (Fig. 19.19). The main reason for development of cataracts is ageing, but certain diseases of the eye may predispose to secondary cataract development. Important predisposing factors include ultraviolet B exposure, diabetes mellitus and cigarette smoking. Those affected commonly present with symptoms of blurring of vision and experience haloes seen around bright lights.

Fig. 19.19 Cataracts. **(a)** Schematic view of lens structures and corresponding types of cataracts. Slit lamp examination of affected persons showing **(b)** nuclear cataract, **(c)** wedge-shaped cortical cataract and **(d)** subcapsular posterior cataract. The cataracts appear as ill-defined white areas in the lens. Most patients have more than one type of cataract. (From Liu Y-C, Wilkins M, Kim T, et al. Cataracts. *Lancet*. 2017; 390[10094]:600–612. ISSN 0140-6736, https://doi.org/10.1016/S0140-6736(17)30544-5 with permission.)

The aqueous then filters through a network of spaces lined by endothelium, the **trabecular meshwork** (see Fig. 19.12), which runs around the circumference of the root of the iris, at the periphery of the anterior chamber, and enters the **canal of Schlemm** (Fig. 19.20). This canal runs around the whole circumference of the limbus within the sclera. From the canal of Schlemm, the aqueous enters venous vessels.

The angle between the margin of the cornea and the iris root where the trabecular meshwork lies is the **iridocorneal drainage angle**.

There is a normal resistance to the flow of aqueous at the level of the trabecular meshwork, such that continued secretion and resorption of the aqueous result in a normal intrinsic resting pressure within the globe (intraocular pressure) of 10–22 mmHg.

Fig. 19.20 Canal of Schlemm and Trabecular Meshwork. (a) The canal of Schlemm runs around the circumference of the cornea at the limbus and communicates with the trabecular meshwork, which runs around the circumference of the root of the iris. The aqueous from the anterior chamber of the eye filters through the trabecular meshwork into the canal of Schlemm and thence drains into venous vessels. **(b)** Micrograph showing the trabecular meshwork (T) as an area of slit-like spaces with the canal of Schlemm (CS) within the sclera. The aqueous filters from the anterior chamber (A) just above the iris (I).

CLINICAL EXAMPLE

Glaucoma

Abnormalities in the drainage pathway of aqueous humour result in a rise in the intra-ocular pressure (glaucoma) which, if untreated, damages the nerve cells of the retina and causes blindness.

KEY FACTS

The Eye

- Aqueous humour is produced by the ciliary body, goes through the pupil and drains through the trabecular meshwork into the canal of Schlemm.
- The cornea is kept translucent by the action of the ion-pumping endothelial cells on its inner surface.
- The uvea contains melanocytes and comprises the choroid, ciliary body and iris.
- The photoreceptor layer of the retina is maintained by its close contact with the retinal pigment epithelium.
- The retina is supplied by a single artery that runs through the optic nerve.
- The nerve fibres in the optic nerve originate from the retinal ganglion cells.
- Cones are concentrated in an area of the macula termed the *fovea*, which is responsible for high-resolution colour vision.

ACCESSORY COMPONENTS OF THE EYE

The conjunctiva is composed of a mucin-secreting columnar epithelium.

The normal conjunctiva is a translucent membrane that lines the inner surface of the eyelids (palpebral conjunctiva) and reflects onto the globe (bulbar conjunctiva) to cover its anterior surface up to the margin of the cornea (limbus).

The conjunctiva is covered by layers of stratified columnar epithelium, which give way to a flattened squamous epithelium toward the limbus. Goblet cells (see p. 57) are present in this epithelium but mainly in the medial portion, being scarce in the temporal bulbar conjunctiva (Fig. 19.21).

Beneath the epithelium, the conjunctival stroma is composed of loose fibrocollagenous support tissue with small blood vessels and lymphatics running through it. With ageing, there is loss of collagen in this tissue.

Fig. 19.21 Conjunctiva. Micrograph showing conjunctival epithelium with goblet cells (G) containing mucin overlying the subepithelial support tissues, which contain vessels and a few lymphoid cells.

The eyelids contain many different secretory glands.

The structure of both upper and lower eyelids is similar and comprises the following four layers:

- Skin
- Orbicularis muscle (a layer of skeletal muscle)
- Tarsal plate (a plate of dense fibroelastic tissue)
- Conjunctiva
  Within these layers are various types of glands (Fig. 19.22):
- Meibomian glands, sebaceous in type and secreting a lipid-rich substance that delays evaporation of the tear film that lubricates and protects the cornea
- Glands of Zeis, small sebaceous glands associated with the eyelashes
- Glands of Moll, apocrine sweat glands at the margin of the eyelid
- Glands of Krause, accessory lacrimal glands in the fornix of the conjunctiva
- Glands of Wolfring, accessory lacrimal glands just above the tarsal plate

---

The lacrimal glands produce tears, which drain via a duct system into the nose.

Tears are produced by the main lacrimal gland, which is located beneath the conjunctiva on the upper lateral margin of the orbit, and by the accessory glands of Krause and Wolfring (see Fig. 19.22). The glands secrete a serous fluid, the tears, and have a complex branched structure with secretory acini and ducts (Fig. 19.23). There are three main cell types. Glandular acini are composed of secretory columnar epithelial cells. Ducts leading from acini are lined by cuboidal ductal epithelial cells. Both acini and ducts are surrounded by myoepithelial cells, which function to expel the watery secretions produced by the gland into the lacrimal ducts.

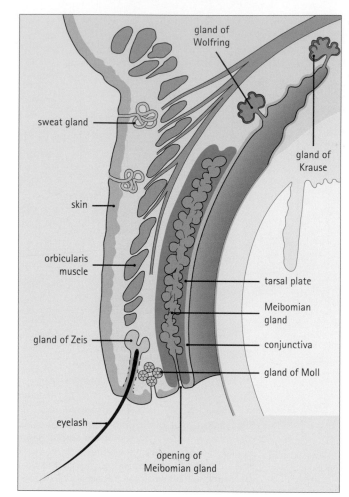

Fig. 19.22 Structure of the Eyelid. The eyelid, which is composed of skin, orbicularis muscle, tarsal plate and conjunctiva and contains various types of glands.

Fig. 19.23 Lacrimal Gland. This micrograph shows the acinar structure of the lacrimal gland. Each acinus is lined by a secretory columnar epithelium. The gland is surrounded by collagenous tissue.

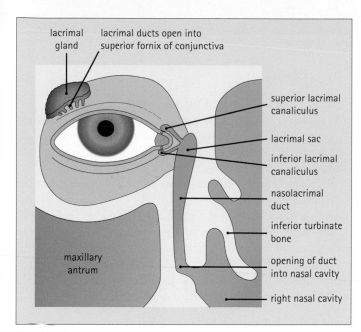

lacrimal gland lacrimal ducts open into superior fornix of conjunctiva

superior lacrimal canaliculus

lacrimal sac

inferior lacrimal canaliculus

nasolacrimal duct

inferior turbinate bone

opening of duct into nasal cavity

right nasal cavity

maxillary antrum

Fig. 19.24 Lacrimal Apparatus. The lacrimal gland discharges tear fluid onto the conjunctiva. Drainage from the conjunctival surfaces is via superior and inferior lacrimal puncta, located at the medial ends of the upper and lower eyelids. These open into small ducts (canaliculi) that unite to drain into the lacrimal sac. The lacrimal sac drains into the nasal space by the nasolacrimal duct, most of which runs within the bone.

The main lacrimal gland drains into the upper fornix of the conjunctiva via a series of about 10 small ducts. Tears then wash over the surface of the eye and drain via two canaliculi located at the medial end of the eyelids. These passages, the superior and inferior lacrimal canaliculi, drain into the lacrimal sac; this empties via the nasolacrimal duct into the nasal cavity through an opening beneath the inferior turbinate bone (Fig. 19.24 and see Chapter 10).

The superior and inferior lacrimal canaliculi are lined by stratified squamous epithelium, whereas the lacrimal sac and nasolacrimal duct are lined by respiratory-type pseudostratified ciliated columnar epithelium.

CLINICAL EXAMPLE

Dry Eye Syndrome

Disorders of the lacrimal gland can cause failure of production of tears, leading to so-called *dry eye syndrome*. Patients experience eye discomfort, redness of the eyes and, when severe, damage to the cornea may occur. In most patients with mild symptoms no cause is found, and symptomatic treatment with eye drops to lubricate the eye surface (artificial tears) is effective.

Several diseases caused by autoimmunity may affect the lacrimal gland and cause reduced tear production, including systemic lupus erythematosus, rheumatoid disease, and Sjögren's syndrome (Fig. 19.25). In these conditions destruction of glandular acini is associated with infiltration of the gland by lymphoid cells as part of an immune-mediated process.

Fig 19.25 Lacrimal Gland Sjögren's Syndrome. This micrograph shows part of a lacrimal gland in which only the dark-stained ducts remain, surrounded by pink-stained fibrous scar tissue infiltrated by blue-staining chronic inflammatory cells. No secretory glandular acini remain. This is the result of an immune-mediated destruction of the acinar cells in the lacrimal gland (compare with Fig. 19.23). Sjögren's syndrome is of unknown causation. The salivary glands can also be affected leading to dry mouth. (Micrograph from digital pathology whole slide image provided by the University of Leeds Virtual Pathology Project https://www.virtualpathology.leeds.ac.uk. Reproduced with permission.)

For online review questions, please visit https://studentconsult.inkling.com.

CHAPTER 2

Case 2.1   A Child With Muscle Weakness

A 2-month-old child is admitted to hospital because his parents are concerned that he has been experiencing difficulty with feeding and becoming breathless. Examination reveals proximal muscle weakness. There is no clinical evidence that the peripheral nerves are involved. Routine blood investigations are normal. In particular, serum creatine kinase levels are normal (the enzyme is released from muscle fibres as they undergo cell death).

A biopsy of skeletal muscle shows excessive glycogen in muscle fibres, with large numbers of lysosomes also containing glycogen. Assay of muscle showed a greatly reduced level of acid alpha-glucosidase (GAA), a lysosomal enzyme. Subsequent echocardiogram shows abnormally thick cardiac muscles.

Q. Describe the functional and structural basis of this case. In particular, classify this type of disease within the spectrum of causes of disease. Why do you think the heart is found to be abnormal?

Case 2.1   Answer

Lysosomes are membrane-bound intracellular organelles and are part of the acid vesicle system. These contain hydrolases that operate at the acidic pH found within the lysosome. In the acid vesicle system there are more than 30 defined and specific acid hydrolases, which not only degrade abnormal large molecules but also recycle or process normal cell constituents. Lysosomes internalize material that is degraded by hydrolases. Among the many substances broken down within the lysosome is glycogen. The enzyme responsible for the breakdown of glycogen is GAA (formerly called *acid maltase*).

In this case, GAA activity is greatly reduced in association with the accumulation of glycogen within muscle. This has led to muscle disease with clinical features of proximal muscle weakness and poor ability to feed.

This type of disease is called a **lysosomal storage disorder** and is caused by a genetic defect that leads to lack of activity of one of the enzymes normally found within lysosomes. The substance that would normally be broken down by the missing enzyme accumulates within the cells and causes damage. Clinical manifestations of lysosomal storage diseases are mostly related to damage to cells that are non-dividing permanent populations such as neurons, skeletal muscle and liver tissue.

The heart is abnormal because the cardiac muscle cells are also affected. Were an endomyocardial biopsy to be performed, this would also show abnormal accumulation of glycogen within cells.

Other causes of abnormal glycogen storage are also the result of genetic defects that lead to reduced activity of enzymes involved in glycogen metabolism.

This disease is defined as the following:
- A storage disorder – The disease is associated with abnormal accumulation and storage of a substance within cells.
- A lysosomal storage disease – The disease is caused by absence of a lysosomal enzyme.
- A glycogenosis – The disease is associated with the abnormal handling of glycogen.

Muscle diseases that are associated with abnormalities of skeletal muscle fibres are termed **myopathies**. In this case, the patient's condition would be classified as a metabolic myopathy.

Cardiac diseases that are caused by primary defects in myocardial muscle fibres are termed **cardiomyopathies**. This child would be classed as having a cardiomyopathy.

Case 2.2   A Tumour of Unknown Origin

A 37-year-old man has been referred to hospital for investigation. He had noted a swelling in his neck, and his doctor felt that this was because of enlarged lymph nodes. On examination, the man had several palpable enlarged lymph nodes in the right lower cervical region. Detailed imaging confirmed enlarged lymph nodes but no obvious associated lesions in other organs. A surgeon has removed an enlarged node and sent it for histological examination to determine the cause of disease. A poorly differentiated tumour is discovered but its origin is not clear from initial histology.

Q. How might immunohistochemical assessment using antibodies to different cell constituents help in diagnosis? Concentrate on how expression of intermediate filaments could help with the diagnosis. What other cellular markers might be considered?

Case 2.2   Answer

When a biopsy shows a tumour, optimal treatment depends on characterizing the type of tumour, which requires ascertaining its cell of origin. In most instances, this is not a diagnostic problem, and routine histological examination allows for a diagnosis to be made based on morphology alone. However, in some patients, histological examination using haemoxylin and eosin (H&E) staining does not allow the cell of origin of a tumour to be determined. The case under discussion is a common clinical problem: metastatic disease (i.e. a malignant tumour that has spread from its organ or tissue of origin to another site such as a lymph node or the liver) is discovered in the absence of any known primary site.

In such cases, standard histological examination is supplemented by immunohistochemical assessment of the tumour to detect markers that might point to the cell of origin. It is common to perform immunohistochemical staining using a panel of antibodies capable of detecting a wide range of possible tumours.

The intermediate filaments are composed of protein subunits and form part of the cytoskeleton. Different types of intermediate filaments characterize different cell types. The main types are as follows:

Cell Type	Intermediate Filament
Mesenchymal cells and other cell types	Vimentin
Epithelial cells	Cytokeratins
Neurons	Neurofilament proteins
Glial cells	Glial fibrillary acidic protein (GFAP)
Muscle cells	Desmin

If immunostaining is performed using antibodies against specific intermediate filament proteins, it is possible to determine the cell of origin of a tumour.

In this case, expression of cytokeratins would lead to the conclusion that the tumour was of epithelial origin and was therefore some sort of carcinoma (**carcinoma** is the term used to refer to malignant tumour of an epithelial tissue).

Epithelial cells from different tissues can also express specific proteins useful in diagnosis. For example:

- Tumours derived from prostatic epithelium may be detected by immunostaining for prostate-specific antigen or prostate-specific acid phosphatase.
- Tumours derived from the thyroid may be detected by immunostaining for thyroglobulin.
- Tumours derived from the breast may express oestrogen receptor.
- Tumours derived from the gastrointestinal tract may express carcinoembryonic antigen (CEA).
- Tumours of lymphoid tissues express markers of normal lymphoid cells.
- Tumours of muscle often express desmin, the intermediate filament of muscle.

It would be very unusual for a tumour of the nervous system to spread to lymph nodes. However, tumours that arise in the nervous system can be characterized by immunostaining for GFAP and neurofilament proteins to determine their cell of origin.

Any tumour of neuroendocrine type can be characterized by detecting proteins expressed on neurosecretory granules, such as synaptophysin or chromogranin A.

Vimentin is expressed by so many cell types that it is not particularly helpful in diagnosis.

In some patients, a tumour becomes so poorly differentiated that no diagnostically helpful pattern of expression of any protein is seen. Such anaplastic tumours generally carry a very poor prognosis.

CHAPTER 3

Case 3.1   Nodules in the Liver

A 62-year-old man is admitted to hospital with abdominal pain. On examination, he has an enlarged liver, and investigations show multiple nodules in the liver. Although a diagnosis of cancer spreading to the liver is strongly suspected, detailed imaging reveals no obvious site for a primary tumour. Under image guidance, a needle biopsy of one of the liver lesions is performed. This reveals unusual cells in the liver that are characterized by large, densely stained nuclei, variation in nuclear size and many mitoses.

Q. What do the histological features suggest as a likely diagnosis? What other histological assessments could be done to help refine the diagnosis? Concentrate on why these features do not fit with normal histology. What stains can be used to help determine cellular differentiation?

Case 3.1   Answer

Normal cells and tissues are characterized by a uniformity of cytology and a coherence of tissue architecture.

Cell division is usually restricted to a specific part of a tissue, for example, the basal layer of the epidermis of the skin or the crypts in the intestinal mucosa. Cells are usually of uniform size within any given tissue and tend not to show much variation in size or shape. In normal cells, the intensity of nuclear staining is related to the activity of the cell.

Neoplastic cells from malignant tumours are often found to have nuclei that are more darkly staining than in normal tissues (hyperchromatism). They also show variation in nuclear size and shape (pleomorphism), and evidence of cell proliferation exists in the form of mitoses.

In this case, the finding of cells with variable size and shape, mitoses and darkly stained nuclei suggests a neoplastic process and raises the possibility that the lesions in the liver are tumours.

In any tissue, a malignant process can be caused by a tumour arising locally (primary tumour) or spreading to the tissue from another site (metastatic tumour).

Histological assessment of a tumour is an important part of diagnosis and may be the investigation that suggests the original site of origin. This is important because prognosis and therapy of tumours are related to the site of origin and histogenesis.

Differentiation of tissues can be detected by conventional stains, immunohistochemical staining, electron microscopy and molecular genetic testing.

Conventional stains such as Alcian blue or periodic acid–Schiff (PAS) can detect the presence of mucin, which in this case would suggest that the tumour was epithelial in origin and of glandular differentiation; therefore the tumour would be classified as an adenocarcinoma.

Immunohistochemistry can be used to detect proteins expressed by cells that are specific to different cell types (see details as described in answer to Case 2.2). The majority of tumours that involve the liver are secondary, metastatic tumours that have spread from another site. Common sites of origin include carcinomas arising from the stomach or colon, lung and breast.

Primary malignant tumours may develop in the liver either arising from hepatocytes or from bile duct epithelium. In such cases markers can be applied using immunohistochemical staining and are related to the cell lineage of the tumour. As an example, a panel of antibodies might be used to investigate whether a tumour was a primary hepatocellular carcinoma derived from hepatocytes. Positive staining might be expected for cytokeratins 8 and 18, Hep Par1, glutamine synthetase, glypican-3, alpha-fetoprotein and CD10.

The key concept to take away from this case is that histological examination using a panel of antibodies using immunohistochemistry provides important clinical diagnostic information.

CHAPTER 4

Case 4.1   Infant With a Broken Femur

Parents bring their 1-year-old daughter to the hospital as an emergency. They give a history that after a bath she had been pulling up to stand, when there was a 'popping' noise and she collapsed, screaming out in pain. She lay on the floor crying with pain. Her leg looked deformed and appeared broken.

An x-ray confirms a fractured femur. In the hospital, there was an initial suspicion of possible non-accidental injury. However, further detailed investigation showed that the child had a genetic abnormality in type I collagen formation of the type known to be associated with 'brittle bones'.

Q. Explain how this molecular defect relates to abnormal bone fragility. Knowing that there are many types of collagen, each with a different gene and tissue distribution, predict which organs and tissues may be affected by genetically abnormal collagen.

Case 4.1   Answer

The strength of bone is determined by its extracellular matrix proteins and its mineralization. Osteoblasts elaborate the support matrix of bone, osteoid, which subsequently calcifies to form bone.

Osteoid is composed mainly of type I collagen, which is associated with the extracellular glycosaminoglycans (GAGs) chondroitin sulphate and keratin sulphate. Two glycoproteins, sialoprotein and osteocalcin, are mainly found in the bone matrix and bind calcium; therefore they may have a role in bone mineralization. In children, several types of so-called 'brittle bone disease' are recognized, properly called **osteogenesis imperfecta** (OI).

OI is a dominant inherited condition that leads to a disorder of type I collagen, which is the main extracellular matrix protein of bone. Several forms of OI have been described, and only the most common types (I–IV) are presented here.

Type I

- Most common and mildest form
- Bones predisposed to fracture
- Most fractures occur before puberty
- Triangular face
- Sclerae have a blue or grey tint
- Patients may have spinal curvature
- Bone deformity absent or minimal
- Collagen structure is normal, but the amount is less than normal

Type II

- Fractures are numerous and severe, resulting in bone deformity
- Most severe form

- Often lethal at or shortly after birth
- Small stature develops
- Collagen is improperly formed

Type III

- Bones fracture easily
- Fractures are often present at birth
- Short stature develops with bone deformity
- Triangular face
- Sclerae have a blue or grey tint
- Patients may have spinal curvature
- Collagen is improperly formed

Type IV

- Intermediate in severity between types I and III
- Bones fracture easily, most before puberty
- Triangular face
- Sclerae normal in colour
- Generally only moderate bone deformity
- Patients may have spinal curvature (scoliosis)
- Collagen is improperly formed

CHAPTER 5

Case 5.1   Sudden Cardiac Death

A 24-year-old male is brought into hospital by ambulance, having collapsed while running in a half-marathon. Paramedics had attended, and he was found to have no cardiac output and was in asystole. He was pronounced dead, and an autopsy was requested to establish the cause of death.

The pathologist found that the heart was greatly enlarged and showed hypertrophy of the left ventricle. The left ventricular wall was much thicker than normal. Histology showed that myocardial cells were greatly enlarged and had an abnormal pattern of myofibres. A diagnosis of hypertrophic cardiomyopathy was made. Further genetic testing showed a mutation in one of the genes coding for cardiac-specific myosin.

Q. Explain the relationship between the mutation in the gene and cardiac disease.

Case 5.1   Answer

Cardiac muscle is a form of striated muscle. Individual cardiac muscle cells are joined end to end at intercalated discs to form long fibres. Nuclei are typically in the centre of each cardiac muscle cell.

The term **hypertrophic** refers to the fact that the mass of the heart is enlarged by an increase in the size of individual cardiac muscle cells. The term **cardiomyopathy** implies that heart disease has resulted from a primary defect in the cardiac muscle.

The main contractile proteins in cardiac striated muscle are actin and myosin. Myosin interacts with several other proteins to form a regular array of contractile proteins arranged in striations.

The proteins involved in muscle contraction may be abnormal because of a mutation in the coding gene. In some patients with mutation in a gene form of cardiac myosin, contraction of muscle fibres is inefficient, leading to cardiac hypertrophy (enlargement of individual muscle cells that causes an increase in total mass of the myocardium).

It is now recognized that mutation in the genes coding for several muscle proteins, each of which is part of the contractile mechanism, can lead to hypertrophic cardiomyopathy. Mutations in the genes for cardiac myosin-binding protein C (MYBPC3) and β-myosin heavy chain (MYH7) account for about 80% of families with identified mutations.

CHAPTER 6

Case 6.1   Possible Epileptic Seizure

A 52-year-old man is admitted to hospital because he has collapsed with a possible epileptic seizure. Clinical examination suggests that he has mild weakness of the right side of the body. A computed tomography (CT) scan shows an abnormal area in the left cerebral hemisphere, which is felt to be a possible brain tumour.

Q. What cells can give rise to tumours affecting the brain?

Case 6.1   Answer

The main cell types in the brain are neurons and glial cells comprising astrocytes, oligodendrocytes, ependymal cells and microglia. Outside the brain are epithelial cells associated with the meninges; such cells are called **meningothelial cells**. Tumours can arise from any of these cell types.

The most common primary tumours arise from glial cells (gliomas) in the form of astrocytic tumours. Less common are tumours of oligodendrocytes (oligodendrogliomas) and ependymal cells.

Tumours that contain neurons are not very common compared with those that are purely glial.

True tumours of the resting phagocytic cells of the brain, the microglia, are extremely rare. However, lymphoid cells that migrate through the brain can cause tumours – so-called **cerebral lymphomas**.

One of the most common tumours that affect the brain is derived from the epithelial cells of the meninges, which form **meningiomas**.

In childhood, tumours arise from small primitive cells that are believed to be related to the primitive neuroectoderm. Such tumours can have a variety of patterns of differentiation.

In adults, a common cause of a mass lesion (tumour) in the brain is metastasis of a malignant tumour arising from a primary site elsewhere in the body.

Magnetic resonance (MR) imaging often shows features which narrow the diagnosis to either a primary or metastatic tumour. Neurosurgical intervention and taking a biopsy of a tumour is usually required to get a histological diagnosis. As with other cases, immunohistochemical assessment of a biopsy is performed in order to characterize the histogenesis of any brain tumour. Increasingly, molecular assessment to determine genetic changes is also used to define the specific type of primary brain tumour and determine subsequent further treatment.

Case 6.2   Diabetes-Related Neuropathy

A 45-year-old patient with diabetes mellitus complains of numbness in the hands and feet. He has developed ulcers on the toes that are painless. Clinical examination shows reduced sensation to pain, touch and vibration in the hands and feet. A nerve conduction study shows a reduced speed of conduction (low-conduction velocity). A diagnosis of peripheral neuropathy is made.

Q. Describe the structural elements of peripheral nerve that may have become abnormal. Given that there is a reduced nerve conduction velocity, what component is most likely to be affected?

Case 6.2   Answer

A peripheral nerve is composed of the following:
- Axons
- Schwann cells, which make myelin
- Spindle-shaped fibroblast support cells, which produce fibrocollagenous tissue
- Blood vessels

There are three types of support tissue in a nerve trunk: the endoneurium, the perineurium and the epineurium.

Endoneurium is composed of longitudinally oriented collagen fibres, extracellular matrix material rich in glycosaminoglycans and sparse fibroblasts. It surrounds the individual axons and their associated Schwann cells, in addition to capillary blood vessels.

Perineurium surrounds groups of axons and endoneurium to form small bundles (fascicles). It is composed of seven or eight concentric layers of epithelium-like flattened cells separated by layers of collagen. The cells are joined by junctional complexes, and each layer of cells is surrounded by an external lamina.

Epineurium is an outer sheath of loose fibrocollagenous tissue that binds individual nerve fascicles into a nerve trunk. The epineurium may also include adipose tissue, along with a main muscular artery supplying the nerve trunk.

In a peripheral neuropathy, the structures most likely to be damaged are the axons or the myelin and Schwann cells. In some cases, disease is caused by abnormalities in blood vessels that lead to local ischaemia of a nerve.

The speed of conduction along nerves is limited by the electrical capacitance and resistance of the axon. Because wide axons have a lower capacitance than narrow ones, increasing the diameter of axons is a useful means of increasing the speed of nerve conduction. This is inefficient, however, because giant axons require high metabolic upkeep. The speed of conduction along axons is increased by myelination, with conduction taking place at the nodes of Ranvier. The abnormal reduction in conduction velocity seen in this patient suggests that the main problem is loss of myelin from nerves (demyelination).

Diabetic patients are especially prone to development of peripheral neuropathy.

CHAPTER 7

Case 7.1   A Man Who Was Tired and Weak

A 62-year-old man is admitted to hospital for investigation. He had gone to his family physician feeling generally unwell and tired. A full blood count had shown a greatly reduced red cell count, together with a reduction in the number of circulating white cells and platelets. Red cells were of normal size (normocytic) and contained normal amounts of haemoglobin (normochromic).

The neutrophil count was 0.5×10^9/L.

The platelet count was 20×10^9/L.

A diagnosis of pancytopenia was made, and further investigations were performed. A biopsy of the bone marrow was taken and showed a low cellularity affecting all precursors. A diagnosis of aplastic anaemia was made.

Q. Describe the structural and histological background to this case. Concentrate on describing the normal formation of the cells in the blood, and describe the functional complications that may be expected from disease.

Case 7.1   Answer

In aplastic anaemia, the quantity of all cellular elements in the blood is reduced because of failure of the bone marrow to manufacture cells.

In normal bone marrow, stem cells divide and produce committed progenitor cells that produce the various cell lineages.

All cellular elements of the blood originate from a common pluripotential progenitor stem cell (haemopoietic stem cell, HSC). These pluripotential stem cells are present in very small numbers at sites of blood cell formation, and even fewer of them can be found in the peripheral blood. Histologically, they resemble lymphocytes but can be identified by the use of immunohistochemical techniques because they have distinctive cell surface antigens. The pluripotential cells divide and give rise to cells with a more restricted line of growth.

It is possible to divide blood-forming cells into four groups, depending on capacity for self-renewal, cell division and ability to form different cell types. Pluripotential stem cells are capable of forming any type of blood cell; multipotential progenitor cells are capable of forming a specific but wide range of blood cells; committed progenitor cells are capable of forming only one or two types of blood cells; and maturing cells are undergoing structural differentiation to form one cell type and so are incapable of division.

Growth control of blood stem cells is through secreted growth factors and local cell contacts.

The best understood mechanism of control of growth of the different types of HSCs is through the action of growth factors. These substances are secreted systemically or locally and modulate three aspects of cell growth:

- Proliferation
- Differentiation
- Maturation

Less well understood in the control of blood cell formation is the role of local cell–cell contacts. Stromal cells in the bone marrow appear to be important in the control of differentiation and maturation; however, the signals involved are at present uncertain.

Aplastic anaemia can be associated with a variety of conditions and can be encountered as a disease of unknown cause:

- Reduction in platelets leads to increased tendency to bleed, with ease of bruising and bleeding from gums often being described by an affected person.

- Reduction in red cells leads to clinical features of anaemia, with tiredness, fatigue and breathlessness often being described by an affected person.
- Reduction in white cells leads to susceptibility to infection.

In this case, a bone marrow biopsy showed a lack of precursor cells for all formed elements in the marrow. This indicates that the reduced cellularity of all elements in the blood is caused by a failure of marrow production rather than a process of increased peripheral consumption or loss of cells.

CHAPTER 8

Case 8.1   A Boy With Big Lymph Nodes

A 12-year-old boy is admitted to hospital for investigation of enlarged lymph nodes in the neck. He had been complaining of being unwell for about 6 weeks and had lost weight. He had what his mother described as drenching sweating attacks at night that often woke him up. On examination, he had palpable enlarged lymph nodes in the neck.

Surgical excision of a lymph node was performed so that it could be looked at histologically. The reporting pathologist noted the following: 'There is expansion of germinal centres associated with extensive expansion of deep cortical areas. There are multiple aggregates of epithelioid macrophages with multinucleate forms within the lymph node. These are surrounded by zones of activated T cells. The appearances are those of granulomatous inflammation. In the centre of many granulomas are areas of necrosis. These features suggest that tuberculous infection is the most likely cause'.

Q. Describe the anatomical and histological background to the case. Concentrate on describing the normal structure of a lymph node.

Case 8.1   Answer

This clinical case illustrates a common problem: an enlarged lymph node of uncertain cause. The lymph node is a bean-shaped organ with a fibrocollagenous capsule from which fibrous trabeculae extend into the node to form a supporting framework.

Lymph nodes contain three functional compartments:

- A network of endothelial-lined lymphatic sinuses continuous with the lumina of the afferent and efferent lymphatic vessels
- A network of small blood vessels, where circulating lymphocytes enter the node
- A parenchymal compartment composed of superficial cortex, deep cortex and medulla

The superficial cortex of the lymph node contains the densely staining spheroid aggregations of lymphocytes (lymphoid follicles). Some of the follicles (primary follicles) are of fairly uniform staining density; however, most of the follicles that respond to antigen have less densely staining germinal centres and are described as secondary follicles. The lymphocyte population of the follicles consists predominantly of B cells, but there are smaller populations of TH cells, macrophages and accessory cells.

The cell population of the deep cortex consists of lymphocytes and accessory cells, which constantly move in and out of the region. T cells dominate the deep cortex, entering the node from the blood via the high endothelial venules (HEVs) and leaving via the efferent lymphatics. When activated, T cells enlarge to form lymphoblasts. These then proliferate to produce an expanded clone of activated T cells. In a T-cell–dominated immunological response, the deep cortex may expand into the medulla, producing a so-called 'paracortical reaction'. Activated T cells are then disseminated via the circulation to peripheral sites, where much of their activity occurs.

In this case, the lymph node is characterized by expansion of both cortex (B-cell) and deep cortical (T-cell) areas. One aspect of the function of activated T cells is the secretion of cytokines and the recruitment and activation of macrophages. This is the functional background to the formation of aggregates of histiocytic cells to form structures called **granulomas**.

Several disorders trigger T cells to activate macrophages and cause a granulomatous inflammatory response. Histological features of the granuloma can point to a likely cause. When associated with necrosis, granulomatous inflammation in a lymph node is likely to have been caused by tuberculous infection. Further investigation to characterize the presence of mycobacteria would normally be performed.

CHAPTER 9

Case 9.1   Sudden Death in an Obese Woman

A 57-year-old obese woman collapses with acute breathlessness, becomes blue in the face and dies within a few minutes. According to her husband, she had been unwell with flu for about 4 days, most of which time she had spent in bed. The family practitioner explains to the distraught husband that the death must be referred to the coroner for the district and that an autopsy will be necessary. He undertakes to meet the widower after the autopsy to explain to him the cause of death, and few days later the husband arrives with a death certificate issued by the coroner, which states:

Cause of death   1(a)   Massive pulmonary thromboembolism
                 (b)   Deep vein thrombosis (Rt leg)

The family practitioner explains that a blood clot had formed in the veins deep in the muscles of the right calf and had probably enlarged over a few days. A piece of the blood clot had then broken off and passed into the main blood vessel of the lung that it blocked off, leading to sudden death.

Q. Describe the structural and anatomical background to this case.

Case 9.1   Answer

A vein is lined by endothelium. Under normal circumstances, endothelial cells express proteins that prevent platelet adhesion and activation. However, changes in the composition of the blood can shift the balance and render it more prone to coagulate. Amongst other predisposing factors are dehydration and infection. Obstruction or reduction in the flow of blood through veins can predispose to activation of coagulation, and bed rest can be sufficient to predispose to activation of blood coagulation

The local activation of blood coagulation in a vein is a pathological process called **thrombosis**. You can refer to a pathology textbook for a thorough discussion of this topic. Thrombosis is the pathological process in which a solid thrombus forms within the blood circulatory system. A thrombus is composed of aggregated blood platelets meshed together with strands of fibrin, an insoluble polymeric protein molecule derived from the soluble blood protein fibrinogen. In simple terms, platelets aggregate on a damaged endothelial surface and release factors that, with other factors from the damaged vessel wall, initiate the so-called **coagulation cascade**, a sequence of stepwise chemical reactions that ultimately catalyses the conversion of soluble fibrinogen (a normal plasma protein) into insoluble fibrin. The fibrin meshes with the original aggregated platelets, and additional masses of platelets become adherent, stimulating yet more fibrin formation. Thus in certain circumstances, a thrombus may grow relentlessly until it is big enough to completely block the lumen of a vessel. Fragments of thrombus may break off from the original site of formation and pass to another site in the blood circulation. This is called **thromboembolism** and is the cause of death in this case.

Anything solid that forms in the leg veins and breaks off will be carried in the venous flow into the right side of the heart and from there into the pulmonary artery system. In detail, the route leads from the deep veins in the right calf into the right femoral vein, the right external iliac vein, the right common iliac vein and the inferior vena cava. The mass passes up the inferior vena cava and into the right atrium, through the tricuspid right atrioventricular valve into the right ventricle and out of the heart through the pulmonary valve into the large common pulmonary artery trunk.

So far, the mass of thrombus has passed through vessels that are increasingly large in bore. However, at the division of the common pulmonary trunk into right and left main pulmonary arteries, the vessels begin to have a smaller bore. Eventually, the solid mass meets a blood vessel that is too small in bore to permit further passage, and an impaction occurs, completely blocking off the blood vessel. The clinical effect on the patient depends on the size of vessel obstructed. When both main pulmonary arteries are blocked, cardiac output fails and sudden death occurs.

Case 9.2   A Man With Central Chest Pain

A 62-year-old cab driver is admitted to hospital as an emergency with a central crushing chest pain, persisting for 14 hours. It came on while he was gardening but did not go away when he rested, nor overnight with complete bed rest. On examination, he was severely breathless, with white froth on his lips, cyanosed and in distress. He had a weak rapid pulse and was hypotensive (low blood pressure). The examining physician could hear widespread crepitations over both lung fields and could hear a scratching noise over the heart area in time with each systole; he explains to some attending students that this represents a pericardial friction rub. An electrocardiogram (ECG) carried out in the emergency room (ER) shows changes that the physician explains as indicative of an anteroseptal myocardial infarction of the left ventricle.

After emergency treatment in the ER, the patient is transferred to a coronary care unit, where his cardiac activity is continuously monitored and treatment is maintained.

He appears to be making a good recovery, but on the eighth day he suddenly collapses and dies. At postmortem, his pericardial cavity is found to be greatly distended by blood.

Q. Describe the structural and anatomical background that explains this case. Include an explanation for the pericardial friction rub and the postmortem findings in the pericardium.

Case 9.2   Answer

The diagnosis in this case is anteroseptal myocardial infarction of the left ventricle. The anatomy can be broken down as follows:

- Left ventricle – This is the most substantial and bulky component of the heart. The chamber receives oxygenated blood from the lungs via the left atrium and pumps it throughout the body at high pressure. Therefore it has a thick wall of contractile cardiac muscle lined by smooth endothelium and covered externally by the smooth epicardium. Because it has a large work output, the muscle of the left ventricle has a high demand for oxygenated blood, supplied by coronary arteries.
- Anteroseptal part of the left ventricle – This part of the left ventricle consists of the anterior wall of the left ventricle and the anterior half of the interventricular septum. This part of the heart is usually supplied by the anterior descending branch of the left coronary artery.
- Myocardial infarction – This is the name given to the pathological process in which death of myocardium (cardiac muscle) results from an abrupt interference with its oxygenated blood supply. It usually follows sudden complete obstruction of a branch of a coronary artery.

In this case, complete obstruction of the anterior descending branch of the left coronary artery has led to necrosis of the myocardium in the anteroseptal part of the left ventricle.

The following symptoms displayed by this man are typical of myocardial infarction:

- Central crushing pain in the chest, which persists and does not improve with rest
- Breathlessness (see later)
- Distress

The following physical signs, elicited on examination, are also typical:

- Shock (weak rapid pulse, low blood pressure)
- Cyanosis (see later)
- White froth on the lips (see later)
- Widespread crepitations over both lung fields (see later)
- Pericardial friction rub (see later)

The clinicopathological correlation of myocardial infarction can be briefly summarized as follows: The damaged left ventricle is unable to contract efficiently, so the left ventricular output is reduced; this produces the low blood pressure and a weak pulse, and the heart rate increases in an attempt to augment the cardiac output. The pulse rate is rapid.

Another manifestation of the failing function of the left ventricle is its inability to empty completely with each systole. With each diastole, the same amount of blood pours into the left ventricle from the left atrium, to be added to the blood remaining in the left ventricular chamber at the end of systole. After the development of left ventricular wall failure, the left ventricle begins to dilate. The filling pressure rises in the left ventricle and is eventually transmitted backward into the left atrium and from there into pulmonary veins and back into the pulmonary capillaries. The increase in pulmonary capillary pressure has important clinical and pathological consequences.

High pressure in the extensive pulmonary capillary network leads to transudation of some of the fluid content of the blood in the capillaries into the alveolar air sacs. (The pulmonary capillaries are in intimate contact with the alveolar air sac wall.) The consequence of this is that the air sacs become filled with watery fluid, which interferes with gas transfer (pulmonary oedema), and this reduces oxygenation of the blood, producing breathlessness and cyanosis, both of which (combined with the severe chest pain) produce distress. The white froth around the lips is oedema fluid originating in the alveoli of the lungs and being coughed up through the main airways – an indication of severe widespread pulmonary oedema. On auscultation of the lungs, the movement of inspired air trying to get into the alveoli containing watery fluid gives rise to the physical sign called **crepitation**.

Infarction of the full thickness of the left ventricular wall also leads to damage to the inner endocardium and the outer epicardium, both of which can produce major complications. An indication that the epicardium has been affected is the presence on auscultation of a pericardial friction rub, a high-pitched scratching noise that occurs in time with each systolic heartbeat caused by inflammation of the epicardium. An acute inflammatory reaction in response to the presence of dead cardiac muscle leads to deposition of fibrin within the pericardial sac. The final fatal complication, filling the pericardial sac with blood, has been rupture of the myocardial wall. The dead muscle layer becomes soft, and under systolic pressure the heart wall ruptures, filling the pericardial sac with blood and leading to sudden death.

CHAPTER 10

Case 10.1   A Case of Anosmia

A 24-year-old man was involved in a drunken fracas outside a nightclub, during which he was thrown to the ground and banged his head on a concrete slab. He was admitted to hospital unconscious with profuse nosebleeds, and investigations showed a crack fracture of the base of the skull in the anterior cranial fossa. For 2 hours, watery fluid also passed down the nose, and tests showed characteristics of cerebrospinal fluid. He was treated conservatively, recovered consciousness and made a good recovery. His only long-term impairment was total anosmia (loss of sense of smell).

Q. Describe the structural background to this case.

Case 10.1   Answer

This man's total loss of the sense of smell followed an episode of severe trauma to the skull, during which he sustained a crack fracture to the base of his skull in the anterior cranial fossa. The olfactory nerves and bulb lie on the floor of the anterior cranial fossa on either side of the midline, running in an anterior-posterior direction. They may be transected in a transverse fracture across the floor of the anterior cranial fossa, resulting in loss of the sense of smell. Posttraumatic anosmia has been found in around 20% of persons after head injury. It may be related to damage to the olfactory nerves or olfactory cortex, as suspected in this case because of the location of the skull fracture. In other patients, damage to other cortical areas, especially the insular cortex, can be associated with disturbance of the perception of smell rather than loss of the sense of smell.

Case 10.2   A Case of Hoarse Voice

A 69-year-old man is referred to an otorhinolaryngologist because of progressive loss of voice for 3 weeks, getting worse daily. On direct laryngoscopic examination, the surgeon finds a small, warty malignant tumour growing on the free edge of the left true vocal cord. It does not seem to have spread anteriorly or posteriorly to the commissures. Biopsy shows a carcinoma, a malignant tumour of the epithelium, originating from the epithelium covering the true cord.

Q. Describe the structural background to this case. Explain why the lack of involvement of commissures is important, and speculate whether this man's prognosis would have been better if the tumour had originated in the false cords instead of the true cords.

Case 10.2   Answer

This man's loss of voice is the result of a structural abnormality in the laryngeal region, and the loss of voice means that the true cords are involved. Loss of voice has many causes, including bacterial or viral infection ('laryngitis'), but long-standing and progressive loss of voice means that a tumour must be excluded, particularly in elderly smokers. Phonation (voice production) is dependent on vibration of the freely moving true vocal cords under the control of the vocalis muscle and laryngeal nerves.

Even benign tumours can affect the structure of the true cord enough to produce symptoms such as hoarseness, but invasive malignant tumours so disrupt the anatomy of the true cord that progressive hoarseness eventually leads to complete loss of voice. This malignant tumour is derived from the stratified squamous epithelium that covers the outer surface of the true cord.

Malignant tumours can spread away from the site of origin by various mechanisms, including invasion into the lumen of a lymphatic vessel at the original tumour site, and clumps of tumour cells can break off and pass through the lymphatic vessels to regional lymph nodes. Spread to the lymph nodes in the side of the neck is common in carcinoma of the larynx. The true cords contain no lymphatic vessels except at the commissures, so spread to distant sites is common only when the primary tumour in the true cord extends to involve the commissures.

The other parts of the laryngeal apparatus, such as the false cords, are well supplied with lymphatic vessels, so tumours originating in these sites are much more likely to spread away from the primary site to regional lymph nodes than tumours confined to the true cord, with a correspondingly poor prognosis.

Case 10.3   A Case of Deteriorating Chest Infection

A 78-year-old woman, a resident in a care home, became ill during an influenza epidemic, with fever, malaise, runny nose, sore throat and a cough. Whereas the other members of the care home who had also contracted influenza showed evidence of improvement after 5 or 6 days, this lady did not improve, becoming increasingly short of breath and mentally confused. She is admitted to hospital, where physical examination indicates that the bases of both lung fields are solid, with little or no air entry. Urgent chest x-ray confirms that there is consolidation of the lungs in the basal parts of the lower lobes, indicating pneumonia.

Q. Describe the structural background to this case. Explain how infecting organisms can spread through the lung.

Case 10.3   Answer

Pneumonia has developed in both lungs, but it is confined to the basal parts of the lower lobes. In bacterial pneumonia, bacteria gain access to the alveolar air sacs in two main ways: by being carried down in bronchial mucus from higher up the respiratory tree in situations in which the normal mucociliary ladder does not work or by being inhaled directly into the air sacs.

In this older adult woman who has recently had an upper respiratory tract infection, the bacteria have initially colonized an upper respiratory tract that has been damaged by a preceding viral infection (influenza) that severely damaged the surface epithelium of the trachea and main and branch bronchi, destroying in particular the surface cilia normally responsible for sweeping the thin sheet of bronchial mucus upwards. In the absence of these defence mechanisms, the bronchial mucus slides down the bronchial tree under the influence of gravity, and the bronchioles in the distal respiratory tree become obstructed with mucus. As they pass downwards, the bacteria infect the trachea (tracheitis), the bronchi (bronchitis) and the bronchioles (bronchiolitis), and when they reach the thin-walled terminal and respiratory bronchioles, the bacteria can pass out through the walls to infect the alveolar air sacs around the bronchioles. This pattern of spread of bacterial lung infection is called **bronchopneumonia**.

CHAPTER 11

Case 11.1   An Obese Man With Heartburn

An obese man of 56, a heavy smoker, is seen by his family practitioner because of severe intermittent pain in the centre of his lower chest. It is particularly bad at night when he first goes to bed and lies down. His doctor takes a full history and makes a diagnosis of gastrooesophageal reflux disease (GORD); he prescribes drugs to reduce gastric acid production and recommends weight loss and stopping smoking. However, the patient returns 2 weeks later saying that his symptoms have not improved and is anxious that he may have angina, a work colleague of his age having recently collapsed and died at work from a myocardial infarct. The doctor suspects noncompliance with his advice, but refers the patient to hospital for investigation. At hospital, the patient gives exactly the same history. Investigation shows no evidence of myocardial ischaemia. An endoscopy shows inflammation and ulceration at the lower end of the oesophagus, termed *reflux oesophagitis*.

Q. Describe the structural and anatomical background to this case. Explain the differences between the normal lining epithelium of the oesophagus and that lining the upper part of the stomach.

Case 11.1   Answer

This patient is thought by his family practitioner to have GORD because of the history he gives, especially the fact that the pain is particularly frequent and severe at night when he lies down in bed. The basis of this disorder is that the acid secretions in the lumen of the stomach pass up into the lower oesophagus. Here, they cause inflammation to the stratified squamous epithelium of the lower oesophagus, which is not resistant to the effects of acid (unlike the tall, columnar epithelium lining the stomach, which has a protective layer of mucus secreted by the gastric mucous cells).

Reflux of gastric acid into the oesophagus is normally prevented by the gastroesophageal sphincter, which is partly structural (a ring of sphincteric smooth muscle in the wall at the gastrooesophageal junction) and partly functional, with extrinsic pressure from the muscles of the diaphragm and the normal angulation at the gastrooesophageal junction both playing a part. To understand the role of the diaphragm, read about hiatal hernia in your surgical textbook.

During an upper gastrointestinal endoscopy, it is common for small biopsy samples to be taken of the oesophageal and gastric epithelium. Histological examination can confirm oesophagitis. In some patients, prolonged exposure of the lower oesophageal epithelium to gastric acid causes metaplasia and transformation to a glandular-pattern epithelium, when it is termed *Barrett's oesophagus*.

Case 11.2   A Young Man With Persistent Severe Diarrhoea

A 26-year-old man is referred urgently to the hospital by his family practitioner because of severe bloody diarrhoea, present for 3 days. He had been passing about 10–15 very liquid blood-stained stools per day and was particularly distressed by the extreme urgency of defecation with little or no warning, leading to embarrassing incontinence.

On examination, he was anxious and distressed, with a fever (38.5°C) and a rapid pulse rate (105/min). He complained of lower abdominal discomfort but did not have a distended abdomen and gave no history of vomiting. Full blood count showed anaemia (9.8 g/dL) with some hypochromic microcytic red cells, polychromatic red cells and increased platelet count; his erythrocyte sedimentation rate (ESR) was 45 mm/hr. A stool sample was sent to microbiology for urgent direct microscopy and culture, and he was admitted for further urgent investigation and treatment. Sigmoidoscopy showed redness of the large bowel mucosa, and a biopsy was taken; this showed superficial

ulceration of the large bowel mucosa with loss of surface epithelium associated with infiltration by neutrophils, indicating focal acute inflammation. No infective condition was identified.

A diagnosis of ulcerative colitis is made, and further management is planned.

Q. Describe the structural and anatomical background to this case. What clinical effects can be explained by loss of the bowel surface epithelium through ulceration?

Case 11.2   Answer

The patient cites a very short history of severe uncontrollable diarrhoea, the stools being very watery and blood-stained. A biopsy shows loss of the mucosa with extensive superficial ulceration, and a diagnosis of the condition termed *acute ulcerative colitis* is made.

The mucosa of the colon and rectum is lined by tall columnar epithelium arranged in straight tubular glands, and the majority of the epithelial cells are either absorptive or mucus secreting. The major function of the large intestine is to absorb water from the liquid small intestinal contents, which pass into it through the ileocaecal valve. Thus the liquid small intestinal contents are converted into semisolid faeces by concentration through massive reabsorption of water, and the passage of the semisolid faecal mass along the distal colon and rectum is eased by the mucus added to it from the colonic mucus-secreting goblet cells. At the bottom of the tubular glands are also neuroendocrine cells and stem cells; the latter are important in the healing process in this disease.

Extensive loss of mucosa of the large intestine in severe ulcerative colitis significantly interferes with the function of the large intestine; loss of so much absorptive epithelium means that the ileal contents pass through largely unchanged because the water is not absorbed, and no semisolid faeces is formed. Because the disease destroys and erodes much of the mucosa, the underlying submucosa, which contains abundant thin-walled blood vessels, is exposed and significant bleeding occurs, producing iron-deficiency anaemia, as in this case. The sphincter mechanism in the anus (internal anal sphincter and external anal sphincter) has a very limited capacity to retain the liquid contents of the colon and rectum, and faecal incontinence is a problem.

Case 11.3   A Woman With Abdominal Discomfort, Diarrhoea and Weight Loss

A 32-year-old woman is referred to hospital by her family practitioner because of almost constant abdominal discomfort, sometimes with more severe pain, and frequent diarrhoea. She also complained of feeling generally unwell and had become excessively tired over the previous few months and had lost considerable weight, despite an almost normal appetite. On examination, she was pale and thin, with a slightly bloated abdomen, which was somewhat tender on palpation. On more detailed questioning about her diarrhoea, she stated that there was no bleeding, and the stools were not often fluid, but very soft and pale, with a tendency to float and difficult to flush away. The physician recognized this as a description of steatorrhoea. Full blood count showed that she had a moderate iron-deficiency anaemia but with a normal platelet count, suggesting that there had been no recent blood loss. A barium meal and small bowel follow-through showed mild dilation of the small bowel but no major structural abnormality. She underwent a jejunal biopsy, and the pathologist's report said that the changes were suggestive of gluten enteropathy (coeliac disease), with loss of the normal villous pattern and replacement of the small bowel by a flattened epithelium.

Q. Describe the structural, functional and anatomical background to this case. Describe the likely clinical and functional consequences of losing the small bowel villous pattern.

Case 11.3 Answer

The mucosa and submucosa of the small bowel are thrown up into a large number of folds, or plicae, arranged circularly around the lumen. These are most prominent in the jejunum. The surface of the plicae is further arranged into villi, which protrude into the intestinal lumen. Tubular glands or crypts extend down from the base of the villi to the muscularis mucosae.

The small bowel mucosa is formed of enterocytes, which are tall columnar cells with round or oval nuclei in the lower third of the cell. The luminal surface of enterocytes is highly specialized; each cell bears 2000–3000 tightly packed, tall microvilli, which are coated by glycoproteins, the glycocalyx. The glycocalyx contains a number of enzymes (brush border enzymes, e.g. lactase, sucrase, peptidases, lipases and alkaline phosphatase), which are important in digestion and transport.

In coeliac disease, an immune response to ingested gluten found in wheat flour leads to death of cells in the small bowel epithelium. In response to cell death, there is increased production of epithelial cells by the crypts. The crypts become longer than normal. However, cell death of formed epithelial cells continues, and the bowel mucosa does not form a villous pattern.

A consequence of losing the villous pattern is that the surface area of small bowel for absorption is reduced. This leads to small bowel malabsorption. Fat is especially not absorbed, so it remains in the stool, making them greasy, pale and difficult to flush away (steatorrhoea). The absorption of iron, vitamin B_{12} and folate can also be affected, leading to anaemia.

Another consequence of having a rapid turnover of small bowel epithelial cells is that they do not have time to achieve full differentiation. The expression of surface enzymes such as lactase and sucrase may not occur, and so absorption of these sugars may not happen, as they cannot be broken down into simple sugars.

In patients with coeliac disease, a gluten-free diet is advised. Immune-mediated damage ceases, and the epithelial architecture of the small bowel returns to normal.

CHAPTER 12

Case 12.1 A Man With a Bad Liver

A 62-year-old man is admitted to hospital having been found collapsed in the street. He is unresponsive and smells of alcohol. On examination, he is found to be hypoglycaemic, and glucose is administered. His abdomen is distended, and it is felt that he has ascites. He also has oedema of the ankles. His spleen

appears enlarged on palpation. Blood tests show an elevated bilirubin level and a low serum albumin.

Q. How do all these clinical findings relate to the normal structure and function of the liver? What pattern of liver disease is suggested by this case?

Case 12.1 Answer

In this patient, collapse is likely to be related to a high blood ethanol level and low blood glucose level. Alcohol is a recognized hepatotoxin and can interfere with normal liver function and cause liver cell damage. The main functions of the liver are as follows:

- Bile synthesis and secretion – The liver produces bile, which contains water, ions, phospholipids, bile pigments (mainly bilirubin glucuronide) and bile acids (glycocholic and taurocholic acids).
- Excretion of bilirubin – Bilirubin is produced in the spleen from the breakdown of the haem component of haemoglobin. In the liver, the bilirubin is conjugated with glucuronic acid, and the conjugate (bilirubin glucuronide) is excreted in the bile and thence the faeces.
- Protein synthesis – The liver synthesizes many proteins, including albumin, and blood clotting factors, such as fibrinogen and prothrombin.
- Gluconeogenesis – Lipids and amino acids are converted into glucose in the liver by gluconeogenesis.
- Storage – Triglycerides, glycogen and some vitamins are stored in the liver.
- Deamination of amino acids – In the liver, amino acids are deaminated to produce urea, which is excreted by the kidney.
- Conjugation and chemical breakdown of toxins – The smooth endoplasmic reticulum of the liver possesses large numbers of enzymes that break down or conjugate toxic substances (e.g. alcohol, barbiturates) to convert them into other metabolites.

In this patient, the following three aspects of liver function have been found to be abnormal:

- Low blood sugar – Possibly related to failure of gluconeogenesis
- Elevated bilirubin – Possibly related to failure of bile synthesis and excretion
- Low serum albumen – Related to failure of protein synthesis by the liver

An additional clinical feature that is observed is ascites – the accumulation of fluid within the peritoneal cavity. The patient may be predisposed to this condition by a low serum albumen, with a corresponding low plasma oncotic pressure. Another factor that can cause ascites is a raised blood pressure in the portal venous system – portal hypertension. In the normal liver, blood from the portal vein runs through the liver in vessels in portal tracts, then into liver sinusoids. If a disturbance of liver structure occurs because of disease, then the flow of blood through the sinusoids may be impaired, leading to backpressure in the portal venous system and portal hypertension.

A disease that can result in all these features is cirrhosis, in which long-standing damage to liver cells leads to fibrosis (deposition of collagenous scar), death of liver cells and, through attempted regeneration, formation of nodules of liver cells. This disturbed architecture of the liver leads to distur-bance of the vascular arrangement and portal hypertension. Reduction in liver cell mass and abnormal anatomy lead to failure of liver cell function, with elevated bilirubin, impaired gluconeogenesis and failure of secretion of serum proteins. This pattern of disease is termed **chronic liver disease**, as it results from long-standing damage.

In this instance, it is most likely that chronic alcohol abuse has led to liver cell damage and eventual development of cirrhosis.

CHAPTER 13

Case 13.1   A Case of a Road Traffic Accident

A 23-year-old man, an amateur soccer player, sustains a com-pound fracture of his tibia and fibula in a road traffic accident while riding his motorbike. After the fractures have been treated surgically by insertion of pins and plates, and after the fracture and surgical site have been fully healed, he persists with having difficulty with weight-bearing on the affected leg and has not been able to return to playing football. His muscle mass has decreased, and he enters a prolonged period of rehabilitation, which involves physiotherapy to his thigh and calf muscles of the affected leg.

Q. Explain the structural basis of this case. Why is physio-therapy necessary?

Case 13.1   Answer

When bones are so severely fractured that displacement occurs, normal bone fracture repair cannot take place because the frac-tured bone ends are too far apart. The aim of surgical treatment is to put the ends of the fractured bone together ('fracture re-duction') and hold them in close apposition ('fracture fixa-tion'), so that speedy healing can occur. Given that this fracture required fixation with metal pins and plates, one can assume that considerable displacement was present.

Even when the fracture is reduced and fixed in this way, it takes at least 8 weeks for the fracture to repair, during which time the movement of the limb is limited, and the patient is unable to bear weight on it for some weeks. During this time, the muscles of the limb are significantly underused, and they can undergo atrophy as a result of disuse, leading to reduction in the muscle mass and weakness in the limb when it is eventu-ally fully mobilized. These changes can be minimized by a pro-gramme of physiotherapy to keep the muscles in use, even if they are not used for walking.

Physiotherapy to the thigh and calf muscles is essential from the outset for the following two reasons:

- It is essential for minimizing disuse atrophy of the muscle, which develops because of physical inactivity during the period of fracture healing.
- It minimizes the risk for leg vein thrombosis (see Case 9.1).

Case 13.2   Muscle Weakness in Childhood

A 2-year-old boy is seen in a neurology clinic because he has been delayed in achieving his motor development and is clearly weak. There is a family history of similar problems, with a cousin dying after progressive muscle disease in late adolescence. A muscle biopsy shows death of many muscle fibres, with evi-dence of muscle fibre regeneration and fibrosis. No expression of the protein dystrophin is seen. Genetic investigation shows a mutation in the gene coding for dystrophin.

Q. How does lack of expression of dystrophin relate to mus-cle disease?

Case 13.2   Answer

Dystrophin is a protein that is associated with the cell mem-brane of skeletal muscle fibres and is responsible for providing a link between the intracellular proteins that mediate contrac-tion and the extracellular proteins in the external membrane surrounding each muscle fibre.

If dystrophin is not expressed, then forces generated by con-traction of muscle fibres are not transmitted efficiently to the extracellular matrix. In normal muscle, contraction forces are coordinated and transmitted uniformly through the extracel-lular matrix to allow the muscle to behave as a single mass.

In patients without expression of dystrophin, a condition called *Duchenne muscular dystrophy,* contraction causes tearing of the cell membrane, leading to death of muscle fibres. Al-though some regeneration of muscle fibres can occur, over time fibres are lost and fibrosis develops in muscle, manifesting as permanent muscle weakness. Dystrophin is also expressed in cardiac muscle, and patients with Duchenne muscular dystro-phy also develop cardiac disease.

It is now realized that mutation in genes coding for other membrane-linking proteins can also result in muscular dystrophy.

Case 13.3   A Man With a Limp

A 68-year-old man is referred by his family practitioner be-cause of difficulty with walking owing to pain in his right hip, gradually getting worse over about 3 years. He is now walking with a limp, favouring his left leg and supporting his right leg with the use of a walking stick. On examination, movement at the right hip is limited, mainly by pain. Imaging shows nar-rowing of the hip joint cavity, with flattening of the head of the femur and outgrowth of new bone (osteophyte formation) around the rim of the femoral head. A diagnosis of osteoar-thritis is made.

Q. What joint structures are likely to be involved in this process, and how do you think the clinical features relate to deranged function of the joint?

Case 13.3   Answer

The hip joint is a typical synovial joint between the head of the femur and the cup-like acetabulum of the pelvis, into which the femoral head fits in the form of a ball-and-socket joint. Because it is a synovial joint, both articular surfaces are normally coated by a layer of articular cartilage, and the smooth and virtually friction-free movement of the two articular surfaces is assisted by the presence between them of a thin film of slippery lubri-cating synovial fluid produced by the synovial lining of the internal surface of the joint capsule.

In the normal structure of the femoral head, a thick coat of smooth articular cartilage on the articular surface rests on the dense compact cortical bone, from which the complex interfac-ing network of trabecular bone struts run to occupy the medul-lary cavity of the bone.

In the disease suffered by this patient (osteoarthritis or osteoarthrosis), degeneration of articular cartilage occurs over many years, leading to progressive erosion and thinning of the articular cartilage on the two opposing surfaces of the two bones participating in the joint. Eventually, much of the articular cartilage is eroded away, and the cortical bone of the head of the femur is in constant contact with the lining of the acetabular cup. The cortical plates of the two bones undergo thickening to withstand the extra forces they must resist once the cushioning effect of the cartilage has gone. The cortical bone not only becomes thickened, but it becomes even more compact as a result of progressive degenerative changes, and the constant friction of the two hard cortical bone surfaces leads to the bone surfaces becoming very compact and highly 'polished' (a process called **eburnation**). The vertical compressive forces on the femoral head lead to variable degrees of flattening of the usually round head because some of the bone trabeculae under the reinforced cortical plate may buckle.

A further structural change that occurs in the femoral head is the formation of protuberant spurs of bone termed *osteophytes* at the periphery of the head. This occurs because of reactive new bone formation as a result of degenerative and inflammatory changes altering the structure of the femoral head with the progression of the disease.

Production of osteoarthritic changes. As described previously, the main changes that occur are the result of progressive excessive wear and tear, and most can be explained purely by the physical forces involved. Osteoarthritis is common in the hip in the elderly but also occurs in joints that are heavily used, for example, in the fingers of keyboard operators and the knees of athletes such as soccer players. However, development of the disease is not inevitable, and evidence suggests that genetic factors may have an influence, particularly on the function and response of the chondrocytes in the articular cartilage to trauma.

Case 13.4   A Woman With Back, Buttock and Leg Pain

A 35-year-old woman developed sudden onset of severe pain in the lumbar region while pruning a large rose bush. She hobbled into the house and lay down on her back on the bed, the only position in which she could tolerate the pain. She had a restless night despite taking analgesics. The next morning, the pain in her back had abated somewhat, but she had pain in the left buttock, radiating down the back of the left thigh, and by the following day, the pain also affected the back of the calf and the foot. Despite 2 days of bed rest, her symptoms persisted and she contacted her family practitioner, who visited. He found that she had some sensory loss on the sole and posterior calf and was unable to raise her left leg when the knee was straight. She also had some weakness of ankle and toe flexion on the left. A diagnosis of prolapsed intervertebral disc was made.

Q. Describe the histological and anatomical basis for this condition.

Case 13.4   Answer

This patient gives a clinical history suggestive of an intervertebral disc protrusion, causing symptoms of back pain ('lumbago') and pain in the buttock and down the back of the leg with neurological symptoms ('sciatica').

The bony vertebral bodies are separated from one another by intervertebral discs, which act as both shock absorbers and as non-synovial joints, allowing limited anteroposterior and lateral flexion and extension of the spine.

Each intervertebral disc is composed of fibrocartilage with a central area of soft gelatinous fibromyxoid tissue called the **nucleus pulposus**, around which the denser fibrocartilage is arranged as a surrounding shell, called the **annulus fibrosus**. In disc protrusion, the central nucleus pulposus material bulges out through the lateral wall, barely restrained by the thin annulus fibrosus. The cause of this is not certain, but extruded disc material removed at surgery for the treatment of disc protrusion shows the annulus fibrosus to be thinned and partly disrupted by rather pale, disorganized nucleus pulposus material that looks degenerate.

The bulging disc material presses on spinal nerves as they emerge from the spinal cord on their way to the pelvis and lower limbs. This physical pressure on the nerves produces the neurological symptoms and signs of sciatica.

CHAPTER 14

Case 14.1   A Woman With Multiple Symptoms

A 37-year-old woman was referred to hospital by her family practitioner for investigation and treatment. For about 6 months, she had noticed that she had become increasingly clumsy in the home, dropping many things and becoming very irritable and 'stressed'. At times of great 'stress' she noticed that her hands trembled and her palms were often hot and sweaty. She slept badly and described 'palpitations', where she felt her heart was racing. A major problem was her constant restlessness, being unable to complete a task before moving on to another, and this caused her great distress, as she felt she was losing her focus at work and antagonizing her workmates. On direct questioning, she admitted to diarrhoea and irregular periods over the preceding few months and considerable loss of weight. Blood tests showed features of thyrotoxicosis, and further investigations were arranged to look at the likely cause.

Q. Describe the functional and histological background to this case. Concentrate on describing the normal control of thyroid hormone production, and speculate where this may become deranged, leading to oversecretion.

Case 14.1   Answer

To understand the answer to this question, you need to be familiar with the normal histology of the thyroid gland, the structural and functional relationships of the thyroid acinar cells and the feedback control of thyroid hormone secretion.

The surgeon was particularly interested in the palpation of the front of the neck because he suspected the thyroid gland was the source of the problem, and there was a good chance that the entire gland or part of it would be sufficiently enlarged that it would be easily palpable. Sometimes, the gland is so enlarged that it is easily visible (goitre).

This patient has thyroid hyperplasia, in which the thyroid acini contain increased numbers of thyroid epithelial cells. Normally, a high proportion of the epithelial cells lining the thyroid acini are small and in an inactive phase; only a few cells at any one time are actively involved in synthesizing thyroid hormone or reprocessing formed thyroglobulin from the stored thyroid colloid to produce active thyroid hormone. The proportion of active to inactive thyroid cells varies according to the body's requirement for thyroid hormone, controlled by a feedback mechanism involving thyroid-stimulating hormone (TSH) secreted by the anterior pituitary gland. In thyroid hyperplasia, this feedback mechanism is circumvented; an abnormal circulating antibody stimulates the thyroid epithelial cells directly. This can be detected on blood tests and is part of establishing a diagnosis. In response to stimulation, thyroid epithelial cells increase in number, and a much higher proportion becomes actively involved in synthesizing and mobilizing thyroid hormone, irrespective of the body's needs. This leads to the clinical syndrome of thyrotoxicosis, in which constant excessive output of active thyroid hormone increases the body's metabolic rate, leading to increased appetite, weight loss, irritability, restlessness, sleeplessness, clumsiness, physical hyperactivity, palpitations, diarrhoea and heat intolerance.

This patient suffers from many of the listed symptoms as a result of the continuous high output of active thyroid hormone by her histologically abnormal thyroid gland.

Case 14.2   A Man Who Became Obese and Hypertensive

A 56-year-old man is referred to hospital for investigation. At a recent well-man clinic, he had been found to be hypertensive, and the community doctor noted that he was obese, with abdominal striae. A possible diagnosis of Cushing's disease, caused by the effects of excessive corticosteroid, was considered. Investigations show an elevated cortisol level, and further tests are considered to investigate the cause.

Q. Describe the structural and functional background to this case. Concentrate on describing the normal regulation of cortisol production and speculate where this could go wrong to produce disease.

Case 14.2   Answer

This patient was thought to have Cushing's disease. Many patients have upper body obesity with a rounded face and increased fat deposition around the neck and shoulders. Abdominal striae are purple-red stretch marks that can appear on the abdomen, arms, breasts, buttocks and thighs. High blood pressure is common. Many patients also complain of fatigue and have muscle weakness. Impaired glucose tolerance may result in diabetes mellitus.

The disease is caused by excessive levels of the hormone cortisol. Cortisol is produced by the cells of the adrenal cortex. This is regulated by secretion of adrenocorticotropic hormone (ACTH) by the adenohypophysis of the pituitary gland, which stimulates production. The release of ACTH is in turn regulated by influences from the hypothalamic region of the brain and the secretion of corticotropin-releasing factor (CRF), which stimulates secretion.

When levels of cortisol in the blood reach appropriate levels, the hypothalamus and pituitary release less CRF and ACTH.

This feedback system regulates the amount of cortisol released by the adrenal glands.

The possible causes of excess secretion of cortisol could reside in the hypothalamus, the pituitary gland or the adrenal gland.

Excessive CRF secretion may lead to overproduction of cortisol. In practice, this does not commonly explain cases of Cushing's disease; when it does happen, its origin is not the hypothalamus, but rather it has an ectopic cause, usually a lung tumour.

Excessive secretion of ACTH may happen in the presence of a tumour of the pituitary gland (pituitary adenoma). In this situation, the tumour continues to secrete ACTH independently of any regulation by levels of CRF. In some patients, ACTH can be secreted from an ectopic site, for example, a lung tumour.

Excessive cortisol may be the result of autonomous secretion by an abnormality in the adrenal gland. The usual cause is a tumour of the adrenal cortex. In most cases, this is an adenoma (benign), but in some patients, it can be an adrenal cortical carcinoma (malignant).

CHAPTER 15

Case 15.1   A Child With Blood in the Urine

A 6-year-old boy is admitted to hospital because his mother noted that he had been passing reduced amounts of concentrated dark brown urine. He had also been unwell, lethargic and tearful, and she noticed that his face had become puffy. She had taken a sample of the child's urine to the family practitioner, who applied a simple test, which showed that the dark brown colour was caused by the presence of blood (haematuria), and the urine also contained abundant protein. On admission, the test was repeated and severe haematuria confirmed. The paediatrician also noted the facial puffiness, particularly around the eyes, and found that the child had high blood pressure. Laboratory tests showed that he had a raised blood urea. A clinical diagnosis was made that the child was developing renal failure, and the possibility that this was caused by glomerular disease was considered, termed *glomerulonephritis*. It was felt that the child had developed nephritic syndrome. Further investigations were planned to explore the underlying cause.

Q. Describe the structural and functional background to this case. Concentrate on describing the normal structure of the glomerulus and what normally prevents blood and protein from entering the urine. Speculate how the glomerular structure can become abnormal in disease to cause leakage of red cells in the urine and reduced glomerular filtration leading to uraemia. Why do you think there is associated hypertension?

Case 15.1   Answer

This child shows the features of nephritic syndrome (acute glomerulonephritis), which is composed of the following:

- Haematuria and passage of reduced amounts of urine (oliguria)

- Transient rise in blood pressure
- Transient rise in blood urea
- Oedema, particularly periorbital

The features are the result of structural abnormalities in all the glomeruli in both kidneys. Normally, blood is able to pass through the glomerular capillaries. If the endothelial cells are damaged in a disease process, the cells of the normally thin endothelial layer lining the glomerular capillaries proliferate so that the lumina of the capillaries are blocked and prevent the passage of blood through them. This reduced glomerular blood flow stimulates the renin–angiotensin–aldosterone system, leading to a rise in blood pressure. Because little blood passes through the glomeruli, little ultrafiltration occurs across the glomerular filtration barrier; the volume of urine passed is greatly reduced (oliguria), and the blood urea rises.

The pathogenesis of nephritic syndrome is complex, but the basic abnormality is an immunological injury to the glomerulus, with the deposition of immune complexes in the membrane, the presence of which stimulates the proliferation of the endothelial cells.

Fortunately, in most cases, nephritic syndrome in children is short-lived. The immune complexes in the glomerular basement membrane are cleared, and the proliferated endothelial cells regress until the capillaries are again lined by a thin layer of flat endothelial cells. As the capillaries regain their lumen, blood flows through them once more; the blood pressure falls and ultrafiltration resumes, so that urine output increases and the blood urea level falls.

A range of disorders can affect the structure of the glomerulus, leading to loss of protein, loss of red cells or both. Inherited conditions, leading to defects in glomerular structure, are found to be a cause in a proportion of cases. Immune-mediated damage associated with a range of diseases is another common cause of glomerular disease. In these cases, immune complexes are filtered in the glomerulus and stimulate inflammatory responses, leading to damage and structural changes. Metabolic causes of glomerular disease often have a common factor in causing damage to podocytes as an initial focus for developing structural changes. Irrespective of initial causation, another common structural component of glomerular disease is proliferation of mesangium and deposition of mesangial matrix, often called *glomerular scarring*.

Case 15.2 A Middle-Aged Man With Severe Proteinuria

A 46-year-old man who had had diabetes mellitus since his teens developed proteinuria (excessive protein loss in the urine), as noted by his family practitioner, and an appointment was made for him to see his diabetic physician. In hospital, the presence of severe proteinuria was confirmed, but it was also noted that he had puffy swelling (oedema) of his hands, feet, fingers and toes. Laboratory tests also showed that he had a low serum albumin. He was admitted and transferred to the care of a renal physician for further investigation of his nephritic syndrome.

Q. Describe the structural and functional background to this case. Concentrate on describing how the renal glomerulus normally prevents protein loss into the urine. Speculate what structural or functional changes may have developed to cause disease.

Case 15.2 Answer

This man has the combination of symptoms, signs and laboratory findings that constitute nephrotic syndrome:

- Excessive protein loss in the urine (proteinuria)
- Low serum albumen levels (hypoalbuminaemia)
- Oedema, particularly of the hands and feet

Because of an abnormality in the glomerular filtration barrier, large amounts of protein pass out from the blood plasma in the glomerular capillary lumen into the urinary space. The normally functioning glomerular filtration barrier holds back most of the plasma protein. The protein (particularly the smaller protein molecules such as albumen) passes down the tubular system in the glomerular filtrate. Normally, any small amounts of protein that pass through the normally functioning glomerular filtration barrier are reabsorbed in the proximal convoluted tubule, so that the urine eventually contains no protein at all. However, in nephrotic syndrome, the amount of protein in the glomerular filtrate far exceeds the tubule's capacity to reabsorb it, so protein is present in the final concentrated urine. This is called **proteinuria**.

When protein loss (particularly albumen) in the urine has been severe and prolonged, the amount of protein loss exceeds the capacity of the liver to synthesize new albumen. When the blood is tested for protein content, it is found that the level of albumen is low. This is called **hypoalbuminaemia**.

With a low serum albumen, the forces that control the balance of fluid between the intravascular and extravascular (tissue) fluid are disturbed. One of the important factors that draws fluid into the intravascular space at the capillary level from the interstitium of the tissues is the osmotic (oncotic) pressure exerted by the high levels of protein in the plasma within the capillaries; this sucks in fluid from the extravascular space. When the plasma protein levels are low, this oncotic pressure is reduced, and less interstitial fluid is drawn into the capillary lumina. Therefore fluid accumulates in the tissue interstitium, leading to tissue oedema.

Case 15.3 A Young Man With Multiple Injuries

A 23-year-old man was involved in a road traffic accident and was trapped in the car for some hours. An intravenous infusion was set up by paramedics, but his blood pressure remained low and he lost consciousness while he was being extricated from the wreckage by fire officers with metal-cutting equipment. It was obvious that he had sustained compound fractures of the tibia and fibula in both legs, and it was suspected that he had internal bleeding from either a fractured pelvis or a ruptured internal organ. Despite intravenous plasma expanders and blood transfusion, he remained hypotensive and hypovolaemic in the ambulance. In the emergency room, it was considered that his persistent hypotension was the result of intra-abdominal bleeding, and emergency laparotomy showed a ruptured spleen. This was removed and good haemostasis was obtained at the site; with the aid of blood transfusion, his hypotensive and hypovolaemic state improved sufficiently that the orthopaedic surgeons operated on the compound fractures of tibia and fibula in the same operation. After the operation, he remained hypotensive for a further 24 hours despite blood transfusion. It was noted that he was not passing urine, and blood samples were sent for analysis. This showed that he had a raised hydrogen ion concentration in his blood (acidosis) and that his serum potassium level was raised (hyperkalaemia). It was thought that he had acute renal failure.

Q. Describe the structural and functional background to this case. Concentrate on describing how which part of the kidney regulates hydrogen ion and potassium levels and speculate what might have happened to cause disease.

Case 15.3   Answer

The component of the nephron damaged in this case is the tubule system, particularly the metabolically active proximal and distal tubules, which are so important in fluid and ion exchange and therefore in maintaining homeostasis. The persistently low blood pressure has resulted in poor perfusion of the kidneys, and he has developed acute kidney injury (AKI).

The capillaries that supply the tubules (peritubular capillaries) are at the end of a long and complicated vascular supply to the kidney: renal artery, main renal artery branch, segmental artery, interlobular artery, arcuate artery, afferent arteriole, glomerular capillary network, efferent arteriole and peritubular capillary network. Perfusion of blood through this very distal capillary system is always likely to be compromised if any central loss of perfusion pressure occurs, and the cells that they supply (i.e. the epithelial cells of the tubules) are likely to suffer from hypoxia. Unfortunately, these cells have a very high oxygen requirement, as they are so rich in mitochondria because of their high metabolic activity.

In this case, the patient suffered multiple injuries involving severe loss of blood (from a ruptured spleen and bone fractures) and was hypotensive and hypovolaemic for a long period. During such a time, perfusion through the most peripheral blood vessels such as the peritubular capillaries is greatly reduced and oxygenation of tissues (including the tubular epithelial cells) becomes inadequate for normal cell function. The ion-pumping activities cease, and many of the tubular epithelial cells therefore die (acute tubular necrosis). The failure of their function leads to severe disorders of electrolyte balance, with metabolic acidosis and hyperkalaemia being the first to manifest on blood testing. Reduced blood perfusion through the glomerular capillaries leads to reduced ultrafiltration, with consequent reduction in the production of glomerular filtrate and therefore urine. In this case, perfusion of blood through the kidney vessels was so greatly reduced that no urine was produced at all (anuria).

This man has an excellent chance of recovery once his blood loss is stopped. He will then cease to be hypovolaemic and hypotensive, and the blood flow through his peripheral blood vessels will return to normal. Normal perfusion through the glomerular capillaries will allow ultrafiltration to occur, and urine will be produced again. Normal perfusion in the peritubular capillaries will allow adequate oxygenation of any tubular epithelial cells that have survived, and they will begin to pump

ions again in a small way. The tubular epithelial cells have a great capacity to regenerate; the tubules soon become completely repopulated by functional epithelial cells, and normal homeostatic mechanisms return.

CHAPTER 16

Case 16.1   A Man With Urinary Problems

A 63-year-old man presented with a 1-year history of problems with micturition. After a period when his only problem was increasing nocturia (having to get up to pass urine in the night), he then found that he needed to go more frequently day and night, had a poor stream and often dribbled when he thought he had finished. He also sometimes had to wait a long time before the stream started. The urological surgeon performed a rectal examination and found that the prostate gland was enlarged.

Q. Describe the histological and structural background to this case. What might happen to the bladder if the prostate gland is enlarged?

Case 16.1   Answer

After leaving the bladder, the male urethra passes through the prostate gland before running through the penis. As it passes through the prostate, the urethra can become compressed if the prostate gland becomes enlarged. Enlargement of the prostate gland is common in men older than 60 years and results from hyperplasia of the glands in the mucosal (inner periurethral) and submucosal (outer periurethral) groups. This proliferation of glands leads to enlargement of the entire gland, and the normally tubular prostatic urethra is squashed into a narrow slit-like shape, producing partial obstruction. This leads to difficulty in emptying the bladder during micturition. The symptoms experienced by this man (urinary frequency, poor stream, difficulty in starting and stopping) are typical of those resulting from prostatic obstruction of the urethra.

As a result of this obstruction of the urethra, some urine is always left behind in the bladder at the end of micturition (residual urine); the amount retained increases with the severity of the obstruction, and the bladder may become permanently distended. The bladder has to work harder than normal to empty against the obstruction, and as a result, the smooth muscle in the wall of the bladder undergoes work hypertrophy. The bladder wall becomes thicker as the three muscle layers undergo hypertrophy, and the enlarged muscle bands can be seen through the mucosa (trabeculations).

Case 16.2   A Couple With Subfertility

A young married couple is being investigated for subfertility. In a semen analysis, the male partner is found to have no spermatozoa, and both testes are smaller than normal and rather firm. It transpires that as a young boy, he had surgery for bilateral undescended testes.

Q. Describe the structural and functional background to this case. Concentrate on describing what one would normally expect in the postpubertal testis, and speculate on what you might find histologically in the testis in a patient who has no spermatozoa in his ejaculate.

Case 16.2 Answer

The testes develop high on the posterior abdominal wall during early embryological development and migrate down into the scrotal sac before birth. It is believed that the lower temperature in the scrotum is essential for normal development of the germ cells and their subsequent maturation into spermatozoa in the process called **spermatogenesis**. The normal mature testis is composed of seminiferous tubules lined internally by germ cells (spermatogonia), which, under the influence of testosterone secreted by the Leydig cells lying in the interstices between seminiferous tubules, undergo the division and maturational processes known as **spermatocytogenesis** and **spermiogenesis** to produce motile spermatozoa. This process begins with the onset of puberty. Formed spermatozoa pass into the rete testis, then into efferent ductules and into the epididymis. From there, they pass into the long tubular vas deferens (ductus deferens), which runs in the spermatic cord from the epididymis into the ejaculatory ducts, which run through the prostate gland and open into the prostatic urethra at the utricle. At the beginning of the ejaculatory ducts, the vas deferens is joined by short ducts from the seminal vesicles, the secretions of which provide nutrients for the spermatozoa.

Absence of spermatozoa in the ejaculate means that either the testes are not making spermatozoa or the passage of spermatozoa from the testes to the urethra is completely obstructed on both sides. In this case, the most likely cause is that the testes are not making spermatozoa as a result of failure of the testes to descend into the scrotum during intrauterine life (cryptorchid testes). In such circumstances, the germinal epithelium does not develop, even though the testes are often drawn down into the scrotal sac surgically in childhood. Once all the germ cells are non-viable, there does not seem to be any capacity for regeneration once conditions improve. Without germinal epithelium to form the internal lining of the seminiferous tubules, the only cells present are the Sertoli cells. The tubules remain small, with thick basement membranes, and the testis as a whole remains small, showing little of the enlargement that normally occurs at puberty. The testosterone-secreting Leydig (interstitial) cells are not damaged in undescended testes and continue to secrete hormone, so secondary sexual characteristics develop normally.

Other causes of germ cell destruction in the testes exist, including viral infection in mumps. If the cause of absence of spermatozoa in the ejaculate is not apparent, a needle biopsy of the testis can be performed.

CHAPTER 17

Case 17.1 A Woman Who Cannot Become Pregnant

A 26-year-old woman is seen because she has not been able to become pregnant despite trying with her partner for 2 years. She has normal regular periods, and endocrinological investigations suggest that ovulation is taking place normally. Investigations have excluded a likely male factor.

Q. Describe the structural and functional features that allow successful fertilization and implantation. Speculate where abnormalities may develop that might explain infertility.

Case 17.1 Answer

In order for an ovum to be fertilized and become implanted after its release from the ovary, it must pass down the uterine (fallopian) tube. The fertilized ovum then must implant itself in the endometrium of the uterus at the correct phase.

Ovarian factors are a common cause of female infertility. It is possible that endocrine factors prevent maturation of the follicle and release of an ovum; however, this appears to be excluded in this case on investigation.

The next most common group of disorders relates to problems in the uterine tubes. The uterine tubes convey ova from the ovary to the lumen of the body of the uterus (endometrial cavity). They are also the usual sites of fertilization of the ovum by spermatozoa. After fertilization, the tube transmits the fertilized ovum to the endometrial cavity, where implantation can take place. Each uterine tube is 10–12 cm long and extends from a dilated open end close to the ovary to a narrow portion that passes through the myometrial wall of the uterus before opening into the uterine cavity.

The infundibulum of the uterine tube is surrounded by a fringe of epithelial-coated fimbriae. In some diseases, the fimbriae become densely adherent to the surface of the ovary, such that it is not possible for a released ovum to enter the tube. The uterine tube is a muscular tube lined by specialized epithelium that is variably folded and plicate, differing in appearance at different sites. In the presence of disease of the tube, such as that causing narrowing, or disease of the lining epithelium, the ovum may be impeded in its passage down the tube. Two types of epithelial cells line the uterine tube: ciliated cells and secretory cells. The ciliated cells may be responsible for movement of the ovum through the infundibulum and ampulla, although tubal peristalsis probably plays a greater role. Ciliated cells may also have a role in propelling the spermatozoa in the opposite direction. Rare genetic conditions in which cilial motility is impaired may be associated with impaired fertility.

Endometrial or uterine factors may also lead to infertility. Implantation has to take place in the endometrium in the secretory phase. If endocrine factors are such that the endometrium is not in a secretory phase, then implantation may not occur. Inflammatory conditions and anatomical abnormalities of the endometrium, such as polyps, may also interfere with implantation. In some women, scarring and narrowing of the endometrial cavity may prevent implantation.

CHAPTER 18

Case 18.1 A Man With Blisters

A 62-year-old man is seen in the clinic because he has developed a tense blistering skin rash, most evident in the flexures of the arms. A skin biopsy is performed, which shows that the blistering is based at the epidermal-dermal junction, associated with an infiltrate of eosinophils.

Immunofluorescence staining shows a linear band of deposits of autoantibody IgG and C3 at the dermoepidermal junction. A blood sample from the patient shows circulating antibodies, which are shown to bind to the epidermal-dermal junction of a normal skin sample.

A diagnosis of bullous pemphigoid is made, an autoimmune condition in which autoantibodies are directed against a normal component of the hemidesmosome.

Q. Describe the structural and functional background to this case. Focus on the structural features of the epidermis that facilitate its anchorage to the dermis and how disruption of hemidesmosomes predisposes to blistering. Speculate which other structural defects may lead to blistering skin diseases.

Case 18.1   Answer

This disease (bullous pemphigoid) is caused by an abnormal process located at the epidermal basement membrane, so it is important to know its structure.

The basement membrane between epidermis and dermis has three main layers: an electron-lucent lamina lucida on the epithelial side; an electron-dense lamina densa beneath it; and, on the dermal side of the lamina densa, an ill-defined layer called the *fibroreticular lamina,* through which various anchoring fibrils (type VII collagen) and microfibrils (fibrillin) pass and connect to collagen and elastin fibres in the dermis. These firmly tether the basement membrane to the underlying dermis. On the other (epidermal) side of the basement membrane, the basal cells of the epidermis are firmly bound to the basement membrane through specialized structures called **hemidesmosomes**, which connect to the lamina densa by anchoring filaments that pass from the hemidesmosome to the lamina densa through the lamina lucida.

At least 17 different antigens have been identified in the various layers of the basement membrane, 2 of which are known as the **bullous pemphigoid antigens** (BP230 and BP180, also called *BPAG1* and *BPAG2*). One of these resides in the hemidesmosome, and the other is located in the lamina lucida. In the disease bullous pemphigoid, autoantibodies develop against these two antigens, and an antigen–antibody reaction occurs at the site of the antigens, that is, in the hemidesmosomes and lamina lucida. The damage to the antigen molecules by this autoimmune process leads to weakness of the epidermal basement membrane, and separation of the epidermis from the dermis occurs in the plane of the lamina lucida. Fluid accumulation in this separation space leads to the lifting of the epidermis to form a fluid-filled blister. Electron microscopy of an early blister shows that the separation occurs in the lamina lucida, the lamina densa being left behind on the surface of the dermis at the base of the blister.

The blood test demonstrates the presence of antibodies against the bullous pemphigoid antigens (BP230 and BP180) circulating in the bloodstream, and the immunofluorescence staining of the skin biopsy shows the presence of antibodies confined to the basement membrane.

Other blistering diseases are associated with different abnormalities in the way in which epidermal cells adhere to each other and the methods by which the basement membrane is stuck firmly down onto the dermis.

Case 18.2   A Girl With a Blistering Rash

A 6-year-old girl is referred to a dermatology clinic because she has developed a recurrent blistering rash. It seems that she has always developed blisters on the hands and feet in response to mild friction. A skin biopsy shows intraepidermal separation forming small blisters in the suprabasal layer. Further investigation shows mutation in the gene coding for one of the keratin intermediate filaments.

Q. Explain the possible structural basis for blistering in this condition. Concentrate on how cytokeratin filaments normally stabilize the epithelium and anchor skin via basement membrane. What other molecular/structural defects in the basement membrane/epidermis might be responsible for blistering disease?

Case 18.2   Answer

The normal skin is a tough structure specifically designed to provide a resilient outer layer with important barrier functions. The toughness is provided by a variety of adhesion mechanisms that unite cells and the extracellular matrix into a single structure.

In normal skin, epidermal cells are tightly held together by intercellular junctions called **desmosomes**. The desmosomes are linked to the intermediate filament cytoskeleton of epidermal cells (called **keratins**). The basal layer of the epidermis is strongly linked to the basement membrane by hemidesmosomes, which also link into the cytokeratin intermediate filament cytoskeleton.

As the cells differentiate and move up the stratified epithelium, they remain tightly bound by desmosomal junctions, but the cytokeratin proteins change to higher molecular weight forms. Cells in the upper part of the epithelium express genes coding for a variety of specialized proteins that interact with the cytokeratin filaments and the cell membrane to produce a resilient and mechanically robust compact mass (keratin). Small granules (keratohyaline granules) contain some of these specialized proteins. Desmosomes are converted to corneodesmosomes such that anchorage is maintained between non-living corneocytes at the skin surface.

Both desmosomes and hemidesmosomes are composed of multiple link proteins responsible for cell anchorage.

The basement membrane is anchored to the extracellular matrix of the dermis by several anchoring proteins and glycoprotein interactions.

In this case, one of the keratin intermediate filament proteins is abnormal because of a mutation in a coding gene. The consequence of this is to prevent complete anchoring of cells to one another. Although the desmosomes and hemidesmosomes bind cells together, within the cells no cross-linking exists, which is normally mediated by keratin filaments. Trauma is associated with separation of cells that literally tear apart in the absence of a bracing network of keratin intermediate filaments. This leads to clinical blistering.

The blistering skin condition called *epidermolysis bullosa simplex* (EBS) is caused by keratin gene mutations, and further details of different clinical variants can be found online. One variant of localized EBS presents in childhood, mainly affecting the hands and feet.

Case 18.3   A Woman With a Lump in the Breast

A 46-year-old woman presents to her doctor with an intermittently tender lump in the breast. Examination shows an irregular mobile lump with a rubbery texture in the lower medial quadrant of the left breast approximately 2 cm in diameter. There is no attachment to other structures and no enlargement of local lymph nodes. Further investigation by imaging and histological sampling is planned.

Q. Describe the structural and histological background to this case. Concentrate on normal structures in the breast that may be the origin of neoplastic growth.

Case 18.3   Answer

The functional unit of the female breast is the **mammary lobule**, composed of a series of blind-ending terminal duct lobular units (TDLUs). The terminal ducts carry secretions to a larger duct that lies outside the lobule – the extralobular duct; this then connects with extralobular ducts from adjacent lobules before opening into a series of increasingly larger ducts, the largest of which open to the exterior at the nipple. Each TDLU is embedded in a loose fibrous support tissue, the specialized lobular fibrocollagenous stroma, which is hormone sensitive. The epithelium of the TDLU is also endocrine sensitive, responding to hormone secretion (by the ovary and pituitary) by synthesizing a lipid- and protein-rich fluid (milk). This reaches maximum effectiveness during late pregnancy and lactation, when the lobules increase enormously in size as a result of hyperplasia of the secretory epithelium as they increase the amount of milk synthesized under the influence of continued secretion of lactation-stimulating hormones by the ovary and the pituitary gland. The glandular component of the lobules then undergoes hyperplasia, and the breast enlarges as a whole. When lactation ceases, the lobules slowly return to their normal size.

Neoplastic growth may originate in the epithelial structures of the TDLU or in the stromal component. A common benign tumour is called a *fibroadenoma* and is composed of both epithelial and stromal elements. The most common malignant tumour of the breast is derived from the epithelial component, termed an *adenocarcinoma*. Two common histological patterns are recognized, termed *lobular carcinoma* and *ductal carcinoma*.

Another common reason for a lump to be present in the breast is the result of hyperplastic and cystic changes. This is non-neoplastic. Over a period of many years, the cyclical changes of enlargement and shrinkage during menstruation, pregnancies and lactation can lead to distortion of the normal architectural arrangements of the lobules and ducts. In particular, the fibrous stroma (both the extralobular and the specialized intralobular) increases in amount, and bands of collagenous tissue develop, which split up some lobules and constrict and obstruct some of the ducts so that they become blocked and distended.

Such fibrocystic change is understood to be a consequence of repeated cyclical endocrine stimulation of glandular and hormone-responsive breast stroma. The area of fibrocystic change is composed of collagenous fibrosis, distortion and growth of the lobular glandular tissue (adenosis) and dilatation of obstructed ducts (cystic change). On palpation, such an area in the breast is typically irregular in outline, rubbery, not adherent to overlying skin or underlying muscle and may be tender.

Given that clinical examination alone is not a reliable way of ascertaining whether a breast lump is neoplastic or not, mammography and ultrasound imaging would be used to characterize such an area. Using a syringe and needle, fluid may be aspirated from large cysts and sent for cytological examination. A needle biopsy may also be taken under ultrasound guidance and a sample submitted for histological examination to determine the cause of a breast lump.

CHAPTER 19

Case 19.1   Gradual Onset of Deafness

A 58-year-old man has been referred to a hearing assessment unit because he has experienced increasing difficulty with hearing. Physical examination of the tympanic membrane is normal, and it is planned to perform audiography to determine the pattern of hearing loss.

Q. Describe the functional and structural background to this case. Concentrate on structural aspects of hearing that may be abnormal and lead to deafness.

Case 19.1   Answer

There are three main groups of causes of deafness, categorized as conductive, sensorineural and mixed.

Conductive hearing loss occurs when sound vibrations are impeded in transmission from the outer ear through to the middle ear structures, affecting hearing before the sound reaches the cochlea and the nerve receptors of the inner ear. Causes include blockage in the auditory canal, accumulation of secretions in the middle ear and abnormalities in the arrangement or mobility of the auditory ossicles.

Sensorineural hearing loss results from damage to the neural receptors of the inner ear (the hair cells in the organ of Corti of the cochlea), the nerve pathways to the brain (auditory nerve) or the areas of the brain that process sound information.

Some causes of sensorineural deafness are birth related or involve diseases in early childhood, for example, Rh incompatibility or birth anoxia. Feto-maternal infections, such as rubella, measles and cytomegalovirus infection, may be associated with deafness.

In many conditions that lead to sensorineural deafness, the root of disease is genetic. In many instances, the genes for these conditions have been discovered and the gene products linked to abnormal function of cochlea hair cells.

In adult life, toxic substances, including some medicines, may lead to sensorineural deafness. Continued exposure to loud noise, as in certain industries, can result in damage to the inner ear and lead to permanent hearing loss. An uncommon cause of sensorineural deafness is a tumour of the acoustic nerve, derived from support cells of the nerve, called an **acoustic neuroma**. Trauma to the skull base involving the inner ear can also result in deafness.

Mixed hearing loss is a combination of conductive and sensorineural hearing losses.

Case 19.2   A Woman With Deteriorating Vision

A 63-year-old woman is seen in the clinic, having been referred because of deterioration in her vision. Ophthalmoscopic examination shows some cupping of the optic disc, and the intraocular pressure is elevated. A diagnosis of glaucoma is made.

Q. Describe the structural and functional background to this case. Focus on structural changes in the eye that might cause an increase in the intraocular pressure.

Case 19.2   Answer

Intraocular pressure is determined by the secretion and drainage of the aqueous humour. The anterior and posterior aqueous chambers lie anterior to the lens, on each side of the iris, and communicate with each other via the aperture of the pupil.

The aqueous humour is a watery fluid resembling cerebrospinal fluid and is secreted at a rate of approximately 2 mL per minute by the epithelial cells of the ciliary body in the posterior chamber. The aqueous filters through a network of spaces lined by endothelium, the trabecular meshwork, which runs around the circumference of the root of the iris and at the periphery of the anterior chamber and enters the canal of Schlemm. This canal runs around the whole circumference of the limbus within the sclera. From the canal of Schlemm, the aqueous enters venous vessels. The angle between the margin of the cornea and the iris root where the trabecular meshwork lies is the 'iridocorneal drainage angle'.

There is a normal resistance to the flow of aqueous at the level of the trabecular meshwork, such that continued secretion and resorption of the aqueous result in a normal intrinsic resting pressure within the globe (intraocular pressure) of 10–22 mmHg.

If the structures involved in the drainage of aqueous are abnormal, drainage may be impaired, leading to an increase in the intraocular pressure, called **glaucoma**.

Conditions that lead to glaucoma include the following:
- Physical blockage of the drainage angle by particulate matter in the anterior chamber, proliferating blood vessels or trauma that literally blocks the trabecular meshwork
- Blocking of the drainage angle and entrance to the trabecular meshwork by close apposition of the iris to the back of the cornea

In many cases, no physical blockage of the drainage angle can be demonstrated, and there is a functional blockage of drainage of the aqueous. Some causes of glaucoma have a familial basis. Some forms of glaucoma are congenital and are present in early childhood.

REVIEW QUESTIONS

CHAPTER 1 HISTOLOGY

1. Which of the following are types of empirical staining methods? *Select all that apply*.
   A. van Gieson
   B. Haematoxylin and eosin (H&E)
   C. Periodic acid–Schiff (PAS)
   D. Alkaline phosphatase enzyme histochemistry
   E. Immunoperoxidase

2. Which of the following are characteristics of resin-embedded histology? *Select all that apply*.
   A. Allows a higher resolution than other preparations for use in routine light microscopy
   B. Cannot be used for hard tissues such as bone
   C. Used for assessment of tissue as part of transmission electron microscopy
   D. Is applied to fresh-frozen material
   E. Toluidine blue staining is commonly used

3. Which of the following statements about histology and tissues are correct? *Select all that apply*.
   A. Histological examination is seldom used outside of the area of biological research
   B. Epithelial tissues are the basis of some solid organs
   C. Connective tissues are characterized by a high cellularity and a low volume fraction of extracellular material
   D. A compound tissue is composed of one dominant cell type
   E. The skin can be considered an organ

4. Read the following statements about tissues and histological stains and choose which are correct. *Select all that apply*.
   A. Cells with a similar function but widely distributed in several anatomical sites can be described as a system
   B. To examine tissues by routine histology, the material is first embedded in wax
   C. H&E staining of a tissue section causes cell cytoplasm to appear orange, whereas nuclei are stained a deep pink colour
   D. The PAS staining method can be used to detect glycogen in histological sections
   E. Immunocytochemistry relies on the availability of antibodies used as reagents that can specifically bind to a protein or related structure within a tissue section

5. For each of the statements, select the most appropriate option from A to K. Each option may be used once, more than once or not at all.
   A. Tissue
   B. Histology
   C. Epithelium
   D. Organ
   E. System
   F. Cell
   G. Light microscopy using wax-embedded sections
   H. Fixation
   I. Electron microscopy
   J. Embedding
   K. Histochemistry

   1. The study of the microscopic structure of biological material and the ways in which individual components are structurally and functionally related
   2. A discrete, organized collection of cells with similar morphological characteristics
   3. Cells which cover surfaces, line body cavities or form solid glands
   4. The main technique used in the microscopic study of cells and tissues
   5. The immersion of tissue in a solution of formaldehyde

CHAPTER 2 THE CELL

1. Which of the following are correct statements in relation to the cell nucleus? *Select all that apply*.
   A. Contains cellular DNA
   B. Braced by lamins
   C. Site of creation of ribosomal RNA
   D. Acidophilic in tinctorial stain preparations
   E. Continuous membrane establishes isolation from cytosolic space

2. Which of the following are correct statements in relation to cell cycle and cell division? *Select all that apply*.
   A. G0 cells are non-dividing
   B. S-phase cells are synthesizing proteins for cell division, having completed DNA synthesis
   C. G2 cells have a double complement of cellular DNA
   D. The nuclear membrane breaks down in prometaphase
   E. The nuclear membrane reforms in telophase

3. Which of the following are features of membranes found in cells? *Select all that apply*.
   A. Structurally based on a lipid bilayer
   B. Contain proteins that only act as enzymes
   C. Surround the nucleus in a single layer
   D. Surround individual ribosomes within the cell
   E. Maintained by vesicles derived from the Golgi

4. Which of the following are features of mitochondria? *Select all that apply*.
   A. Replicate independently from cell division
   B. Are the main site for oxidative phosphorylation
   C. Have a highly impermeable outer cell membrane

D. Vary in morphology between different cell types

E. Contain their own genetic material

5. Which of the following features are present in lysosomes? *Select all that apply.*
   A. Lysosomes have a membrane H^+-ATPase capable of maintaining an acidic environment
   B. The enzymes contained in lysosomes are also present in peroxisomes
   C. Vesicles from the Golgi take acid hydrolases to lysosomes
   D. Fusion of an endosome with a vesicle containing acid hydrolases forms an endolysosome
   E. Lysosomal storage diseases are caused by lack of specific lysosomal enzymes leading to accumulation of a metabolic product

6. Which of the following are seen in dividing cells? *Select all that apply.*
   A. The nuclear membrane is fragmented during separation of chromosomes
   B. The nucleolus is involved in ribosomal biogenesis and is a prominent structure in dividing cells
   C. Prophase and metaphase both occur in the S phase of the cell cycle
   D. The final daughter cells that derive from meiosis are haploid
   E. Control of the overall cell population may be regulated by apoptosis

7. The following functions can be delivered by cell membrane proteins. *Select all that apply.*
   A. Attach cytoskeletal filaments to cell membrane
   B. Transport molecules in or out of cells
   C. Limit the movement of adjacent phospholipids to make the cell membrane more stable
   D. Act as receptors for chemical signalling
   E. Act as an enzyme to catalyse a biochemical reaction

8. Which of these statements about caveolae are correct? *Select all that apply.*
   A. They are external protrusions of the cell surface membrane
   B. Associated with a bracing protein termed clathrin
   C. Can transport substances into the cell in a process termed potocytosis
   D. Have a cell membrane bearing surface proteins that function as signal receptors
   E. Can translocate substances from the extracellular space on one side of the cell to the extracellular space on the other side of the cell

9. Which of the following are present in the cytosol of cells? *Select all that apply.*
   A. The glycolytic pathway enzymes
   B. Cytoskeletal filaments
   C. Free lipids
   D. Basement membrane
   E. Glycocalyx

10. Which of the following statements about cell structure are correct? *Select all that apply.*
    A. In the bilayer cell membrane, the composition of the inner and outer lipid layers is the same
    B. Exocytosis leads to material from the extracellular space being internalized into the cell
    C. Exosomes and ectosomes act as transport vesicles that can move material between cells by migrating through the extracellular space
    D. The inner nuclear membrane is braced by proteins called lamins
    E. The nucleolus is darkly stained and is the site of condensation of chromatin in an inactive conformation

11. For each of the statements about transport in and out of cells, select the most appropriate option from A to I. Each option may be used once, more than once or not at all.
    A. Endocytosis
    B. Exocytosis
    C. Pinocytosis
    D. Phagocytosis
    E. Caveolae
    F. Receptor-mediated endocytosis
    G. Clathrin
    H. Caveolin
    I. Actin

    1. Braces coated pit membranes
    2. Invagination of a coated pit brings substances from outside the cell to the inside of the cell
    3. Internalization of fluid and small molecules into a cell
    4. A bacteria attaches to receptors on the cell surface and is internalized into a vesicle
    5. Fusion of a cell vesicle with the surface membrane to discharge contents into the extracellular space

12. For each of the statements about cell components, select the most appropriate option from A to K. Each option may be used once, more than once or not at all.
    A. Ribosome
    B. Nucleolus
    C. Nucleus
    D. Mitochondrion
    E. Rough endoplasmic reticulum
    F. Golgi apparatus
    G. Lysosome
    H. Peroxisome
    I. Actin
    J. Smooth endoplasmic reticulum
    K. Cytosol

    1. Main location of glycogen within the cell
    2. Contains acid hydrolases
    3. Main location of cellular DNA
    4. Release of contents acts as a trigger for programmed cell death
    5. Main site of synthesis of ribosomal RNA

13. For each of the statements about the cell membrane, select the most appropriate option from A to G. Each option may be used once, more than once or not at all.
    A. Phospholipid
    B. Cholesterol
    C. Glycolipid
    D. Glycerol
    E. Membrane protein
    F. Microtubule
    G. Fatty acid

    1. Attach cytoskeletal filaments to cell membrane
    2. Limits movement of phospholipids and makes membrane less fluid and more mechanically stable
    3. Found exclusively in the outer leaflet of the cell membrane
    4. Act as receptors for cell signalling
    5. Present in both faces of the cell membrane with a hydrophilic and hydrophobic polarity

14. For each of the statements about the cytoskeleton, select the most appropriate option from A to D. Each option may be used once, more than once or not at all.
    A. Actin
    B. Microtubule
    C. Centriole
    D. Intermediate filament

    1. Braces cell membrane
    2. Mediates axonal transport in neurons
    3. The basal body in motile cilia
    4. Mediates cell motility
    5. Example includes cytokeratin
    6. Maintains extended tubular arrangement of the endoplasmic reticulum
    7. Organizes aggresomal response

CHAPTER 3 EPITHELIAL CELLS

1. Which of the following are distinct features of epithelial cells? *Select all that apply.*
   A. Squamous epithelial cells are flat and plate-like
   B. A pseudostratified epithelium has all its cells in contact with the underlying extracellular matrix
   C. A simple columnar cell is typically two to three times higher than its width
   D. Cell division occurs at all layers in a stratified squamous epithelium
   E. Transitional epithelium is a characteristic cell type lining the urinary tract

2. Which of the following features are present in epithelial cell junctions of varying types? *Select all that apply.*
   A. Occluding junctions prevent lateral diffusion of membrane proteins
   B. Adherent junctions interact with the actin filaments in cells

   C. Desmosomal junctions interact with the actin filaments in cells
   D. Hemidesmosomes anchor cells to basement membrane
   E. Gap junctions have a role in intercellular communication

3. Which of the following features are seen in epithelial cells? *Select all that apply.*
   A. Microvilli have a centriole at their base
   B. Membrane plaques are a feature of transitional epithelium
   C. Cilia are based on a cytoskeleton of intermediate filaments
   D. The glycocalyx is seen within the rough endoplasmic reticulum
   E. Cytokeratin is a type of intermediate filament

4. Which of the following is true for the secretory role of epithelial cells? *Select all that apply.*
   A. Endocrine secretion occurs when a cell enters the bloodstream
   B. Mucin-secreting cells have a well-developed Golgi, this being the main site of protein glycosylation
   C. Ion-pumping cells have many lysosomes to export transported solutes
   D. Merocrine secretion occurs when a secreted product is exocytosed from the cell onto a surface or into a lumen
   E. Apocrine secretion occurs when the whole cell is shed as the secreted product

5. Which of the following statements about epithelial cells are correct? *Select all that apply.*
   A. Occluding junctions prevent lateral migration of specialized cell membrane proteins, thus delineating and maintaining specialized cell membrane domains
   B. The shape of microvilli is maintained by a bundle of microtubules
   C. A striated epithelial cell is one that has developed characteristics of muscle
   D. The acinus of a gland is composed of collagen
   E. Some basement membrane components are produced by the epithelial cells

6. For each of the statements about epithelial cells, select the most appropriate option from A to K. Each option may be used once, more than once or not at all.
   A. Simple squamous epithelium
   B. Simple cuboidal epithelium
   C. Simple columnar epithelium
   D. Stratified epithelium
   E. Straight tubular gland
   F. Holocrine secretory cells
   G. Ciliated epithelial cells
   H. Protein-secreting cells
   I. Mucin-secreting cells
   J. Steroid-secreting cells
   K. Ion-pumping cells

1. Cells with a complex folded surface membrane associated with numerous mitochondria, linked together by tight (occluding) junctions
2. Cells lining the air-conducting passages of the upper respiratory tract
3. The type of cell lining blood vessels, abdominal and pleural cavities
4. Cells with an extensive smooth endoplasmic reticulum, free cytoplasmic lipid and mitochondria with tubular cristae
5. Cells with large, open, nuclei and abundant rough endoplasmic reticulum

CHAPTER 4 SUPPORT CELLS AND THE EXTRACELLULAR MATRIX

1. Which of the following statements about collagen are correct? *Select all that apply.*
   A. Type I is the main collagen in skin
   B. Type IV is the main collagen type in bone
   C. Type III is the main collagen type in reticulin
   D. Is secreted by fibroblasts as procollagen molecules
   E. Is one of the matrix components of osteoid

2. Which of the following statements about glycosaminoglycans are correct? *Select all that apply.*
   A. Are composed of repeating sugar residues
   B. Are weakly hydrophilic
   C. May be attached to proteins to form proteoglycans
   D. Include hyaluronic acid, dermatan sulphate, heparin and fibronectin
   E. Have a very dense folded structure that gives turgor to the tissue extracellular matrix

3. Which of the following statements about basement membranes are correct? *Select all that apply.*
   A. Contains type I collagen
   B. Contains laminin
   C. Contains glycosaminoglycans
   D. Links to epithelial cells via integrin receptors
   E. Acts as a permeability barrier

4. Which of the following features are seen in the specific types of support tissue listed? *Select all that apply.*
   A. Fibrocollagenous tissue is the major support tissue in most organs
   B. Chondroblasts elaborate the specialized extracellular matrix of cartilage
   C. Hyaline cartilage forms the main component of the auricle of the ear
   D. Unilocular adipose tissue is important for thermogenesis in the neonatal period
   E. After severe tissue damage, fibrocollagenous tissue is formed in healing to produce a fibrous scar

5. For each of the statements about support cells and extracellular matrix, select the most appropriate option from A to K. Each option may be used once, more than once or not at all.
   A. Fibroblasts
   B. Chondrocytes
   C. Osteoblasts
   D. Myofibroblasts
   E. Elastin
   F. Basement membranes
   G. Hyaline cartilage
   H. Fibrocartilage
   I. Elastic cartilage
   J. Multilocular adipose tissue
   K. Unilocular adipose tissue

   1. Forms the initial skeleton in fetal development
   2. Produces osteoid
   3. Anchored to hemidesmosomes
   4. Assists with wound shrinkage in tissue repair after injury
   5. Found in the auricle of the ear

CHAPTER 5 CONTRACTILE CELLS

1. Which of the following statements about skeletal muscle are correct? *Select all that apply.*
   A. Cells have thin filaments made of actin which are anchored to the Z band
   B. Cells have thick filaments made of desmin
   C. Contraction is regulated by control of calcium release from the sarcoplasmic reticulum
   D. Individual cells are surrounded by an external lamina
   E. Each cell contains multiple nuclei

2. Which of the following statements about cardiac muscle cells are true ? *Select all that apply.*
   A. Cells are mononuclear and linked by intercellular junctions to form a fibre
   B. Are striated in a similar way to skeletal muscle
   C. Normally regenerate after cell damage
   D. Regulate contraction by release of calcium from the sarcoplasmic reticulum
   E. Have communicating junctions linking fibres to propagate contraction

3. Which of the following statements about smooth muscle cells are correct? *Select all that apply.*
   A. Have a single nucleus
   B. Use actin and myosin to develop contractile forces
   C. Are surrounded by an external lamina
   D. Have membrane receptors for hormones
   E. May generate their own level of rhythmic contraction

4. Which of the following statements about myofibroblasts, pericytes and myoepithelial cells are correct? *Select all that apply*.
   A. Myoepithelial cells are found in exocrine glandular tissue such as the breast
   B. Myoepithelial cells are stellate cells, with multiple processes, which surround secretory units of glands
   C. Myoepithelial cells are controlled by autonomic innervation
   D. Pericytes may assume the role of primitive mesenchymal cells
   E. Myofibroblasts proliferate and are involved in repair after tissue damage

5. For each of the statements about contractile cells, select the most appropriate option from A to G. Each option may be used once, more than once or not at all.
   A. Skeletal muscle
   B. Striated muscle
   C. Smooth muscle
   D. Cardiac muscle
   E. Myofibroblast
   F. Pericyte
   G. Myoepithelial cell

   1. Expels secretions from exocrine glands
   2. Seen in association with capillaries and venules
   3. After tissue damage, participates in angiogenesis
   4. Characterized by the presence of desmosomal-type, junctional-type and communicating-type junctions
   5. Provides the contractile function in the walls of hollow viscera

CHAPTER 6 NERVOUS TISSUE

1. Which of the following features are seen in neurons? *Select all that apply*.
   A. Dendrites carry signals away from the cell body
   B. They have few lysosomes
   C. The smooth endoplasmic reticulum is termed 'Nissl substance'
   D. Slow anterograde transport down the axon is mediated by microtubules
   E. The terminal bouton is located at the end of the axon

2. Which of the following statements about synapses are correct? *Select all that apply*.
   A. Synaptic vesicles are derived solely from transport down the axon
   B. Release of neurotransmitter is mediated by voltage-sensitive calcium channels in the nerve terminal
   C. Release of transmitter substance is via diffusion through the presynaptic membrane
   D. The postsynaptic membrane is fused to the presynaptic membrane by cell adhesion proteins
   E. Membrane from synaptic vesicles becomes transiently incorporated into the presynaptic membrane

3. Which of the following statements about myelin are correct? *Select all that apply*.
   A. Myelin completely unsheathes myelinated axons throughout their length
   B. Is formed by Schwann cells in the central nervous system (CNS)
   C. May regenerate after damage in the peripheral nervous system (PNS)
   D. Reduces the conduction speed in very large-diameter axons
   E. In the PNS myelin has a different biochemical composition from that in the CNS

4. In the PNS which of the following are true? *Select all that apply*.
   A. The perineurium surrounds a group of nerve fascicles
   B. The epineurium is composed of flattened, epithelial-like cells
   C. Axons are all myelinated
   D. Nodes of Ranvier are areas of bare axon between segments of myelination
   E. Ganglia contain neuronal cell bodies, axons, Schwann cells and satellite cells

5. Which of the following statements about myelin are correct? *Select all that apply*.
   A. Oligodendrocytes form myelin in the spinal cord
   B. The major dense line in myelin is formed by the fusion of inner surfaces of the cell membrane of the myelinating cell
   C. Schmidt–Lanterman incisures are devoid of cytoplasm
   D. The intraperiod line is formed by the fusion of the outer surfaces of the cell membrane of the myelinating cell
   E. P0 protein is a main component of CNS myelin

6. Which of the following statement about astrocytes are correct? *Select all that apply*.
   A. The main intermediate filament in astrocytes is neurofilament protein
   B. Astrocytes contribute to the structure of the blood–brain barrier
   C. Astrocytes have a bipolar morphology
   D. After damage to the CNS, repair takes place by proliferation of astrocytes
   E. Astrocytes play an important role in maintaining ion and fluid balance within the CNS

7. For each of the statements about the cells of the central nervous system, select the most appropriate option from A to K. Each option may be used once, more than once or not at all.
   A. Purkinje cell
   B. Sensory neuron
   C. Motor neuron
   D. Oligodendrocyte
   E. Ependymal cell

F. Astrocyte
G. Microglial cell
H. Meningothelial cell
I. Choroid plexus
J. Lymphocyte
K. Monocyte

1. Ciliated cell arranged in coherent sheets lining ventricles
2. In wax sections, seen as a rounded nucleus with a peripheral 'halo' of vacuolation and seen especially in the white matter
3. In wax sections, seen as rod-shaped nuclei in both grey and white matter and having an immune-surveillance function
4. Cells with a microvillar surface, arranged on vascular papillae
5. Inconspicuous cells found in the dura, arachnoid and pial layers

8. For each of the statements about the PNS, select the most appropriate option from A to K. Each option may be used once, more than once or not at all.
A. Schwann cell
B. Epineurium
C. Perineurium
D. Endoneurium
E. Fascicle
F. Ganglion cell
G. Satellite cell
H. Neuron
I. Oligodendrocyte
J. Astrocyte
K. Monocyte

1. The compartment immediately surrounding axons in a peripheral nerve, composed of collagen fibres, extracellular matrix and fibroblasts
2. The largest cells seen in a peripheral ganglion
3. Support cells seen adjacent to neuronal cell bodies in peripheral ganglia
4. The structure composed of several layers of cells with epithelial structural properties grouping and delineating a bundle of axons
5. The cell that surrounds non-myelinated axons in a peripheral nerve

CHAPTER 7 BLOOD CELLS

1. Which of the following statements about red blood cells are correct? *Select all that apply.*
A. A biconcave shape that maximizes the surface/volume ratio for gas transfer in capillary vessels
B. No mitochondria
C. A membrane-associated cytoskeleton that maintains its shape
D. A lifespan in peripheral blood of about 20 days
E. They are removed, when aged, by cells located in the spleen

2. Which of the following statements about neutrophils are correct? *Select all that apply.*
A. They have a regular, spherical nucleus
B. They perform their main functions in the peripheral blood
C. Contain the enzyme myeloperoxidase, which is important for bacterial killing
D. Express cell adhesion molecules on their surface to allow them to adhere to endothelium in blood vessels
E. Express receptors on their surface that recognize foreign material for internalization by phagocytosis

3. Which of the following statements about specialized roles of white blood cells are correct? *Select all that apply.*
A. Basophils emigrate into tissues and form plasma cells
B. Monocytes have a main role as a phagocytic cell
C. Lymphocytes of certain types can secrete immunoglobulin
D. Eosinophils are increased in number in the tissues and blood in allergic reactions
E. Neutrophils have a long half-life of about 30 days once they are activated and have entered tissues

4. Which of the following is true regarding the blood cells generated by haemopoiesis? *Select all that apply.*
A. All blood cells derive from a common haemopoietic stem cell
B. Both granulocytes and monocytes derive from a common committed progenitor cell
C. Each of the cytokines that control and modulate haemopoiesis acts specifically on one cell line
D. Platelets are formed from dendritic cells
E. Committed progenitor cells do not divide

5. For each of the statements, select the most appropriate option from A to K. Each option may be used once, more than once or not at all.
A. Megakaryocyte
B. Normoblast
C. Monocyte
D. Metamyelocyte
E. Neutrophil
F. Eosinophil
G. Basophil
H. Mast cell
I. Tissue resident macrophage
J. Natural killer cell
K. B lymphocyte

1. Matures to a cell that secretes immunoglobulin
2. A precursor of an erythrocyte
3. A cell type seen in granulocyte maturation
4. The precursor cell of blood platelets
5. A tissue-resident cell that has densely basophilic granules

6. For each of the statements, select the most appropriate option from A to K. Each option may be used once, more than once or not at all.
   A. Stromal cell
   B. Mast cell
   C. Erythrocyte
   D. Lymphocyte
   E. T cell
   F. B cell
   G. NK cell
   H. Macrophage
   I. Neutrophil
   J. Eosinophil
   K. Plasma cell

   1. Has a rounded nucleus with a prominent nucleolus, basophilic cytoplasm (caused by abundant rough endoplasmic reticulum [RER]) and a pale-stained area seen adjacent to the nucleus
   2. Increased in peripheral blood in response to bacterial infections
   3. Characterized by primary, secondary and tertiary granules in cytoplasm
   4. Characterized by a bilobed nucleus
   5. Dominant phagocytic role and also responsible for presenting antigen to the immune system

CHAPTER 8 IMMUNE SYSTEM

1. Which of the following features are indicative of B lymphocytes? *Select all that apply.*
   A. Mature into plasma cells and secrete immunoglobulin
   B. Are derived from cells that originate in the bone marrow
   C. Are the main cell type in the paracortex of lymph nodes
   D. Have receptors for antigen on their surface
   E. Can be seen as small lymphocytes in peripheral blood

2. Which of the following statements about T lymphocytes are correct? *Select all that apply.*
   A. May be seen as small lymphocytes in peripheral blood
   B. May express CD4 or CD8
   C. Secrete antibodies and cytokines
   D. May be divided into groups on the basis of expression of distinct types of T-cell receptors
   E. Are the main cell responsible for the cell-mediated immune response

3. Which of the following statements about the thymus gland are correct? *Select all that apply.*
   A. Is divided into red and white areas
   B. Contains epithelial cells that interact with developing T cells
   C. Contains structures called Hassall's corpuscles, which are vessels wrapped by surrounding macrophagic cells
   D. Undergoes involution after puberty
   E. Becomes completely replaced by adipose tissue in adult life

4. Which of the following statements about lymph nodes are correct? *Select all that apply.*
   A. The germinal centres are found in the superficial cortex and are predominantly composed of B cells
   B. The majority of lymphocytes gain entry to the node via the high endothelial venules in the paracortex
   C. Antigen-presenting cells are not found in germinal centres, but are concentrated in the paracortex
   D. Lymph enters the subcapsular sinus via afferent lymphatics
   E. Plasma cells are mainly concentrated in the medullary sinuses

5. Which of the following statements about the immune system are correct? *Select all that apply.*
   A. The main cell types involved in the immune response are lymphocytes, macrophages, and dendritic cells
   B. The primary organs of the immune system are the bone marrow and the thymus gland
   C. The secondary organs of the immune system are lymph nodes, spleen, and mucosa-associated lymphoid tissue (MALT)
   D. The three main types of lymphocytes are termed B cells, T cells and monocytes
   E. The main antigen-presenting cells are dendritic cells and macrophages

6. Which of the following statements about lymphoid cells are correct? *Select all that apply.*
   A. Naïve T cells express either CD8 or CD4 together with CD3
   B. CD4+ cells interact with MHC class I
   C. CD8+ cells interact with MHC class II
   D. Gamma delta T cells (γδ T cells) are mainly seen in the bowel
   E. T cells mature in the thymus gland

7. Which of the following statements about macrophages are correct? *Select all that apply.*
   A. Tissue resident macrophages form a population of cells able to phagocytose and process dead or damaged cells
   B. Macrophages may be stimulated by T cells to secrete cytokines
   C. Macrophages are not able to present antigen to the immune system
   D. Küppfer cells are a form of specialized tissue-resident macrophage
   E. Thymic nurse cells are a special form of tissue-resident macrophage

8. Which of the following statements about dendritic antigen-presenting cells are correct? *Select all that apply.*
   A. They phagocytose antigenic material, process it through proteolytic systems and present the resulting fragments to lymphocytes
   B. They have surface expression of class II major histocompatibility molecules

C. They are derived from precursor lymphoid cells

D. Langerhans' cells are a form of dendritic antigen-presenting cell

E. The lymph nodes and spleen are two sites that do not contain a resident population of dendritic antigen-presenting cells

9. For each of the statements about the immune system, select the most appropriate option from A to H. Each option may be used once, more than once or not at all.
   A. Bone marrow
   B. Nodal sinus
   C. Deep cortex of lymph node
   D. Splenic sinusoid
   E. Splenic red pulp
   F. Splenic white pulp
   G. Thymic cortex
   H. Thymic medulla

   1. Composed mainly of mature lymphoid cells including some germinal centres
   2. Site of origin of all T cells and B cells
   3. Contains mainly mature T lymphocytes
   4. Site of acquisition of immune self-tolerance
   5. Site of so-called nurse cells

CHAPTER 9 BLOOD AND LYMPHATIC CIRCULATORY SYSTEMS AND HEART

1. Which of the following statements about the heart are correct? *Select all that apply.*
   A. The main coronary arteries run in the epicardium
   B. Myocardial cells have central nuclei and are striated
   C. The endocardium contains elastic tissue
   D. The valves are composed of dense collagenous tissue and lack an endocardial covering
   E. The pericardial sac is lined by mesothelial cells

2. Which of the following statements about the arterial system are correct? *Select all that apply.*
   A. Large elastic arteries do not contain smooth muscle in their media
   B. Muscular arteries have both an internal and external elastic lamina
   C. Muscular arteries do not have an intimal layer
   D. The tone of smooth muscle is regulated by factors secreted by the endothelium in addition to innervation by the autonomic nervous system
   E. Vasa vasorum supply blood to the walls of large arteries

3. Which of the following statements are true regarding the cardiac conducting system? *Select all that apply.*
   A. Cardiac contractions originate in the sinoatrial node
   B. Internodal atrial muscle carries signals directly to the left and right bundle branches
   C. Purkinje fibres are structurally indistinguishable from adjacent myocardial cells

D. The atrioventricular node gives rise directly to the bundle of His

E. The atrioventricular node is the only part of the conducting system composed of neuronal tissue

4. Which of the following statements about the lymphatic circulatory system are correct? *Select all that apply.*
   A. Lymphatic capillaries take fluid from the extracellular space
   B. The term 'chyle' is used to describe lipid-containing lymph draining from the intestines
   C. Large lymphatic vessels have smooth muscle in their walls
   D. Valves assist the flow of lymph in lymphatic vessels
   E. Lymph that goes to the lymph nodes returns to the venous system via a main lymphatic vessel such as the thoracic duct

5. Which of the following statements about the structure of blood vessels are correct? *Select all that apply.*
   A. The tunica intima is lined by endothelial cells
   B. The intimal layer contains myointimal cells that have contractile, phagocytic and secretory roles
   C. The media is composed predominantly of smooth muscle but is devoid of elastic tissue
   D. The elastic lamina separating the tunica media and the tunica adventitia is called the internal elastic lamina
   E. The tunica adventitia is composed largely of fibroblasts and collagen

6. Which of the following statements about endothelium are correct? *Select all that apply.*
   A. The cytoplasm of most endothelial cells is barely visible in routine histological sections
   B. Endothelial cells are attached to an underlying basal lamina
   C. Endothelial cells have prominent tight junctions that prevent diffusion between cells
   D. A prominent feature of endothelial cells are lysosomal vesicles
   E. Endothelial cells contain Weibel–Palade bodies

7. Which of the following statements about endothelium are correct? *Select all that apply.*
   A. Endothelial cells can sense changes in blood pressure, oxygen tension and blood flow
   B. Activated endothelium becomes thinner and flatter than normal
   C. Activated endothelium can express cell adhesion molecules for neutrophils
   D. Under the effects of histamine, endothelial cells lose attachment to each other and fluid and proteins can diffuse out into the local tissues
   E. Endothelial cells can secrete thromboxane (TXA_2) and endothelin-1 to cause vasoconstriction

8. For each of the statements about vessels and the heart, select the most appropriate option from A to K. Each option may be used once, more than once or not at all.
   A. Tunica intima
   B. Tunica media
   C. Vasa vasorum
   D. Endothelium
   E. Arteriole
   F. Capillary
   G. Small muscular artery
   H. Vein
   I. Atrial cardiomyocyte
   J. Purkinje fibre
   K. Sinoatrial node

   1. Secretes factors that regulate the tone of vascular smooth muscle
   2. The layer of a vessel wall adjacent to its lumen
   3. Vessel mainly responsible for vascular peripheral resistance
   4. Has neuroendocrine granules responsible for hormone secretion
   5. May be of continuous or fenestrated type

CHAPTER 10 RESPIRATORY SYSTEM

1. Which of the following statements about the true vocal cords of the larynx are correct? *Select all that apply.*
   A. They are covered by ciliated columnar epithelium
   B. They are rich in lymphatics
   C. They are rich in capillaries
   D. Contain fibres of the vocal ligament
   E. Contain fibres of the vocalis muscle

2. Arrange the following components of the respiratory tract in correct anatomical order moving from proximal to distal.
   A. Alveolar duct
   B. Terminal bronchiole
   C. Alveolus
   D. Respiratory bronchiole
   E. Alveolar sacs

3. Which of the statements about type 1 pneumocytes are correct? *Select all that apply.*
   A. They are more numerous than type 2
   B. Are joined to each other by tight junctions
   C. Are rich in mitochondria
   D. Have prominent surface microvilli
   E. Are very resistant to inhaled toxins

4. Which of the following statements about type 2 pneumocytes are correct? *Select all that apply.*
   A. They have surface microvilli
   B. Are flat, plate-like cells
   C. Are stem cells that can produce new type 1 and type 2 pneumocytes
   D. Can become detached to act as intra-alveolar macrophages
   E. Contain multilamellate bodies in their cytoplasm

5. Which of the following statements about the histology of the nasopharynx are correct? *Select all that apply.*
   A. The nasal mucosa is lined by a simple columnar epithelium
   B. Beneath the nasal epithelium, the lamina propria contains secretory glands
   C. The lamina propria of the nasal mucosa contains lymphocytes, plasma cells, macrophages and eosinophils
   D. The nasopharynx is lined by columnar ciliated epithelium
   E. The eustachian or auditory tubes are lined by stratified squamous epithelium, like the pharynx

6. Which of the following statements about the histology of the olfactory epithelium are correct? *Select all that apply.*
   A. The olfactory mucosa is lined by a pseudostratified columnar epithelium
   B. The glands of Bowman associated with the olfactory epithelium are of the mucus type
   C. The basal cells of the olfactory epithelium are stem cells
   D. The olfactory vesicle bears cilia
   E. The proximal process of olfactory cells connects to the first cranial nerve

7. Which of the following statements about the histology of the bronchial tree are correct? *Select all that apply.*
   A. The bronchial tree is lined by a ciliated columnar epithelium, which is pseudostratified in the larger bronchi
   B. Goblet cells are present in the respiratory mucosa and secrete mucin
   C. The lung is an organ that does not have a local population of neuroendocrine cells
   D. In the intrapulmonary bronchi, smooth muscle is located in the submucosal region
   E. The bronchial tree is the site of one component of mucosa-associated lymphoid tissue

8. Which of the following statements about the peripheral part of the lung are correct? *Select all that apply.*
   A. Respiratory bronchioles are lined by cuboidal ciliated epithelium
   B. Each alveolar duct terminates in alveolar sacs
   C. Pores of Kohn link small bronchi directly to alveolar sacs
   D. The alveolar walls are devoid of elastin, allowing for effective alveolar ventilation on inspiration
   E. Alveolar walls are of uniform thickness throughout their structure to allow for gas exchange over the whole of their surface area

9. For each of the statements, select the most appropriate option from A to H. Each option may be used once, more than once or not at all.
   A. Pseudostratified ciliated columnar epithelium
   B. Ciliated columnar epithelium
   C. Cuboidal epithelium
   D. Squamous epithelium

E. Pneumocytes
F. Transitional epithelium
G. Endothelium
H. Mesothelium

1. The epithelium lining the pleura
2. The epithelium lining the trachea
3. The epithelium covering the false vocal cords
4. The epithelium covering the true vocal cords
5. The lining of alveoli

CHAPTER 11 ALIMENTARY TRACT

1. Which of the following statements are true of the oral cavity? *Select all that apply*.
   A. The surface of the anterior two-thirds of the tongue is raised in a series of elevations called papillae
   B. Taste buds are found around the base of circumvallate papillae and in fungiform papillae
   C. The tongue muscle is composed of a complex interlaced pattern of non-striated smooth muscle fibres
   D. The periodontal ligaments tether the teeth in the alveolar sockets of the mandible or maxilla
   E. The floor of the mouth is lined by non-keratinized stratified squamous epithelium

2. Which of the following statements about salivary glands are correct? *Select all that apply*.
   A. They secrete a watery solution that contains amylase and lysozyme
   B. The submandibular glands have a mixed population of serous and mucous cells
   C. The parotid glands are composed of mucus-secreting cells
   D. They have striated ducts that are lined by ion-pumping cells
   E. They are found on the inner surface of the lips and in the submucosa of the dorsal tongue

3. Which of the following statements about the stomach are correct? *Select all that apply*.
   A. Acid is produced by chief (peptic) cells
   B. Enzyme-producing cells secrete pepsinogen
   C. The mucosa in the body is characterized by long, straight, tubular glands containing acid-producing, enzyme-producing, mucin-producing and neuroendocrine cells
   D. The mucosa in the pylorus has relatively few acid-producing cells compared with the body region
   E. Enteroendocrine cells secreting gastrin are concentrated in the cardiac region

4. Which of the following statements about the small bowel are correct? *Select all that apply*.
   A. Villi are seen macroscopically as large folds arranged circularly around the lumen
   B. Enterocytes have a well-developed microvillus surface that forms the brush border

C. Paneth cells are seen as large, vacuolated, pale-staining cells and are found mainly in the neck region of intestinal crypts
D. Brunner's glands are serous in type and are found in the duodenum
E. All mucosal epithelial cells are derived from common specialized stem cells located in the crypts

5. Which of the following statements about teeth are correct? *Select all that apply*.
   A. The mature tooth has five main components
   B. The pulp cavity of the tooth is composed of collagen and fibroblasts embedded in an acellular matrix
   C. The outer surface of the pulp cavity is lined by odontoblasts that produce enamel
   D. Enamel is composed almost entirely of the mineral hydroxyapatite
   E. A layer of cementum covers the root of the tooth

6. Which of the following statements about the alimentary system are correct? *Select all that apply*.
   A. The oesophageal mucosa is composed of non-keratinizing stratified squamous epithelium, lamina propria and muscularis mucosae
   B. The submucosa of the oesophagus contains acid-secreting glands
   C. The muscle layers in the lower third of the oesophagus are composed entirely of smooth muscle
   D. At its upper end, the anal canal is lined by columnar epithelium
   E. The small and large bowel are characterized by an inner longitudinal layer and an outer circular layer of smooth muscle

7. Which of the following statements about the alimentary system are correct? *Select all that apply*.
   A. The adventitia is the outer coat of the digestive tract and surrounds the external layer of muscle
   B. The peritoneal cavity is lined by mesothelial cells
   C. Peyer's patches are covered by a mucin-secreting, tall, columnar epithelium
   D. The myenteric nerve plexus of the gut lies in the submucosal layer
   E. Interstitial cells of Cajal are gut neuroendocrine cells that secrete peptide hormones

8. For each of the statements, select the most appropriate option from A to K. Each option may be used once, more than once or not at all.
   A. Paneth cell
   B. Interstitial cell of Cajal
   C. Gamma delta T cell
   D. M cell
   E. Enteroendocrine cell
   F. Gut stem cell
   G. Pancreatic exocrine cell
   H. Brunner's gland cell
   I. Submucosal ganglion cell

J. Myenteric plexus ganglion cell
K. Smooth muscle cell

1. Overlies Peyer's patch
2. Produces urogastrone and an alkaline secretion
3. Pacemaker cell for peristalsis
4. Produces defensins
5. Produces serotonin and cholecystokinin

CHAPTER 12 LIVER

1. Which of the following statements are true for the blood entering the liver through the hepatic portal vein? *Select all that apply*.
   A. Is highly oxygenated
   B. Contains material absorbed from food in the small intestine
   C. Contains haemoglobin breakdown products from the spleen
   D. Enters the hepatic sinusoids
   E. Contains formed bile for metabolic breakdown by hepatocytes

2. Which of the following statements about the liver lobule are correct? *Select all that apply*.
   A. The terminal branch of the portal vein is at the centre of the lobule
   B. The portal tracts are located at the periphery of the lobule
   C. Blood passes from the periphery to the centre of the lobule
   D. Bile passes from the hepatocytes to the centre of the lobule
   E. The hepatocytes of the limiting plate are at the periphery of the lobule

3. Which of the following statements about bile are correct? *Select all that apply*.
   A. Contains products derived from haemoglobin breakdown in the liver
   B. Is stored and concentrated in the gallbladder
   C. Accumulates in the liver and blood when the common bile duct is blocked
   D. Passes into the duodenum at the duodenal papilla (ampulla of Vater)
   E. Is acidic and augments the effects of gastric acid in digestion

4. Which of the following statements about hepatocytes are correct? *Select all that apply*.
   A. Are rich in peroxisomes
   B. Have a canalicular surface that is involved in bile secretion
   C. Are separated from the sinusoid endothelium by the space of Disse
   D. Contain glycogen
   E. Rest on a reticulin scaffold

5. Which of the following statements about the liver are correct? *Select all that apply*.
   A. The terminal parts of the hepatic portal and arterial systems run in a connective tissue framework called portal tracts
   B. The hepatic sinusoids are lined by fenestrated endothelium
   C. Phagocytic cells partly line sinusoids
   D. Hepatic stellate cells are a specialized form of hepatocyte
   E. The liver has no lymphatic system

6. Which of the following statements about hepatocytes are correct? *Select all that apply*.
   A. The hepatocyte sinusoidal surfaces are characterized by microvilli
   B. Hepatocytes have coated pits responsible for internalization of material from sinusoidal blood
   C. The canalicular surfaces of hepatocytes are involved in the absorption of bile precursors from the blood
   D. Hepatocytes close to the portal tracts contain many esterases, being involved in conjugating and detoxifying reactions
   E. Hepatocytes are capable of regeneration after injury

7. Which of the following statements about the gallbladder are correct? *Select all that apply*.
   A. The submucosa is separated from underlying tissues by a muscularis mucosae
   B. The lining epithelium is specialized for fluid secretion
   C. The lining epithelium is a tall columnar pattern
   D. The wall of the gallbladder has a defined muscle layer composed of smooth muscle
   E. Part of the gallbladder has an adventitial surface covered by mesothelial cells

8. For each of the statements, select the most appropriate option from A to K. Each option may be used once, more than once or not at all.
   A. Hepatocytes
   B. Küppfer cells
   C. Centrilobular hepatocytes
   D. Periportal hepatocytes
   E. Portal tracts
   F. Central veins
   G. Space of Disse
   H. Stellate cells
   I. Biliary canaliculi
   J. Gallbladder
   K. Hepatic sinusoid

   1. Location of enzymes involved in oxidative reactions
   2. Site of production of bile
   3. Site of storage of glycogen
   4. Site of storage of vitamin A
   5. Location of material phagocytosed from sinusoids

CHAPTER 13 MUSCULOSKELETAL SYSTEM

1. Which of the following statements about osteoblasts are correct? *Select all that apply.*
   A. Are derived from blood monocytes
   B. Synthesize and secrete osteoid collagen
   C. Produce matrix vesicles important in mineralization of bone matrix
   D. Have abundant rough endoplasmic reticulum
   E. Have a characteristic ruffled border on the surface closest to the bone

2. Which of the following statements are true for osteoclasts? *Select all that apply.*
   A. Are derived from osteoprogenitor cells
   B. Erode bone
   C. Are stimulated by parathyroid hormone
   D. Are stimulated by calcitonin
   E. Are rich in alkaline phosphatase

3. Which of the following statements about skeletal muscle are correct? *Select all that apply.*
   A. Develops from primitive rhabdomyoblasts
   B. Contains type 1 fast-twitch fibres
   C. Contains satellite cells that are phagocytic
   D. Contains stretch receptors called muscle spindles
   E. Contains motor nerve twigs that terminate in motor endplates

4. In bone development, which of the following features are seen? *Select all that apply.*
   A. Chondroblasts develop in primitive mesenchyme and form an early perichondrium and cartilage model
   B. The term diaphysis refers to the shaft region
   C. The term epiphysis refers to the club-shaped expansion at the end of long bones
   D. The epiphyseal plate can be divided into periosteum, bone collar, and osteoprogenitor zones
   E. Postnatal increase in length is the result of endochondral bone formation near the end of long bones

5. Which of the following statements about the musculoskeletal system are correct? *Select all that apply.*
   A. Cells which are differentiating into muscle express a transcription factor in the nuclei called myod1
   B. The cell membrane of a skeletal muscle fibre is called the sarcolemma
   C. Muscles with a role in maintaining posture have a high proportion of type 1 fibres
   D. Individual skeletal muscle fibres are surrounded by the perimysium
   E. An anatomically defined muscle composed of many fascicles is surrounded externally by the epimysium

6. Which of the following statements about the musculoskeletal system are correct? *Select all that apply.*
   A. Weight training results in an increased number of muscle fibres developing, increasing the mass of muscle

B. Individual skeletal muscle fibres contain multiple nuclei
C. If a skeletal muscle fibre has nuclei in the centre of the fibre, it is an indication of regeneration in adult life
D. The activity of acetylcholine in a motor endplate is curtailed by the enzyme acetylcholinesterase, which is bound to the basement membrane in the junctional folds
E. Intrafusal muscle fibres are involved in sensing the stretch of a muscle

7. For each of the statements, select the most appropriate option from A to K. Each option may be used once, more than once or not at all.
   A. Fibroblasts
   B. Monocytes
   C. Osteoprogenitor cell
   D. Rhabdomyoblasts
   E. Satellite cell
   F. Lamellar bone
   G. Woven bone
   H. Trabecular bone
   I. Osteoid
   J. Osteoclast
   K. Osteocyte

   1. Regulate bone remodelling by secretion of several factors that act on other cell types
   2. Multinucleate cells derived from blood monocytes
   3. Precursors of osteoblasts
   4. The specialized matrix produced by osteoblasts
   5. Stimulated by parathyroid hormone to resorb bone

CHAPTER 14 ENDOCRINE SYSTEM

1. Which of the following statements about follicular epithelial cells of the thyroid acinus are correct? *Select all that apply.*
   A. Synthesize and secrete calcitonin
   B. Can convert iodide into iodine
   C. Can process thyroglobulin with the release of active thyroid hormones
   D. Are controlled by thyroid-stimulating hormone (TSH) from the hypothalamus
   E. May proliferate and produce a hyperthyroid state

2. Which of the following statements are true of parathyroid glands? *Select all that apply.*
   A. Are always four in number
   B. Secrete parathormone in response to a high serum calcium
   C. Contain chief cells, which are the main hormone secretors
   D. Contain a variable amount of adipose tissue
   E. May develop benign tumours that lead to bone destruction

3. Match the components of the adrenal with the relevant major secretion product.
   A. Zona reticularis
   B. Medulla
   C. Zona fasciculata
   D. Zona glomerulosa
   1. Cortisol
   2. Aldosterone
   3. Androgens
   4. (Nor)epinephrine ([nor]adrenaline)

4. Which of the following statements about the pituitary gland are correct? *Select all that apply.*
   A. Is divided into two parts: anterior (neurohypophysis) and posterior (adenohypophysis)
   B. Is supplied by blood vessels that run from the hypothalamus
   C. Secretes antidiuretic hormone (ADH) from the adenohypophysis
   D. Has most of the growth hormone (GH)–secreting cells in the lateral wings of the adenohypophysis
   E. Is located in the sella turcica

5. Which of the following statements about the neuroendocrine cells are correct? *Select all that apply.*
   A. Neuroendocrine cells secrete their product by exocytosis
   B. The secretory pole of endocrine cells faces away from capillary vessels
   C. Synaptophysin can be used as a marker of neuroendocrine cells in histology
   D. Ultrastructural examination of neuroendocrine cells shows a dense core and clear membrane-bound vesicles
   E. Islets of Langerhans are an example of clusters of neuroendocrine cells in an exocrine organ

6. Which of the following statements about the pituitary gland are correct? *Select all that apply.*
   A. Lactotrophs produce growth hormone
   B. Ultrastructural examination of cells of the anterior pituitary shows abundant lysosomes responsible for metabolizing precursor products of hormones
   C. Cells identified as acidophils in the anterior pituitary secrete prolactin and growth hormone
   D. Cells identified as basophils in the anterior pituitary secrete TSH, luteinizing hormone (LH), follicle-stimulating hormone (FSH), and adrenocorticotropic hormone (ACTH)
   E. Lactotrophs increase in size and number during pregnancy

7. For each of the statements, select the most appropriate option from A to K. Each option may be used once, more than once or not at all.
   A. C cells
   B. Thyroid epithelial cells
   C. Adrenal medulla
   D. Adrenal cortex
   E. Zona glomerulosa
   F. Zona fasciculata
   G. Chief cells
   H. Oxyphil cells
   I. β cells
   J. Enterochromaffin cells
   K. Sustentacular cells

   1. Site of production of steroid hormones
   2. Site of production of parathormone
   3. Age-related development in an endocrine gland
   4. Site of production of calcitonin
   5. Have prominent smooth endoplasmic reticulum and elongated mitochondria, with tubular cristae

CHAPTER 15 URINARY SYSTEM

1. The glomerular filtration barrier comprises which of the following? *Select all that apply.*
   A. Endothelial cells
   B. Podocyte cytoplasm
   C. Bowman's capsule epithelium
   D. Capillary basement membrane
   E. Endothelial glycocalyx

2. Which of the following features are seen in the proximal convoluted tubule epithelium? *Select all that apply.*
   A. Shows extensive microvilli on the luminal surface
   B. Shows extensive basal interdigitation
   C. Reabsorbs water from the glomerular filtrate
   D. Excretes glucose into the glomerular filtrate
   E. Is partly controlled by the level of antidiuretic hormone (ADH) secreted by the posterior pituitary

3. Which of the following features are seen in the juxtaglomerular apparatus? *Select all that apply.*
   A. Is located in the glomerular mesangium
   B. Contains highly specialized myoepithelial cells that also contain neuroendocrine granules
   C. Secretes angiotensin
   D. Secretes renin
   E. Is important in maintaining plasma volume and blood pressure

4. Which of the following features are present in the lower urinary tract? *Select all that apply.*
   A. The renal pelvis, ureter and bladder are lined by transitional epithelium
   B. The ureter has two muscle layers
   C. The bladder has two muscle layers
   D. The male urethra is lined by a pseudostratified columnar epithelium throughout its length
   E. The female urethra is lined mainly by a stratified squamous epithelium

5. Which of the following statements about the kidney are correct? *Select all that apply*.
   A. The renal cortex forms columns that lie between the units of the medulla
   B. The tip of the medullary pyramid is known as the papilla
   C. The nephron is composed of the glomerulus and cortical tubular systems only and excludes the medullary tubular system
   D. The kidney produces both of the hormones erythropoietin and renin

6. Which of the following statements about the renal vascular system are correct? *Select all that apply*.
   A. Each glomerular tuft receives blood from multiple afferent arterioles
   B. Efferent arterioles in the superficial cortex divide into a capillary system that runs in the interstitial spaces between the cortical tubules
   C. The efferent arterioles leaving glomeruli situated deep in the cortex form the vasa recta
   D. The vasa recta remove urea from the blood
   E. The capillary system in the glomerular tuft does not transfer the majority of its contained oxygen to the tissues

7. Which of the following statements about the glomerulus are correct? *Select all that apply*.
   A. The epithelial cells lining the parietal component of Bowman's capsule are thin and flat
   B. The epithelial cells coating the glomerular capillary tuft are transitional epithelium
   C. The epithelium-lined space between the coated glomerular capillary network and the parietal shell of Bowman's capsule contains ultrafiltrate
   D. The glomerular basement membrane is produced by the fusion of podocyte and capillary endothelial cell basement membranes
   E. The mesangium supports the glomerular capillary loop system

8. For each of the statements, select the most appropriate option from A to L. Each option may be used once, more than once or not at all.
   A. Bowman's capsule
   B. Fibroblast
   C. Podocyte
   D. Afferent arteriole
   E. Proximal convoluted tubule
   F. Distal convoluted tubule
   G. Loop of Henle
   H. Lacis cell
   J. Mesangial cell
   K. Interstitial cell
   L. Macula densa

   1. Absorbs water under control of ADH
   2. Forms the stroma around which the glomerulus is organized

3. Major structural component of the glomerular filtration barrier
4. Associated with filtration slits
5. Produces erythropoietin

CHAPTER 16 MALE REPRODUCTIVE SYSTEM

1. Which of the following statements about the germinal epithelium of the testis are correct? *Select all that apply*.
   A. Lines the seminiferous tubules and rete testes
   B. Produces haploid male gametes
   C. Is dependent on testosterone for its functional integrity
   D. Is supported by Sertoli cells
   E. Is an example of a renewing stem cell population

2. Which of the following statements are true for the spermatozoon? *Select all that apply*.
   A. Contains the haploid nucleus in the head region
   B. Has an acrosomal cap that contains several enzymes believed to help with penetration of the ovum
   C. Contains an axoneme that is based on actin filaments
   D. Is rich in mitochondria in the middle piece
   E. Is formed by maturation of spermatids, which takes place adjacent to the luminal surface of Leydig cells

3. Which of the following statements about the prostate gland are correct? *Select all that apply*.
   A. Discharges its secreted products into the seminal vesicles
   B. Has three zones of glands termed mucosal, submucosal and main prostatic glands
   C. Has both glandular and fibromuscular components
   D. Has glandular elements lined by transitional epithelium
   E. Is sensitive to endocrine stimulation, especially from testosterone

4. Which of the following statements about the penis are correct? *Select all that apply*.
   A. There are two dorsal corpora spongiosa and one ventral corpus cavernosum
   B. Blood is supplied to the erectile tissue by the helicine arteries
   C. The urethra runs through the corpus spongiosum
   D. The urethra is lined by squamous epithelium in its distal portion in the glans penis
   E. There are small mucous glands that secrete into the urethra

5. Which of the following statements about the male reproductive system are correct? *Select all that apply*.
   A. The tunica albuginea is composed of multiple layers of epithelial cells
   B. The testis is separated into lobules by fibrous septa
   C. Leydig cells are located within seminiferous tubules
   D. Haploid spermatids give rise to spermatozoa
   E. The vas deferens has two muscular layers

6. Which of the following statements about the male reproductive system are correct? *Select all that apply.*
   A. Spermiogenesis occurs while the spermatids are embedded in the surface of Sertoli cells
   B. The acrosomal cap is composed of closely aggregated mitochondria
   C. The axoneme, which is responsible for spermatozoon motility, is based on an extension of the actin cytoskeleton in the spermatozoa
   D. Occluding junctions between Sertoli cells form the blood–testis barrier
   E. Sertoli cells phagocytose any residual cytoplasm (residual bodies) shed by maturing spermatids during spermiogenesis

7. For each of the statements, select the most appropriate option from A to K. Each option may be used once, more than once or not at all.
   A. Seminal vesicle
   B. Testis
   C. Rete testis
   D. Vas deferens
   E. Prostate gland
   F. Seminiferous tubule
   G. Sertoli cell
   H. Leydig cell
   I. Epididymal duct
   J. Ejaculatory duct
   K. Germinal epithelium

   1. Secrete inhibin
   2. Synthesize testosterone
   3. Contain Reinke crystalloids
   4. Site of maturation of spermatozoa (develop motility and the capability to fertilize an ovum)
   5. Production of alkaline fluid secretion

CHAPTER 17 FEMALE REPRODUCTIVE SYSTEM

1. Which of the following statements about the transformation zone of the cervix are correct? *Select all that apply.*
   A. Is the site where endometrium changes to endocervix at the internal os
   B. Is the result of vaginal acid acting on the lower endocervical epithelium
   C. Is an important site for the development of cervical cancer
   D. Results in Nabothian follicles
   E. Develops shortly after birth

2. Which of the following statements about the sexually mature endometrium are correct? *Select all that apply.*
   A. Is the site of implantation of the fertilized ovum
   B. Is shed every month at the time of ovulation
   C. Is regenerated every month from its basal portion after menstruation
   D. Undergoes atrophy after menopause

   E. Undergoes the process of decidualization after implantation

3. Which of the following statements about the corpus luteum of the ovary are correct? *Select all that apply.*
   A. Develops from a ruptured tertiary Graafian follicle
   B. Secretes progesterone but not oestrogen
   C. Undergoes involution at the end of each menstrual cycle
   D. Converts into a corpus fibrosum after involution
   E. Persists as a progesterone-secreting source in the first 3 months of pregnancy

4. Which of the following statements about the ovary are correct? *Select all that apply.*
   A. The cortex consists of a spindle-cell stroma that surrounds the gamete-producing structures
   B. Most primordial follicles undergo atresia
   C. A primary follicle is composed of an oocyte surrounded by granulosa cells and Sertoli cells
   D. A tertiary follicle is also called a Graafian follicle
   E. The thecal cells that surround the secondary follicle are derived from stromal cells

5. Which of the following statements about the female reproductive system are correct? *Select all that apply.*
   A. The skin of the mons pubis is characterized by the presence of oblique hair follicles
   B. The skin of the labia majora contains many apocrine glands
   C. The labia minora are covered by a keratinized squamous epithelium
   D. The glans of the clitoris is devoid of hair follicles, sebaceous glands, eccrine glands and apocrine glands
   E. The vagina has a layer containing bundles of smooth muscle

6. Which of the following statements about the female reproductive system are correct? *Select all that apply.*
   A. The ectocervix is covered by stratified, squamous non-keratinizing epithelium
   B. The endocervical canal is lined by a single layer of tall, columnar, mucus-secreting epithelium
   C. The cervix has a stroma of smooth muscle fibres embedded in collagen
   D. The myometrial smooth muscle is arranged in a single layer
   E. The ciliated tubal epithelial cell in the uterine tube is responsive to oestrogen

7. For each of the statements, select the most appropriate option from A to K. Each option may be used once, more than once or not at all.
   A. Decidua
   B. Syncytiotrophoblast
   C. Hofbauer cells
   D. Corpus luteum
   E. Blastocoele

F. Endometrium
G. Corpus albicans
H. Granulosa cells
I. Graafian follicle
J. Theca interna
K. Primary follicle

1. Have a phagocytic function
2. Transformed endometrial stroma after implantation
3. Secretes human chorionic gonadotropin (hCG)
4. Secrete oestrogen
5. A mature tertiary follicle

CHAPTER 18 SKIN AND BREAST

1. Which of the following statements about the basal layer of the epidermis are correct? *Select all that apply.*
   A. Is responsible for the constant production of keratinocytes
   B. Is composed of cuboidal or columnar keratinocytes
   C. Is attached to the basement membrane by desmosomes
   D. Contains scattered melanocytes
   E. Contains keratinosomes

2. Which of the following statements about melanocytes are correct? *Select all that apply.*
   A. Are pigmented because of the melanin they contain
   B. Have long cytoplasmic processes that extend between keratinocytes
   C. Are greatly increased in number in dark-skinned races
   D. Contain characteristic spherical premelanosomes
   E. Are neural derived and also act as mechanoreceptors

3. Which of the following statements about skin appendages are correct? *Select all that apply.*
   A. Sebaceous gland units usually open directly on to the skin surface
   B. Apocrine glands secrete sweat
   C. Eccrine glands are particularly frequent on the palms and soles
   D. The internal root sheath of the hair follicle produces the hair shaft
   E. Erector pili muscles control the position of the hair shafts

4. Which of the following statements about terminal duct lobular units are correct? *Select all that apply.*
   A. They are embedded in endocrine-responsive, loose, fibrous support tissue
   B. Are composed of a lobule and its associated terminal duct
   C. Terminal ductule epithelium cells show secretory activity in the second half of the menstrual cycle
   D. Contains myoepithelial cells
   E. Undergo structural and functional atrophy after menopause

5. Which of the following statements about the breast are correct? *Select all that apply.*
   A. The areola contain large sebaceous units that form small nodular elevations called Montgomery's tubercles
   B. Breast ducts are lined by epithelium with an outer layer of myoepithelial cells
   C. If pregnancy occurs, progesterone stimulates proliferation and secretory activity in the breast lobule
   D. The male breast has a system of simple nipple ducts
   E. The lobular stroma of the breast is hormone responsive

6. For each of the statements, select the most appropriate option from A to K. Each option may be used once, more than once or not at all.
   A. Apocrine gland
   B. Eccrine gland
   C. Sebaceous gland
   D. Merkel cell
   E. Langerhans cell
   F. Melanocyte
   G. Keratinocyte
   H. Keratohyaline granule
   I. Tonofilaments
   J. Rete ridges
   K. Pilosebaceous unit

   1. Produce sweat
   2. Contain profilaggrin
   3. Mainly located in axillary skin and inguinal region
   4. Responsible for immune surveillance
   5. Composed of cytokeratin

CHAPTER 19 SPECIAL SENSES

1. Which of the following statements about the ear are correct? *Select all that apply.*
   A. The pinna is composed of elastic cartilage
   B. The ceruminous glands are modified apocrine glands
   C. The tympanic membrane is lined on one side by cuboidal epithelium
   D. The middle ear cavity is lined by ciliated pseudostratified epithelium
   E. The auditory ossicles articulate by syndesmoses

2. Which of the following statements about the inner ear are correct? *Select all that apply.*
   A. Hair cells have cilia on their surface to detect movement
   B. The ampullae of the semicircular canals detect acceleration
   C. The macula of the saccule detects sound
   D. The vestibular and tympanic cavities contain perilymph
   E. The basilar membrane is continuous with the organ of Corti

3. Which of the following statements about the eye are correct? *Select all that apply.*
   A. The posterior chamber lies behind the lens
   B. The lens is suspended from the ciliary body
   C. The inner part of the cornea is lined by endothelium
   D. The aqueous humour drains through the trabecular meshwork
   E. Aqueous humour is produced by the epithelium of the ciliary body

4. Which of the following statements about the retina are correct? *Select all that apply.*
   A. Retinal pigment epithelial cells are responsible for phagocytosis of photoreceptor membranes
   B. Cones are concentrated at the periphery of the retina
   C. The photoreceptor layer is isolated from the rest of the retina by a belt of adherent junctions forming the external limiting membrane
   D. The macula contains the fovea
   E. The optic disc is devoid of photoreceptors

5. Which of the following statements about the ear are correct? *Select all that apply.*
   A. The tympanic membrane has five layers
   B. The auditory ossicles are covered by periosteum
   C. The mastoid sinuses are lined by non-keratinizing squamous epithelium
   D. The stapedius and tensor tympani muscle are composed of striated muscle
   E. The auditory tube is lined by ciliated epithelium

6. Which of the following statements about the ear are correct? *Select all that apply.*
   A. The cochlear duct, the saccule and the utricle are part of the osseous labyrinth
   B. Deflection of microvilli causes electrical depolarization of the hair cell membrane
   C. Hair cells are found in the macula of the utricle
   D. Hair cells in the organ of Corti have a kinocilium in addition to stereocilia
   E. Hair cells in the inner ear are supported by satellite cells

7. For each of the statements, select the most appropriate option from A to K. Each option may be used once, more than once or not at all.
   A. External ear
   B. Auditory tube
   C. Saccule
   D. Utricle
   E. Tectorial membrane
   F. Ampulla of circular canal
   G. Cochlear duct
   H. Osseous labyrinth
   I. Vestibular cavity
   J. Modiolus
   K. Spiral ligament

   1. Location of the organ of Corti
   2. Lined by periosteum
   3. Linked to hair cells
   4. Contains perilymph
   5. Surrounds the cochlear nerve

8. For each of the statements, select the most appropriate option from A to K. Each option may be used once, more than once or not at all.
   A. Sclera
   B. Bowman's membrane
   C. Descemet's membrane
   D. Corneal lamellae
   E. Uvea
   F. Bruch's membrane
   G. Ciliary body
   H. Pigment epithelium
   I. Vitreous
   J. Anterior chamber
   K. Canal of Schlemm

   1. Lies between the sclera and retina
   2. Consists of pars plica and pars plana
   3. Surrounds keratocytes
   4. Covered by endothelial cells
   5. Drains aqueous from the eye

REVIEW ANSWERS

CHAPTER 1 HISTOLOGY

1. A, B
2. A, C, E
3. B, E
4. A, B, D, E
5. 1. B. Histology, 2. A. Tissue, 3. C. Epithelium, 4. G. Light microscopy using wax-embedded sections, 5. H. Fixation

CHAPTER 2 THE CELL

1. A, B, C
2. A, C, D, E
3. A, E
4. A, B, D, E
5. A, C, D, E
6. A, B, D, E
7. A, B, D, E
8. C, D, E
9. A, B, C
10. C, D
11. 1. G. Clathrin, 2. A. Endocytosis, 3. C. Pinocytosis, 4. D. Phagocytosis, 5. B. Exocytosis
12. 1. K. Cytosol, 2. G. Lysosome, 3. C. Nucleus, 4. D. Mitochondrion, 5. B. Nucleolus
13. 1. E. Membrane protein, 2. B. Cholesterol, 3. C. Glycolipid, 4. E. Membrane protein, 5. A. Phospholipid
14. 1. A. Actin, 2. B. Microtubule, 3. C. Centriole, 4. A. Actin, 5. D. Intermediate filament, 6. B. Microtubule, 7. C. Centriole

CHAPTER 3 EPITHELIAL CELLS

1. A, B, C, E
2. A, B, D, E
3. B, E
4. B, D
5. A, E
6. 1. K. Ion-pumping cells, 2. G. Ciliated epithelial cells, 3. A. Simple squamous epithelium, 4. J. Steroid-secreting cells, 5. H. Protein-secreting cells

CHAPTER 4 SUPPORT CELLS AND THE EXTRACELLULAR MATRIX

1. A, C, D, E
2. A, C
3. B, C, D, E
4. A, B, E
5. 1. G. Hyaline cartilage, 2. C. Osteoblasts, 3. F. Basement membranes, 4. D. Myofibroblasts, 5. I. Elastic cartilage

CHAPTER 5 CONTRACTILE CELLS

1. A, C, D, E
2. A, B, D, E
3. A, B, C, D, E
4. A, B, C, D, E
5. 1. G. Myoepithelial cell, 2. F. Pericyte, 3. F. Pericyte, 4. D. Cardiac muscle, 5. C. Smooth muscle

CHAPTER 6 NERVOUS TISSUE

1. E
2. B, E
3. C, E
4. D, E
5. A, B, D
6. B, D, E
7. 1. E. Ependymal cell, 2. D. Oligodendrocyte, 3. G. Microglial cell, 4. I. Choroid plexus, 5. H. Meningothelial cell
8. 1. D. Endoneurium, 2. H. Neuron, 3. G. Satellite cell, 4. C. Perineurium, 5. A. Schwann cell

CHAPTER 7 BLOOD CELLS

1. A, B, C, E
2. C, D, E
3. B, C, D
4. A, B
5. 1. K. B lymphocyte, 2. B. Normoblast, 3. D. Metamyelocyte, 4. A. Megakaryocyte, 5. H. Mast cell
6. 1. K. Plasma cell, 2. I. Neutrophil, 3. I. Neutrophil, 4. J. Eosinophil, 5. H. Macrophage

CHAPTER 8 IMMUNE SYSTEM

1. A, B, D, E
2. A, B, D, E
3. B, D, E
4. A, B, D, E
5. A, B, C, E
6. A, D, E
7. A, B, D
8. A, B, D
9. 1. F. Splenic white pulp, 2. A. Bone marrow, 3. C. Deep cortex of lymph node, 4. H. Thymic medulla, 5. G. Thymic cortex

CHAPTER 9 BLOOD AND LYMPHATIC CIRCULATORY SYSTEMS AND HEART

1. A, B, C, E
2. B, D, E
3. A, D

4. A, B, C, D, E
5. A, B, E
6. A, B, C, E
7. A, C, D, E
8. 1. D. Endothelium, 2. A. Tunica intima, 3. E. Arteriole, 4. I. Atrial cardiomyocytes, 5. F. Capillary

CHAPTER 10 RESPIRATORY SYSTEM

1. D, E
2. B, D, A, E, C
3. B
4. A, C, E
5. B, C, D
6. A, C, D, E
7. A, B, D, E
8. A, B
9. 1. H. Mesothelium, 2. A. Pseudostratified ciliated columnar epithelium, 3. B. Ciliated columnar epithelium, 4. D. Squamous epithelium, 5. E. Pneumocytes

CHAPTER 11 ALIMENTARY TRACT

1. A, B, D, E
2. A, B, D, E
3. B, C, D
4. B, E
5. A, B, D, E
6. A, C, D
7. A, B
8. 1. D. M cell, 2. H. Brunner's gland cell, 3. B. Interstitial cell of Cajal, 4. A. Paneth cell, 5. E. Enteroendocrine cell

CHAPTER 12 LIVER

1. B, C, D
2. B, C, E
3. A, B, C, D
4. A, B, C, D, E
5. A, B, C
6. A, B, E
7. C, D, E
8. 1. D. Periportal hepatocytes, 2. A. Hepatocytes, 3. A. Hepatocytes, 4. H. Stellate cells, 5. B. Küppfer cells

CHAPTER 13 MUSCULOSKELETAL SYSTEM

1. B, C, D
2. B, C
3. A, D, E
4. A, B, C, E
5. A, B, C, E
6. B, C, D, E
7. 1. K. Osteocyte, 2. J. Osteoclast, 3. C. Osteoprogenitor cell, 4. I. Osteoid, 5. J. Osteoclast

CHAPTER 14 ENDOCRINE SYSTEM

1. B, C, E
2. C, D, E
3. 1 (C), 2 (D), 3 (A), 4 (B)
4. B, D, E
5. A, C, D, E
6. C, D, E
7. 1. D. Adrenal cortex, 2. G. Chief cells, 3. H. Oxyphil cells, 4. A. C cells, 5. D. Adrenal cortex

CHAPTER 15 URINARY SYSTEM

1. A, B, D, E
2. A, B, C
3. B, D, E
4. A, B, E
5. A, B, D
6. B, C, E
7. A, C, D, E
8. 1. F. Distal convoluted tubule, 2. J. Mesangial cell, 3. C. Podocyte, 4. C. Podocyte, 5. K. Interstitial cell

CHAPTER 16 MALE REPRODUCTIVE SYSTEM

1. B, C, D, E
2. A, B, D
3. B, C, E
4. B, C, D, E
5. B, D
6. A, D, E
7. 1. G. Sertoli cell, 2. H. Leydig cell, 3. H. Leydig cell, 4. I. Epididymal duct, 5. E. Prostate gland

CHAPTER 17 FEMALE REPRODUCTIVE SYSTEM

1. B, C, D
2. A, C, D, E
3. A, C, E
4. A, B, D, E
5. A, B, C, D, E
6. A, B, C, E
7. 1. C. Hofbauer cells, 2. A. Decidua, 3. B. Syncytiotrophoblast, 4. J. Theca interna, 5. I. Graafian follicle

CHAPTER 18 SKIN AND BREAST

1. A, B, D
2. B
3. C, D, E
4. A, B, C, D, E
5. A, B, C, D, E
6. 1. B. Eccrine gland, 2. H. Keratohyaline granule, 3. A. Apocrine gland, 4. E. Langerhans cell, 5. I. Tonofilaments

CHAPTER 19 SPECIAL SENSES

1. A, B, C
2. B, D, E
3. B, C, D, E
4. A, C, D, E
5. D, E
6. B, C, D
7. 1. G. Cochlear duct, 2. H. Osseous labyrinth, 3. E. Tectorial membrane, 4. I. Vestibular cavity, 5. J. Modiolus
8. 1. E. Uvea, 2. G. Ciliary body, 3. D. Corneal lamellae, 4. C. Descemet's membrane, 5. K. Canal of Schlemm

INDEX

Page numbers followed by 'f' indicate figures, 'b' indicate boxes, and 't' indicates tables.